Dr L. W. Svihlik D.C.
3439 Grand Blvd.
Brookfield, ILL. 60513
485-7112

Chiropractic Management of Sports and Recreational Injuries

SECOND EDITION

Chiropractic Management of Sports and Recreational Injuries

SECOND EDITION

R. C. SCHAFER, DC, FICC

Review Editors

Leonard W. Schroeder, DC, CCTP, FICC
James F. Ransom, DC, FICC
George J. Goodheart, DC, DICAK, FICC
Michael A. Sabia, Jr., DC, PhD
Jan M. Corwin, DC
Paul A. Jaskoviak, DC, FICC
Brian M. Davis, DC, DACBR, FICC
W. Heath Quigley, DC, MS, FICA
Charles Brandstetter, DC, ND
Faye B. Eagles, DC, FICC
M. Wayne Brown, DC

Developed in cooperation with
THE COUNCIL ON SPORTS INJURIES
of the
AMERICAN CHIROPRACTIC ASSOCIATION
and
ASSOCIATED CHIROPRACTIC ACADEMIC PRESS

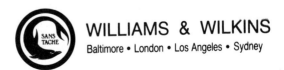

WILLIAMS & WILKINS
Baltimore • London • Los Angeles • Sydney

Editor: Jonathan W. Pine, Jr.
Associate Editor: Carol Eckhart
Copy Editor: S. Minton
Design: JoAnne Janowiak
Illustration Planning: Lorraine Wrzosek
Production: Anne G. Seitz

Printed in the United States of America

Library of Congress Cataloging-in-Publication Data

Main entry under title:

Chiropractic management of sports and recreational injuries.

Includes bibliographies and index.
1. Chiropractic. 2. Sports—Accidents and injuries. 3. Wounds and injuries—Treatment. 4. Sports medicine. I. Schafer, R. C. II. American Chiropractic Association. Council on Sports Injuries. [DNLM: 1. Athletic Injuries—therapy. 2. Chiropractic—methods. 3. Sports Medicine. QT 260 C539]
RZ275.S65C47 1986   617′.1027   85-29470
ISBN 0-683-07583-7

Composed and printed at the
Waverly Press, Inc.

86 87 88 89 90

10 9 8 7 6 5 4 3 2 1

PREFACE TO
THE SECOND EDITION

Although it has been less than 4 years since the first edition of this book was introduced to the field, this new edition became necessary because of the widespread and enthusiastic reception to the topics presented. Coupled with this has been the many rapidly evolving approaches and techniques being utilized in the management of sports-related injuries that deserve broad communication.

Several topics within the first edition were directed to a wide audience—almost anyone interested or involved in the health care of the student, professional, or weekend athlete. However, because many of the important advances in sports medicine have been of a technical or therapeutic nature, this edition has given emphasis to the concerns of the professional health-care provider. The reader will find that about 100 pages of new material have been included in this edition. To accomplish this while keeping the book within an economical price range, a number of less pertinent topics have been presented in abstract form.

The first edition has long been recognized as a "best seller," and the pride surrounding such recognition must be shared by many dedicated physicians and instructors. I am most grateful for the cooperation of so many chiropractic educators who supported this work by sharing their thoughts and opinions during this and the initial edition. In addition to this broad support, I would be remiss if I did not call special attention to the suggestions and encouragement of Dr. Paul A. Jaskoviak of the National College of Chiropractic, Dr. John Nash of the Texas Chiropractic College, and Dr. Tuan A. Tran of the Los Angeles College of Chiropractic during the development of this edition.

—R.C.S.

PREFACE TO
THE FIRST EDITION

This manual has been designed for the physician and student who desire a reference to the proper management of sports-related disorders—whether it be one who occasionally cares for athletes or one who desires to build a specialization in this area of interest. Thus, one's involvement may take various forms from that of strictly in-office health care, to that within small community clubs, to that as a professional team physician, and the many levels between such as intramural activities and those conducted for personal pleasure by the weekend athlete or vacationer.

Many sections will also be of vital interest to athletic trainers, coaches, and administrators. Each chapter summarizes traumatology and its background according to the current state-of-the-art within athletic and recreational activities. Concern has been given to both background theory and the practical aspects involved in the management and prevention of sports-related injuries and disorders.

Participation in this area will show that there are some unique disabilities found in competitive athletics that are rarely, if ever, encountered in private practice. Each sport requires a different type of history-taking and examination emphasis; and each age group (children, adolescents, adults) presents specialized problems. Preadolescent participation in sports offers unique risks and professional challenges. Likewise, an increasing number of senior citizens maintain a degree of fitness through tennis, golf, bowling, jogging, volleyball, and other sports—activities that are not without risk. These factors are added to the usual variations seen in general practice such as degree of maturation, body type, past illnesses and surgery, congenital abnormalities, sexual variances, and so forth. As a rule, athletic rehabilitation must be carried beyond the usual range considered to be full function. Last, but far from least, is the particular athlete's motivation and career aspirations which must be carefully appraised in terms of fitness and short-term and long-range goals.

By applying one's discipline to sports injuries and related disorders, any doctor can find a vast range of clinical challenges at hand. The demand for alert health counsel and health management is insatiable. The broadening of a variety of sports available on the inter-scholastic and community level is increasing, as is the incidence of sports-related disorders. Of necessity, the on-site physician is often challenged to analyze, differentiate, diagnose, treat, or refer "on the spot" without aid of x-ray and laboratory reports. Such a skilled doctor must work solely with the basic tools of the physician: eyes, ears, and hands.

On first glance, a reader may question why certain degenerative conditions are mentioned in a text on traumatic injuries. While it is obvious that a person suffering a serious disability would not be engaging in sports, quite often an accident suffered during the early stages of pathology may be the initiating factor in bringing the process into clinical view. For this reason, differentiation must be made between acute trauma and trauma superimposed on a previously subclinical entity.

This text is divided into four parts. The first three parts offer a foundation for appreciating the role of professional health care within sports-related activities and the theory behind modern application. The fourth part offers a carefully researched compendium of the case management of sports-related injuries on a regional basis. These sections have been designed for ready reference to quick answers to common problems and techniques.

Part 1 offers an introduction to the role of the athletic physician, accident prevention and conditioning factors in sports, and the importance of athletic equipment and safety gear. Communicable diseases and their prevention are discussed, along with skin diseases associated with sports. The special considerations involved in female athletics, nutrition and physical activity, and the clinical assessment aspects of physical fitness offer a comprehensive foundation of understanding health care within athletics.

The scope of Part 2 is one of basic examination and evaluation considerations. Unique factors in examining procedures, anthropometric considerations, biomechanics, and body structure are discussed in relation to the participating athlete. A section on physical performance and the typical training rationale offers insight into the practical applications of physiologic mensuration upon which much clinical judgment must be based. This section is followed by a discussion of the various environmental influences on athletic performance, with emphasis upon the myriad effects of heat and cold. Inasmuch as the athlete is more than tangible tissue, an overview of the psychodynamic aspects of athletics is offered. And to complete the discussion on examination and evaluation a section on basic roentgenology in sports care is offered.

Part 3 discusses the general aspects of trauma, including first aid and emergency care; basic physiologic therapeutic procedures; skin and soft-tissue injuries; muscle, fascia, and tendon injuries; and peripheral nerve injuries. Part 3 concludes with a discussion on spinal subluxation considerations, with emphasis upon the neurologic implications.

Part 4 offers the practical aspects of examination, symptomatology, rapid differential diagnosis, prognosis, common complications, and conservative therapeutics (primary and ancillary) involved in alert health care. Specific sections are offered for head and facial injuries, traumatic eye and ear disorders, neck and cervical spine injuries, upper extremity disabilities, thoracic and abdominal injuries, pelvic and spinal injuries, and lower extremity disabilities. The best of the recognized methods of articular correction, taping, muscle therapy, trigger-point therapy, physiotherapy, physical support, and other rehabilitative procedures are discussed. In many instances, alternative techniques are offered to meet special needs. For clarity, adjustive and taping procedures are illustrated to support text descriptions.

It should be kept in mind that while many techniques are discussed, a technique is an art, and an art is interpreted by human standards. Thus, an art is not "the way" to do something, but "one way" to do something. Twelve excellent chiropractic physicians may adjust a spinal listing a different way, and twelve expert trainers may tape an ankle a different way—but each will do what is necessary to obtain a correction efficiently.

—R.C.S.

ACKNOWLEDGMENTS

Deep appreciation is expressed to the members of the ACA Council on Sports Injuries, as well as scores of reputable practitioners and educators. Because of their specialized ability and acknowledged expertise, the scope of this text has been enhanced by their contributions to the basic manuscript and their constructive review refinements.

Board of Review and Technical Assistance

While space does not allow mention of all contributors and reviewers, special gratitude must be extended to the following, in alphabetical order:

Charles Brandstetter, DC, ND
   President, American Council on Chiropractic Physiotherapy
M. Wayne Brown, DC
   President, Council on Mental Health of the ACA
Robin Canterbury, DC, DACBR
   Chairman, Department of Roentgenology, Palmer College of Chiropractic
Jan M. Corwin, DC
   Team Chiropractor, University of California (Berkeley)
   Member, American College of Sports Medicine
Brian M. Davis, DC, DACBR, FICC
   Secretary, Council on Roentgenology of the ACA
Faye B. Eagles, DC, FICC
   President, Council of Women Chiropractors of the ACA
George J. Goodheart, DC, DICAK, FICC
   Charter Diplomate, International College of Applied Kinesiology
   Member, Commission on Sports Medicine Modalities of the US Olympic Council
Paul A. Jaskoviak, DC, FICC
   President, Council on Neurology of the ACA
   Dean, National-Lincoln School of Postgraduate Education
Scott J. Murray, DC
   Member, Department of Roentgenology, Northwestern College of Chiropractic
John M. Nash, DC
   Dean of Students, Texas Chiropractic College
Shu Yan Ng, DC
   Director, Chiropractic Clinic of Hong Kong
Reed B. Phillips, DC, MSCM, DACBR
   Research Director, Foundation for Chiropractic Education and Research
W. Heath Quigley, DC, MS, FICA
   Director of External Affairs, Cleveland Chiropractic College (Los Angeles)
James F. Ransom, DC, FICC
   First Vice President, Council on Sports Injuries of the ACA
Michael A. Sabia, Jr., DC, PhD
   Lecturer; Ringside Physician, New Jersey Boxing Commission
Leonard W. Schroeder, DC, CCTP, FICC
   President, Council on Sports Injuries of the ACA
Neil Stern, DC, DACC, FACC, FICC
   Acting President, New York Chiropractic College

Tuan A. Tran, PhD
  Vice President for Research, Los Angeles College of Chiropractic

Cooperating Professional Organizations

American Chiropractic Association (ACA)
Council on Mental Health of the ACA
Council on Neurology of the ACA
Council on Physiotherapy of the ACA
Council on Roentgenology of the ACA
Council on Sports Injuries of the ACA
Council of Women Chiropractors of the ACA
Foundation for Chiropractic Education and Research (FCER)

Cooperating Chiropractic Colleges

Los Angeles College of Chiropractic (LACC)
New York Chiropractic College (NYCC)
Northwestern College of Chiropractic (NWCC)
Palmer College of Chiropractic (PCC)
Texas Chiropractic College (TCC)
Western States Chiropractic College (WSCC)

Cooperating Service Organizations

Associated Chiropractic Academic Press (ACAP)
Behavioral Research Foundation (BRF)
Chattanooga Corporation
Contour Comfort Company
Flex-Wedge Company
Gebauer Chemical Company (GCC)
Ohio Chiropractic Equipment & Supplies (OCE&S)
Smith Truss Company, Inc. (STC)
VRB, Inc.
Widen Tool & Stamping, Inc.

Illustration and Photography Credits

Unless credited to other sources, all drawings and photographs incorporated in this book have been reproduced with the permission of Associated Chiropractic Academic Press (ACAP).

CONTENTS

PART 1
INTRODUCTION

PART 2
EXAMINATION AND EVALUATION

PART 3
GENERAL ASPECTS OF TRAUMA

PART 4
INJURY CASE MANAGEMENT

Part 1

INTRODUCTION

CHAPTER 1

Introduction to Sports-Related Health Care

If you were to ask the average coach about the responsibilities of an athlete, he would most likely reply that he or she was to conduct one's self to the credit of the team, play fair, obey the officials, keep in training, be a credit to the sport, follow the rules, and enjoy the game: win or lose. This is the rhetoric commonly spooned to the naively inclined. If it were true, fewer sports injuries would be suffered.

With rare exception, even the Little Leaguer is commonly taught to WIN, drilled to disguise foul play from the eyes of the referees and umpires. Even in so-called noncontact sports, emphasis if often placed on getting the other team's stars out of the game without causing injury to your own team. While conditioning is emphasized, the motivation is frequently on the preservation of a potential winning season rather than on prevention of a personal injury to a human being.

These words are harsh, but realistic. Yet, doctors handling athletic injuries must have a realistic appraisal of sports today if they are in good conscience to properly evaluate disability and offer professional counsel.

THE ART OF EVALUATION

All people participating in vigorous sports should have a complete examination at the beginning of the season. Re-evaluation is often necessary at seasonal intervals and is always necessary with cases where the candidate has suffered a severe injury or illness or has had surgery.

Evaluation begins with questioning. Because of drilled routine, any doctor is well schooled in the taking of a proper case history. But, with an athletic injury, both obvious and subtle questions often appear. How extensive was the preseason conditioning? How much time for warm up is allowed before each game or event? What precautions are taken for heat exhaustion, heat stroke, concussion, and so forth? Does the coach make substitution immediately upon the first sign of disability so that proper evaluation can be made? How adequate is the protective gear? How many others on the team have suffered this particular injury this season?

Who, what, when, where, how, and WHY? These are the questions which must be answered before any positive course of health care can be extended. A detailed history of past illness and injury is vital. In organized sports, an outline of the regimen of training as well as a record of performance should be a part of the history. Most sports will require a detailed locomotor evaluation of the player. Special care must be made in evaluating the preadolescent competitor because of the wide range of height, weight, conditioning, and stages of maturation. A defect may bar a candidate from one sport but not another, or it may be only a deterrent until it is corrected or compensated. Many famous athletes have become great in spite of a severe handicap.

THE PHYSICIAN'S RESPONSIBILITIES

If a doctor only had to concern himself with injury prevention, care, and rehabilitation, his role would be much easier. But many other factors are involved. For instance, consider motivation. The average coach has many pressures upon him, as do the players. These pressures may blind a coach to the fact that a player is participating with an injury, playing beyond the point of exhaustion, or playing with an injury where further trauma may lead to permanent injury. Players too, in their enthusiasm, may avoid reporting injury or even try to hide its effects.

The attending physician should mentally

target that he is only responsible to the patient and his professional code of conduct. He is not responsible to the coach, trainer, ticket buyers, fans, school board, administrators, or the alumni association. Thus the question must be asked: Who has the authority to return a injured player to play or to practice—the physician, the trainer, or the coach? Obviously, no athlete should be allowed to risk permanent damage, regardless of the circumstance. In terms of preassessment before participation or competition, the physician should:

1. Determine the fitness of the individual by a thorough history and examination relative to a particular type of activity, and, when necessary, arrange for evaluation and treatment. During the interview, take note of any previous injuries or weaknesses from prior competition. Check each complaint thoroughly, as some athletes have a tendency to be stoic. Carefully check new team members for pre-existing disorders that may compromise an athletic career. In addition, the physician and coach may wish to determine minimum standards of strength and fitness before letting someone participate.

2. Conduct basic clinical tests. A routine full blood count and urinalysis are essential, a standard resting ECG is often important, and a chest x-ray film is desirable. Take comprehensive tests when clinical symptoms or signs appear. The physical examination should always include a spinal analysis, posture check, and neurologic and orthopedic evaluations.

3. Advise the candidate with an atypical condition of suitable sports or modifications. While all sports involve some risk, advise, or if necessary restrict, the candidate with overt or covert limitations from activities presenting great risk. Offer professional counsel which would contribute to optimal health and development.

4. Consider a psychologic assessment as to the athlete's goals, attitudes, desires, motivation, and reasons for participation. Make all physical, laboratory, and psychologic assessment tests with the permission of parents or a guardian in the case of a minor.

AREAS OF NECESSARY COOPERATION

The doctor must demand a degree of con-

trol equal to his responsibilities, and this is often difficult during the heat of competition. The physician's decisions will not always be treated with respect by the nonprofessional. Thus, it is imperative that the doctor do his best to establish areas of cooperation and an atmosphere of mutual rapport.

A sport is a game, and a game should not unduly jeopardize a person's health or safety. However, the coach and the athlete justifiably expect both serious and minor disabilities to be treated with readiness, skill, and efficiency because any handicap has serious consequences. Both coach and athlete must feel that the doctor understands the problem and is as interested in quickly returning the athlete to competition as they are. Honest, open communication is the cornerstone from which to build trust and confidence.

The Athlete

No rule exists that the athlete must confide in a doctor or accept his recommendations when there is a lack of confidence. The need for sympathetic understanding of the athlete and his particular problems and aspirations cannot be overemphasized. Creating an atmosphere of mutual confidence and trust is vital to establishing control. Likewise, the development of the athlete's confidence in the doctor will help to prevent "doctor shopping" by the athlete to get the opinion the athlete wants. Without confidence in the doctor, the athlete may not report possible masking or harmful do-it-yourself or over-the-counter remedies or devices.

All disabilities are important, and all must be dealt with individually: not by rote or preference for a favorite "star" or influenced by pressures where each prediction of potential disability may be publicized. Each athlete presents a variance as to strength and weakness, attitudes, motivations and goals, pain threshold, development, body type, the specific acute trauma, etc. In a squad of two dozen, there are 24 unique people. These factors must be analyzed and differentiated and a therapeutic solution applied (Fig. 1.1).

The Trainer

The ego of a physician is often deflated

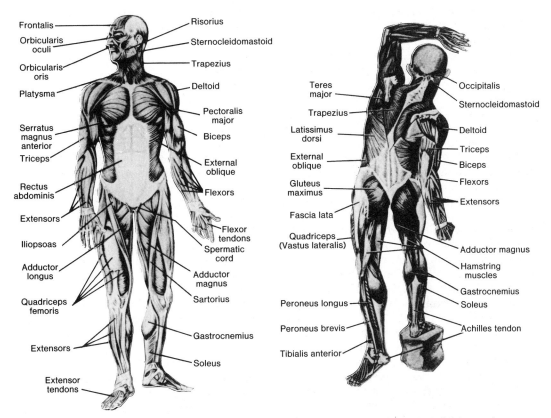

Figure 1.1. Artist's rendering depicting the overall relationship of the superficial muscles.

when he learns that the trainer is held in higher respect. If a team had to choose between a team physician or a trainer, the physician would usually lose. And this respect is usually well earned. The trainer's entire life has been devoted to the care of sports injuries. Loyalty also builds respect. Trainers have often been with the team for many seasons, while physicians have come and gone.

Many trainers and coaches possess a remarkable memory which can recall in detail a similar injury occurring many years ago, its efficient treatment, the exact duration of the rehabilitation process, and the capabilities of the athlete on recovery—to the dismay of a young doctor (and with a blow to his professional pride), who must at least match the record.

While the trainer is commonly seen at the college and professional level, his aid is usually missing at the secondary and primary levels—and this lack makes the phy-

sician's role overly demanding and sometimes impossible. The reason for this is that a trainer must be an expert at applying bandages, splints, dressings, slings, specialized athletic taping, and other first-aid measures. He is an expert at evaluating, ordering, fitting, and maintaining equipment, and he is often called upon to custom design a special piece from available material. The skilled trainer is an expert in physical conditioning, in physical rehabilitation, and in a large variety of physiotherapeutic applications and their contraindications.

The experienced trainer "knows his people" for he lives daily with their complaints, hopes, opinions, personality quirks, and the unchecked locker room shop talk which few doctors are allowed to hear. He knows the art of listening to feelings rather than words and thus gains an insight into capabilities that others do not have. This insight is invaluable to both physician and coach, who do not enjoy the closeness with the athlete that the trainer is allowed.

A good trainer is more than an assistant to the doctor; he often serves somewhat as a mentor to the new team physician. On the other hand, an unskilled trainer must be carefully judged and evaluated as to his capability of carrying out delegated duties and his willingness to perform. Is there a definite plan for handling a serious injury or health emergency both at games and at practice? Planning ahead is imperative. Duties and procedures must be cordially discussed and mutually agreed upon, not proclaimed. The doctor and trainer have different yet parallel roles, and each should respect the experience and limits of the other. Few young doctors can tape a sprained joint as skillfully as an experienced trainer. The handicap of little mutual confidence is an impossible situation.

Hirata reminds us that "The doctor who runs out on the field at the slightest provocation on heavily attended game days, but leaves the trainer to sink or swim during weekday practice, may impress the crowd and himself but certainly not the trainer or the team. Far worse, he exhibits little respect for the trainer's integrity and in turn will receive very little."

The Coach and Staff

As with the doctor-trainer relationship, the physician and coach also have different yet parallel roles. The coach wants a winning team; the doctor wants a healthy team. Obviously, it is often impossible to "charm" an entire athletic staff or every athlete. Here lies the necessity of administrative power to cope with poor cooperation, else each disagreeable decision will be met with increasing subversion. While it is important to develop firm friendships with athlete, coach, and trainer, the doctor must take care that such cordial relationships do not cloud his professional principles.

Sometimes the physician is forced to be a scrutinizing evaluator of the coaching staff. Has conditioning been developed progressively? Are tactics with a known high rate of injury discouraged? Are such safety factors as failure to use mouth protectors being ignored in practice as well as during games? Are the causes for injury determined? Does shortcuts to optimum athletic fitness? Does conditioning take into consideration individual differences of structure and function: inherited or acquired? Are old wives' tales such as no water during practice being advertised on the field? Are adequate precautions being taken to safeguard against heat exhaustion or heat stroke? The questions appear endless.

To build respect between coach and physician, the doctor must be empathetic with the coach's position. A coach is under pressure from both within and without and looks to the physician as the usual bearer of bad news. A coach cannot be expected to be happy with any bad news, even if it's clinically minimal, and he can be expected to argue at times with professional opinion. Regardless, it is the doctor's responsibility to calmly inform the coach, with certainty, of any athlete's diagnosis, the prediction of future performance capabilities, prognosis, and the progress during recuperation and rehabilitation. Without accurate information, free from medical jargon, the coach cannot do his job. He wants the facts made simple. How bad is the injury, how long will it take to bring the athlete back to the pre-injury or peak performance level? When can the athlete participate again? How permanent is the damage? With this information, he must modify his squad and game plan, often minute-by-minute during competition.

In organized sports, the physician should provide the coach with a written disability list which is revised daily if necessary. The Athletic Department (eg, college) should receive a copy of the list if such a department is involved. This list should name the player and offer a brief description of medical status and performance capability. A prediction of when the athlete can be expected to return to full activity is helpful to the coach in planning his substitution strategy.

In community sports such as Little League, the neighborhood ex-jock or volunteer coach is rarely thoroughly trained in safety precautions, first aid, proper field conditions, physical conditioning, or protective equipment and its fitting. Often, all he wants for his boys or girls is to win and maintain a boastful win-loss record. In some states, any certified teacher may be employed as a high school coach, regardless of experience.

The Family Physician

The development of cooperation between team physician and family physician or consulting specialist helps to reduce the bugbear of conflicting opinions, often delivered to an already confused athlete. While disagreements and differences are to be expected, prompt referral for primary care or surgical attention is vital to assure mutual respect. The typical family doctor has little knowledge of the practicalities involved in specialized sports injury management and should accept logical procedures and recommendations when explained.

The Press

Publicity surrounding health decisions is common in organized sports. It is an area to be confronted which is usually unknown in private practice. No disability should be reported to the press without the coach's knowledge because such news may give an opposing coach an advantage. Inaccurate or ill-timed reporting can destroy a team's morale. Information must always be given sparingly, and without a named source to emphasize the team approach.

Being quoted out of context or misquoted in the local media or on national wire services is often embarrassing. It is unfair, but it happens, and more so with those inexperienced in handling the press. Some reporters carefully check their facts, others do not and rely much on romanticized teammate hearsay or speculation. There are many sports reporters who deem themselves experts in all phases of coaching, training, doctoring, and playing. Inaccuracies must be directly communicated to the coach, the athlete, and the athlete's family. All involved must have faith in the doctor's personal statements, not what appears widely publicized in the paper or on the air.

Terminology

It is granted that an injury may be recognized and treated regardless of what label we place on it. By the same token, the subject of sports injuries is frequently confusing when misinterpreted lay terms are used to replace accurate anatomic and pathologic descriptions. This should not imply that lay people should be forced to use health science terminology, but it does emphasize the need for good intra- and intercommunication among doctors, athletic administrators, trainers, coaches, sports writers, and insurance personnel.

Such colorful terms as "black eye," "cauliflower ear," "charley horse," "cramp," "glass" arm or jaw, "hip pointer," "jock itch," "little league arm," "muscle soreness," "pinched nerve," "shin splints," and "tennis elbow" are often bantered about with ambiguous meanings and interpretations. It is not uncommon to hear erroneous expressions referring to a "sprained muscle" or a "strained joint." In this text, care will be taken to associate scientific terminology with the colloquialisms of sports jargon in a practical, precise manner which will consider cause, symptoms, signs, extent of severity, management, complications, and prognosis.

THE CLUB OR TEAM PHYSICIAN

The opportunity of being a team physician is often quite unique for the typical doctor in that he is dealing, as a rule, with patients who are usually healthy and physically fit. This is rare in general practice. Young athletes are often in the peak of physical condition and motivation, accounting for a rapid rate of recovery. While the professional prerequisites are obtained in regular health care education, on-site athletic care is often a far different experience than that of general practice.

Responsibilities of the Team Physician

Innumerable cranial, spinal, and extremity contusions, strains, sprains, fractures, subluxations, dislocations, and soft-tissue trauma must be immediately recognized (Fig. 1.2). In addition, injuries to the kidneys, spleen, liver, stomach, and intestines are not uncommon. The dangers of cardiorespiratory failure and shock are always a threat. When on the field, the team physician does not have the advantage of laboratory reports and x-ray films or even the simpler diagnostic instruments.

Parameters

It is rare that the team physician is al-

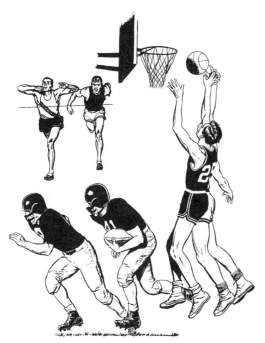

Figure 1.2. A physican treating sports injuries must be thoroughly skilled in the recognition of athletic injuries and in first aid in all its aspects. Knowledge of how an injury is caused is vital to developing optimal diagnostic, prognostic, and rehabilitative procedures.

lowed to take full responsibility for any player-patient. This role is generally that of the player's family physician, whether it be a doctor of chiropractic, allopathy, or osteopathy or a Christian Science practitioner. An athlete's right to "freedom of choice in health care" should never be obstructed, regardless of a particular doctor's preference.

The role of the team physician is inevitably to render only those therapeutic measures necessary to bridge the period from injury or the recognition of disease until the player's family physician can be reached. It is not the role of the team physician to utilize some type of cavalier treatment which may be thought questionable by another practitioner for being beyond the scope of the team doctor's specialty or legal or ethical code of conduct. While the ultimate course of case management of a particular injury or ailment is the responsibility of the player's family physician, the decision as to whether an athlete is fit, with or without

reservations, or not fit to play should inevitably rest with the team physician.

Acute Injury on the Field

The athlete who is acutely injured on the field of play must be managed as any accident victim would be handled. If symptoms warrant it, transportation to the sidelines, the locker room, or the nearest hospital is ordered. Notify the player's parents immediately in cases of severe injury. Do not let the excitement of the moment rush objective appraisal. If the player is unconscious, do not be in a hurry to use smelling salts. After evaluating the possibility of fracture, determine if the player is ambulatory. If there is any doubt, use a litter, regardless of the player's spartan protests. A football helmet should never be removed on the field until the possibility of head or neck injury has been eliminated. Even then, it must be removed with extreme caution.

GOOD HEALTH CARE

Proper care implies doing needful and helpful things for the injured or sick individual to restore him or her to the best possible state of physical and mental health in the shortest time. These needful and helpful things include environmental, hygienic, therapeutic, and supportive measures to protect against contracting any additional pathologic condition, physical or emotional. Body, mind, and spirit must all receive attention.

In the larger athletic oganizations, several members of a health care team may be involved, where each person contributes something toward the patient's welfare. Each member of such a health team must understand and appreciate the other's role. Each must know where he fits in, what he is to do, to whom he is responsible, and how he is to do his part. Otherwise, function is impossible, and an injured player is in danger of being neglected.

All personnel and all players, regardless of social status or diagnosis, should be recognized as potential carriers of pathogenic organisms. It is thus essential to consider strict hygienic practices that prevent the transfer of these organisms from one person to another.

The majority of players seeking health care do so because of minor illness, injury, or concern over personal health. If these individuals are returned to competition from the dispensary or the attending doctor's office without adequate examination, treatment, and reassurance, they continue to worry about their health, lose confidence in the health care extended, and become less effective in their assignments. On the other hand, if they are needlessly referred to specialized care, time is lost unnecessarily and professional time and facilities are used needlessly.

The Athletic Dispensary

A dispensary is a treatment facility designed primarily to provide care of ambulatory athletes and to arrange for referral to another practitioner, hospital, or specialized clinic. Athletic dispensaries also perform various administrative, preventive, and sanitary activities related to sports and the personnel served. An athletic dispensary is often referred to as an "aid station." Most dispensaries are fixed and usually located close to a stadium, arena, or field of play. Some, however, are mobile and can move or be moved from place to place to provide health care support at tactical locations.

Function

A well-organized and efficiently operated facility is one of the most effective means of providing and extending health service to the club or team. Some of the more important activities carried on by an aid station involve (1) sudden sicknesses, (2) emergency treatment, (3) continuing routine treatments or a series of treatments for players who do not need external care, (4) physical examinations, diagnosis, and disposition of players receiving health care, (5) sanitary inspections related to health of personnel and players served, (6) administration of dispensary records, property, and supplies, and (7) supervision of subordinate personnel.

Emergency care

Emergency treatment in a dispensary is the early care given to the injured, wounded, or sick by a trained professional prior to referral. Specific measures to be applied at the scene will be discussed later in the section concerning first aid.

In the dispensary, the doctor in charge is usually the first professional to see the patient who has come or been brought to the dispensary for emergency treatment. He or she must be prepared to receive emergency situations and maintain proficiency in applying first-aid measures. Emergency equipment should be ready for use, in its proper location, and immediately available (not locked up). Trained personnel must be available who know how to operate all necessary emergency apparatus and how to use all items on an emergency basis. There is no time to look up a technique in a procedure manual or to review an instruction booklet. All emergency equipment should be inspected, maintained, and tested at regularly scheduled intervals.

Doping: A Dangerous Practice

While an exact definition of doping has not been universally accepted, doping is usually considered the act of using chemical substances with the deliberate goal of altering athletic performance, usually with the intent to gain an unfair advantage over a rival. To help control abuses in major competition, dope detection methods have been developed to identify such substances. Most substances taken to act during active competition can be detected by some type of chromatography.

The four major types of drugs commonly used to modify performance are stimulants, sedatives, anabolic steroids, and anti-inflammatory agents and analgesics.

1. Stimulants are used to delay fatigue and enhance feelings of alertness, strength, and aggressiveness. The two major types of stimulants used are (a) the psychotonics such as the amphetamines, which act upon the central nervous system, and (b) the analeptics such as adrenaline and ephedrine, which influence the cardiac and respiratory regulating mechanisms. Caffeine is both a mild psychotonic and an analeptic. Among the side effects of the strong stimulants are psychologic dependence, hypertension, cardiac arrhythmias, hostile behavioral changes (eg, paranoid reactions), and cardiovascular collapse from impaired temper-

ature regulation (ie, cutaneous vasoconstriction).

2. Sedatives are used to develop a "calmness" in a player whose performance depends greatly on precision and control such as in archery and rifle matches.

3. Anabolic steroids are troublesome drugs used to promote muscular development, especially during preseason development programs, where great power is necessary (eg, weight lifting, shot put). The side effects of water retention, various forms of glandular suppression and exaggeration, and osteoporosis make them quite dangerous. Any drug that is sufficiently potent to alter metabolism in the healthy athlete is also likely to produce manifold undesirable effects.

4. Certain substances are used primarily to reduce pain. Anti-inflammatory agents (eg, salicylates, cortisone) and analgesics (eg, procaine) compromise the body's normal response to painful stimuli. When pain is eliminated, the benefit of muscle spasm to splint an injured part is lost, and further motion contributes to greater injury. The long-term effect is often traumatic arthritis.

SPECIAL CONSIDERATIONS IN FEMALE ATHLETES

For the sake of optimum health, both sexes should be allowed to participate in a wide variety of athletic events. Girls and women are now taking an increasing role in sports participation as various taboos and culturally imposed restrictions give way. While women have long been active in such sports as tennis and golf, they have recently increased their participation in such violent activities as wrestling, boxing, football, and demolition derbies.

Growth, Development, and Function

The capacity for physical activity during childhood is equal for both sexes. Strength, cardiovascular endurance, and motor skills exhibit few differences between the sexes up to the age of 12 years. After adolescence, however, males develop faster physically, allowing for greater power and potential, but the capacity to develop motor skills remains about equal.

The ratio of lean body mass to fat is one of the most obvious physical differences. Males present greater bone strength and density, greater muscle bulk and broadness in the shoulder area, and greater subcutaneous fat in the upper half of the body.

At maturity, females are generally shorter in height, have more flexibility in their joints, have more delicate ligaments and tendons, have more subcutaneous fat in the hips and lower body regions, have less erythrocyte and hemoglobin mass, exhibit a greater degree of pelvic tilt and obliquity; the female elbow offers a greater carrying angle and tendency toward cubitus valgus. The female has smaller lungs, heart, liver, and kidneys than does the male. Schroeder points out that female joints are more subject to injury in sports which require the expulsive effort, sudden stopping, sudden checking of speed and turns, and landing in jumps.

Special Sports Concerns

Contrary to common opinion, women have been shown to achieve much greater muscle strength without an appreciable change in muscle bulk. Weight lifting, with proper techique, will not necessarily cause undue hypertrophy.

To ensure optimal endurance and performance, adequate iron is necessary in the diet to carry oxygen to the cells. Iron deficiency is the most common nutritional fault in American females. A female loses from 5 to 45 mg of iron/day during menstruation. Thus, most female athletes require supplementation and frequent monitoring of iron content in the blood.

Participation During Menstruation

With the exception of an athlete who is experiencing unusual discomfort or excessive flow, there is no physiologic reason why training or competition should be avoided during menstruation. Statistics show that most Olympic sportswomen do not interrupt training during menstruation, although the type of training and the intensity of training may be modified. About 1 out of 4 sometimes interrupt training, and only 1 out of 20 do not train during menstruation.

Although the majority of females prefer tampon protection during some phase of menstrual bleeding, the recent controversy about "toxic shock syndrome" deserves caution and suggests frequent changes. Caution must also be given relative to diaphragms continually worn and to intrauterine devices which might complicate an abdominal blow.

The female athlete usually exhibits less colic, less premenstrual headaches and tension, and greater regularity than the nonathlete. In fact, physical exercise appears to be a distinct aid in the treatment of dysmenorrhea. Neither the menarche nor conditions for future pregnancy are disturbed by active participation in sports, and no detrimental long range gynecologic effects from vigorous physical activity have been determined. However, many female athletes report disruption or even cessation of their periods during intensive training. This has been shown to be related to lowering of the percentage of body fat which has a direct effect on hormonal levels and the menstrual cycle.

The influence of menstruation on athletic performance is a highly individualized effect. The female athlete who is distinctly disadvantaged by the physiologic function of menstruation can have her menstrual cycle medically adjusted so that competition will occur at the optimum time of her cycle, but this is not usually advisable. F. M. Eagles, DC, cautions against the numerous, and often serious, side effects from hormone therapy such as the potential for emboli formation following small foot fractures and the visual changes some females experience while on this type of medication. Headaches and fluid retention are other common complaints detected from cycle alteration.

Pregnancy

Except with a poor obstetric history, there is no evidence that a normal pregnancy will be threatened by exercise. Of all athletics, swimming appears to be the best physical activity for the expectant mother. On the other hand, there is evidence that physical fitness during pregnancy contributes to ease of labor, and postpartum light exercise assists the process of involution. Following delivery, intense competition is usually contraindicated for several months, especially if the mother is breast feeding.

Pregnant women should avoid increasing body temperature, especially during the 1st and 2nd trimesters. Overtraining in environments of high humidity and heat (along with the practice of utilizing hot tubs, saunas, and jacuzzi baths) can be responsible for raising body temperature for longer than 10 minutes. This can cause irreversible neurologic damage to the fetus. The personnel of spas and health clubs involved with the pregnant women should be aware of this situation.

The Breasts and Genital Organs

A metal breast protector is necessary in all contact sports and in some noncontact sports, such as volleyball, to prevent contusions and pain (Fig. 1.3). Breast injury may lead to a localized hematoma producing a region of fat necrosis characterized by a firm and painless lump developing several weeks or months after the accident. This is impossible to differentiate from breast cancer except by biopsy.

Haycock et al. have proved that lack of an adequate supportive bra can cause discomfort as well as injury to the breast when walking and running. Their controlled-study data suggest that women without proper breast support experience trauma to the breasts and supporting ligaments, es-

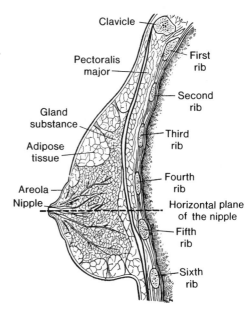

Figure 1.3. Right breast in sagittal section; inner surface of outer segment.

pecially when the breasts are large or pendulous. Thus, the need for a properly engineered athletic bra is obvious. A sports bra should cover the breasts, prevent slapping or lateral shifting during activity, and offer enough support without undue restriction or abrasiveness, that there are no signs of ache or tenderness after activity. Metal parts, seams, and allergenic effects may present problems.

The activity itself and the size of the breasts, along with the tone of the supporting muscles and ligaments, determine whether a special athletic bra, a regular bra, or no bra is adequate. In modern dance or swimming for instance, the no bra situation may occur when the participants are small breasted because the stretch material in leotards and swim suits (plus water support) provides adequate support.

The most common female direct-trauma genital injuries are those involving vulval lacerations and hematomas (eg, vaulting, hurdles). Forceful douching occurs in inexperienced water skiers that can result in serious gynecologic problems. This can be prevented by wearing rubber pants.

Dermatologic Problems

Female skin is more delicate than that of the male. Many dermatologic problems can be prevented if conditioning and participation progresses slowly enough to allow the skin to accommodate to the acquired demands of excessive exposure to perspiration, dirt, and bumps.

During menstruation, large and bulky external sanitary napkins may irritate inner thighs during prolonged vigorous competition to the extent that a severe dermatitis develops.

Hair and fingernails also present special consideration. In may sports, hair must be either cut short or pulled out the way of vision through tight braiding pulled into buns or ponytails. This traction, however, may occasionally cause some degree of hair loss and balding. Traumatized fingernails may result in nail breaking and splitting which may lead to secondary infection.

Ovulatory Patterns

Temperature patterns occur in the menstruating female that reflect the effects of ovulation. There is a fall in morning temperature just prior to menstruation that continues until midpoint between the two periods. In about 24–36 hours before ovulation, the morning temperature rises and stays at a somewhat higher level until just before the next menses.

Temperature Responses in Sportswomen

Because a female has fewer functional sweat glands, body temperature in the female rises 2–3°C higher than that of the male before the cooling process of perspiration becomes significant. Thus, acute heat stress is a greater concern in female athletes. However, studies show that during prolonged activity in normal or hot weather females have less change in body temperature as compared to the male. While males sweat more, females cool quicker after muscular activity in hot weather. Females appear to adjust their perspiration rate more efficiently to the required loss of heat. This suggests that females present more efficiency in body temperature regulation and have a greater cardiovascular component of thermoregulation.

CHAPTER 2

Accident Prevention and Conditioning

Each particular sport, the player's position, and his or her degree of physical capabilities and skill all contribute to injury incidence. Many specific injuries seem peculiar to certain sports and occupations and are rarely met elsewhere, and some injuries are met both in sports and elsewhere. Nevertheless, specific steps can be taken to help reduce the quantity of acute injuries and prevent the formation of chronic disability.

ACCIDENT PREVENTION

When a player running at full speed collides with a wall, a goal post, or another player, a force may develop equal to hitting a concrete wall at 20 mph. Many injuries and accidents can be prevented with proper officiating, coaching, matching, equipment, facilities, health care, self-control, and conditioning. The maxim of "prevention is better than cure" is nowhere more important than in sports. All too many athletic injuries are unnecessary.

Officiating

Game rules and regulations are designed (a) to preserve the character and spirit of the sport and (b) to protect an athlete from both himself and his competitors by minimizing risk. Without proper officiating and disciplinary action, players lose a fundamental protection based on game experience. Unnecessary violence should never be left unpenalized. It is vital that all officials be both technically and emotionally qualified. Unless players and coaches have confidence in the officials, the officials' decisions will not be respected. The less the respect, the greater the injury incidence and the less the competition will be enjoyed by the participants.

The doctor must be familiar with the rules and procedures concerning each sport to be alerted to the possible and probable mechanisms of injury. Identical disabilities and injuries have a different effect on different types of athletes. A specific injury may be less important in terms of performance in one position than another; eg, a sprained thumb of a guard as contrasted with that of a center in football.

Coaching

One goal of good coaching is the improvement of skill, as the improvement of performance lowers the incidence of injury. Skill development should be made progressively to allow for physical and functional adaptation. If the incidence of injury is to be minimal, tactics with a high injury risk must be avoided. When any player shows signs of disability, substitution should be made immediately so that proper evaluation can be made.

In a good preventive program, all injuries should be analyzed for cause and corrective coaching measures should be applied. It is the coach's responsibility to see that every player wears the proper type of well-fitting apparel and keeps in optimum physical fitness.

Helpful information by itself does not guarantee compliance. Written instructions and oral recommendations are rarely meaningful by themselves. Effective behavioral change requires reasons for change, motivation, instruction, illustration, individualization, repetitive practice, and insistence.

Matching

Proper matching allows for greater safety and participation and for more equitable competition. In neighborhood programs, as well as in elementary and junior high school programs, players are often grossly overmatched against much faster, larger, stronger, taller, and heavier opponents in contact (collision) sports. If not in the games themselves, then this often happens in practices or scrimmages. Each sport determines the criteria (eg, height in basketball, weight in wrestling). A youth's age and maturation are always a consideration. Bony prominence measurements (eg, the Tipton-Tcheng method) have proven helpful wherein measurements are taken of standing height, chest width and depth, hip width, and ankle width. However, more controlled studies in a variety of sports are needed for accurate matching criteria.

Disability Prevention

As mentioned, good health care is founded on thorough evaluation and the development of confidence between doctor and trainer, coach, player, and family physician. All should be educated as to the benefits of injury prevention, good nutrition, conditioning, and body heat balance. Towards this end, whenever possible the doctor should attend practice sessions as well as official games, not only to be available to offer professional attention and counsel, but also to witness the cause of injury or potential injury and to try to offer suggestions on preventive measures.

Chronic disability can often be prevented by following established safety principles.

1. Players should never be allowed to play until an injured part is adequately healed. The risk of repeated injury leading to serious chronic disability must be well weighed. When an athlete enters game or practice competition with a minor injury, the part should always be well taped, supported, padded, or wrapped to protect it against further injury. It is well established that when an athlete returns to competition under the influence of a pain killer, the risk to injury aggravation and chronic disability is extremely high.

2. To compensate for joint-ligament weakness, the strength in an injured limb *and* the opposite limb should be redeveloped to a degree stronger than the preinjury level. Voluntary resistance exercises, specifically designed for the sport and position involved, are most helpful in developing joint strength. Especially in cases of ligamentous damage, the development of overall muscle power of a limb can increase

residual strength to enhance resistance against twists and blows. A knowledge of applied kinesiology is helpful here to better evaluate muscular imbalance.

CONDITIONING FUNDAMENTALS

To maintain acquired conditioning, each team member and prospective member should be given a regimen for preseason conditioning, and each player should be required to adequately warm up before each competition or practice. As a general rule, at least 3 weeks of practice should be held prior to the first competition. During the off season, two or three moderate workouts a week are usually enough to prevent much deterioration. When an athlete is physically capable of performing a sport with optimal efficiency, he or she can meet both the physiologic and biomechanic demands placed upon the body, not only for typical performance demands but also for critical situations.

General Fitness

One of the most important factors in preventing injuries is the development of an appropriate level of physical fitness. Haycock feels that "conditioning is the equivalent of physical fitness." In the last analysis, to be "fit" is to be equal to the demands. But, to be physically fit for one sport or position does not imply fitness for another. Yet, a conditioned athlete will have greater endurance, strength, and stamina than the nonathlete.

Certain sports require greater levels of fitness of different anatomic parts, and this must also be realized. A marathoner will traditionally have poor upper body development as compared with a discus thrower who will have superior upper body fitness.

A low level of physical fitness leads to fatigue that tends to break down the conditioned reflexes involved in physical skills. However, skill alone won't protect an athlete against the effects of overexertion if activity is carried beyond the limit of his/her level of physical fitness. Conditioning enhances flexibility, agility, speed, endurance, and strength—all safeguards against injury, which have positive benefits to an athlete's level of general fitness and performance (Fig. 2.1).

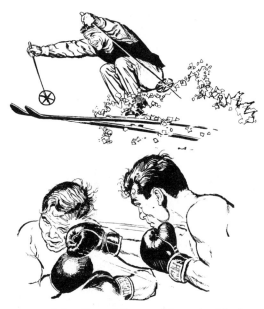

Figure 2.1. One of the most important factors in preventing injuries is the development of an appropriate level of physical fitness.

Conditioning Components

To develop good athletic performance, conditioning programs should have four major components: (1) warm up and stretching, (2) the development of muscular strength, (3) the development of joint flexibility, and (4) the development of endurance (both somatic muscular and cardiorespiratory).

Warmup and Stretching

The value of calisthenics has long been debated from a physiologic standpoint, and the final answer is still not known. The weight of evidence is empirical. However, we do know that properly designed and performed exercises call into action little used muscle groups, strengthen them reasonably, and contribute to flexibility. Repetition increases muscle tone and enhances cardiovascular efficiency.

A warmup period, as a ground work in training, consists first of the entire body being put through stretching or flexibility exercises and then exercising specific body parts vital to the sport and position. The duration of a warmup period varies with the individual. Usually, it is said to be sufficient when perspiration arises. Warmup should never result in fatigue, but it should present a renewed sense of joint "freedom." Careful supervision should be maintained during the warmup to prevent the eager athlete from overdoing and becoming discouraged, sore, or strained. Acclimatization to a change in environment or altitude, temperature changes, and humidity changes also influence an athlete's performance. In general, the well-trained athlete adapts faster than one out of condition.

Strength

Strength can be said to be the effect of one's all-out effort against resistance. It is specific to a muscle or muscle group and specific to that angle at which the training occurs; thus, to be strong at every angle, training must be throughout the range of joint motion. As motion requires synchronized body parts, all parts must be trained to be strong and have adequate endurance. Strength is acquired through training that requires repetition against increasing resistance.

Weight lifting is quite helpful in enhancing muscular strength and endurance when judiciously applied, but it has little effect on developing flexibility or cardiorespiratory endurance. With weights, sets of about a dozen repetitions per bout are typical. A "bout" is one exercise series or program. Training with weights has both its zealot adherents and opponents, and both are well-armed with empirical evidence.

Certain exercises should be discouraged. For instance, deep-knee bends and the duck-waddle, both used for many years with several sports, exert severe stress on the cruciate ligaments of the knee, far outweighing any benefit to the quadriceps muscles.

Care must be taken for gradual progression in any exercise program. Regardless of an athlete's enthusiasm, the beginning level should be comfortably below that which may cause injury. Progression at any stage should be to a comfortable point which requires moderate effort. Stress should be felt, but pain should not be. An ideal program should be well balanced and conducted on a daily basis with varying intensity on alternate days, depending on how often and when the athlete competes.

An intense workout the day before competition is usually not wise.

ATHLETIC EQUIPMENT AND SAFETY GEAR

Clothing and other gear worn by athletes can be divided into two categories: basic clothing and protective equipment. Basic clothing consists of such items as shirts, sweaters, jackets, pants, skirts and dresses, underwear, socks and tights, gloves, and footwear. These items help to protect the skin from injury and often aid in holding interior padding in place. With the increase of female participation in sports, new designs for protective equipment must be created or adapted when established male designs are not satisfactory.

All sports have developed protective equipment uniquely adapted to particular requirements. The need for gloves, catcher's pads and masks, and batting helmets is obvious in baseball. The hockey goalie's bulky padding and fiberglass mask are a must, as is the fencer's mask and the shin guards used in soccer. Likewise, we see the shoulder pads, arm guards, helmets and face guards used in lacrosse, field hockey goalkeeper toe boots, and fail-safe ski bindings. While space does not permit a discussion of all protective gear utilized in sports, the need, use, and fitting of some models will be briefly explained in this section so that pertinent principles may be underscored.

Corwin warns that an athlete at times may forego protective clothing or padding in the interest of increasing speed or flexibility. This practice must be discouraged.

Design Considerations

Poorly designed protective equipment presents two hazards: it is dangerous in itself and it can instill in its wearer a false sense of security. Williams and Sperryn offer four basic requirements for athletic clothing which are worthy of repetition here. They state that protective clothing should do the following:

1. Provide complete or adequate protection to the appropriate part of the body under the conditions of use. It should withstand any foreseeable impact, and any distortion which may take place under stress should be within clearly defined limits.

2. Be made of such a material as to allow proper cleansing and retain its properties for a reasonable period of time. Protective clothing is not acceptable if it progressively loses its capacity to protect.

3. Be so designed and made as to allow the wearer an appropriate freedom of action and not interfere with his activities in such a way as to constitute a source of danger to him.

4. Be so designed and made that its use does not in any way constitute a source of danger to anyone with whom the wearer comes into contact. In general, this later requirement should be fulfilled by any item of sportswear.

Adrian also points out the necessity for such features as nonrestrictive movement, nonabrasive and nonirritating characteristics, heat loss and heat retention balance, light weight, and the initial level of protection.

1. *Nonrestrictive movement:* Test clothing by having the wearer vigorously swing limbs up and down and across the body, bending side to side, backward and forward, rotating, twisting trunk right and left, reaching high and low, squatting—covering the major joints' full range of motion, especially those concerning typical position postures. Check that tight clothing does not bind at the armpit, elbow, neck, or chest. Undergarments should not creep with vigorous movements. Check shoes by prancing, jumping, stamping, rising on toes, pushing off, making quick turns, and putting the ankle and foot joints through their full range of motion. Check gloves by flexing and extending fingers and palms, then put the wrist through its full range of motion.

2. *Nonabrasive and nonirritating characteristics:* Most athletic clothing made today is a blend of manmade and natural fibers that is soft and nonabrasive. Heavy or poorly sewn seams and thick hems, as seen in "bargain" sportswear, often cause chafing. In addition, some clothing which features wash-and-wear nonwrinkle benefits, odor prevention qualities, and water repellency characteristics may be abrasive to sensitive skin. Some athletes may be allergic to wool or sensitive to the chemicals or electrostatic charges within clothing.

3. *Heat loss and heat retention balance:*

Synthetic materials have a tighter and more elastic weave than natural fibers. They do not allow easy passage of air, and this inhibits heat loss and interferes with proper perspiration evaporation. Because of their low permeability to moisture and air, noniron finishes and waterproofing processing especially inhibit heat loss. Manmade materials used in modern footwear rarely allow for proper air passage; they restrict heat loss and encourage the growth of fungi and bacteria.

4. *Light weight:* The less weight the less effort necessary for activity; however, the low-weight feature must not overlook the need for adequate padding, warming or cooling, and other safeguards. Adrian believes that athletes without lightweight clothing are probably putting out 10% more effort than they would otherwise need.

5. *Initial level of protection:* Basic clothing should offer the first level of protection against both extrinsic and intrinsic forces. This protection is made by smooth, nonabrasive clothes covering the skin, protecting against skidding, abrasion, sliding, falling, and colliding irritations.

Skull, Face, and Eye Protection

Protective equipment for the skull, face, and eyes should be so designed that it moves with the head without loosening, is lightweight, and protects the vital areas of the scalp, ears, eyes (without affecting peripheral vision), cheekbones, face, nose, mouth, teeth, chin, and neck.

Safety Glasses

Safety glasses come in both plastic and heat-treated lenses. The heat-treated lenses are usually preferred because the resin type easily scratches. The bridge of the nose should be cushioned to prevent possible trauma. Temple bars should comfortably wrap around the ears and be stabilized on the head by an elastic band.

Contact Lenses

Contact lenses are available in two sizes. One size (scleral or haptic) covers the entire white of the eye. The other size (corneal) covers only the colored part of the eye. Both hard (acrylic) and soft types are available. Contact lenses offer distinct disadvantages

and advantages over conventional spectacles with safety lenses and frames.

The major disadvantages are that in contact sports they may become dislodged and lost, and, in several sports, dust or sand often works its way under the lens, becomes trapped, and sets up an irritating abrasion of the cornea. Contributing to this is the fact that after contacts are worn for about a month, the cornea loses some of its normal sensitivity and the early warning sign of pain is diminished. The resulting abrasion may produce corneal scars which contribute to visual loss. It is almost impossible for a swimmer or diver to keep a corneal contact in place, but the scleral type usually can be held by squinting. In addition, contact lenses require frequent removal, cleaning, storage, and reinsertion to avoid irritation or infection. Many ophthalmologists suggest that athletes allow a 2-month break-in period before competition is tried with contact lenses.

The distinct advantages with contacts are that irregular astigmatism is more readily corrected, peripheral vision is enhanced, and contacts do not cloud up as do spectacles. Another benefit is the tinting attribute of contact lenses that offers special advantages in particular sports. For example, in skiing a grey or dark blue tint helps to reduce snow and sun glare, while in hockey a yellow tint reduces ice glare. In wrestling, contacts are possible and spectacles are not, but even contacts should not be worn unless vision is severely impaired.

Mouth Protectors and Face Guards

One of the most serious problems in athletes has been injuries to the head and face. Doland and Holladay point out that tooth damage runs from 45–55% of a body-contact-sport squad's injuries. The proper use of mouth protectors in both contact and noncontact sports is invaluable to injury-prevention goals. It is now mandatory that each high school and college football player wear an occlusal and labial protector. However, use is increasing in such sports as basketball, polo, glide flying, hockey, skating, judo, karate, lacrosse, parachuting, skiing, snowmobiling, soccer, surfing, and touch football. It takes the typical athlete about 10 days to get accommodated to wearing a mouth piece, yet the benefits are large.

A face guard is a great asset in deflecting severe blows from the orbital, frontal, and mandibular areas of the face—any of which may result in a fatal injury. Experience has shown that face guards and mouth protection greatly cushion the teeth, lips and cheeks and reduce jaw fractures and concussion if the condyle head of the lower jaw is jammed posterior-superior against the skull.

Two types of mouth protectors are recommended. (1) Custom-designed protectors, fitted by a dentist and constructed from an impression mold of the athlete's own teeth; this type offers the best fit, comfort and protection and affords the best ease of speech and breathing when worn. (2) Mouth-formed protectors, self-fitted to the individual by clenching the teeth into the protector itself; it is first treated with a chemical or boiled, then impressed and allowed to harden. A third stock-variety type is not recommended, but is available with or without the safety-release helmet strap. Each type must be examined frequently for damage and cleaned daily with a disinfectant.

When teeth are damaged in the absence of a face or mouth guard, the athlete should be warned not to apply finger pressure to test the degree of tooth looseness. Only liquids should be consumed until he or she has seen a dentist. A paraffin or wax, heated to a chewing gum consistency, can be molded around the base of a loosened tooth as a temporary support. Sometimes teeth completely knocked out can be replanted by a dentist if care is obained within 3 hours. Such "replanted" teeth may last 10–15 years.

Chest, Torso, and Scrotal Protection

Protection for the chest and torso is frequently inadequate because the large variance in body size makes standard sizing inefficient. Another factor is that proper protection is often bulky and reduces speed, which is abhorred by many athletes. Protection must be given to all vital areas, offer impact absorption, and yet allow free motion (Figs. 2.2–2.4).

An inadequate supportive bra can cause discomfort as well as injury to the breast of

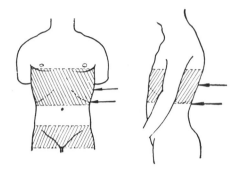

Figure 2.2. The figure at the *left* shows the three zones of incidence of abdominal contusions. The uppermost zone indicates the area commonly affected by abdominothoracic wounds. When injury occurs on the left side (*arrows*), rupture of the ribs, spleen, kidney, or all three may result. The figure on the *right* indicates the area commonly affected by posterior injury, in which case the spleen, kidney, or both may be involved.

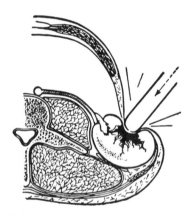

Figure 2.3. Schematic compression of a kidney against the spine and adjacent musculature by an external force.

the athletic female when walking or running. Women without proper breast support experience trauma to the breasts and supporting ligaments, especially when the breasts are large or pendulous. A metal breast protector is necessary in all contact sports and in some noncontact sports, such as volleyball, to prevent contusions and pain.

The genitourinary (GU) area is subject to many minor injuries during sports. This area, often called "the vital zone" by coaches, calls for effective protection, espe-

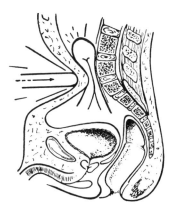

Figure 2.4. The compression of bowel against the sacral promontory by an external force.

cially for a boy 12 years of age or older. The major purpose of an athletic GU supporter is not, as popularly believed, to protect the athlete from being hit in that area. The main purpose of the "jockstrap" is to help keep the cremaster muscles from being overextended. The function of the cremaster muscles is to retract the testicles and safeguard their normal position within the scrotum; however, their poor blood supply and resulting poor tone make them readily susceptible to stretch during sports which might lead to a twisted spermatic cord.

Arm and Hand Protection

Long sleeves and elbow guards are recommended in such sports as roller skating, skate boarding, hockey, fencing with sabres, and volleyball or for any person who has suffered an elbow injury. Bulky forearm and hand protection is necessary in lacrosse and for field and ice hockey goalkeepers. The T-shirt style is much better than the underwear-style uniform in basketball.

Special gloves are necessary in many sports to reduce blister formation, to offer added traction, to support, and/or to prevent the effects of trauma. Examples are baseball mitts, fencing gloves, gymnastic gloves, handball gloves, bowling gloves, and ski gloves.

Football Gear

Basic clothing in football, as in any sport, should allow unrestricted movement, be lightweight and nonabrasive, be nonirritating, provide adequate heat loss/retention

balance, and offer optimal protection to a player without being a hazard to an opponent. Any type of padding should be of a quality shockabsorbing material which is large enough to fully cover the intended part. The positioning of knee and thigh pads is determined by careful fit of the pants. Hip and sacral pads safeguard the pelvis best when they are on a one piece belt which is separate from the pants, that is, not manufactured in the pants themselves.

The Helmet

Most football protective equipment has a dual purpose: to protect the player, and to protect the opponent. Likewise, well-designed equipment should afford good protection for the player without adding danger to an opponent. It is this latter point which has subjected the modern hard-shelled helmet to criticism.

A poorly designed helmet will do little to reduce the severity of head injuries, but that is not the only factor which must be considered. A long thin neck with poor musculature, improper helmet fitting, improper tackling techniques, and a poor face guard or mouth protector are other factors that contribute to unnecessary injury. To avoid a mixup after careful fitting, the player's name should be entered in each helmet.

All helmets manufactured today do not meet optimum safety standards. Yet, the modern helmet is able to withstand G-forces that few except those working in the field believed possible. A good helmet will lessen the severity of many head injuries if it is properly engineered, fitted, and worn.

Shoulder Protectors

By necessity, proper engineering must be a compromise between good stability and guaranteed arm mobility—with the helmet, the shoulder-pad apparatus, and the jersey working as a trinity for shoulder protection. The jersey should be porous to allow for heat dissipation, durable, somewhat elastic, and tight to help secure the shoulder pads. The shirt tail should be long enough that it can be pulled from the back and buttoned in the front to prevent slippage.

Shoulder pads are a complicated product of engineering research. They come in various sizes and body arch to meet the needs

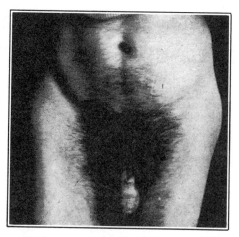

Figure 2.5. Trochanteric bursitis following a fall on the hip.

of different positions. Fit must be done carefully and individually to accommodate for body size, thickness of the neck, and shortness of the neck.

Hip, Thigh, Knee, and Leg Protection

A good hip pad should protect the posterior iliac spines and sacrococcygeal area, the trochanteric bursae and entire iliac crest laterally, and the anterior iliac spines in front if painful injuries are to be prevented (Fig. 2.5). In football, the "pro" type of hip pads are usually too light to afford the protection necessary. As bulk at the waist decreases speed, most athletes have a bad habit of wearing their hip pads too low. Hip

pads worn too low also force an improper position on the shell pant and thigh pad.

Thigh and knee pads cannot do what they are designed to do if the pants are improperly fitted. A loose fit allows the thigh and knee pads to slide about, and external taping rarely can make proper compensation. The knee pad used in volleyball, for instance, must be slick so that impact force can be reduced by sliding. In such sports as hockey, rugby, and soccer, shin guards are important. It is highly advised that basketball players wear long socks to help protect the legs from kicks suffered near the basket.

Footwear and Foot Protection

There is great need for improvement in the design of sports footwear to provide greater safety and efficiency. Athletic footwear should possess three main features: good shock-absorbing characteristics, good traction features, and good lateral support under stress. Keep in mind that jogging creates vertical forces from two to four times body weight.

While "low cut" models of football shoes have become popular because they are lighter and allow greater speed, the older "high top, high lace" type affords added protection against ankle injuries. In track, emphasis has been on shoe lightness at the expense of firm soles and freedom of toe movement. Special orthotic devices are often required. Repeated hard trauma during infancy and childhood has an especially injurious influence.

CHAPTER 3

Communicable Diseases and Their Prevention

Infection is associated with many sports-related injuries. One of the vital conditions for infection is lowered tissue resistance. The resistance of tissues may be lowered by mechanical, chemical, thermal, and electrical stimuli that are of a degree to be injurious. It is also lowered by altered innervation, and this may be caused by interference with the transmission and expression of nerve energy.

BACKGROUND

Skin lesions may be caused by a primary infection or superimposed on another skin disease. No skin infection should be considered minor, especially with the grime and sweat associated with athletic activities. Secondary infection is always a danger to the person afflicted as well as to an athlete's teammates. Poor general health, low resistance, and excessive fatigue encourage such infections. Recurrent infections suggest possible underlying systemic disorder.

The presence of bacteria in the human body does not always constitute infection, nor does it always indicate the existence of an infectious disease. Various types of bacteria are found in many organs of the body in perfectly healthy people.

Before an infection takes place (1) the bacteria must be pathogenic; (2) they must be present in large numbers; (3) they must possess a sufficient degree of virulence; (4) they must enter the body by a path or avenue adapted to their requirements; (5) they must find an environment suitable to their nutritional requirements; and (6) there must be lowered tissue resistance.

Basic Hygiene Education

No responsibility requires more vigilance in sports than the prevention of skin diseases. While athletic health management is rarely concerned with the contagious exanthems, it is openly concerned with several skin diseases of bacterial, viral, mycotic, and parasitic etiology.

Although "team spirit" and cooperation enhances team morale, it should never lead to the interchange of clothing or equipment. Cross-infection often occurs by interplayer use of athletic supporters, combs, drinking cups, bottles and ladles, elastic bandages, hats and helmets, socks, slippers, T-shirts, towels, side-line blankets, and other basic clothing and protective equipment.

Craig offers the constant reminder that if all minor infections are recognized and treated during their early stage, healing will be faster, and the risk of cross-infection among the team will be greatly reduced. Thus, immediate attention is required for all blisters and skin infections.

Basic hygienic practices must be adhered to in all sports. For example, swimmers must preshower before entering the pool to minimize contamination and cross-infection. They should also reshower if they leave the pool to defecate. Wrestling mats must be kept scrupulously clean (eg, herpes, impetigo). Towels pick up more than perspiration; they pick up nose and mouth secretions. Pants, sweatshirts, socks, shorts, and athletic supporters must be laundered frequently in a clorox-like bath to decrease the chance of infection. Hands should be scrubbed after urination and defecation and before eating. Strict hygienic measures must be taught and used with disinfecting mouth protectors.

Dermatological Cautions

Four dermatological cautions should be kept in mind. (1) Don't form an opinion from the history of the case. Note the eruption and all other symptoms, then substantiate it by the history. (2) Don't depend upon any one symptom, but let your opinion be guided by the general makeup of the disease as a whole. (3) Don't forget that many conditions of the skin are dependent upon disturbances in the general health of the patient. Therefore, (4) don't forget to inquire into the performance of the various organs.

Immunization

As scientific evidence is conflicting, the American Chiropractic Association (ACA) has not taken a position for or against immunization practices. The ACA has, however, constantly approved guidelines for national health planning goals which guarantee the health consumer "freedom of choice."

It is granted that vehement arguments have taken place for decades among enthusiasts on both sides. Thus, we shall not be forward enough to take a stand here, feeling the decision is a personal one and respecting individual beliefs. Some practitioners favor all commonly accepted immunization practices, others a select number, and still others are against all forms of immunization because of the inherent risks. It appears from the literature reviewed that few clinicians argue against tetanus immunization when spores may be forced into a wound during injury. Many feel that the incidence of small pox is so rare that immunization is no longer advised; even most proponents of immunization feel that immunization for typhoid and yellow fever are only important if the athlete is traveling to a region where these diseases remain endemic.

Antibiotics

Antibiotics frequently reduce the severity and effects of many bacterial disease processes, yet they have distinct disadvantages and many limitations as well. As life-saving as they may be in some cases, they are far from the panacea once claimed. Their widespread use tends to develop new resistant strains of bacteria, to destroy normal intestinal bacteria, and to encourage inactive intestinal fungi to become active. Antibiotics have no effect on viral illnesses such as hepatitis, influenza, or the common cold. They commonly cause side effects, producing symptoms of dizziness, rash, and iatrogenic allergies. Indiscriminate use frequently creates a sensitivity which prohibits

the person from a later use which could be beneficial.

PARASITIC INFESTATIONS

Two groups of animal parasites cause the most trouble in athletics: scabies (the "7-year itch"), and the various forms of pediculosis (lice, crabs).

Scabies

This intensely itchy contagious skin disease begins with the female mite (Fig. 3.1) boring its way into the skin after she has been impregnated. Within the next 2 months, tunnels (cuniculi) are dug through and along the epidermis, during which time she lays two or three larvae daily which hatch in a few days. The tunnels are observed as thin black lines about ¼ inch in length.

Transmission is via close skin-to-skin physical contact such as with teammates, family members, lovers. It is not spread through bedding or clothing. Common entry sites into the body are at the finger webs, the thin-skinned flexor surface of the wrists or elbows, the axillae, the nipples, the penis, lower buttocks, and the belt line. The mite's entering site is early evidenced by a red spot with a minute vesicopapule at the open end, but it might take 2 months (rarely) before skin irritation and itching occur. Warmth, such as from bed blankets, stimulates the mites activity and increases the itching. Scratching may lead to eczema or a secondary infection leading to impetigo, dermatitis, or boils. Untreated scabies has resulted in impetigo quickly spreading through an entire team, cancelling several weeks of competition.

A prompt first-aid control used by many trainers consists of thoroughly scrubbing the host with soapy hot water and then using a

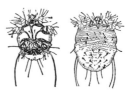

Figure 3.1. The itch mite which produces scabies in humans and mange on some animals. Male shown on the *left*, female on the *right*.

preparation such as 25% benzyl benzoate or 1% gamma benzene hexachloride over the entire skin surface from the neck down. This bath and preparation should be repeated the next day only. As a rule, prompt results occur in 5 days.

Pediculosis

There are three types of lice (Fig. 3.2): capitus (head), corporis (body or clothing), and pubis (groin). Head lice and pubic crabs live directly on the host; body lice live in the undergarments. Scratching the wheals often produces a secondary infection of impetigo. Itching worsens when the lice are feeding.

Pediculosis Capitus

Head lice are witnessed with a lens as firm pear-shaped little "bugs" which are translucent gray-green or whitish in color, strongly clinging to the base of scalp hair shafts. They cannot be easily dislodged like scales. Intense itching results when the crab is feeding upon the scalp. The section of the scalp usually infected is the occipital area, but the lice may spread throughout the scalp and into the eyebrows, eyelashes, and beard. Swollen lymph nodes behind the ears may be detected, and a dermatitis or a secondary infection is not uncommon. Transmission is often through the interchange of combs and hats.

As grease will smother pediculi, first aid may consist of a grease or larkspur cap. A stocking cap is placed on the head after the scalp has been loaded with vaseline petroleum jelly. After 12 hours, the scalp is shampooed with a hot vinegar solution. Another method used by trainers is to apply a solution of 50% odorless castor oil and 50% kerosene to the hair and cover with a stocking cap before the athlete retires at night. In

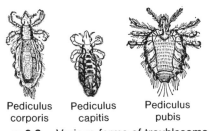

Pediculus   Pediculus   Pediculus
corporis   capitis   pubis

Figure 3.2.   Various forms of troublesome lice.

the morning, the dead pediculi are combed out and the hair is thoroughly shampooed with shaving cream and then rinsed thoroughly with warm water. Some feel that a DDT dusting powder is quite effective in killing the pests.

Pediculosis Corpus

This type of lice, uncommon with good hygienic practices, lives in clothing seams and bites only when seeking food. They are an important vector of those organisms which cause epidemic typhus, relapsing fever, and trench fever, as seen in environments promoting unclean clothing and poor personal hygiene.

A series of small papules with blood-crusted tips associated with linear scratch marks appear where the host has been bitten. Urticaria or a superficial bacterial infection may be associated. Occasionally, furunculosis is a complication. In chronic conditions, the skin especially around the belt line is colored a dirty brown (Vagabond's skin). The upper part of the back and shoulders are also prime targets. There appears to be a distinct relationship between the attack and a host's thiamine deficiency.

One method of first aid used by trainers is to rub the body thoroughly with thick cold cream for at least 10 minutes. Another method is to apply Cuprex to the affected area, wait a half hour, remove the preparation, reapply the Cuprex, wait for another half hour, then thoroughly scrub the body with hot soapy water. For prevention, the athlete's clothing should be pressed with a hot iron, especially at the seams.

Pediculosis Pubis

Pubic nits are difficult to see unless the pubic hair is shaven. The crabs clutch the skin strongly. The biting causes intense itching, sometimes associated with chills. Transmission contact is from benches, toilet seats, combs, hats, bedding, and using another's clothing, but the common method is venereally. Excoriation and secondary dermatitis (often from self-medication) develop early. Recurrence is not uncommon.

Effective first aid by trainers has been for many years with "blue ointment," a parasiticide preparation of mercury and mercury oleate in solid bases. Cuprex is popular, but certain precautions must be taken. Improvement is rapid with 1% gamma benzene hexachloride cream or lotion applied once a day for 2 days, then once again in 10 days to kill remaining pests.

FUNGAL INFECTIONS

Dermatophytosis is an extremely broad term referring to a collection of dermatoses induced by sundry fungus species with three features in common: (1) mycotic etiology; (2) superficial morbid effects—the fungi do not invade tissue deeply as do certain other, more dangerous, fungi (eg, sporotrichosis, actinomycosis); and (3) the prognosis is usually good. It affects many different regions of the skin and has a wide range of morbid anatomical expressions, but it hardly ever enters the blood or metastases viscerally. As a group, fungus infections represent the most frequent skin conditions in America (Figs. 3.3 and 3.4).

A multitude of synonyms are in use, depending upon the area affected. It is often seen on the foot and called athlete's foot, ringworm, bathmat itch, cracked toe, dyshidrosis, or toe itch; in the groin as tinea curis, red flap, jock itch, gym itch, or Y-itch; and, less often, on the hands.

Background

Fungi thrive best in an environment that is warm and moist. According to Weidman, males are much more commonly affected than are females, and this may be because of greater cleanliness or less "sweaty" activities. It is preeminently a disease of young adults, yet is occasionally seen in the very young and very old, and the incidence is higher in the southern states. The predominating fungus species vary in different parts of the world and even between the northern (trichophyton interdigitale) and southern

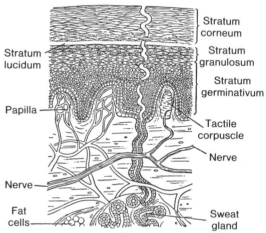

Figure 3.3. Diagram of a skin section showing its structure. The epidermis consists of the strata corneum, lucidum, granulosum, and germinativum. The corium lies below the epidermis.

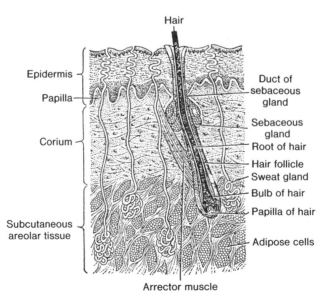

Figure 3.4. Vertical section of the skin showing sebaceous glands, sweat glands, hair, and follicle.

(trichophyton purpureum) United States. A diabetic state is a predisposing factor.

Pathogenic forms of fungi have been demonstrated on apparently normal skin, and thus are somewhat comparable to the ubiquity of streptococci in apparently normal tonsilar crypts or skin. Some athletes appear to have an individual susceptibility to fungus infection, while others are rarely bothered even under adverse conditions. Intermittent remissions and exacerbations of a gradually extending lesion are not uncommon. Such a lesion features scaling with a slightly raised border.

Signs and Symptoms

The fungus is invariably confined to the epiderm. In simple infection, it is noted as a minor grade of edema and corium round-cell infiltration in uncomplicated cases. In advanced cases, epidermal hyperplasia and hyperkeratosis are superimposed. Constitutional symptoms are almost unknown, with symptoms being restricted to local or regional burning, itching, and pain when fissures develop. Scratching and rubbing can quickly lead to secondary bacterial complications that may offer a diagnostic problem.

Regional Manifestations

Toe Ringworm. Tinea pedis (athlete's foot) is a common chronic superficial fungal infection of the skin of the foot, especially between the toes and on the soles when local skin resistance is low (Fig. 3.5). It may spread to or originate at the bearded parts (t. barbae), scalp (t. capitis), or perineal folds (t. cruris). Itching varies from nil to extreme. Its progression can be described as (a) beginning as a mild, interdigital erythema with some possible fissuring; (b) an added white, sodden, parchment-like hyperkeratosis, especially between the 4th and 5th toes; (c) spreading of the infection to other toes on the same foot, to the toes of the other foot, and then extending to the space between the toe base and the sole. A related lymphangitis is rarely associated with inguinal adenopathy. Acute episodes with many vesicles and some bullae are common during warm weather. It is extremely important that careful inspection of the toes be made in every case presenting ringworm of the

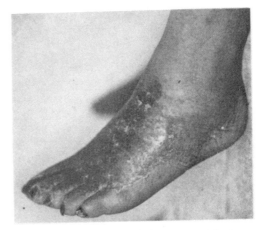

Figure 3.5. Eczematoid ringworm of foot, extending to the dorsum from position between the toes.

groin or of the axilla. The word of the patient should never suffice. Ringworm of the nails (tinea unguium), especially the toenails, is frequently secondary to tinea pedis. The nails appear thick and lusterless, debris accumulates under the free edge, and the nail plate becomes separated if not destroyed. A state of autosensitization self-infection is typical where the small blisters break and the exudate travels to adjacent areas of healthy skin where new ulcers develop. The infection may also be transported solely via the host's local blood and/or lymph vessels. Extension to the hands is rare, but secondary extension to the groin and/or axilla may take place.

The Soles. Eczematoid exacerbations may spread to the dorsum of the foot and more rarely to the leg. The most common manifestation are dyshidrotic lesions producing thickening and scaling of the soles. Lesions may expand beyond the plantar surface into a "moccasin-type" distribution. Inflammation and vesiculation vary from slight to severe. When hyperkeratoic forms are seen, they are usually on the soles.

Tinea Cruris (jock itch). When an athlete sweats, the acid within perspiration reduces natural agents on the skin which might destroy fungi, thereby allowing the mold to thrive. The saprophyte that causes jock itch is a plant which has become unable to manufacture chlorophyll and thus loses its ability to extract nourishment from the air. It attaches itself to a host to live on dead organic material. As the mold grows, it gives off a toxin that kills healthy skin cells upon which the fungi further thrive. The groin reaction to the mold is comparatively uniform, characterized by fine scaling, sharp circinate margination, clearing in the center. It is relatively dry in the early stages, with oozing and crusting appearing in the more severe forms. Extreme itching may lead to sleeplessness and neurasthenia. Large domed, extremely itchy, papules may appear on the scrotum. Recurrence is common. The axillary or umbilical picture is almost identical to that described for the groin.

Anal and Vulvar Forms.   Rarely, cases of pruritis ani and vulvae can be traced to a fungus. The anal lesions are smaller with larger papules located a short distance from the anus.

The Hands.   Erythematous manifestations, similar to those of tinea cruris, can occur between the fingers and spread to the palms and nails (Fig. 3.6); however, dyshidrotic vesicles may be the only expression, or the vesicles and erythema may be combined. Deeper vesicles may transform into pustules. The subcutaneous tissues may become edematous, resembling severe cellulitis with lymphangitis. Secondary bacterial infection is common, leading to severe eczematoid development which may progress to lymphangitis, axillary adenopathy, and constitutional symptoms.

Disseminated Forms.   Generalized forms are seen as singular or multiple lesions distributed anywhere on the body surface (tinea corporis). Their appearance may be either erythematous and marginate or circle-like and marginate as in the groin. Peripheral vesicles may be seen; in fact, the condition seems to expand peripherally and

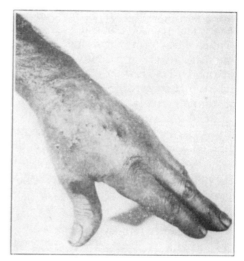

Figure 3.7.   Clinical picture of pustular dermatophytosis.

clear centrally. The circinate form is more common to the armpit, groin, and toe regions. In the chronic phase, infiltration, scaliness, and a psoriasiform appearance is noted.

Intertrigo.   This disorder is characterized by erythematous skin eruptions occurring on apposed skin surfaces, and thus is seen in athletes who are obese and have folds of warm moist skin which encourage the development of fungi. The common sites of this dermatitis are the armpits, groin, navel, and under female breasts, but rarely on the chest or abdomen. It begins as a mild inflammation which evolves into a series of vesicles which rupture easily, leaving a "strawberry-like" glazed surface on the tender skin. The weight of heavy equipment such as football pads over the lesion is quite painful.

The Scalp.   Ringworm of the scalp (tinea capitis) affects mainly children. It is contagious and can become epidemic. The lesions are small and scaly. The scalp presents lusterless hair with semibald patches of broken hair. The lesions begin in a small confined area, then coalesce and involve the entire scalp.

Diagnosis

Dermatophytosis should be the first suspicion in any superficial erythematous disorder because it is so common (Fig. 3.7).

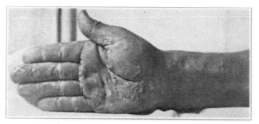

Figure 3.6.   Hyperkeratoic form of ringworm on a hand.

Other conditions should not be considered until fungus has been ruled out. Eczemas are not marginated; they are a comparatively diffuse process. The fungi are associated with minute vesicles or pustules at the advancing margins; however, the unequivocal evidence is supplied by microscopic examination of scrapings.

Scrapings are taken at the active margin, not the center of the lesion. Collect a good quantity of material on small squares of black paper such as photographic negative wrapping. Check with your local laboratory as to how they wish the specimen to be collected, preserved, and transported (eg, 10–30% potassium hydroxide), as each lab has its preferred method.

Examination of dyshidrotic lesions from fungus of the soles is not accomplished by taking scrapings, but by excising the roof of a vesicle and examining it in toto upside down under the microscope. An efficient way to secure the sample is to transfix the roof of the vesicle with a needle and then snip off the roof by quickly inserting curved scissors under the needle at the same time that the roof is pulled upward by using the needle as a handle.

Treatment and Prevention

Weidman points out that each patient must be treated individually, depending upon the part infected and the stage the process has reached. Generally, bland lotions are used by trainers in the acute stage and stimulating ones in the chronic stage. Every dermatologist has his favorite medicaments. An example is 2% salicylic acid in 70% alcohol during the acute stage and 10% during the chronic stage, with desired results in 10–14 days. Some DCs get good results with ultraviolet light as an adjunctive therapy. The chronic reservoirs on toes and nails usually require prolonged treatment after the acute condition has been checked.

Prevention includes frequent use of an antifungal agent; keeping the body dry, especially between the toes and the groin, after swimming, showering, or bathing; wearing well-fitted ventilated or perforated shoes which prevent heat buildup; and using nonrestricting uncolored cotton socks and underwear, which appear to be more absorbent than pure wool or synthetic materials. Socks and underwear should be changed frequently in warm weather. It is not good practice to dry the feet first and then the groin. Generally, athletes find that an antifungal agent in powder form is better than one in a spray or liquid.

Dolan and Holladay state that some trainers control ringworm of the feet by spraying a solution of formaldehyde in athletic shoes from inside tip to heel. The archaic "public footbath" to "sterilize" feet is useless, as is disinfecting floors with strong chemicals. Griseofulvin is reported to be effective in most cases, but added fat must be ingested for this medication to be properly absorbed by the intestinal tract. A first-aid measure for jock itch often used by trainers is a lotion of 25% tincture of iodine and 75% alcohol, applied four times each day. Because ordinary washing will not kill fungi, athletic supporters and underwear should be soaked in Clorox to oxidize (free oxygen) the mold and poison (chlorine) the spores prior to washing.

COMMON VIRAL INFECTIONS

Many viral infections are spread by coughing, sneezing, close talking, and physical contact, one or more of which are quite common to most sports. Most uniforms cannot accommodate a simple handkerchief. The athlete who appears "in shape" is not immune by this factor alone. On the other hand, it is generally recognized that proper nutrition, general resistance and tone, and sensible health practices are beneficial.

Respiratory Infections

Minor respiratory viral infections (eg, common cold) should never be discounted as they often include a myocarditis in their infiltration repertoire. The commonly seen respiratory viruses lead to influenza, acute bronchitis, viral pneumonia, croup, mumps, viral conjunctivitis, infectious mononucleosis, and the common cold, all of which can quickly spread throughout a team. Fever is a contraindication to athletic exertion; however, some authorities feel that exercise during the recovery phase of a mild viral infection is helpful. Over-the-counter medications have little effect except to mask symptoms.

Herpes

The word "herpes" is a general term which refers to any inflammatory skin disease characterized by clustered small vesicles. Herpes is a viral exanthem whose category includes, besides herpes, such disorders as measles, chickenpox, and smallpox. In practice, the term is usually restricted to those diseases caused by the herpesviruses (any of a group of DNA viruses) such as herpes simplex (cold sores) seen around the lips or nose and herpes progenitalis of the groin area. Eruptions may appear almost anywhere on the body. Fever, fatigue, headache, upset stomach, and chills are commonly associated with primary infections. There is always a rare risk of visceral or cerebral involvement, and a psychosomatic relationship is frequently noted. Scratching can lead to impetigo or some other secondary infection.

A first-aid treatment of herpes simplex used by many trainers to promote healing and reduce itching consists of dabbing the lesion about four times each day with a Q-tip saturated with phenolsulfonic acid. Pool chlorination appears to lessen the virus's effect, but it does not deactivate it. Immunization offers only a temporary protection. Prevention comes from good hygienic practices and early detection, isolation, treatment, and good resistance.

Herpes zoster (shingles) is a painfully acute unilateral self-limited vesicular and/or ulcerative inflammatory disease of the cerebral ganglia, the ganglia of posterior nerve roots, and peripheral nerves segmen-

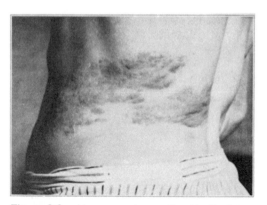

Figure 3.8. Herpes zoster confined to the lower left quadrant of the trunk.

tally (Fig. 3.8). It is caused by the chickenpox virus. Symptoms of chills, fever, malaise, and gastric disturbances usually arise 3–4 days prior to the vesicular eruption and neuralgic pain. As a back injury is often in the history, a careful spinal analysis should be made. Fatigue, either mental from worry/stress or physical from low endurance, also appears to be a factor.

Two rarer viral disorders should be briefly mentioned. (1) Herpes zoster ophthalmicus painfully involves the ophthalmic nerve with a vesicular erythematous rash along the nerve path, leading to keratitis and corneal numbness. It is first noticed along the forehead, eyelid, and cornea. (2) Herpes zoster oticus of the geniculate ganglion is characterized by pain, motor involvement, and vesicular lesions of the external ear, auditory canal, and drum.

Wrestler's Rash

This is a infection of herpes simplex, carried by approximately 75% of the population, which may spread rapidly throughout a wrestling team. Breaks in the skin appear to be the mode of transmission. Infection usually occurs during early childhood, with the carrier subject to possible recurrent attacks activated by some stimulus (environmental, physical, emotional). The common skin abrasions, sweaty contact, and repeated skin trauma associated with wrestling offer a unique predisposition to transmission of the infection. Also, the fatigue, weight problems, and spinal strains associated with wrestling may have a bearing upon an athlete's resistance.

There are two major preventive recommendations. (1) Immediately remove any infected athlete from competition until his skin is healed (2–3 weeks). (2) Educate wrestlers and coaches of the danger of herpes and how to recognize it and of the absolute need to report any suspicions immediately before the whole team is infected.

Molluscum Contagiosum

This is a poxvirus skin disease, more common in the mature athlete, featuring round, firm, smooth, waxy, translucent, skin-colored, crateriform papules (2–10 mm in diameter) containing casseous matter and peculiar capsulated bodies. The condition resembles large "whiteheads," often appearing on an athlete's genitals, pubic area, eyelids, or buttocks as a small asymptomatic patch containing about a dozen lesions. Sometimes a large single molluscum may grow to 30 mm in diameter. An area of dermatitis may surround the lesion patch. Transmission is by direct contact, often venereal. Treatment requires referral for freezing, cauterization, or surgical removal.

Verrucae

Verrucae (warts) are often considered a contagious viral infection, but clear evidence has not been established. Athletes often present numerous warts on their hands, wrists, and arms at trauma sites which may become irritated by further trauma, but they may spread elsewhere.

A first-aid measure used by many trainers for common warts is the application of Freezone, or an equivalent, daily for 6 days, after which time the part is soaked in 118°F water for 30 minutes. If troublesome warts are stubborn, referral is advised for cryotherapy, cauterization, electrodesiccation, fulguration, etc.

Plantar Warts

Plantar warts are internal common warts usually surrounded by a callus formation on the sole of the foot which become flattened by body weight. They are frequently intensely tender and greatly impair athletic performance (eg, running, jumping). Characteristics include horny layers on the sole of the foot that contain a core. This sets up an area of friction between bone and the inside layer of adjacent skin. Differentiation is made from corns and calluses by carefully paring away the surface and noting the tendency to pinpoint bleeding. Plaques of many small closely set plantar warts are called mosaic warts.

Plantar warts usually occur near the metatarsal heads, thus a metatarsal pad or crescent on the shoe's sole helps to reduce pain during activity. Frequent use of a whirlpool bath at 108°F helps the plantar wart to soften, extrude, and disappear. Ultrasound has been found to be beneficial in dislodging plantar warts, but it takes several applications a week for a few weeks. Other common methods use liquid oxygen or nitrogen.

Viral Hepatitis

Hepatitis refers to any inflammation of the liver, regardless of cause. Infectious hepatitis is an acute IH viral disease which is usually transmitted by ingesting infected material (eg, feces) and rarely by blood transfusion (serum h.), a contaminated needle (eg, drug addict), or unhygienic tattooing. Incubation takes about 25 days. It is characterized by fatigue, fever, anorexia, vague gastrointestinal symptoms, jaundice, itching, pale stools, dark urine, and a tender enlarged liver. It is not uncommon for the disease to quickly spread throughout a team or community (eg, poor water supply and/or sewage system).

Infectious Mononucleosis

This is an acute infectious disease, widespread in young adults, associated with the Epstein-Barr virus. The incubation period is from 5–15 days. An excess of mononuclear leukocytes and atypical lymphocytes resembling monocytes manifest in the blood with overt symptoms of sore throat, fever, chills, headache, malaise, and signs of a generalized lymphadenopathy. From 5–14 days after the onset of the illness in about 15% of cases, a skin eruption appears which is most prominent over the trunk, characterized by a scarlatiniform, morbilliform, or vesicular rash.

A player should not be allowed to return to competition until the fever, lymph nodes, spleen size, and lab reports are normal. Return to competition should be gradual, relative to the athlete's health status. High protein and high B-complex supplements are helpful to speed recovery.

TYPICAL BACTERIAL INFECTIONS

Pathogenic staphylococci are normally carried in the nostrils of 50% of the population and on the skin of one out of five healthy adults. Common clinical pictures of staphlococci infection include boils, pneumonia, and staph infection of the heart lining, bone, and stomach and intestinal linings.

Streptococcal infections are grouped clinically into three categories: the carrier state; the acute illness state which is often suppurative; and the state of delayed nonsuppurative complications (eg, rheumatic fever). During the carrier state where there is no outward evidence of infection, streptococci within the digestive and respiratory tracts have a covert opportunity to be transmitted.

Boils

The most commonly seen bacterial infection associated with athletics is furuncles (boils), an infection of a hair follicle, especially where clothes may rub dirt and perspiration into the skin such as on the neck, buttocks, and armpits (frequently predisposed by using strong antiperspirants). A multicored carbuncle is severely painful, and almost never self-limited. Septicemia is always a threat with boils and carbuncles. Boils occurring on the head, face, or neck are of particular concern because of their association with possible brain abscess.

Referral for a wide-band antibiotic is much preferred over contraindicated squeezing or lancing that may spread the infection. First aid is often done by trainers by applying a compress of ichthyol ointment on the affected area to help the infection "head." Another method is to pack the core area with streptokinese-streptodornase jelly, leave in place for half an hour, then remove with a loop curet. Prevention is accomplished by prohibiting the exchange of clothing or equipment, cleaning equipment and laundering clothing frequently, and using soap liberally while showering or bathing.

Impetigo

Impetigo is characterized by distinct, superficial vesiculopustules, especially around the mouth, which crust and rupture. The three types of impetigo seen in athletics are *Ecthyma*, *Impetigo contagiosa*, and *Bockart's*. *Ecthyma* invades the deeper skin, often producing ulcers which result in scars. The common site is on or near the legs as a complication of scabies. *Impetigo contagiosa* arises as a small red spot which evolves into a nonitchy, flat, raised sac filled with fluid having a straw-like color. When the sacs break, the oozing fluid carries the infection to adjoining areas and new lesions appear. Rather than breaking, the sacs more commonly dry into a yellow crust. Large blister-like lesions, about the size of a quarter, are called bullous impetigo. *Bockart's impetigo* is characterized by small pustules at the base of hairs, no larger than a pin head and thus often missed. If left untreated, secondary infection may occur leading to a severe septicemia. The first signs of any form of impetigo demand immediate referral to the family physician.

Sycosis Barbae

This unsightly disorder is a superficial bacterial papulopustular inflammation of hair follicles, especially of the beard, often called "barber's itch." The nonspreading lesions are the size of a penny and capable of returning several months after apparent cure. Contact with wool should be avoided until recovery is complete. Referral to a medical physician usually results in a prescription for a hydrocortisone ointment. This helps to control the infection but does nothing to correct the probably associated lowered resistance and poor hygienic practices.

CHAPTER 4

Miscellaneous Skin Disorders

Skin has unique functions and characteristics. It provides an interface between internal and external environments, it is selectively permeable, it serves as a homeostatic mechanism, and it regulates temperature despite external extremes. It contains the same basic elements as do the major organs: connective tissue, blood and lymph vessels, nerves and glands. It has excretory, secretory, absorptive, synthetic, and sensory functions.

BACKGROUND

Common symptoms involving the skin in sports include pain, itching, and rashes. They are associated with such dysfunctions as skin dryness, scaling, follicular plugging, acne, and excessive or diminished sweating. New symptoms or asymptomatic lesions are compared to the norm. Question date of onset, proneness to spreading, rate of progression, location, seasonal relationship, environmental exposure to irritants, and associated symptoms. Skin is usually the first organ to show side effects from drugs and many systemic diseases.

Examination of the skin includes color, texture, moistness, and lesions, along with mucous membranes, hair, and nails. While the skin is the largest body organ in terms of surface area and the most visible, it is often the most overlooked.

A noticed change in pigmented nevi may offer an important diagnostic clue. Such change may be an alteration in color, an increase in growth, pain, bleeding, itching and inflammation, or recent development. Recently developed moles, the development of a sudden brown or black band in a fingernail or toenail of a Caucasian, or a history of black spots in the mouth suggest metastatic melanoma.

Pain and Pruritus

Painful skin lesions are common in sports because the skin is richly innervated. Such pain is often the result of inflammation and edema. The lack of pain or its diminished perception is also an important clue. Both diseases of the nerve proper and diseases involving the neurovascular bundles in the skin can produce anesthesia. In evaluating the physiopathology involved, keep in mind that the same pathways are involved in the transmission of pain, touch, itching, hot, and cold.

Pruritis is a disagreeable cutaneous dysesthesia which demands attempted relief through voluntary or involuntary scratching. Intense itching is associated with obstructive hepatobiliary disease, poison ivy and oak, and a large variety of allergic, inflammatory, and idiopathic skin conditions. As vasodilation commonly aggravates itching, a patient may report that heat increases (eg, hot shower) and cold decreases pruritus.

When pruritus is a complaint, determine whether the itching disturbs sleep, if scratching can be controlled, or what situations appear to aggravate or ease the itching, such as certain clothing, temperatures, etc. Objective evidence of the effects of scratching may be noted during the physical examination, such as whealing, erythema, excoriations, lichenification, or pigmentation.

Pruritus can be related to a systemic disease, to a primary skin disease, or to neither. It may be generalized with or without skin eruptions, or it may be localized with or without evident pathology. A severe generalized pruritis may be the result of a disease and (1) may occur without skin lesions from dry or dirty skin, contact sensitivity, allergies to foods (Fig. 4.1) or drugs, psychogenic factors, metabolic disorders, and malignant conditions; or (2) it may occur with skin eruption such as in urticaria, contact dermatitis, atopic dermatitis, neurodermatitis, dermatitis herpetiformis, scabies, and lichen planus.

Examples of localized pruritis associated

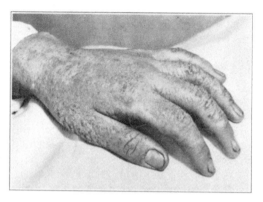

Figure 4.1. Subacute dermatitis on a hand of a person known to be sensitive to asparagus.

with evident local pathology are those related to (1) skin disorders, (2) genitourinary disorders, and (3) certain rectal disorders. Localized pruritis associated without evident local pathology is characteristic of a parasitic infestation, a psychogenic origin, a contact sensitivity, or a systemic condition.

Rash

The word "rash" is a vague term. When a rash is a part of the clinical picture, questions should probe onset, first location and changes, initial appearance and changes, relationship to clothing or environmental exposure, relationship to known allergies, family history, personal habits, relationship to cosmetics, prescribed drugs, and proprietary medications. Associated symptoms such as fever, malaise, joint and other pains, itching, oozing, or the formation of hives, blisters, and blebs should be questioned. A history of a rash is often the first clue of a primary dermatologic disease or a serious systemic disease, of a common infectious process, or of serious drug reactions.

TRAUMA-ASSOCIATED DISORDERS

Legal files are filled with many cases of disease which have followed trauma so closely that it may appear that the disease was a direct result of the injury. This poses major medicolegal problems if it can be demonstrated that an injury precipitated a disorder or that the disease was purely coincidental.

Trauma and Disease

As almost everyone has many relatively serious accidents sometime during his or her life, it is impossible statistically to make any one disease appear to be the result of injury. Davidson points out that some clinical researchers have definitely recognized that (1) injury, by increasing vessel permeability, may activate a dormant disease; (2) trauma may set up a point of diminished resistance in which microorganisms may lodge; and (3) the emotional stress of injury may accelerate a previously latent psychosis.

Trauma may induce many types of skin eruptions, and this trauma may be a microtrauma from wind, dust, sunshine, etc. Mosquito bites cause hive-like itchy areas, and biting flies and wasps can cause painful stings. The athlete is also exposed to numerous bacteria, fungi, viruses, poison plants, parasites, dusts, dyes, temperatures, and chemicals, in addition to dirt, perspiration, scratches, and many allergy-producing substances.

Tetanus

Tetanus is an acute, often fatal (50% in the unimmune) illness characterized by tonic muscular spasm and hyperreflexia, resulting in lockjaw, general muscle spasm, opisthotonus, glottal spasm, convulsions, and seizure attacks. It is caused by a neurotoxin whose spores enter the body through a wound. An athlete involved in contact sports is thus frequently exposed due to the high incidence of injury. The incubation period is 1–3 weeks.

Erysipelas

This debilitating condition, more common in basketball elbow blows than in other sports trauma, can attack an athlete with low resistance who has received a head injury. A bright red, hot lesion (St. Anthony's fire) appears in the infected skin, peaking 4–8 days after injury and infection. Upon suspicion of erysipelas, immediate referral to a medical physician should be made. The typical immediate treatment is a wide-band antibiotic.

While the infection is active, the athlete's vision and timing are impaired (up to 3 months) to some degree, some balding may occur, and associated apathy and listlessness are common. It usually takes an athlete about 6 weeks to recover his full competition strength, but symptoms begin to ebb after 3 weeks. A high-protein, high-vitamin/mineral diet is usually recommended during recuperation.

Sporotrichosis

This is a chronic fungal disease occurring in three forms: a disseminated form, a pulmonary form, and a cutaneous lymphatic form. The latter type is seen sometimes in football linemen (forearm shiver-block bumps) because of their forearm-type blocking. The disorder is caused by repetitive trauma to the forearms or fingers in which blows cause dirt to enter a wound. This state evolves into a series of nodular swellings or abscesses, sometimes ulcerative, just under the skin near the area of injury along the lymphatic draining course, especially at the elbow joint or bend of the wrist. Suspicion warrants immediate referral to a medical physician; a common prescription is a potassium iodide saturated solution taken orally.

Paronychia

Acute, sometimes chronic, bacterial infection of folds of skin near a fingernail or toenail is not uncommon, especially if an ingrown nail, wound, or chronic irritation (eg, detergents) is present. Biting the fingernails encourages the infection, as does repeated trauma as seen with baseball catchers.

One first-aid treatment used by many trainers consists of soaking the digit in a hot 1% Lysol solution for several minutes and then painting 3% thymol in chloroform beneath the nail fold. Surgery may be required in severe cases. A method of prevention is cutting the toenail's tip square rather than rounded and bathing the feet at least once daily, drying them thoroughly.

Hidradenitis

Hidradenitis is an inflammation of sweat glands, often resembling furuncles (Fig. 4.2). Signs of severe chronic recurrent suppurative hidradenitis are pea-like lumps of the axillae or groin sweat glands and rarely around the nipples or anus. It is characterized by an intensely painful inflammatory process resulting in obstruction and rupture of the sweat ducts. Discharge and sinus tract

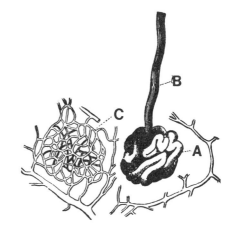

Figure 4.2. Coiled end of a sweat gland; A, the coiled end; B, the duct; C, the network of capillaries inside of which the sweat gland lies.

formation are common. First aid requires absolute cleanliness and immediate referral to the family physician. In fact, any growth in the axillae or groin demands immediate referral.

Stomatitis

Stomatitis is a generalized inflammation of the oral mucosa. In general practice, canker-sore lesions of the mouth are commonly associated with systemic disease, vitamin C or riboflavin deficiency, drug allergy, denture irritation, or of a visceral-reflex nature. In athletics, stomatitis can usually be traced to a poor-fitting mouthpiece (eg, football, boxing) that causes the gums to become red, swollen, and sore and the tongue to become large and thick. Salivation is usually marked. A football helmet's chin strap can exert considerable pressure upon an ill-fitted mouthpiece. First aid requires a bland mouthwash. Underlying systemic conditions should be treated appropriately, and dental referral should be made to determine proper mouthpiece adjustment.

Stasic Eczema

Venous insufficiency may arise in the ankles or lower legs as a result of tight ankle wraps or binding from high shoes. The result is congestion, brownish pigmentation, and later scaling and weeping. Repeated injury leads to edema and phlebitis. Chronic scratching leads to secondary infection; and, if left unmanaged, cellulitis, with or without ulceration, develops. Varicose veins, ulceration, thrombophlebitis, and secondary infection are always a threat. First aid by many trainers consists of elevating the limb and using a paste (eg, 3% ichthyol in Lassar's paste) on the lesions.

Nummular Eczema

This disorder is often induced by the trauma of winter temperatures. It is sometimes seen in sports played outdoors in cold weather, such as football, and is most common in linemen who play without gloves or warm socks. It usually begins as a mild itchy skin infection of the hand, characterized by coin-shaped patches of vesicles and papules, which progress to a widespread secondary dermatitis characterized by oozing and crust formation, especially during cold weather. Lesions are commonly sited on the extensor aspects of the extremities and on the buttocks. First-aid management is the same as for any dermatitis; ie, wet dressings applied by the trainer during the acute stage, pastes and ointments used during the chronic stage.

Keloid

A keloid is a benign tumor featuring a smooth, pink, shiny (often dome-shaped) overgrowth of fibroblastic tissue that arises from tissue injury. These tumors are more common in Blacks. Occasionally, a keloid may develop without a history of injury. Suspicion requires investigation by a surgeon.

Decubitus Ulcers

These pressure sores, seen most often on the feet, are sometimes experienced by the athlete early in the season, especially when resistance is low. They are caused by pressure and encouraged by mild trauma. The clinical picture is one of ischemic necrosis and ulceration in an area overlying a bony prominence where prolonged external pressure has been applied. It begins as soft red skin whose redness disappears on pressure. It then progresses to a deeper redness, induration, edema, and sometimes blistering and desquamation are seen. In the later stages, the skin is necrotic and the lesion extends through fat, muscle and bone with typical complications.

To aid granulation and healing, an early first-aid measure used by many trainers is to coat the lesion with a fresh 5% aqueous solution of tannic acid and then cover the coat with adhesive plaster. Other recommendations are to coat with gentian violet, bismuth violet, or Vaseline irradiated with radon B, and then to cover with an adhesive pad. Recurrence can often be guarded against by protecting against pressure; ie, padding the shoe's counter with foam rubber about ¼ in thick.

Corns

Corns are round or cone-shaped localized callosities of skin which possess a horny core. The picture is one of a circumscribed area of hypertrophied skin resembling a small shell containing a harder core which presses on nerves of the foot in the weight-bearing position. The cause can usually be attributed to atypical bone formation or position (frequently requiring adjustment), to undue external pressure, or to repeated trauma. There are two types: soft corns and hard corns.

Soft corns form in areas where skin touches skin (eg, between the toes) in an area where heat is poorly released, perspiration has difficulty in evaporating, and an adjacent bone puts pressure on the skin. Prevention is aided by keeping the feet clean and dry, wearing round-toed shoes with metastarsal cresents, wearing nylon undersocks, and performing exercises to strengthen the metatarsal arch. First aid consists of the above prevention measures plus using an alcohol foot wash frequently, drying thoroughly, and applying a foot powder. Another method used by many trainers is to dust between the toes with a powder such as sulfomerthiolate or bismuth formic iodide.

Hard corns are firm, rigid, and dense. They arise over prominent protuberances on parts of the foot where sport shoes exert considerable pressure such as on the lateral side of the small toe and the top of the middle toes. Many trainers use a first-aid measure to eliminate pressure on the area with pads and rings and frequently cover the corn with an effective "corn paint." Stubborn cases should be referred to a chiropodist.

NONTRAUMA-ASSOCIATED DISORDERS

Miliaria

"Prickly heat" or "heat rash" manifests as a series of pink, pruritic, papulovesicular lesions under protective gear (eg, shoulder pads, rib pads) worn during warm-weather activities. It is not uncommon to football linemen. No protective uniform can be considered "cool" for the overweight athlete. The disorder is brought on by excessive sweating, a distinct lack of perspiration, or a partial obstruction (eg, congenital) to the ducts of the sweat glands that forces sweat to escape into the epidermis.

One first-aid measure recommended by many is to freely dust the body with talcum before exercise and follow exercise with an alcohol rub. Preventive measures include keeping the skin cool and dry and avoiding excessive perspiration, which are almost impossible in athletics.

Eczema

Eczema is a general category under which are classed various forms of dermatitis, and the classification varies with different authorities. In general practice, the term applies to a superficial acute, subacute, or chronic inflammatory process of the skin characterized by early redness, burning and itching, minute vesicles and papules, which lead to weeping, oozing, pustules, crusting, late scaling, lichenification, and sometimes pigmentation. Unmanaged infections unrelated to dermatitis frequently cause a dermatitis because of secondary infection (eg, ringworm infection progressing into dermatitis).

The cause may be exogenous (eg, adhesive tape, wool, cosmetics) or endogenous (eg, food allergy, drugs, neurosis). The more common causes are external irritants, especially with a person who has inherited sensitive skin; yet, the skin of most people is potentialy sensitive to an irritant after long and repeated exposure. Some researchers feel, because the dermatitis appears most often on the exposed skin surfaces (ie, face, neck, arms, hands), that some type of microtrauma is the exciting cause (eg, soaps, sunlight, dust, plants, wind, or environmental chemicals).

Sometimes the area of sensitivity is far removed from the site of contact: ankle tape or a knee painted with benzoin as a base for tape has been shown to be the cause of irritated eyelids. In some people, lesions appear immediately after exposure; in others, several days may pass; in still others, several exposures may be necessary to lower resistance enough to obtain a reaction.

Sensitivity Test

A patch test can determine an individual's degree of sensitivity to various irritants. First, have the player prepare a careful record of everything he touches and uses as part of his athletic activities. Second, hold the material (eg, wool patch) on a tender area of skin, cover it with Saran Wrap, and secure it with adhesive tape. Remove the patch in 2 days and examine for a sensitivity reaction. The tender skin just above or below the inner elbow is usually used. If the irritant is suspected to be a powder, chalk, dust, or a noncaustic liquid (eg, benzoin), saturate a gauze square with the substance and secure it as described.

Hyperhidrosis

Excessive feet sweating (usually associated with scales, fissures, maceration, and a strong odor) can often be managed with an antiperspirant powder. It is more often seen with the overweight athlete. The fetid odor (bromhidrosis) is the result of perspiration and cellular debris being decomposed by yeasts and bacteria. The patient's perspiration often contains a high amount of urea.

Sweat gland overactivity may also occur in the palms, axillae, groin, inframammary region, or have a general distribution. The cause of localized excessive sweating is unknown. Hyperhidrosis of the palms and soles is often considered psychogenic. Generalized hyperhidrosis may have an endocrine, febrile, or central nervous system basis. A rash that can be confused with ringworm may be associated.

Scrupulous cleanliness must be maintained. Socks should be undyed and laundered frequently. Alternate three sets of athletic shoes which are dusted frequently with a fungitoxic powder. Some trainers recommend that when the feet are involved, saline or alcohol foot baths followed by a soothing astringent (eg, 25% aluminum chloride each night for 3 weeks) usually bring relief. If there is an axillary problem, the hair should be shaven and a nonirritating antiperspirant applied after bathing.

TOXIC ERUPTIONS

Toxic signs vary from a simple sneeze, to tearing eyes, to indigestion, to a severe skin eruption, and/or to diarrhea. Toxic eruptions often show a clear history of recent exposure to some type of new clothing material, insect bite, drug, or food known for its reactive capabilities. Typical manifestations are acne, urticaria, and poison-plant irritations.

Acne

The pimples of acne are especially common to adolescent and young adult male athletes (Fig. 4.3). It is an inflammatory disorder of the skin resulting in the formation of papules and pustules which are often mixed with comedones (blackheads). In athletes, acne occurs commonly on the face, neck, and shoulders. There is always a danger that trauma may irritate the lesions and cause a secondary infection (eg, impetigo). Basketball players with shoulder acne should be advised to wear the T-shirt type of garment rather than the undershirt type of uniform. This will help to both protect and hide the lesions.

Nutritional control is the first preventive measure to be considered. Fats, chocolate, malt, eggs, milk, yeasts, carbonated beverages, candy and pastry, and "junk foods" are to be avoided. Fluids and bulk foods should be increased, and the overall diet should be nutritionally well balanced. Drugs containing iodine or bromine should be avoided.

A trainer's first-aid measures may include pH controlled soaps, mild bactericide lotions, and calamine lotions. Treatment is a challenge to the dermatologist.

Urticaria

Acute or chronic hives (nettle rash) is a vascular reaction featured by often itchy, transient, pink or white, slightly elevated welts or weals. The exciting cause usually arises from some food allergy (eg, berries, chocolate, seafood); drugs (u. medicamentosa) such as phenolphthalein; insect bite (u. papulosa); infection (leading to pustules); or emotional stress. Dust, animal danders, plants, light, cold, chalk, exercise, and heat are less common causes. Thus, a careful history is vital. Prevention is aided by keeping a player out of contact with a known irritant. First aid is restricted to normalizing physiologic tone and applying an antipruritic lotion.

Poison-Plant Irritations

All field sports not played on artifical turfs subject an athlete to such irritants as poison ivy, poison oak, and poison sumac. These plants contain a poison, urushiol, which is extremely long lasting after the plant has died. Contact produces early signs of itching and skin reddening. Small water blisters, which later enlarge and become puffy, appear within a few hours and spread rapidly to adjacent areas. If blisters rupture, oozing sores manifest and become subject to secondary infection which increases the patient's temperature and restlessness.

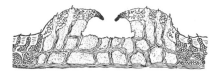

Figure 4.3. Diagram of a carbuncle.

CHAPTER 5

Nutrition and Physical Activity

For centuries diet has played an important role in athletics, although much has been based on tradition and old wives' tales rather than on science. History shows that, as long ago as the first Olympic game, athletes were concerned with their diet. While coaches for ages have noted a relationship between an athlete's performance and the food eaten, it has only been recently that poor performance could sometimes be associated with something *not* eaten.

NUTRITIONAL REQUIREMENTS

The athlete's requirements are the same as the average person's for a balanced diet, except that the athlete's demands are greater. Both the athlete and the nonathlete require an adequate supply of proteins, fats, carbohydrates, vitamins, basic minerals, trace elements, and water in adequate proportions and at suitable times to meet individual needs. It must be kept in mind, however, that digestion and assimilation are not mechanical acts which produce the same results in all human beings.

Basic Considerations

Except for the increased need for food energy and the replacement of fluids and electrolytes lost through perspiration, studies have shown that intense or prolonged exercise does not increase the need for any specific nutrient. The major goals of a team physician in regard to nutrition as it particularly relates to athletic performance are offering guidance and encouragement to (1) achieve a competing weight, (2) enhance the basic diet, (3) meet the athlete's energy needs, (4) meet the athlete's fluid and electrolyte requirements, and (5) monitor body weight 2–3 times each week during the training and competitive season. In competitive events where dehydration may be a problem, body weight should be checked before and after each vigorous session.

Altering body composition by either in-creasing lean body mass or reducing body fat is an important and frequently voiced concern of many athletes. N. J. Smith reports that excessive body fat can limit endurance and quickness. However, athletes should be warned of the pitfalls that result from fad diets, starvation, and nutritional abuses that lead to dehydration and deficiencies. In most sports, the minimal level of body fat is 5–7%. When weight gain is desired, it should be noted that no specific amino acid, drug, food, hormone, mineral, nutrient, or vitamin will increase muscle tissue in the healthy postpubescent individual. Only muscle work will increase muscle mass and lean body weight.

Energy Requirements

The demands of the sport plus the basic requirements of the body determine an athlete's energy needs. The exact amount of fuel required varies with the duration and the intensity of the particular physical activity involved. Studies have shown that muscle needs only energy provided essentially by carbohydrates and by fats to a lesser extent. Of all sweets, honey has the highest caloric value and is turned into fuel rapidly. For this reason, honey is often used as a light between-match snack. While thousands of hours of reserve energy are stored as fat, adipose tissue cannot serve as an adequate resource in anerobic conditions; thus, once glycogen reserves become depleted, exhaution takes place rapidly. Most body fat is some distance from active muscles, and intramuscular lipids soon become depleted.

Protein Requirements

If adequate quantities of essential amino acids are included in dietary protein, other amino acids can be made within the tissues. Most proteins of animal origin are good sources of amino acids, while cereal and legume proteins are less complete. However, many top athletes have been vegetarians.

Exercise does not increase the body's protein requirements, nor is protein lost during exercise. Large amounts of ingested protein increase the fluid necessary for digestion and for the kidney's excretion of protein's nitrogen by-products. In addition, ingestion of excessive protein utilizes greater energy for metabolism. During recuperation from trauma, the body's protein requirements are increased for necessary repair. In demanding athletics, a protein deficiency will be manifested in easy fatigue, weakness, mild depression, and even puffy edema around the knees and ankles in advanced cases.

Energy Expenditure

A calorie is a simple yardstick for measuring the amount of energy needed to meet the body's demands to keep warm and do its work. A food calorie (fuel value in food) is the amount of heat necessary to raise the temperature of 1 kilogram (2.2 lb) of water 1°C. Protein and carbohydrate yield about 4 calories/gram, and fat, about 9 calories/gram. The quantity of calories necessary for daily activities depends upon an individual's activity, age, and weight.

After being ingested, carbohydrates, fats, and proteins (deaminized) are burned to yield energy for external muscles, for internal activity, and for heat. Carbohydrates are also stored as glycogen in the liver and muscles or changed into fat. Ingested fats may be used in the synthesis of tissue lipids, stored as fat, and sometimes changed into carbohydrates. Protein is utilized in tissue building and repair; it is also used in the synthesis of body regulators. Deaminized protein may also be changed into carbohydrate or fat.

In a workload of 75% of maximum oxygen uptake, a high proportion of energy necessary for vigorous effort (eg, 80 minutes) is initially derived from carbohydrate, essentially from glycogen stored within muscle cells. The reserve of liver glycogen can be mobilized slowly, but blood sugar offers a meager energy source for physical work. The extent of postevent fatigue, however, is not necessarily directly proportional to the actual amount of energy expended.

When a diet's caloric value equals the amount of calories expended in physiologic activity, no weight change takes place. Weight gain results when calories taken in exceed the body's demands, and vice versa. In general, when weight loss is desired, a 3500-calorie deficit is necessary to lose 1lb of fatty tissue. Thus, to lose 1 lb/week requires a 500-calorie reduction per day. When weight gain is desired, a 2500-calorie increase plus physical activity is necessary to gain a pound of muscle mass.

Quick Caloric Determination

Here is a simplified method for quickly determining a person's caloric needs:

1. Determine basal calorie level by multiplying body weight (lb) by 3.
2. Determine additional caloric needs for activity: (a) strenuous: desirable body weight (lb) × 10; (b) moderate: desirable body weight (lb) × 5; (c) sedentary: desirable body weight (lb) × 3.
3. Subtract calories for desirable weight loss or add calories for desirable weight gain. Add calories when appropriate for growth, pregnancy, or lactation.

Weight Screening

A simplified method of determining an athlete's optimal weight is to allow 100 lb for the first 5 feet plus 5 lb for every inch over 5 feet. Add or subtract 10% of the total for a large or small build, respectively.

Obesity in athletics often results from eating habits. For example, a football player may require 5,000 calories a day during the active season. If this "football" appetite is carried over to the nonactive months, the effect is excessive fat and an extra load on the heart.

Vitamin Requirements

Vitamins are fundamentally involved in the nutrition of most if not all body cells. An inadequate supply of vitamins over a long period can result in disease and possible death. Fortunately, as enzymes and catalysts, vitamins are needed in extremely small amounts. Evidence does not indicate that exercise significantly increases the body's requirements for vitamins, nor have massive amounts of specific vitamins or combinations been shown to safeguard against infection, prevent injury, improve endurance, or benefit performance for the athlete.

Vitamin D.　Fat-soluble vitamin D plays an important role in strong bone development and stamina. It is also necessary for a healthy heart, skin, teeth, nerves, and thyroid tissue. If the skin is exposed to sunshine, some vitamin D can be synthesized from the ergosterol on or near the skin, thus the term, "the sunshine vitamin." Vitamin D deficiency can make a harmless bone trauma develop into an irritation, causing bone softening. When levels are low, a player may complain about burning sensations in the mouth and throat, diarrhea, insomnia, myopia, nervousness, and signs of poor metabolism. Ingested mineral oil interferes with vitamin D absorption.

Vitamin A.　Vitamin A, another fat-soluble vitamin, is necessary to nourish eyes, skin, and respiratory tissue. Deficiency leads to "night blindness," rough-dry "toad skin," and respiratory troubles. Other symptoms include allergies, appetite loss, skin blemishes, dry hair, fatigue, itching-burning eyes, loss of sense of smell, sinus trouble, dental cavities, and susceptibility to disease. Ingested mineral oil interferes with vitamin A absorption, as does alcohol, coffee, cortisone, excessive iron, and vitamin D deficiency.

Vitamin E.　There is some evidence to guard against a deficiency of fat-soluble vitamin E especially in athletics. The reasoning behind this is that a deficiency of vitamin E results in muscles becoming dystrophic. It has also been shown in animals that resistance to hypoxia and hyperoxia is influenced by vitamin E reserves. Thus, it is not unreasonable to believe that muscles under severe stress have raised demands not met by sedentary requirements, yet reseach has not brought this out. Ingested chlorine, mineral oil, and birth-control pills interfere with vitamin E utilization. It is necessary for the health of blood vessels, the heart, lungs, nerves, skin, and pituitary gland. Deficiency symptoms include muscular deficiency, dry-dull or falling hair, enlarged prostate, gastrointestinal and cardiac symptoms, impotency and sterility.

Vitamin C.　Because of the importance of vitamin C in adrenal metabolism, supplementation would appear advisable in athletics; but again, research has not shown this to be true. Vitamin C, a water-soluble vitamin, is not stored in the body and is readily lost through cooking, especially boiling, and evaporation when foods are left at room-air temperatures. It is necessary for growth, performance, and health maintenance. In addition to its function in the adrenal gland, it is necessary for healthy bone and teeth formation, heart, capillary walls, connective tissue, skin and gums. In athletes, deficiency is often shown by such symptoms as anorexia, tender or painful toes or fingers, irritability, diarrhea and vomiting. Other symptoms include anemia, bleeding gums, capillary-wall rupture (easily bruised), nosebleeds, dental cavities, frequent colds, and poor digestion. Antibiotics, aspirin, cortisone, high fever, stress, diuretics, and tobacco contribute to vitamin C deficiency.

Thiamine.　Thiamine, a water-soluble vitamin, is a member of the B-complex group. It cannot be stored in the body and is readily destroyed during cooking. Thiamine (vitamin B1) requirements are closely related to carbohydrate intake and metabolism. Thus, increased physical work increases thiamine requirements because of the greater energy utilized. While the need to meet necessary carbohydrate metabolism must be provided, any excess ingested will be excreted and not stored. Thiamine is necessary for healthy brain, ear, eye, hair, heart, and nervous tissues. Antifactors to thiamine are alcohol, coffee, fever, raw clams, diuretic, stress, tobacco, and excessive sugar. Irritated by athletic demands, a thiamine deficiency can produce symptoms of constipation, diarrhea, pessimistic outlook, and difficulty in arriving at a rapid decision. Other deficiency symptoms include loss of appetite, fatigue, irritability, precordial aches, shortness of breath, numbness in the hands and feet, and increased sensitivity to pain and noise.

Riboflavin.　Vitamin B2, a water-soluble vitamin, is another member of the B-complex group which cannot be stored in the body and is readily destroyed by cooking. Antifactors to riboflavin include alcohol, coffee, excessive sugar, diuretics, and tobacco. Adequate riboflavin is necessary for healthy eyes, hair, nails, skin, soft tissues of the body, antibody and red blood cell formation. While gross deficiency leading to pellagra is not seen in athletics, milder deficiency symptoms may be seen such as general eye itching, photophobia, and a burning tongue (sometimes ulcerated) (Fig. 5.1). Other symptoms include cataracts, fissures at the corners of the mouth, dizziness, and poor digestion.

Mineral Requirements

Calcium. Calcium is necessary for healthy bone, teeth, blood, heart, skin, and soft tissues. It is the most abundant mineral of the body, 98% of which is stored in bone. Dietary calcium shortage calls for a release of calcium from bone (except teeth) into the blood stream. Calcium is absorbed in the small intestine, and its utilization is facilitated by vitamins C and D. Exercise has not been shown to increase the body's requirements for calcium. However, while osteomalacia is not seen in athletics, calcium deficiency may so weaken bone as to make it more subject to fracture during sports. Antifactors to calcium are excessive stress and lack of exercise, but these would not be a factor in athletics. Deficiency symptoms in-

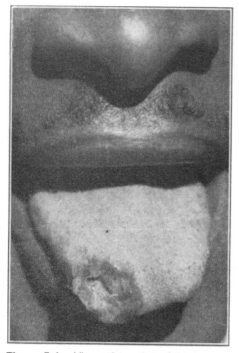

Figure 5.1. Vincent's angina of the tongue.

clude heart palipitations, insomnia, muscle cramps, nervousness, tooth decay, and arm and leg numbness.

Phosphorus. Phosphorus deficiency is a rarity because it is abundant in many foods, and bone contains a large reserve supply. It serves a vital function in skeletal growth, vitamin and enzyme activity, acid-base balance regulation, brain and nerve tissue, and tooth development. A diet containing adequate protein and calcium will never be deficient in phosphorus. Antifactors are excessive intake of white sugar, aluminum, iron, and magnesium. Deficiency symptoms include appetite loss, fatigue, irregular breathing, and nervous disorders.

Iron. Iron is necessary for healthy blood, bones, nails, skin, and teeth. To ensure both endurance and optimal performance, adequate iron is necessary in the diet to carry oxygen to the cells. Iron is vital to the production of hemoglobin and red blood cells. Iron cannot be synthesized, but must be provided within the diet or by supplementation. About 80% of body iron is contained within the blood. Adequate protein and B complex are ncessary along with iron for proper blood formation. Prolonged infections, trauma, bleeding, and chronic "athletic diarrhea" (an emotional reflex disturbance of the intestinal tract) contribute to iron-deficiency anemia. In the United States, iron presents the most common nutritional deficiency, especially in females. Males lose a small amount of iron in hair, skin, and bile loss (1 mg/day), but the female loses an additional amount (5–45 mg/day) during menstruation. Thus, most female athletes require supplementation and frequent monitoring of blood-iron content. Antifactors include coffee, tea, and excessive zinc and phosphorus. Deficiency symptoms include breathing difficulties, brittle nails, iron-deficiency anemia, and constipation.

Marked iron depletion that is *not* associated with demonstrable anemia is not rare, even in affluent socieites, among both males and females. It has been estimated that 15% of American women between the ages of 12 and 45 are found to have some degree of iron deficiency, and such a deficiency may affect athletic performance. Finch has shown that iron-depleted nonanemic rats having well-controlled high concentrations of hemoglobin had their exercise capacity significantly limited. If such a deficiency is suspected, a subanemic condition can be detected by plasma ferritin determination, transferrin saturation, or the level of protoporphyrin concentration in erythrocytes.

Sodium. The habit of taking salt tablets during games and vigorous practice sessions to prevent sodium loss is without scientific support; on the other hand, harm can be done through such practice. Sodium is necessary for healthy blood, lymph system, muscles, and nerves. A lack of chlorine or potassium is an antifactor. Deficiency symptoms include appetite loss, intestinal gas, muscle shrinkage, vomiting, and weight loss.

Potassium. Potassium is necessary for healthy blood, heart, kidneys, muscles, nerves, and skin. Although potassium plays a vital role in muscle function and deficiency exhibits symptoms of fatigue and weakness, large doses of potassium are not warranted. Potassium-rich foods will suffice in fulfilling the body's needs. The antifactors to this mineral are alcohol, coffee, cortisone, and diuretics. Deficiency symptoms include acne, continuous thirst, dry skin, constipation, general weakness, insomnia, muscle damage, nervousness, slow-irregular heartbeat, and weak reflexes.

Magnesium. Adequate magnesium is necessary to convert carbohydrates into energy and in the control of muscular contraction. Although strenuous exercise lowers magnesium reserves through perspiration loss, this loss is easily replaced by a balanced diet. Magnesium is also necessary for healthy bone, muscle, heart, brain, nerves, and arteries. There appear to be no antifactors. Deficiency symptoms include confusion, disorientation, easy arousal to anger, nervousness, rapid pulse, and tremors.

Zinc. Zinc is especially important for healthy blood, heart, and prostate gland tissue. It is present in all body tissues and is multifunctional, but its content in American soils is extremely low. Willis points out two of several of zinc's functions which are of particular interest to athletes; that is, zinc's function as (a) the metalloprotein carbonic anhydrase which facilitates the removal of carbon dioxide from the tissue to lungs and

kidneys where it is expired and excreted; zinc acts to lessen oxygen debt resulting from prolonged effort; and (b) zinc acts as a cofactor in the synthesis and possible proteolysis of collagen which maintains rigidity and cohesion of tissues. Zinc requirements are greatest during periods of growth, stress, healing, and sexual maturation. Willis' study showed that zinc levels in average high school athletes are less than optimal, inferring that the typical high school athlete does not have an optimal diet, let alone one which would enhance athletic performance. Antifactors include alcohol, excessive calcium, and deficient phosphorus. Deficiency symptoms include fatigue, loss of taste, poor appetite, prolonged wound healing, delayed sexual maturity, and sterility.

Iodine. Iodine, like iron, cannot be synthesized in the body and must be provided through dietary or supplemental sources. It is also important for healthy hair, nails, skin, and teeth. To prevent endemic goiter from iodine lack in areas where seafood is not abundant, common table salt is fortified with iodine. Iodine combines with tyrosine, and amino acid, in the thyroid gland to form thyroxine, the active principle of this vital gland. Thyroxine regulates metabolism, thus demands are increased in athletics. Although deficiency symptoms are rare in sports, an athlete's "burned out" signs of weakness, apprehensiveness, lethargy, indifference, chilliness, and constipation may be seen in the iodine-deficient individual, as well as the individual with low motivation and lack of purpose. Other deficiency symptoms include cold hands and feet, dry hair, irritability, nervousness, and obesity. Antifactors are not known.

While not established to date, it may well be that athletes require some additional nutrients, as compared to the nonathlete, which would add a small increment in performance that could make the difference between winning or losing if all else is equal. It should be noted in terms of performance that adverse changes in behavior, mood, and perception result from a low concentration in the brain of any one of the following vitamins: thiamine (B-1), niacin (B-3), pyridoxine (B-6), cyanocobalamin (B-12), pantothenic acid, folic acid, and ascorbic acid (C). Both athletic and nonathletic mental function and behavior may also be affected by changes in the concentration in the brain of other substances that are normally present, such as amino acids and various minerals.

Fads vs the Balanced Diet

Food fads come and go in sports, just as diet fads ebb and flow among the overweight. Fads appeal to human hopes and fears and borrow from superstitions. Many warn against eating seafood and drinking milk, yet clam chowder composed of seafood and milk is considered appropriate. Megavitamin therapy, bee pollen, royal jelly, concentrated or predigested protein, bone meal, wheat germ, kelp, brewer's yeast, desiccated liver, and blackstrap molasses have not been shown to enhance endurance or improve performance. However, a special substance may offer a psychologic advantage to a particular athlete which should not be denied. Some people have an emotional problem associated with their diets which is dangerous to tamper with.

As in any sector of society, athletics has an abundance of faddists. There are the "natural food" faddists, the "rapid reducing scheme" faddists, the "eat more of . . ." faddists, the "eat this only with this" faddists, the "milk shy" faddists, the "fasting" faddists, the "chew every bite 32 times" faddists, etc. As people like to borrow bad habits from each other as well as those which are beneficial, the citadel of nutritional faddism is ignorance. A balanced diet is one which contains a variety of palatable food groups because no one single source provides all the necessary vitamins, minerals, and trace elements necessary for proper metabolism. In general, a balanced diet consists of (1) four daily servings of fruits and vegetables; (2) four or more daily servings of cereals and grains; (3) two or more daily servings (3/4 oz/serving) of meat; and (4) two daily servings of milk or milk products.

MEALS BEFORE, DURING, AND AFTER COMPETITION

Prior to competition, a specialized nutritional plan is often conducted from 48–72 hours before a vigorous contest. Nourish-

ment during and after competition also deserves special consideration.

Pregame Meals

A heavy breakfast of steak and eggs has been traditional in most football squads for many years with the idea that it would aid the later heavy demands for strength and energy. Modern thought, however, states that the pregame meal should be rich in carbohydrates and fruit juices and low in sugar, protein, and fat. Fats delay the stomach's emptying time, and proteins require renal fixed-acid elimination that reduces body fluids.

It usually takes about 2–3 hours for a meal to pass from the stomach and another 2 hours to pass through the small intestines (Fig. 5.2). Milk requires 150 minutes to be evacuated from the stomach, eggs are evacuated in about 160 minutes and beef requires 180 minutes. Thus, at least 3 hours should pass between the pregame meal and participation. Food within the stomach during vigorous competition often results in nausea, vomiting, and intestinal cramps. The cause for this is that the circulation

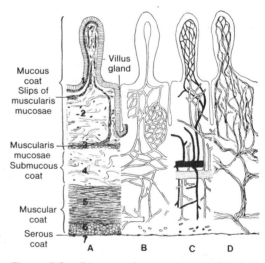

Figure 5.2. Diagram of a cross section of small intestine. *A*, coats of intestinal wall and tissues of coats; *B*, arrangement of central lacteal, lymph nodes, and lymph tubes; *C*, blood supply (arteries and capillaries black, veins stippled); *D*, nerve fibers, the submucous plexus lying in the submucosa, the myenteric plexus lying between the circular and longitudinal layers of the muscular coat.

necessary for digestion is being demanded by skeletal muscles during physical activity.

As gastric emptying time is known to be prolonged by emotional stress (eg, pregame tension), research has shown that a heavy meal taken 3 hours before an event may still be in the stomach as long as 2 hours after the game. Nervous tension decreases circulation to the stomach and intestine, decreases gastric motility, and increases motility in the lower digestive tract (eg, diarrhea). This effect varies considerably with each individual. One solution to this problem is a voluntary pregame liquid meal containing an easily digested well-balanced nutritional formula. Such formulae may be taken up to 3 hours before an event.

Current thought indicates that skipping breakfast may adversely affect performance. Three meals a day should be minimum, and four or five small meals may be better than three large meals.

In planning pregame nutrition, certain fundamentals should be considered:

1. To avoid hunger and weakness during competition, the diet plan should safeguard that there is adequate energy to maintain a normal blood sugar level. For this purpose, fructose is the best sugar source. For at least 2 days before a game, the diet should be well balanced with emphasis on carbohydrates and reduced physical activity to allow for maximum glycogen storage. While carbohydrates should be increased, sugar intake should be reduced to avoid rebound hypoglycemia. Fruit sugar, however, does not offer a rebound effect.

2. A logical state of hydration should be assured through food/fluid intake. Water intake should be a minimum of eight glasses per day. As salt creates excessive fluid retention, sodium-rich foods such as processed meats, salty snacks, and highly-spiced foods should be restricted 24 hours before an event. For vigorous competition, broth or bouillon taken with two or three glasses of water 3 hours before an event provides adequate salt intake.

3. Any specific food or drink that is known to disagree with a particular player should be avoided by that player. Likewise, any logical food or drink desired by a player should not be restricted. Foods considered flatulence-producing (eg, beans, cabbage, brussel sprouts, broccoli) are often restricted for about 48 hours before competition.

4. By game time, the stomach and lower bowel should be empty. High-fiber food such as raw fruits and vegetables and whole grains are normally reduced for about 2 days prior to competition to minimize the need for emptying the bowels during game time.

Nourishment During Competition

Nutrition is often necessary during prolonged competition to prevent dehydration and maintain an optimal energy level. The best solution to this problem is to have the athlete sip fruit juices. Sugar cubes, dextrose, glucose, or candy should be avoided as they attract fluids to the intestinal tract. This contributes to peripheral dehydration.

Postgame Meals

Appetite usually becomes depressed during vigorous physical activity, and there are often psychologic effects of anxiety or depression as the result of personal performance, team performance, travel deadlines, etc. Nevertheless, a light dinner-type meal should be planned that is well balanced and taken in a pleasant environment a few hours after competition.

ATHLETIC CONDITIONING FACTORS CONTRIBUTING TO MALNUTRITION

Continuous participation in athletics increases an individual's caloric and nutrient requirements, just as seen in the effects of a high fever. Thus, a diet adequate under normal sedentary conditions may be far inadequate to meet the needs of athletic activity, growth, or illness. When we combine athletic needs with growth needs in the young athlete, there is a definite nutritional challenge.

Malnutrition within athletics does not happen suddenly; it exhibits during a long, insidious period. In its eary stages, the only symptoms noticed may be tiredness, irritability, low morale, lowered efficiency, and reduced resistance to disease. In this context, the "pregame" meal is not as important as the vast number of pregame meals over several months.

Stages of Malnutrition

Dolan and Holladay describe the development of malnutrition in athletics in four stages.

First Stage: The stage of tissue depletion and weight loss where the tissues become depleted of their stored nutrients. This depletion progresses at a rate relative to the severity and chronicity of the deficiency state.

Second Stage: The stage of biochemical "lesions" where alterations in the normal constituents of the blood occur, exhibited in athletes as a distinct shortness of breath.

Third Stage: The stage of functional changes and overt symptom development. In baseball, for example, a pitcher may require longer warmup periods to loosen muscle tissues of the arm, forearm, or wrist. Postgame soreness lasts longer, and wounds take longer to heal. Peripheral neuritis may result from a thiamine deficiency.

Fourth Stage: This final stage does not occur in athletes as symptoms are so severe that strenuous participation becomes impossible before this stage is reached. Overt clinical signs appear in bones, muscles, and with vision and behavior.

Basic Factors Leading to Athletic Malnutrition

Anything which would interfere with the absorption and utilization of nutrients contributes to malnutrition. Typical examples are gastrointestinal disorders and emotional stress effecting excessive gastric and intestinal activity. Gastrointestinal disorders, emotional disturbances, and food allergies readily interfere with digestion. Excessive perspiration, diarrhea, and polyuria are common factors that cause an increased loss of nutrients. In addition, excessively low or high temperatures during physical activity or high humidity increase nutritive requirements, especially during strenuous physical activity.

CHAPTER 6

Clinical Assessment Aspects of Physical Fitness

Fitness is an attribute of the human organism at its best, differing with culture, social patterns, physical environment, occupation, exercise, daily activities, ethnic background, age, sex, nutritional status, body type, acute illness, chronic disease, and heredity. Nevertheless, Atha points out that when nutritional status is optimal, habitual physical activity seems to be the most powerful factor influencing the activity capacity of a healthy subject.

The role of physical training has still to be accurately defined to the satisfaction of all. Williams and Sperryn look to physical fitness as an "artificial state in so far as it is specially cultivated rather than inherent in the individual." Functional status appears to be able to be increased more in young subjects than the elderly.

ASSESSMENT OF PHYSICAL FITNESS

The development of optimal physical fitness produces changes which increase physical capacity and produces changes at the cellular level in altered metabolism. A reduced level of fitness predisposes injury and likely the extent of injury at both its macroscopic and microscopic aspects. For example, training increases the bulk of muscle fibers and increases muscle interstitial vascularity. Both of these factors have an influence upon the effects of acute muscle strain in that (1) an untrained muscle is more apt to bleed and form a hematoma than is a trained muscle, and (2) the physiologic mechanisms necessary to absorb extravasated fluid is more efficient in a trained muscle than in an untrained muscle.

Personal History

The personal data collected should be similar to that recorded clinically, such as name, address, date of birth, age, sex, pres-ent complaints, present and past occupations, type of work and the number of hours, recreational activities, medical and surgical history, accidents and injuries history, drug and food sensitivities, allergies, congenital difficulties, diet, smoking and drinking habits, insurance data, etc. The athletic history should carefully define type of primary and secondary physical activities, number of hours involved, level of achievement, age at which competition began, etc.

Health Examination

This also is similar to the clinical examination, incorporating the subject's physical examination and laboratory data when necessary. The goal of the examination in assessing physical fitness is to (1) determine the level of health in relationship to freedom from disease, injury, ailment, or abnormality; (2) establish the criteria which indicate the limits of permitted activity for a particular individual; and (3) measure the structural and functional state of a particular individual before participation in a stressful activity.

Physiologic Responses to Exercise

Sometimes it is advisable for a doctor to accurately profile an individual's physiologic response to exercise. Ideally, three basic factors underlie all physiologic tests for physical fitness: (1) maximum oxygen-debt capacity (anaerobic power) which determines the amount of activity possible with all-out effort for approximately 45 seconds through anaerobic release mechanisms; (2) maximum oxygen intake capacity (aerobic power) which determines the amount of activity possible for approximately 15–30 minutes through coordinated circulatory and respiratory adjustments producing the maximum amount of tissue oxygen; and (3) metabolic capacity which determines the amount of activity possible for approximately 2–3 hours through the quantity of energy-yielding substrates maximally available from body reserves during maximum aerobic demands. However, in non-research practice, sufficient data can be obtained about fitness solely by determining aerobic power.

Aerobic power is determined by cardiorespiratory function, intrinsic physical fatigue factors, duration and nature of the physical activity, extra demands on temperature regulation, and intrinsic environmental conditions (eg, altitude, temperature, humidity) (Fig. 6.1).

Apparatus

When a physical activity is conducted against gravity, both basal and working metabolic rates are directly proportional to body weight; thus stepping exercises (at any given stepping frequency and height) and treadmill tests (at any given slope and speed) provide the same relative workloads for all athletes. The apparatus typically used to evaluate physiologic fitness are the motor-driven treadmill, the bicycle ergometer with adjustable mechanical resistance, and the stepping ergometer with adjustable heights.

Intensity and Duration

All tests should begin with a workload low enough to be far below maximum for the individual. The goal is to evaluate the effects of continuous effort at gradually increasing intensities. Duration of testing must also be carefully balanced. Short-duration tests are subject to misinformation, and long-duration tests affect the thermoregulatory mechanisms to such an extent as to cloud aerobic power assessment. In general, intensity levels are maintained for 2 minutes, with the full test ranging from 10 to 16 minutes. For details of testing and scoring procedures, the reader should refer to equipment manufacturers' instructions or to a specific text on the subject.

Contraindications

The examiner must be aware of both the contraindications to testing as well as the indications for stopping a test in process. No adult subject should be placed in a stress test situation who lacks the family physician's approval, has a resting heart rate above 100/minute, has an oral temperature

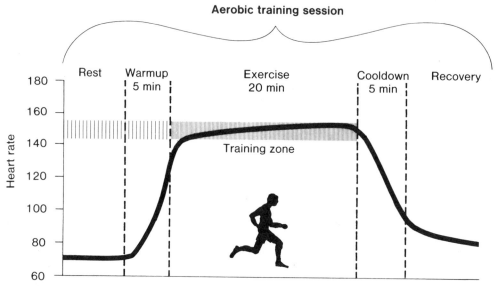

Figure 6.1. Typical aerobic training bout. With regular training session, a previously sedentary adult can expect to see a 20–25% improvement in aerobic fitness and performance in 3–6 months. Improvement depends on level of fitness and age: under 20, 30% improvement; over 70, 10% (with the permission of the Behavioral Research Foundation).

above 99°F, has a history of angina pectoris, has an obvious cardiac malfunction or abnormal ECG, has suffered a myocardial infarction or myocarditis within the past 3 months, or who shows evidence of infection, including the common cold. The effect of menstruation must be judged on an individual basis. All youth must have parental approval.

Repeated blood pressure measurements and cardiac auscultation during frequent testing intervals are mandatory. Testing should be halted immediately when symptoms of distress occur (eg, chest pain, severe dyspnea, intermittent claudication), signs of anoxia occur (eg, cyanosis, pallor, confusion, disorientation), pulse pressure consistently falls when work intensity increases, systolic pressure exceeds 240 mm Hg, diastolic pressure exceeds 125 mm Hg, or when the subject feels he or she is unable to proceed.

Physique and Body Composition

Assessment of physique and body composition should be based on anthropometric measurements, an analysis of body compartments, and an evaluation of maturation. The size and geometry of an athlete's body places individual constraints on the capacity for physical activity. The effects naturally vary with the sport, position, and matching involved. The major areas of concern are the individual's overall size and proportion, weight (Fig. 6.2), height, degree of maturation, degree of symmetry, general body type, and demands of the anticipated activity. It is the physician's role to identify the extent of constraints present and their potential effect on physical fitness during rest and competition. Assessment begins with clues from the subject's history which may indicate genetic, congenital, nutritional, or connective tissue abnormalities.

Overall Size and Proportion

A first consideration is an evaluation of an individual's size and proportion to (1) anticipate physical and functional performance capabilities and potential weaknesses, and (2) isolate a potentially serious health disorder. Normal growth and development involve both an increase in size and a change in proportion. A young athlete is not

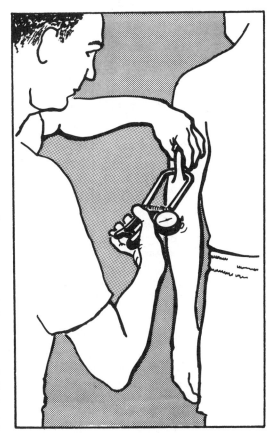

Figure 6.2. Calipering skinfold thickness in back of the triceps to evaluate extremity fatness.

a miniature adult proportionately. Growth and proportion effects are frequently indicators of genetic determinants, hormone balance, connective tissue health, and nutritional considerations.

In review, several hormones influence body habitus. The growth hormone of the pituitary affects somatic growth. Thyroid hormone promotes linear growth and has a direct influence on cartilage ossification, epiphyseal maturation, and thus on skeletal proportions. In the young, an overproduction of androgen stunts growth and an underproduction removes the checks from linear growth. In the adolescent, however, androgens stimulate growth and muscular development and are responsible for the development of secondary sexual characteristics. The sex hormones influence epiphyseal maturation; and if the growth plates in the long bones close too early, longitudinal growth is halted.

Good or poor nutrition also has a distinct influence upon growth and development because of its influence upon hormone and connective tissue quality. Genetics, hormone balance, and nutrition manifest themselves in connective tissue quality as seen in bone, cartilage, collagen, elastin, muscle, and fat.

Abnormal and Subnormal Weight

Weight is both a health and athletic concern (Figs. 6.3 and 6.4). Weight is defined as the total weight of the body, with light or no clothing, and is best measured in pounds or kilograms (2.2046 lb = 1 kg).

The state of being overweight and obesity must be differentiated in physical assessment. Body weight is the total weight of four distinct body substances: protoplasm (50%), extracellular fluid (25%), adipose tissue (18%), and bone (7%). A loss or gain in weight therefore reflects a net loss or gain in one, several, or all of these substances. Obesity implies adipose tissue in excess of 20% above standard and comprises an unnecessary energy loss during motion; a state of overweight may be the result of excessive protoplasm, extracellular fluid, or bone mass as well. As obese people are less dense than the nonobese, body density is a good reference to estimate the contribution of fatty tissue to total body weight.

Body density is ideally calculated by water displacement after removal of nonvital body air, but this is a cumbersome

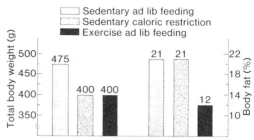

Figure 6.4. Effects of 15 weeks of daily exercise on body composition of adult male rats, portraying the futility of diet alone contrasted with the effectiveness of an exercise program. This test demonstrated that sedentary free-eating animals, representing the typical nondieting inactive American adult, were the heaviest and fattest. Also, the sedentary paired-weight animals, which were physically inactive but restricted in food to match the body weight of runners, were considerably fatter than the runners even though the body weight for both groups was the same. Thus, dieting alone is not an effective way to reduce fatness. Although dieting will cause a reduction in weight, 65% of the weight loss is from muscle mass and only 35% from fatty tissue. Thus, the percentage of body weight is fat (the true indicator of body leanness) can remain about the same in response to weight loss by dieting alone (with the permission of the Behavioral Research Foundation).

research method. The more common means is to caliper skinfold thickness such as back of the triceps (extremity fat) and below the scapula (truncal fat). More than an inch of tissue calipered in these areas is usually considered a sign of obesity. Other areas which may be recorded will be discussed later.

Subnormal body weight is the result of protoplasm, extracellular fluid, or adipose tissue loss, all of which reduce skinfold thickness and weight/height indices. The most common cause is protoplasm loss associated with an abnormal nitrogen and potassium balance. Lean muscle loss is calculated from urinary creatinine excretion and limb-circumference measurements. Protein/caloric malnutrition affects physical performance early, far before results are seen in impaired cellular immunity and infection.

Abnormal and Subnormal Height

Height is a concern in many sports, and abnormal height also has several implica-

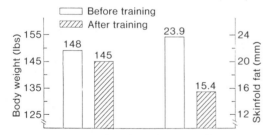

Figure 6.3. Effects of training on body weight and skinfold fat. A recent study viewed the effects of exercise on overweight college women. Eleven females participated in a walk-jog program 6 days per week for 8 weeks. No attempt was made to control diet. Energy expenditure was about 500/day. Both body weight and body fat decreased significantly (with the permission of the Behavioral Research Foundation).

tions for one's health status. Height (length) is the distance from the highest body part to the lowest in the standing position and best measured in inches or centimeters (1 inch = 2.54 cm). Weight and height are related to the body's surface area, and surface area is related to heat dissipation and caloric needs.

Excessive tallness, considered a benefit to the aspiring basketball center, is the result of increased longitudinal growth resulting from either excessive growth stimulation or insufficient growth checks. Proportional measurements aid in evaluation.

Anthropometric Methods

Anthropometry helps in determining patterns of growth and development, helps in the investigation of variations in physique and body composition, helps in defining structural body type, and provides data for a team doctor's referential system. These measurements essentially include measuring body dimensions such as lengths, diameters, circumferences, and skinfold thickness.

The instruments commonly used for conducting anthropometric measurements are weight and height scales, measuring tapes, bilateral (balance) scales, postural plumb line or grid, skinfold caliper, sliding caliper, and steel anthropometer. It is helpful to mark landmarks on the subject with a skin pencil at the beginning of the examination.

Basic Mensuration Technique

For general screening, the examiner may measure (a) the lower body segment by recording the distance from the symphysis pubis to the floor; (b) the upper segment by recording the distance from the symphysis pubis to the highest point on the crown; and (c) the span by recording the distance from the laterally outstretched fingertip to the sternal notch. Normally, these three measurements should be equal after the age of 10. The measurements are made with the patient standing upright. A variation of this technique is to measure total span from fingertip to fingertip of the laterally outstretched upper extremities to arrive at the total span measurement. This should equal the distance from the top of the crown to

the floor when the patient is standing upright.

These measurements offer significant maturation indices. For instance, during early youth, the trunk is normally longer than the limbs. However, as age increases, the extremities increase at a faster rate than the trunk until the limbs and trunk become the same length at about the age of 10 years and remain so throughout adulthood. After the age of 10, it is an abnormal sign when the trunk is longer than the limbs and is usually an indication of hypothyroidism and may be seen in certain chondrodystrophies. If the trunk is shorter than the limbs after the age of 10, gonadal hormone deficiency can be suspected to have removed the checks to long-bone epiphyseal closing at the proper age. Abnormal ratios may be subtle, yet they are distinct diagnostic clues which should be picked up by the examiner.

Minor degrees of atrophy are determined by comparing the circumference at corresponding levels of each arm, forearm, thigh, and calf. Take care that the limbs are in a state of relaxation.

It is also helpful to measure and record the circumference of the head, thorax, abdomen, and obviously asymmetrical parts. If thoracic inflexibility is suspected, it is well to record chest circumference at full inspiration and full expiration. If flexibility is the sole question, one need only record the difference in inches between inspiration and expiration measurements and compare findings periodically to record the degree of improvement.

More Detailed Measurements

When more sophisticated data are sought, the following list of measurements is suggested:

1. *Standing lengths*
   (a) Standing height, from vertex to floor.
   (b) Acromial height, at the most lateral point on the acromion process of the scapula.
   (c) Radial height, at the uppermost border of the radial cup with the arm relaxed in the anatomic position.
   (d) Stylion height, at the most distal point of the styloid process of the radius.

(e) Dactylion height, at the midpoint of the tip of the middle finger.

(f) Trochanterion height, at the uppermost point of the greater trochanter.

(g) Sphyrion height, at the lowest point on the tip of the medial malleolus.

(h) Tibial height, at the upper border of the inner tuberosity of the tibial head at the highest point of its medial border.

2. *Sitting lengths*

(a) sitting height, with hips at right angles, from vertex to floor.

(b) Seated suprasternal height, at the midpoint of the anterior-superior border of the sternum.

3. *Diameter measurements*

(a) Transverse chest width, at the end of normal expiration.

(b) A-P chest width, at the midsternal level.

(c) Biacromial diameter distance, between right and left acromions.

(d) Bicristal diameter, between the most laterally projecting points of the iliac crest.

(e) Humerus biepicondylar diameter, with the elbow bent at a right angle.

(f) Femur biepicondylar diameter, between the lateral and medial epicondyle with the femur bent at a right angle.

4. *Circumference measurements*

(a) Chest circumference, at the lowest point of the sternum where it tapers to the xiphoid process, taken both at maximum inspiration and maximum expiration.

(b) Midarm circumference (contracted and uncontracted), at a point halfway between the acromion and the olecranon.

(c) Forearm circumference, immediately below the elbow joint with the arm hanging loose.

(d) Midthigh circumference, at a point halfway between the greater trochanter and the knee joint.

(e) Midcalf circumference, at the point of maximum thickness.

5. *Skinfold thickness measurements*

(a) Biceps, taken on the ventral of the upper arm, halfway between acromion and olecranon.

(b) Triceps, taken on the dorsum of the upper arm, halfway between acromion and olecranon.

(c) Forearm, taken on the lateral forearm.

(d) Subscapular, taken about 1 cm below the lower angle of the scapula with the subject standing.

(e) Suprailiac, taken about 3 cm above the iliac crest.

(f) Medial thigh, taken halfway between the trochanter and tibia with the subject's knee slightly flexed.

(g) Lateral thigh, taken halfway between the trochanter and tibia.

(h) Calf, taken medially with the subject standing.

Evaluation of Maturation

In addition to height and weight, it is frequently helpful to determine the degree of youth's progression through adolescence for proper matching. This is simply done with males by rating pubic hair, axillary hair, facial hair, and genital development, and with females by rating pubic hair and breast development. Skeletal maturity may be determined by x-ray evaluation of the bones of the wrist and hand and other joints, but exposure for this reason only is contraindicated. It is not unusual for the team doctor dealing with youth to be the first to recognize signs of hormonal imbalance.

General Physical Performance Measurements

Certain tests have been developed to determine the measurable aspects of physical capacity of such activities as power, strength, endurance, speed, flexibility, balance, reaction time, and coordination. Not all tests are considered with all athletes, only those appropriate to the needs at hand. Performance testing is usually the role of coaches or research scientists; the athletic physician is rarely involved. The common performance tests utilized and based against time or distance averages are the meter sprint, distance runs, standing and running long jumps, horizontal beam chinning, sit ups, and grip strength.

BODY TYPES

An analysis of body type is helpful in determining adequacy to certain sports and specific team positions, as well as predispositions to certain types of injury. By general definition, body type (constitution) is the morphologic, physiologic, and psychologic result of the properties of all cellular and humoral influences of the body which are determined by genetic and environmental influences.

Anatomically, physiologically, mentally and emotionally, no two athletes are exactly alike. However, structurally and functionally, three major general body types are recognized and classified: (1) the intermediate, mesomorphic, or normal type; (2) the ectomorphic, asthenic, hypotonic, or carnivorous type; and (3) the endomorphic, hypersthenic, hypertonic, or herbivorus type. The size and location of the various abdominal organs vary considerably from one person to another depending upon the particular body build and posture. Visceral organs are usually placed high in the endomorph and low in the ectomorph as compared to the intermediate build.

The viscera are dynamic, not completely fixed structures as seen on the printed page. They move with the movements of the diaphragm and anterior abdominal wall. They move when posture changes, being highest when the patient is recumbent, lower when he stands and lower yet when he sits. They rise when the anterior wall is voluntarily retracted. These points must be remembered during health examination and performance evaluation. The structures which appear to vary the most are the pyloric stomach (the cardiac orifice is nearly stationary), duodenum, head of the pancreas, liver, spleen and kidneys.

Any close observation of people shows a wide variation in human form. Few will truly fit the anatomy textbooks' descriptions. Of the variations from the so-called normal (intermediate) body form, the two most easily distinguishable types are the ectomorphic (lean) and endomorphic (heavy) types. While most subjects you see will be of mixed types, the basic characteristics of and implications involved with the intermediate, ectomorphic, and endomorphic body types will be briefly described.

The Intermediate Body Type

The intermediate type is characterized by good muscle, fat, and connective tissue development. The trunk is the same length as the limbs after the age of 10 years, and total span is equal to height. Other general proportions are that the arms are three times the length of the outstretched hands; the length of the leg is three times the length of the foot; and the trunk (torso) is three times the height of the head. In the female, the limbs are slightly shorter, the carrying angle of the forearm is greater, and the thighs are more obliquely placed as the result of having a wider pelvis than does the male. The thorax is full and rounded in the intermediate type, and the upper abdomen is rounded. All abdominal viscera, except a small portion of the large and small intestine, are above the umbilicus. The lower abdomen is flat. The stomach is pear shaped and placed well up under the ribs.

The Ectomorphic Body Type

This is the tall and thin, lean and lanky build (Fig. 6.5). The body design is slender, and the physical frame is frail. Musculature, subcutaneous fat, and tissues are often deficient. The neck is long and thin and the larynx protrudes. The clavicles, ribs, and spinous processes protrude because of the deficiency in subcutaneous fat. The extremity bones are long and thin, and the thighs are placed widely apart. The asthenic presents a frail slender physique, light body weight, and delicate body structure, as seen in many sprinters. The thorax is long and narrow, and the abdomen is short. There is disproportion between the pelvic cavity and that of the upper abdomen. The false pelvis is often as wide and capacious as that of an endomorph twice as tall. Chest expansion is limited. The ectomorph's gastrointestinal tract is low. The stomach is long, tubular, atonic, and largely pelvic when the subject is standing. The tone of the gastrointestinal tract is poor and its motility slow. There is a tendency toward visceroptosis. Ectomorphic females are prone to pelvic organ prolapse. This type is best for the runner and noncontact sports.

The Endomorphic Body Type

This is the stocky-sturdy, chubby-heavy

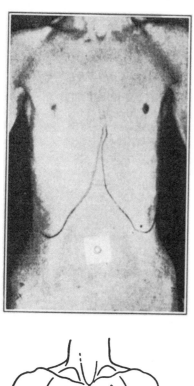

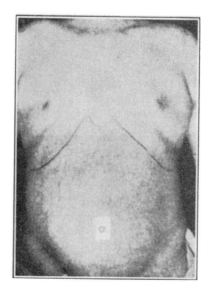

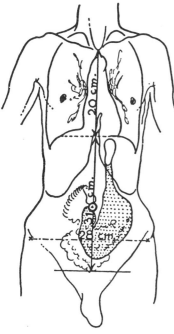

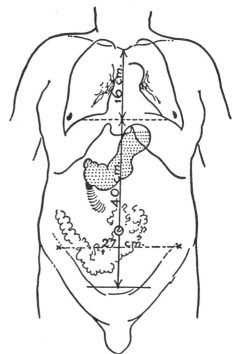

Figure 6.5. *Above*, ectomorphic habitus. *Below*, x-ray film tracings showing typical ectomorphic bowel development.

Figure 6.6. *Above*, endomorphic habitus. *Below*, x-ray film tracings showing typical endomorphic bowel development.

type. (Fig. 6.6). The neck is short and thick. The shoulders and chest are broad, and there is good thoracic expansion. The extremities are large and sturdy. The vertebrae are large and strong, and the lumbar spine

is short. Spinal motion is more restrictive than that seen in the ectomorph or intermediate types. Musculature is well developed and powerful; connective tissue and fat are abundant. The hypersthenic presents a powerful and massive physique, great body weight, and heavy bony framework, as often seen in football tackles and weight lifters. The thorax is short, deep, and wide. The abdomen is long and of great capacity in its upper zone. The endomorph's gastrointestinal tract is high. Gastric and colonic motility is fast, and the whole tract presents marked tone. Strong, short mesenteric attachments hinder the development of visceroptosis. This type is best for the contact or gladiator-type sports.

BODY MECHANICS AND ITS EFFECTS ON ATHLETIC PERFORMANCE

It is unwise to consider the various parts of the body as separate entities. All parts share responsibility in the orthograde posture. Any disturbance in one part causes an immediate and definite functional change in other parts. The center of gravity shifts with each change in body alignment, and the amount of weight borne by the joints and the pull of the muscles vary within reasonable limits with each body movement.

Posture and Body Mechanics

Poor posture from habit, disease, or abnormal reflexes results in constant structural malalignment which allows a disproportionate amount of weight and muscle pull to fall upon some parts. This alters the normal locomotion apparatus and functions of the internal organs as well. While these changes may develop insidiously, the resulting abnormalities produce pathologic changes in the body during standing, sitting, lying, and motion. Such abnormalities are tolerated for a short time, but sooner or later serious, often subtle, maladjustments result when the body's compensation resources become exhausted. These factors, in total, may predispose an individual to injury or hinder performance.

An important factor in athletics is that, with good postural body mechanics, balance is maintained with the least amount of muscular effort, thus encouraging longer endurance, with less strain on any one part. A start can be made with no wasted time or energy. Muscle pull in maintaining an erect carriage is more direct, thus avoiding back

or shoulder strain. A natural balance is maintained between the iliopsoas group and the hip extensors, and a similar condition exists at the knee and ankle joints.

Spinal Deformities and Defects

During health evaluation, overall posture should be inspected for early signs of spinal curvature, subluxations, leg-length discrepancies, and other subtle or gross deformities.

Few if any adult spines are free from defects which involve several vertebrae. In many instances, the entire spinal column labors under the strain of improper balance. In this sense, however, the defects of balance referred to are something less than the classical conditions of clinical kyphosis, lordosis, and scoliosis.

Visceral Implications

Poor body mechanics predisposes certain visceral disorders and injuries; ie, the viscera are held in their optimum position for function in good body mechanics. If mechanics are good, the abdominal cavity is shaped like an inverted pear with adequate space above L4 for the abdominal viscera of an intermediate body type (Fig. 6.7). In the ideal attitude, tissue ledges and shelves exist which partially support the abdominal organs. However, if the lumbar and dorsal curves increase and the abdominal wall relaxes, these vital supports are lost.

Nature provides good support for the abdominal organs when the body is normally erect (Fig. 6.8). For instance, the kidneys normally rest in definite depressions which begin around the level of L4 and are supported by the psoas muscle, quadratus lumborum, and retroperitoneal fat. The liver is generally posterior to the transverse sagittal plane. It is partly supported by the surrounding organs and its attachments to the diaphragm, but most of its weight is borne by the concave space at the side of the spine and by the curves of the lower ribs. With the stomach lying mainly to the left of the spine and supported by a diaphragmatic attachment behind the transverse sagittal plane, there is little tendency for downward displacement if there is no ribcage deformity or abdominal muscle weakness. The spleen is well back and held in place by peritoneal folds, and the pancreas depends chiefly on

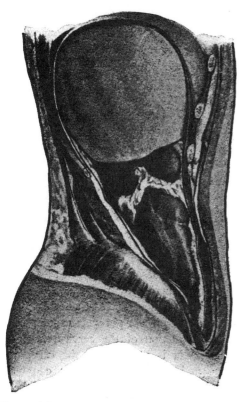

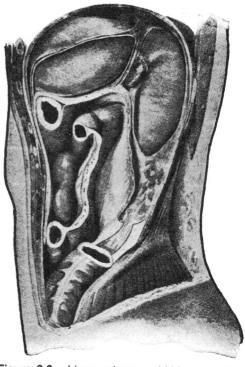

Figure 6.8. Liver, spleen, and kidneys rest on shelves reinforced by adipose tissue and suspended by fibrous bands. In the main, the small and large intestines are suspended; other viscera are shelved.

Figure 6.7. The upper part of the abdomen is roomy, but the lower part is quite narrow due to the dorsal and lumbar spinal curves which give maximum room above and necessary support by the pelvic basin below.

the surrounding organs for support. The attachments of the hepatic and splenic flexures of the colon are external to the kidney and attached to the posterior surface of the abdominal cavity. About seven-eighths of the weight of the abdominal organs is borne by the psoas shelf and the muscles of the abdominal wall.

Respiratory Considerations

Most all sports require good lung capacity. Respiratory balance and the maintenance of proper intra-abdominal pressure are dependent upon good body mechanics (Fig. 6.9). In the ideal attitude, the position of the head well poised and the chest held high is important because the anterior mediastinal ligaments attached to the diaphragm originate in the deep cervical fascia and are attached to the lower cervical vertebrae. When mechanics are poor, a lowered dia-

phragm is the rule, and proper coordination of the muscles of respiration is lost. This abnormal position may decrease vital capacity by more than one half. Venous and lymphatic return is greatly assisted by the rhythmic contractions of the diaphragm. When the diaphragm has been lowered, it has a much shorter range of excursion and is thus much less effective as a circulatory aid.

General Body Balance

Subluxations are often the natural forerunners of balance defects brought about through the effort of the spinal column to compensate for the stress and thus to reduce the more serious effects. Balance defects may also originate from habitual faulty postures in standing, sitting and lying, as well as from activities which too constantly employ the forces of the large muscles in asymmetrical action (eg, shot put, discus, bowling). When created, such defects serve to

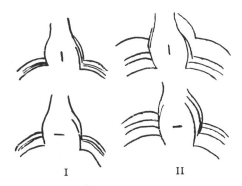

I   II

Figure 6.9. *I*, tracings of diaphragmatic excursion in faulty body mechanics; *II*, tracings of diaphragmatic excursions in the same individual after faulty body mechanics were corrected.

lessen the power of the spinal column to withstand shock and strain and are the natural precursors to subluxations. Other causes for defects of balance are found in the frequent occurrence of unequal lower extremities, in faulty development of the fifth lumbar vertebra and sacrum, and from the effects of abnormal reflexes. The least common cause of balance defects can be attributed to inheritance and disease.

Standing, walking, running, bending, throwing, blocking, hitting, etc, require constant voluntary loss and regain of body balance. The human body tries to maintain an upright posture with the head positioned so that the field of vision is parallel with the horizon and straight ahead. Limb motion or the addition of a load shifts an individual's center of gravity and changes body balance.

While gravity stabilizes the lower extremities in standing and provides friction for locomotion, it also places considerable stress on those body parts responsible for maintaining the upright position. Without appropriate neuromusculoskeletal compensation and accommodation, such actions would result in imbalance and falling. Thus, postural deviations resulting in balance problems lead to frequent strain and injury to antigravity structures.

No two athletes react in an identical manner to actual or potential loss of body balance. All vary somewhat in the accommodation process depending upon one's gross structure and functional capabilities, the momentary potential for redistributing body mass, and the visual efficiency necessary to guide correct accommodations.

In evaluating physical performance, we should understand some of the basic nervous mechanisms which operate both during stance and locomotion to provide distribution of postural tension throughout the musculoskeletal system. With the head erect, the labyrinths are placed in an optimum position to act synergistically with the neck reflexes, and these in turn react with other existing proprioceptive and exeroceptive impulses to supply a symmetrical distribution of tone in proper quantities to the postural muscles throughout the body. Thus, it is not unlikely that proprioceptive impulses combined with the interacting postural reflexes of good body mechanics play a role in the maintenance of good health and optimal performance. Conversely, the maladjustment of nervous impulses within the central nervous system as a result of pressure, irritation, or poor posture may be a causative factor in the production of poor health and hindered performance by contributing to dysfunction from the subtle yet persistent stress involved. It has also been well established that viscerosomatic reflexes can produce hypertonicity of skeletal muscles, thus producing subluxations and/or disturbances in body balance and function.

How one copes with gravitational influences may be witnessed in an athlete's degree of coordination. The center of gravity is a point at the exact center of body mass. Its location will vary somewhat according to body type, age, and sex, and move upward or downward or sideward in accordance with normal position movements and abnormal neuromusculoskeletal disorders. In a model subject, the center of gravity is located in the region of the second sacral segment; ie, 55–58% of the distance from the soles of the feet to the top of the head. The gross and subtle implications of anteroposterior balance, lateral balance, and rotational balance in athletics are manifold.

Balance Scales

To establish the degree of efficiency of spinal balance, a set of balance scales is often helpful. The scale recording the heaviest weight of the patient will be the "long-leg" side during the early stage. Later, chronic muscle stress and weakness, along with the development of a degree of scoliosis, shifts weight from the high side to the low. However, if the scales are placed about 18 inches apart, the heavy side will be the side of the "short leg" because of the weight shift caused by the wider base of support.

Rotational balance defects can be detected in this manner because neither the sacrum nor the spine rotate in a horizontal plane. They rotate obliquely anterior/inferior, thus causing a shifting of weight and an alteration of the center gravity. By such antagonistic rotation, the sacrum compensates for the infinite amount of small, bending, rotary movements of the vertical spine.

One modern application, the Chirotron system, consists of a weighing platform, adjustable for leveling, connected by a 15-foot cable to a remote electronic indicator with an illuminated scale (Figs. 6.10 and 6.11). The subject is first measured for lateral balance, and then rotated on the platform for A-P measurements. The indicator responds only to weight imbalance and not to total weight of the subject. Another mechanism has been developed in recent years that accurately determines, with a single reading, bilateral and anteroposterior

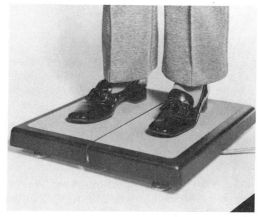

Figure 6.11. The Chirotron weighing platform permits leveling for accuracy. Subject may be rotated on the platform for anterior-posterior measurements.

weight with an accuracy of tolerance in ounces of relationship to body weight (Fig. 6.12). It is adjustable to conform to various foot sizes.

Body Type and Balance Defects

Balance defects tend to differ somewhat in the classic body types (Fig. 6.13). In the lean ectomorph, the anatomical design has a tendency to encourage poor body mechanics. Postural relaxation is the rule unless the person has had specialized training or makes a conscious effort. Habitual relaxation leads to a forward head carriage, flat chest, and narrow subcostal angle. The ribs and diaphragm are low, and the vital capacity is decreased. The abdomen is small above and protrudes just above the symphysis pubis, while retroperitoneal fat is slight. Visceroptosis is usually evident. The spine presents sharp bends in the midcervical and upper dorsal areas. There is a sharp lumbosacral curve with some accompanying lordosis. The pelvis inclines more than 60 degrees, and the knees are often hyperextended.

Such extremes of relaxation do not usually occur in the stocky endomorph because the anatomical construction is not so favorable to strain. However, the endomorph's shorter ligaments and restricted range of joint motion allow symptoms to appear with

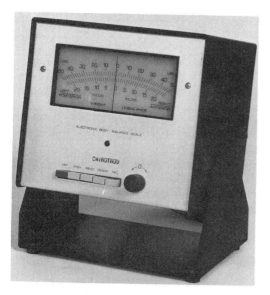

Figure 6.10. Chirotron remote indicator, which responds to weight unbalance, is connected to weighing platform by cable.

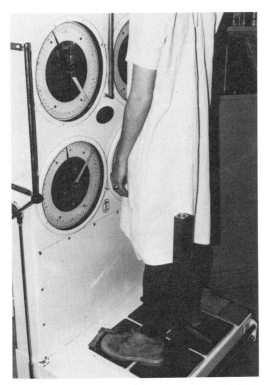

Figure 6.12. Component scales are frequently utilized to record sole and heel weight and determine which quadrant of the body exerts more gravitational weight in a postural defect.

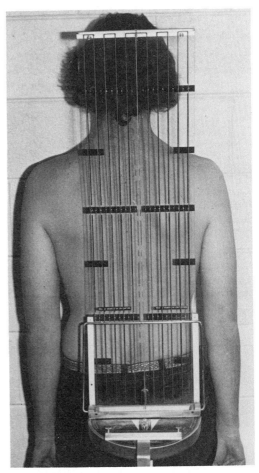

Figure 6.13. A wide variety of equipment is available for arriving at objective data in postural analysis.

only moderate deviations from the ideal. It is common to see sagging of the large, heavy viscera in the poorly conditioned individual, compensated for by a backward inclination of the trunk. Because of the limited range of spinal motion, bending to maintain the center of gravity over the feet usually comes either at the hips or dorsolumbar junction. Thus both areas are common points of stress and fatigue.

Faulty body mechanics also occur in the intermediate body type, resembling either an overly relaxed ectomorph or endomorph, thus difficult to profile.

Suggested Readings: Part 1

CHAPTERS 1–6

Atha, J: Physical Fitness Measurements, in Part VII, *Fitness, Health, and Work Capacity*, New York, Macmillan, 1974.

Adrian, MJ: Proper Clothing and Equipment, in *Sports Medicine for the Athletic Female*, Oradell, NJ, Medical Economics Company, 1980.

American Medical Association: *A Guide to Medical Evaluation of Candidates for School Sports*, Chicago, 1972.

Benenson, AS (ed): *Control of Communicable Diseases in Man*, ed 11, Washington, DC, American Public Health Association, 1970, chapters 1–2.

Berkow, R (ed): *The Merck Manual*, Section 1, ed 13, Rahway, NJ, Merck Sharp & Dohme Research Laboratories, 1977.

Bogert, LJ et al: *Nutrition and Physical Fitness*, ed 9, Philadelphia, W.B. Saunders, 1973.

Cheek, DB (ed): *Human Growth*, Philadelphia, Lea and Febiger, 1968.

Craig, TT (ed): *Comments in Sports Medicine*, Chicago, American Medical Association, 1973, chapters 1, 3, 4, 6, 9–12.

Damon, A et al: *The Human Body in Equipment Design*, Cambridge, MA, Harvard University Press, 1966.

Davidson, HA: Occupational Disorders, in *Cyclopedia of Medicine, Surgery and Specialties*, Vol X, Philadelphia, F.A. Davis, 1949, p. 740.

Dolan, JP and Holladay, LJ: *First-Aid Management*, ed 4, Danville, IL, Interstate Printers & Publishers, Inc, 1974, chapters 10, 13, 16.

Finch, CA et al: Lactic Acidosis Due to Iron Deficiency, *Journal of Clinical Investigations*, 58:447, 1979.

Harris, DV (ed): *Women and Sports: A National Research Congress*, The Pennsylvania State University, H.P.E.R. Series No. 2, University Park, PA, University of Pennsylvania, 1972.

Haycock, CE: *Sports Medicine for the Athletic Female*, Oradell, NJ, Medical Economics Company, 1980, chapters 6–8, 24, 25, 31.

Hirata, I, Jr: *The Doctor and the Athlete*, ed 2, Philadelphia, J.B. Lippincott, 1974, chapters 1–2, 4–6, p. 65.

Jahn, WT: Acceleration-Deceleration Injury, *Journal of Manipulative and Physiological Therapeutics*, Vol 1, No 2, June 1978.

Joyner, G: Parents' Guide to Football Safety, Franklin, NC, Ginseng Press, 1978.

Larcher, AC: Football Helmet Injuries, *Journal of Clinical Chiropractic*, Special Edition: Athletic Injuries, Vol 1, No. 6.

Larson, LA: *Fitness, Health, and Work Capacity*, Part VII, New York, Macmillan, 1974.

Mayer, J: *Human Nutrition*, Springfield, IL, Charles C Thomas, 1972.

Munves, ED: Nutrition, in *Sports Medicine for the Athletic Female*, Oradell, NJ, Medical Economics Company, 1980.

Robinson, CH: *Normal and Therapeutic Nutrition*, ed 14, New York, Macmillan, 1972.

Schafer, RC (ed): *Basic Chiropractic Procedural Manual*, ed 3, Des Moines, IA, American Chiropractic Association, 1980.

Schafer, RC: *Chiropractic Physical and Spinal Diagnosis*, Oklahoma City, OK, American Chiropractic Academic Press, 1980.

Schroeder, LW: Women in Athletics, *Journal of Clinical Chiropractic*, Special Edition: Athletic Injuries, Vol 1, No. 6.

Shephard, RJ: *Endurance Fitness*, Toronto, Ontario, Canada, University of Toronto Press, 1969.

Shierman, G: Conditioning the Athlete, *Sports Medicine for the Athletic Female*, Oradell, NJ, Medical Economics Company, 1980.

Singleton, WT: *Introduction to Ergonomics*, Albany, NY, World Health Organization, 1972.

Smith, NJ: Nutrition and Athletic Performance, in Scott, WN et al: *Principles of Sports Medicine*, Baltimore, Williams & Wilkins, 1984, pp 27–31.

Snyder, D: Chiropractic on the Field, *Journal of Clinical Chiropractic*, Special Edition: Athletic Injuries, Vol 1, No. 6.

Straus, RH: *Sports Medicine and Psychology*, Philadelphia, W.B. Saunders, 1979.

Thorndike, A: Prevention of Injuries in Athletes, *Journal of the American Medical Association*, 162:1126–1132, 1956.

Von Itallie et al: Nutrition and Athletic Performance, *Journal of the American Medical Association*, 162:1120–1126, 1956.

Walczak, M and Ehrich, BB: *Nutrition and Well-being* Reseda, CA, Mojave Books, 1976.

Weidman, FD: Dermatophytosis, *The Encyclopedia of Medicine, Surgery, and Specialties*, Vol IV, Philadelphia, F.A. Davis Co, 1939, p. 861.

Williams, JGP and Sperryn, PN (eds): *Sports Medicine*, ed 2, Baltimore, Williams & Wilkins Co, 1976, chapters 7, 9, 10, 12–13, p. 248.

Willis, JR and JC: Zinc Levels of the Richlands, Virginia High School Basketball Team, *Nutritional Perspectives*, Vol 4, No 1, January 1981.

Wilmore, JH: *Athletic Training and Physical Fitness*, Boston, Allyn and Bacon, 1977.

Womer, WO: Professional Involvement in Athletic Injuries, *Journal of Clinical Chiropractic*, Special Edition: Athletic Injuries, Vol 1, No. 6.

Part 2

EXAMINATION AND EVALUATION

CHAPTER 7

Examination Procedures and Applied Biomechanics

In sports care, "disability" has a profound meaning that includes not only the physical factor of functional impairment but also other considerations such as a player's talent, experience, position, present and future risk to a part or organ, etc.

EXCLUSION CRITERIA

While the scope of this text cannot include all possible types of dysfunction and pathologic structural disorders which would exclude an individual from a specific athletic activity, certain guidelines can be used to base the physician's decision.

1. Whatever the circumstances and pressures, no athlete should be allowed to risk permanent injury.

2. An athlete is either capable from a health standpoint or not. Special consideration on the type of activity, type of intra-team activity, or level of competition should never be made because of health considerations.

3. An athlete should be allowed to participate in the sport of his or her choice if practice and competition can be accomplished without danger to self or squad.

4. As all sports contain some risk, one sport or level of competition (intramural vs varsity) should not be considered safer than another in itself. An impartial viewpoint must be constantly held. However, the risk of a disability must be differentiated between one sport or position, and the demands involved, and another sport or position. For instance, a type of knee weakness may be viewed differently in a running sport than in polo.

THE PHYSICAL EXAMINATION

Specific evaluations will be discussed in future sections. Here we shall outline those aspects common to all athletes and all parts of the body.

Evaluation Criteria

The athletic health examination has a dual function: (1) to assess health status (limits and capacities), and (2) to recognize problems that may only occur during athletic activity. These must be kept in mind for both the professional athlete and the weekend athlete.

Note: If there is undue risk of present injury or future permanent injury or any type under conditioning, practice, or competition situations, the player should be kept from participation regardless of player (or other) objections.

The History Interview

While questionnaires are helpful in obtaining basic data, it is often wrong to delegate the taking of all information to them, for much can be gained by the subtleties occurring during the conversation. Direct conversation may reveal various pressures upon the individual. While the interview process is essentially the same as that seen in clinical practice, there are differences. During the typical physical evaluation, the athlete is neither ill nor in pain, as an office patient might be. Rather than looking at the doctor as a means of relief, the doctor is often viewed by the candidate as a possible obstacle toward athletic goals. Concealment, denial, and inventions are commonly witnessed. And this attitude on the part of a player is not without foundation. An athlete may feel healthy, strong, and well coordinated with good endurance, yet find himself facing permanent disqualification from contact sports. The player may wish to take the risk involved, and this decision may be supported by his parents and others involved. Hopefully, straightforward openness and reasoning by the physician will prevail; if not, the doctor's authority must be utilized.

Scope of Examination

The basic physical examination should evaluate height, weight, sitting blood pressure and pulse, temperature, eyes and vision, ears and hearing, nose, mouth and throat, chest and lungs, female breast, heart, abdomen, rectum and genitalia, feet, and postural mechanics (Fig. 7.1). A pelvic examination should be considered for any female athlete over the age of 20 who has not been examined within a year.

A basic orthopedic evaluation should be conducted on all athletes in regard to limb circumference measurements, joint flexibility, and range of active motion for the cervical spine, shoulders, back, hips, knees, and ankles. Neurologic deep-tendon reflexes and coordination tests should be conducted, with the more sophisticated tests reserved to confirm abnormalities found.

Laboratory tests should be conducted as indicated from the physical examination. However, many feel that all athletes should have as a minimum a blood workup, a urinalysis, and an ECG if possible. X-ray films are not considered routine procedure unless necessary to confirm suspicions. Attempt to avoid collecting information without a clear purpose.

Cautions

Never attempt an examination in the locker room. The ambient noise will not allow adequate auscultation and the lack of privacy may contribute to serious misinterpretations.

In spite of the confidence many place on preseason physicals, such an evaluation cannot be looked upon as the ultimate solution in always filtering the fit from the unfit. Mass physicals lack the detailed, personalized attention sometimes necessary, yet they offer a practical manner to handle the necessary volume in one day. The examination should offer a complete evaluation of health status with special concern given to those body areas directly related without disregard for the "body as a whole." Even when great care is taken, problems will be missed in both history and examination as a complete physical, neurologic, orthopedic workup cannot be given to everyone. This is not to say that all subject movements should not be observed: eg, gait, how garments are taken off and put on again, how the head and trunk are turned during conversation and examination, and the motions used in getting on and off an examining table.

BASIC DISQUALIFICATION FACTORS

Any acute or chronic disease process is reason for disqualification until full health is attained. A weakened palyer is not the equal of a healthy player, and the risk of injury is far higher.

Acquired Disorders

Self-limiting infections require only temporary exclusion. While competition during mild coryza may be permitted, fever is a strict reason for exclusion. A low-grade tonsillitis or dental sepsis may result in a poor performance that can be quickly corrected with proper treatment.

The "step test" can be used for determining if an athlete is ready to return to active competition after an infection. Have the player step on and off an 18-inch platform at a rate of 30 times/minute. Take the pulse rate at 30 seconds, 1 minute, 2 minutes, and 3 minutes after the exercise, then apply the following formula:

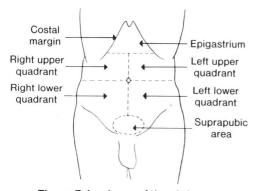

Figure 7.1. Areas of the abdomen.

$$\frac{\text{Duration of exercise in seconds} \times 100}{2 \times \text{sum of any 3 pulse}}$$
counts during recovery

The higher the index, the better the person's condition. An athlete is not ready to return to sports activity if the index is 65 or less.

Surgical and Congenital Disorders

Gross structural deformity, malfunction, traumatic or surgical loss of a major part, a history of extensive pathology, three concussions resulting in unconsciousness of 1 minute or longer, active hernia, or recurring injury of a part are considered by most authorities to be disqualifying in contact sports regardless of body compensation and even if approved by player, parents, family doctor, specialist, psychologist, and coach. The risks are far too great. At the same time, a noncontact sport may be approved.

The postoperative patient must be evaluated not as the average postoperative patient but as one who will be subjected to forces far above those normally encountered. The extent of the pathology and its complications, the extent of the surgery, and the type of incision are all variables which must be evaluated.

In contact sports, a single eye, a limb loss, an undescended testis, or a unilateral renal dysfunction or malformation are usually considered reasons for automatic disqualification regardless of the health status of the functioning part. No athletic activity is worth the consequences of possible injury to the healthy part, although this point is controversial among many. Concern over a single ovary is not as great as the organ is well protected.

Such conditions as recurring glenohumeral dislocations, acromioclavicular separations, and knee instability are usually considered disqualifying. Even with successful surgical repair, wires can break, screws can loosen, and plates can slide from severe stress. The physician's objective must be to avoid the risk of permanent impairment.

Nondisabling congenital defects are judged relative to the risk involved. For example, nonsymptomatic spondylolisthesis without spina bifida features would not bar participation in a contact sport, but severe low back symptoms may be a reason for disqualification even if overt signs are not in evidence.

CARDIOVASCULAR CONSIDERATIONS

Arends points out the axiom that a normal heart under maximum exercise conditions and without environmental extremes of heat or cold will not fail or be the cause of exercise death. As a rule of thumb, there must be some underlying organic disease in any case of exercise death from cardiac failure.

The largest percentage of nontraumatic deaths in sports can be attributed to ischemic heart disease, unsuspected preexisting cardiovascular anomalies, severe myocardial contusion from blunt trauma, and infections having a myocarditis in their repertoire (Fig. 7.2). Occasionally, some conditions are first discovered by the sports physician, such as aortic coarctation, asymptomatic atrial septal defects, dextrocardia, and rarely mitral insufficiency. An abnormal thrill, hum, pulse, blood pressure, murmur, or arrhythmia should be followed by simple exercise tests, and then reevaluated. Transient palpitations, tachycardias, cardiac flutters, and dizziness often cause diagnostic difficulties, and many ectopic arrhythmias will disappear when heart rate exceeds 140. Premature ventricular contractions are frequently noted by a team physician. These

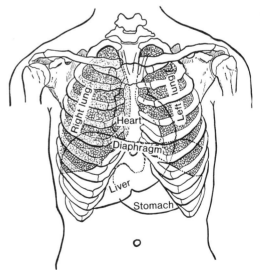

Figure 7.2. Diagramatic of the thoracic and upper abdominal organs.

are often of minor concern and associated with emotional causes, gastrointestinal disturbances, and certain drugs (eg, caffeine).

Heart Disorders

There are wide differences in specific disqualifying criteria. Paroxysmal auricular tachycardia is strictly disqualifying for all competitive sports due to the possibility of unpredictable fainting during stressful activity. This does not include the commonly witnessed psychogenic sinus tachycardia seen prior to competition. Many physicians feel that any significant heart enlargement is the basis for automatic sports exclusion. Compensated or repaired congenital cardiovascular defects must be evaluated on an individual basis according to cardiac reserve, and then only if a written clearance is obtained from the attending cardiologist.

An abnormality within the cardiovascular system of a youth should not cause automatic exclusion from sports. The concept of the need for a strictly normal heart has been proven a fallacy. Records show a champion swimmer with cyanotic heart disease, a famous long-distance runner who had a large aortic aneurysm, a U.S. Olympic skier who participated with a peice of shrapnel imbedded between the pericardium and the pulmonary artery, and many like situations. The goal is to recognize a disorder, evaluate it, and establish the necessary guidelines to prevent serious complications.

Blood Pressure

In healthy athletes, blood pressure will be found in a wide range of short duration. A systolic pressure of 140+ constantly held must be considered abnormal, while pressures of short duration in youth of 150 and college students of 220 are sometimes recorded. Abnormal levels in the healthy return quickly to a normal range with relaxation. Of greater concern is a rise in diastolic pressure, where many feel that a resting pressure over 88 points to kidney disease, a reason for disqualification. Boxing examiners have recorded pressures of 65/40, indicating that hypotension requires a redefinition within sports.

Responses to Exercise

Prolonged strenuous exercise places extraordinary demands on the cardiovascular system's capability to supply oxygen and energy sources and to remove metabolites. Marino and associates report that cardiac output may increase 8-fold, and it may be maintained at 85% of maximum for more than 2 hours in some elite marathon runners. In addition to strenuous exercise, other phases of exercise also cause cardiovascular responses such as seen in just the anticipation of exercise, which produces an increase in arterial pressure, cardiac output, and heart rate and a decrease in venous compliance.

Cardiovascular response to exercise falls into three categories: (1) increased sympathetic stimulation, which produces an increased heart rate, increased cardiac contractility, and constriction of the resistance/capacitance vessels peripherally; (2) vasodilation in the working muscles, graded according to metabolic needs, which decreases the resistance to blood flow and increases oxygen delivery and substrate supply; and (3) appropriate blood shunting and selective vasodilation, which help to maintain body temperature by reducing excessive heat build-up.

While other mechanisms are undoubtedly involved, three main control mechanisms are thought to be involved in regulating cardiovascular responses to exercise:

1. The first and primary factor is hydrodynamic feedback. This feedback is determined by the quantitative sum of venous return and the Frank-Starling law (within limits, the heart will eject all of the blood that is returned to it).

2. The second factor is afferent feedback from working muscles. Contracting muscles send impulses via small myelinated and bare fibers to sympathetic centers at various autonomic levels, which reflexly produces an increase in blood pressure, cardiac output, and heart rate according to physiologic needs.

3. The third factor is thought to be regulatory impulses from the motor cortex to active muscles and the vasomotor centers of the diencephalon and medulla.

RESPIRATORY CONSIDERATIONS

Asthma must be judged on its degree and the sport involved, and some asthmatics receive relief of their bronchiospasm during exercise. Nonasthmatic dyspnea is usually related in the healthy to effort expended during vigorous exercise, and it may be especially noticeable in cold weather.

Mild, occasional hemoptysis is normal with some athletes after strong exertion, but a profuse or commonly bloody sputum demands a full investigation.

ALIMENTARY CONSIDERATIONS

Constipation and abdominal pains are often presenting complaints. Constipation is often the result of preoccupation with body activity, ignorance in the wide range for normal movements, and simple dehydration from inadequate fluid intake. Gastrointestinal "stitches" commonly result from eating shortly before vigorous exercise or from a functional abdominal weakness.

Well-controlled diabetes is not a reason for exclusion by itself, but short-duration sports are preferred to avoid the risks of hypoglycemia.

METABOLIC CONSIDERATIONS

The effects of exercise on the body can be judged by the metabolic patterns produced. During low-level exercise, for example, there is an increased amount of oxygen extracted by the working muscles and an increased production of carbon dioxide, which results in a decreased fraction of oxygen and an increased amount of CO_2 in the air exhaled. As the levels of low-intensity exercise are increased, there is a linear increase in expired CO_2 volume, oxygen consumption, and ventilation. Only insignificant amounts of lactate are produced during low-level activity, and the mechanisms involved are essentially those of aerobic metabolism. This is sometimes referred to as Phase I exercise. During this phase, the active musculature is essentially composed of the slow-twitch, oxidative, skeletal muscle that is richly endowed with myoglobin and mitochondria (giving the fibers a deep red color) and characterized by a high aerobic capacity and a high concentration of isoenzyme H-lactate dehydrogenase (LDH).

There is a nonlinear increase in ventilation and the volume of exhaled CO_2 during moderate (Phase II) exercise, and the ex-

pired air shows an increase in the concentration of oxygen without a decrease in the CO_2 concentration. The lactate level (about 2 mmol/liter) exceeds the anaerobic threshold, which indicates a greater amount of anaerobic than aerobic metabolism. During this phase, some fast-twitch, glycolytic, skeletal muscle tissue is recruited. It has a lower capillary to fiber ratio, is not heavily endowed with myoglobin and mitochondria (giving the fibers a pale color), and thus has a low rate of oxidative metabolism.

During strenuous (Phase III) exercise, ventilation, heart rate, exhaled CO_2 level, and oxygen consumption continue to rise linearly until they plateau near their maximum levels. Lactate levels rise to 4 mmol/liter and above, until maximum oxygen consumption is reached. The continuous rise in expired CO_2 is in compensation for, but inadequate for at maximum levels, the rise in lactic acid. During this phase, which is predominantly anaerobic, both slow-twitch and fast-twitch muscles are active.

RENAL CONSIDERATIONS

During vigorous physical activity, five problems are commonly associated with kidney function: dehydration, athletic pseudonephritis, hemoglobinuria, nephroptosis, and trauma (Fig. 7.3).

Dehydration

Losses of up to 21% of plasma water have been demonstrated after 4 hours of running. During high temperatures and humidity, it is virtually impossible during prolonged exercise to replace fluids from sweat loss, even though it is important to try to keep pace. From 200–300 ml of fluid are suggested for every 15 minutes of strenuous activity. Athletes who present symptoms of chronic dehydration (eg, fatigue, decreased sweating capability, high core temperature) require several quarts of fluid each day in spite of a lack of thirst.

Sodium depletion, often accompanying dehydration, is rarely a problem in temperature climates under normal exercise conditions. It more often arises in very hot climates, with indoor sports, and where restrictive clothing causes increased perspiration. Typical symptoms and signs are thirst,

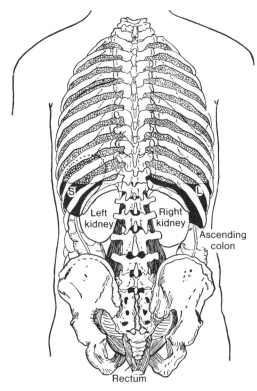

Figure 7.3. The abdominal organs, posterior schematic.

headache, muscle cramps, nausea, apathy, anorexia, sleepiness, postural giddiness, peripheral circulatory failure, and falling blood pressure.

Hemoglobinuria

In the healthy, hemoglobinuria may be noted after prolonged walking or running. It is often associated with boxing, karate, and wrestling, after hard trauma, and in players who assume a forced crouching position (eg, football lineman, baseball catchers). In the latter group, minor renal dysfunction and nephroptosis are often related. Hemoglobinuria or hematuria is rarely seen in females.

Trauma Effects

Dolan and Holladay point out that right nephroptosis has shown in about 22% in boxers as compared to 1–2% in nonboxers. This high incidence is attributed to frequent, strenuous, long-duration crouching and trauma to the supporting bands.

The kidneys are subjected to both macrotrauma and microtrauma in many sports. Repeated minor macrotrauma results in permanent renal scar formation (athlete's kidney), observed late as a pericalyceal and peripelvic deformity. Strenuous exercise, stress, forced crouching, or external blows or forces may produce renal microtrauma, evidenced by painless hematuria. Major kidney trauma is characterized by flank pain, tachycardia, profuse hemorrhage, gastrointestinal symptoms, rigidity of abdominal muscles, fever, and shock.

COMMUNICATION

Sometimes a physician is moved to a decision that is difficult to support by the evidence available. While this is difficult, it is a responsibility faced by all physicians involved in organized sports. A close liaison with the family doctor should be made to communicate abnormal findings. Reports to players, parents, and coaches should be made in terms which are readily understood. Exact scientific terminology is not necessary if it clouds the message we wish to convey to the laity.

CLASSIFICATIONS OF PHYSICAL ACTIVITY

An injury, or potential risk of injury, must be evaluated in relationship to the person as a whole. Human physical activity is a complicated phenomenon which involves all joints, related tissues, and remote sections of the body when movement requires more than singular joint or limb action.

Basic Joint Movements

Regardless of the size or intensity of human motion, the articulations of the limbs constitute the basic elements involved. In this context, as Larson points out, physical activity may be classified according to the basic human movements of various joint flexion, extension, abduction, adduction, circumduction, rotation, and gliding (Fig. 7.4).

Limb Movement Patterns

Fundamental limb movement presents a second method of classification in the patterns of the total organism during motion.

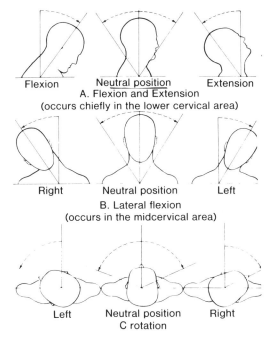

Flexion   Neutral position   Extension
A. Flexion and Extension
(occurs chiefly in the lower cervical area)

Right   Neutral position   Left
B. Lateral flexion
(occurs in the midcervical area)

Left   Neutral position   Right
C rotation

Figure 7.4. Head and neck motion. Top section: flexion and extension occurring chiefly in the lower cervical area. Middle section: lateral flexion occurring chiefly in the midcervical area. Bottom section: rotation occurring essentially between the atlas and axis. Head turning to the right or left is accompanied by a small amount of lateral flexion to the same side.

The basic patterns, for example, would include:
• Locomotion: walking, hopping, skipping, running.
• Friction: starting, stopping, sliding, landing, balancing, skiing, skating, changing direction.
• Manipulation of light objects: throwing, catching, striking a small object (eg, ball).
• Manipulation of heavy objects: lifting, pulling, pushing, bowling, carrying.
• Rhythm: dancing.

Organized Patterns

The strategic application of organized patterns of movement in their basic forms offers a third classification by:
• Application: towards health, preventive, rehabilitation, sports and athletics, leisure and culture, education, institutions, dance, recreation, sports health care.

• Organization: individual, dual, team, group, aquatic, conditioning, remedial forms.
• Objectives: individual health, self-adjustment, effective utilization of the human body during activity, knowledge, goal attainment, social efficiency, leadership/fellowship.
• Development potentials: agility, power, endurance, strength, flexibility, alertness, accuracy, balance, speed, coordination, steadiness, timing, rhythm, reaction time.
• Environment: climate, altitude, geographic location, urbanization, socio-cultural.
• Administrative requirements: outdoor facilities, gyms, stadiums and fieldhouses, recreation buildings, resident facilities.
• Physical environment: land, water, air.
• Academic disciplines: physical sciences, biology, sociology, psychology, philosophy, history.
• Age: birth to 3, 3–5, 6–7, 8–9, 10–11, 12–13, 14–15, 16–17, 18–22, 22–45, 46–65, 65 years and over.
• Maturation: infancy, early childhood, late childhood, adolescence, postadolescence, old age.

Caloric Requirements

Human motion can also be viewed from its workload (caloric) requirements: light (2.5–5.0 kilocalories/minute), moderate (5.1–7.5), heavy (10.1–12.5), exhausting (12.6+).

ANTHROPOMETRIC CONSIDERATIONS

Anthropometry—the science of measurement of weight, size, and proportions of the human body (general anthropometry) and its parts (regional anthropometry)—has many biomechanical implications in athletics. The topics of physique, body composition, and body types, all of which may be considered subdivisions of anthropometry, have been discussed. In this section, we shall further explore anthropometry and goniometry as they apply to evaluation of the athlete (Fig. 7.5).

Human Dimensions

Because of gravitational forces acting on

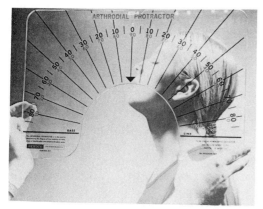

Figure 7.5. Transparent protractors are helpful in screening postural abnormalities and joint function.

the body, body weight in human movement is a significant structural-mechanical variable. Body mass is defined as body weight divided by the gravitational constant (32 feet/sec^2).

Body Mass

In most sports, weight is a vital consideration because of the impact force: the greater the mass, the greater the amount of force required for movement. This may be an advantage or a disadvantage, depending upon motion objectives. For instance, greater mass (dead weight) is a distinct disadvantage in acceleration (eg, runners), and an advantage in being difficult to move (eg, football linemen, wrestlers) or to stop once in motion (eg, football backs).

Dead weight is the weight of the body not involved in locomotion (eg, fat, inactive muscles, viscera). It is for this reason when endurance and acceleration are the primary concerns that resistance exercises are used to develop strength without greatly increasing muscle bulk. Dead weight from inactive muscle mass is as useless as fat. When weight is gained strictly through an increase in muscular weight, the undesirable effects of increasing body mass are offset by the increase in strength available for movement. On the other hand, a football lineman employs his dead weight in gaining momentum (velocity × mass) and uses his fat component to absorb the shock of impact.

Strength is approximately proportional to

the quantity of body muscle. In the well-developed adult male, muscle tissue constitutes about 43% of body weight; in the adult female, about 38%. The relative proportions of the body's fat content and fat-free component (lean body mass) can be determined by offering the regression equation below for estimating body density from fat calipers without applying more sophisticated measures:

$$Y = 1.088468 - .007123X_1$$

$$- .004834X_2 - .005513X_3$$

Where Y is the estimated body density, X_1 is the skinfold thickness of the chest at the midaxillary line at the level of the ziphoid, X_2 is the skinfold measurement of the chest at the juxta-nipple position, and X_3 is the skinfold measurement of the dorsum of the arm at a point midway between the tip of the acromion and the olecranon process.

Body Size

Body length (height), along with the width, and depth of parts are the concern of linear measurements. These dimensions are usually obtained by calipers or gridded photographs. Linear measurements offer us direct evidence of bony framework length.

The rigid bones and mobile joints of the body along with the forces acting upon them represent a system of levers and, as all levers, transmit force and motion at a distance. In the body, contracting muscles normally constitute the force, with resistance being supplied by a body part's center of gravity plus any extra weight which may be in contact with the part. During motor activities, greater height is usually related to longer limb levers (eg, high jump), longer stride (eg, running), greater velocity (eg, discus, javelin), a wider arc of reach (eg, blocking), a larger target (eg, catching), and height dominance over a raised goal such as a basketball hoop or starting at a point further from the ground (eg, shot put). Height presents a disadvantage because of the increased leverage in weight lifting, in activities requiring quick changes in direction, in lack of stability due to the higher center of gravity (eg, judo, wrestling), and in lack of long-limb manipulative balance (eg, soccer). Thus, long limbs are a disadvantage where equilibrium and strength are the priority and an advantage where range of motion and velocity are critical.

Body part depth and width affect motor activity as they affect body mass and relative size. Broadness of hands and feet is an aid to the swimmer, for example. Broad hands are a control advantage to the basketball handler. Large feet offer a wide base of support.

Body Proportions and Build

Evaluation of body proportions in athletics is helpful in determining an individual's center of gravity and body build (type) (Figs. 7.6 and 7.7). A person's common center of gravity is defined as the point of application of the gravitational (vectorial) force acting on the body; in addition to the whole body, each part or segment has its individual center of gravity. Gravitational weight of the body as a whole or its segments differs from subject to subject depending upon body type, height, size, density, age, and sex. The position of a person's normal center of gravity may be slightly changed through the influence of training and conditioning, blood supply, and diet.

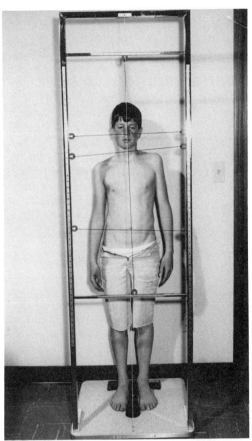

Figure 7.7. Various forms of plumblines can be used to measure faulty body mechanics (with the permission of Dr. R. O. Masters, Sr.).

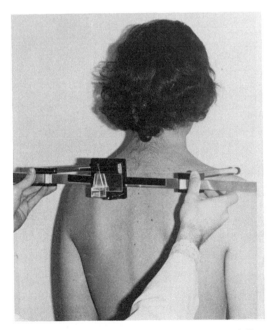

Figure 7.6. Physical analyses help to define physical and bodily structure, organization, development, and body balance.

Physique is defined as the physical and bodily structure, organization, and development (the characteristic appearance or physical power) of an individual or a race. Body type greatly influences performance. It is determined by weight, linear measurements, and girth dimensions. The intermediate type's streamlined physique and lean muscle mass contribute to motor talents in boxers, football backs, and sprinters. The stability of the heavy endomorph is seen in wrestling and football linemen. The advantages of the long-limbed ectomorph is quickly recognized in the basketball center and football end.

Several studies have shown that body type and physical performance in various fields of athletic activity have a close correlation. There are exceptions, but they are rare at the professional level. This means that there are many people striving for high levels of achievement which they probably can never attain. Some authorities feel as high as 80% of the population should never aspire to great heights in terms of purely physical performance. This underscores the fact that the techniques and achievements of champions, commonly used in calculating standards, may not be suitable for different physiques within identical events. One important element which the voluminous literature on somatyping does not include at present is the great variable of personal motivation.

Goniometry

The measurement of joint motion offers an accurate record and extent of disability as part of an athlete's permanent record. The most common method of measurement employs the goniometer, either the 180° system or the 360° system. Both systems depend on the fact that a long bone is like a lever rotating around a fulcrum; when it moves, it describes the arc of a circle. This arc is used in determining the amount of joint motion, and goniometer is used to measure the angle produced between two bony segments when maximum motion in a particular plane has been made.

Measurements are made of movement as it occurs around an axis perpendicular to one of the three body planes: sagittal, coronal, and transverse.

1. Motions in a sagittal plane around a coronal axis include shoulder flexion, extension, internal and external rotation; elbow flexion and extension; wrist flexion and extension, fingers flexion and extension; hip flexion and extension; knee flexion and extension; ankle dorsiflexion and plantar flexion; and thumb abduction.

2. Motions in a coronal plane around a sagittal axis include shoulder abduction and adduction, wrist radial and ulnar deviation, thumb extension, hip abduction and adduction, and foot eversion and inversion.

3. Motions in a horizontal plane around a vertical axis include forearm supination and pronation, and hip internal and external rotation.

BASIC CLINICAL BIOMECHANICS

Biomechanics is the application of the principles of mechanics (the study of forces and their effects) to the body in movement and at rest. Human biomechanics includes the mechanical principles involved, the physiologic considerations of muscle length-tension relations, and an understanding of the controlling neuromotor mechanisms and the sensory feedback apparatus, reflecting both locomotor activity and cerebral function.

The more athletic biomechanics are understood, the better musculoskeletal disorders in sports can be appreciated.The athlete is constantly attempting to improve performance by applying biomechanical principles to specific movements. From the viewpoint of the doctor, knowledge of the mechanisms involved in an injury is necessary to evaluate an injury accurately.

Practical Concepts

All mechanical devices (eg, human body) are subject to wear during use which reflects their history of destructive forces. Unique to living tissue is its ability to heal and strengthen, providing a dialogue between destructive and constructive forces. While machines convert thermal or chemical energy into mechanical energy, muscle tissue transforms nutrients directly into mechanical energy without a thermal intermediary.

Body energy enables it to overcome resistance to motion, to produce a physical effect, and to accomplish work. The body's kinetic energy is reflected in its velocity, and it's potential energy is reflected in its position. Work is the result of a force acting through a distance, while power relates to the time element and the work accomplished. There is a close association in the same unit of time between the work accomplished by a weight lifter and that of a sprinter.

During contraction, muscular work reflects the consumption of mechanical energy. Some of this energy is unproductively used in internal friction, and some is stored for later use within elastic (contractile) tissues. The effect of muscle contraction depends basically upon (1) the unique fiber arrangement which determines the relationship of force that the muscle can produce and the distance over which it can contract; (2) the angle of pull; and (3) the muscle location relative to the joint axis. The resistance offered to the musculoskeletal forces may arise from gravity pull, friction, stationary structures, elasticity of structures, or manual resistance. The effectiveness of resistance or load is determined by the angle of the line of resistance applied and the distance of the load from the axis of the lever system involved. Gravity is the most common load upon the body and provides a line of force in a constant direction.

While forces of all types may cause subluxations, dislocations, fractures, strains and sprains, etc, the biomechanical mechanisms involved determine the type and extent of the injury produced depending upon the applications of force and its resistance. For example, different applications of force may cause bending fractures, stress fractures, or compression fractures. When the examiner understands how an injury was caused, the tissues involved are more readily located and the injury extent is more quickly evaluated.

The Joints

Joints are classified according to the amount of movement they permit—immovable, slightly movable, or freely movable (Fig. 7.8). Thus, articulations are classified according to their freedom of motion. The three basic types are the synarthroses, amphiarthroses, and diarthroses.

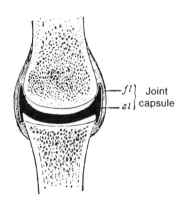

Figure 7.8. Section of a synovial joint: *fl* is fibrous layer and *sl* is synovial layer of joint capsule. The articular cartilages are white, the bone is dotted, and the joint cavity is black.

Joint Mechanics

There are several types of joint motion: gliding and angular, flexion, extension, abduction, adduction, rotation, and circumduction. Attempts to force joints to move beyond their normal limitations can be quite harmful to the integrity of a joint and its surrounding soft-tissue structures.

Some joint disorders are mechanical: the parts of the joint are displaced or subluxated. When the ligaments holding the joint together are partially torn or stretched, but the joint is not excessively displaced, a sprain results. When muscles or tendons are injured by overstretching, a strain results. At some joint locations, the tendon passes over a joint, eg, at the shoulder, elbow, knee, and heel. To reduce pressure, small fluid-containing bursa are formed over and around the tendon, and they may become inflamed as in bursitis.

The Skeletal Muscular System

It is important to think of skeletal muscles (Figs. 7.9 and 7.10) as one part of a three-part nerve-muscle-skeleton unit. For example, a motor nerve is needed to stimulate muscle contraction; the muscle itself must be able to contract and to relax; and the power of the contraction must be transmitted to a bone or other attachment to produce the desired movement. When any one part of this three-part unit cannot function normally, the other two parts also lose their normal functional ability.

Muscle Function

When muscle fibers are stimulated by a nerve impulse to contract, the muscle shortens and pulls against its connective tissue attachment. One attachment is sometimes a fixed joint or anchor, and the direction of action is then toward it. When a muscle contracts, it does so in the direction of the muscle fibers. Movement may take place which reduces the joint angle (concentric contraction) or contraction may take place which increases the joint angle (eccentric contraction). Many normal and abnormal mechanisms can be explained in that a slightly stretched muscle contracts with a great amount of force, whereas a shortened muscle contracts with very little force.

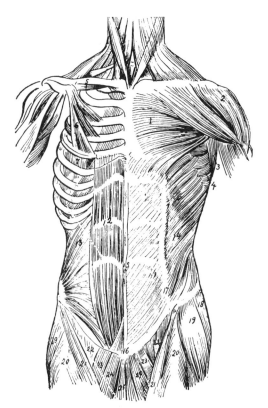

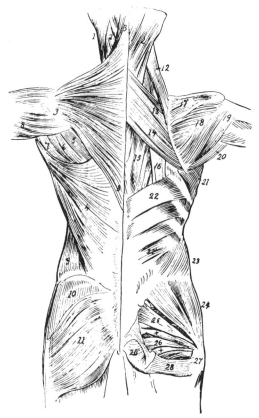

Figure 7.9. Muscles of the trunk from the front (left side, superficial muscles; right side, deep muscles): (*1*) pectoralis major; (*2*) deltoid; (*3*) portion of latissimus dorsi; (*4*) serratus anterior; (*5*) subclavius; (*6*) the pectoralis, sternocostal portion; (*7*) serratus anterior; (*12*) rectus abdominis; (*13*) internal oblique; (*15*) abdominal aponeurosis and tendinous intersections of rectus abdominis; (*16*) over symphysis pubis; (*17*) linea semilunaris; (*18*) gluteus medius; (*19*) tenor fasciae latae; (*20*) rectus femoris; (*21*) sartorius; (*22*) femoral part of the iliopsoas; (*23*) pectineus; (*24*) adductor longus; and (*25*) gracilis.

Figure 7.10. Muscles of the trunk from behind (left side, superficial muscles; right side deep muscles: (*1*) sternocleidomastoid; (*2*) splenius cervicis; (*3*) trapezius; (*4*) latissimus dorsi; (*5*) infraspinatus; (*6*) teres minor; (*7*) teres major; (*8*) deltoid; (*9*) external oblique of abdomen; (*10*) gluteus medius; (*11*) gluteus maximus; (*12*) levator scapulae; (*13*) rhomboideus minor; (*14*) rhomboideus major; (*15*) part of the longissimus dorsi; (*16*) tendons of insertion of iliocostalis; (*17*) supraspinatus; (*18*) infraspinatus; (*19*) teres minor; (*20*) teres major; (*21*) serratus anterior; (*22*) upper and, (*22′*) lower part of serratus posterior inferior; (*23*) internal oblique; (*24*) gluteus medius; (*25*) pyriformis and superior and inferior gemelli; (*26*) and (*26′*) portions of obturator internus; (*27*) tendon of obturator internus; and (*28*) quaratus femoris.

Muscle contraction consumes nutrients and oxygen and produces acids and heat (major source). Acids accumulating as a result of continued activity tend to contribute to fatigue. The quantity of muscle fibers does not vary after birth. Exercise increases muscle quality, not quantity; it allows muscles to become larger, stronger, and better developed.

During examination, it is important to realize that the ligaments play a much greater part in supporting loads than is generally thought. Electromyographic studies in situations involving fatigue from forces act-

ing across a joint prove that muscles play only a secondary role. Such fatigue is basically a form of pain originating in the ligaments rather than in the muscles. Thus, some researchers feel that if muscles involved in a problem are weak to begin with, there is a more immediate strain on the ligaments producing the characteristic fatigue syndrome.

Synergism and Antagonism

Muscles almost always act in groups rather than singly, and the coordinated action of several muscles produces movement; ie, while one group contracts, the other group relaxes, and vice versa. The muscle whose contraction produces the movement is the prime mover. The muscle which relaxes is the antagonist. In flexion and extension of the forearm, for example, the biceps and triceps are alternately prime movers and antagonists.

Muscles which act separately but produce a single movement are synergists; for instance, shoulder adduction produced by contraction of the latissimus dorsi and pectoralis major. Such muscles play a role in both limiting movement and enhancing coordination. Synergism may exist in both simple and complex movements.

Many neuromuscular and musculoskeletal disorders show evidence of disturbed muscle tone such as weakness or spasm, but weakness is the predominating pattern found in muscle testing. This is depicted as a compensatory spasm in the opposite, lateral, or antagonistic muscle.

The central nervous system programs the work of synergist and antagonist muscles through contraction grading in four modes (after Williams and Sperryn): (1) qualitatively, by muscle innervation; (2) intensively, by increasing intrinsic muscle tone; (3) spatially, by action within various optimal zones of contraction; and (4) temporally, by desynchronizing the action of various muscle bundles or muscles within a group.

Note that the concept that there is a form of true antagonism between the muscles that move the joint in one direction as opposed to those that move the joint in another direction is not exact. The action is better termed a reciprocal inhibition because the "antagonistic" muscle relaxes completely. Most muscles which demonstrate a reciprocal pattern do not necessarily have an antagonist role; it is closer to that of a synergistic partner. Nervous coordination is so precise there is no need for muscles to act on antagonism.

Neuromuscular Mechanisms

Healthy muscle is characterized by active contraction in response to the reaction of the nervous system to the environment. This readiness to act, resulting in firing of motor units, as stimuli from the environment impose upon the nervous system is expressed as muscle tone. Muscles that have lost their tone through lack of activity, through primary muscle disease, or through nerve damage become flaccid. The tone of muscles is due to the constant, steady contraction and relaxation of different muscle fibers in individual muscles which helps to maintain the "chemical engine" of the muscle cells. Even minor exercise helps to maintain tone by renewing blood supply to muscle cells.

The nerve cell body, the long axon extending within the motor nerve, the terminal branches, and all the muscle fibers supplied to these branches comprise a nerve "motor unit." Each muscle is composed of a number of motor units that in themselves are several muscle fibers linked to a motor nerve, which in turn is joined to the central nervous system. The motor unit is a functional unit of striated muscle since an impulse descending from its axon causes all the muscle fibers of a particular motor unit to contract simultaneously. With the arrival of nerve impulses, usually below 50/second motor units contract sharply.

When several motor units are stimulated, the attached fibers contract, and body movement occurs. However, because motor units fatigue after several stimulations, other units must be called into play to allow for smooth movement—an asynchronous firing of motor units is made to produce volitional movement. While it appears during normal muscle contraction that all muscle fibers are in a smooth continuous muscle contraction, they are not. This appearance results from a totality of a series of small groups of fibers contracting at the same moment. In the members of these groups, the muscle fibers are supplied by the terminal branches of one nerve fiber or an axon whose cell body is in the anterior horn of spinal gray matter.

Factors Affecting Muscle Contraction

MacDonald and Stanish point out that the mechanical factors governing muscle contraction are (1) the angle of pull, (2) the length of the muscle, and (3) the velocity of muscle shortening. The optimum angle of pull is at a 45° joint angle, and a muscle fiber's contractile force is greatest during extension. Obviously, a long muscle fiber can shorten more than a short fiber. Parallel to this is the fact that a suddenly pre-stretched muscle has an increased contractile capacity. The studies of A. V. Hill showed that the optimum speed at which a muscle can produce its greatest power and efficiency is at approximately one-third its maximum speed.

Besides these mechanical factors, temperature and flexibility should be considered. Hill's studies also showed that a muscle's speed of contraction can be increased 20% by raising body temperature 5°F, thus the benefit of adequate warmup before athletic participation is underscored. Reducing muscle temperature appears to increase the threshold of irritability, which causes weakened and more sluggish contractions. Improved flexibility through static stretching exercises, which does not activate the stretch reflex, appears to reduce soft-tissue restrictions and enhance antagonist relaxation.

Evaluating Strength

Muscle testing demands attention to detail, a working knowledge of anatomy, a comprehensive knowledge of muscle function, joint motion, muscle origin and insertion, muscle antagonistic and agonistic action, and their role in fixation. It is a procedure that depends greatly upon the skill, knowledge, and experience of the examiner.

At the tissue level, the value of strength training includes the following: (1) An increased proportion of active fibers because of the improved neuropathways and impulse transmission. In contrast to a well-conditioned muscle that has 90% activity, a poorly conditioned muscle may have as few as 60% active fibers. (2) An increase in thickness (hypertrophy) of specific slow-twitch and fast-twitch muscle fibers. The greatest reaction is seen in the pale fast-twitch fibers. (3) An increase in the threshold of contraction inhibitory mechanisms (eg, the Golgi sensory receptors). (4) An increase in contraction power and speed. (5)

A decrease of interfiber and muscle surface fat.

Subjective Muscle Testing

Muscle power is measured when there is (1) a complaint of weakness or incoordination, or (2) need for an aid in subluxation analysis and in evaluating correction. The following criteria are used in recording muscle strength:

• Grade 5 (100%, normal)—complete range of motion against gravity with full resistance.
• Grade 4 (75%, good)—complete range of motion against gravity with some resistance.
• Grade 3 (50%, fair)—complete range of motion against gravity.
• Grade 2 (25%, poor)—complete range of motion with gravity eliminated.
• Grade 1 (10%, trace)—evidence of slight contractility, but no joint motion.
• Grade 0 (0%, zero)—no evidence of contractility.

The examiner should strive to evaluate one muscle at a time, thus the subject should be requested not to recruit allied muscles during resistance. The doctor must use extreme caution during resistance to avoid creating cramps, stretch injuries, or excessive fatigue. It should be noted that muscles often test differently in various positions such as from prone or supine to weight-bearing. The trouble with this method is the evaluation rests a great deal upon the subjective skill of the examiner. Thus it is important that the same examiner records initial and follow-up evaluations of the degree of "resistance."

The Hand Dynamometer

Until recently, the hand dynamometer and electromyograph were the only objective clinical instruments available to record the force of muscular contraction; however, recently more practical equipment has been developed. Still, the hand dynamometer does offer the examiner four data: (1) the strength of the grip muscles, (2) the fatigue rate of the grip muscles, (3) the recovery rate of these muscles, and (4) a comparison between the muscles of the right and left hands. While initial readings are helpful in diagnosis, subsequent readings are helpful

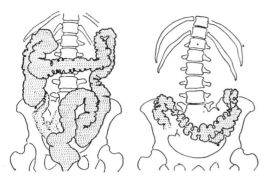

Figure 7.11. X-ray tracings of typical endo-morphic (*left*) and ectomorphic (*right*) intestinal position.

in determining rate of recovery. In dyna-mometry, three readings are taken on each hand in sequence to show strength, fatigue, and recovery rates.

BIOMECHANICS AND TRAUMA

Each year we see athletic performance draw closer to the limits of human capacity. Understanding the biomechanical principles involved helps us to prevent injury and restore functional integrity (Fig. 7.11). While our lever-like extremities transmit forces and motion at a distance, they also favor musculoskeletal injuries by amplifying forces (usually external, occasionally inter-nal) acting on the body's biomechanical sys-tem. Statistics indicate that excessive stress appears greatest on the short arm of first-class levers (eg, elbow, knee).

Forces upon Joints

Joint structure refers to the quality and quantity of the chemical constituents of bone and associated tissues to cope with the action of external and internal forces. A force that is applied which is greater than the structural resistance will fracture a bone or dislocate a joint. Stress is defined as the force exerted. While it requires from about 1,500–3,000 lb to fracture the neck of the femur, a weight of only 20 lb dropped upon it from a few feet will have the same result.

In weight lifting during a dead lift of 200 lb by a 170-lb person, it has been shown that a 2000-lb force is exerted on the lum-bosacral disc. If a deep-squat lift is per-formed exactly as defined in competitive weight lifting, severe stress on inappropriate tissues is frequently inevitable. Thus, the athlete whose goal is solely to strengthen his leg extensors by lifting weights should seek one of the many alternatives to the deep-squat position (eg, partial squat, leg-press machine, Klein bench).

Regardless of what degree of force is in-duced upon a part, there is always a coun-teracting stress because, for every action, there must be a reaction; eg, a downward pressure should equal an opposing upward thrust. A force pulling right should be equal to a pull toward the left, expressed in terms of centropedal and centrifugal force. A twisting force in one direction must be fol-lowed by an equal twisting force in the opposite direction. A force permitting a part to slide downward must be resisted by an adequate upward force. And a force tending to bend a structure along its axis must be resisted by a force equal to prevent such bending.

A pressure always results in a compres-sion stress, and a pull causes a tensile stress which is an action directly opposed to compression. Tensile and compression stresses (axial stresses) operate along the axis of a part without altering it.

A force directed against a structure at an angle to its axis that permits one part to slide over the other is a shearing stress. Both parts may be movable with the parts sliding in opposite directions or one part fixed. A spinal curvature in any direction involves a constant state of abnormal tension and compression of bones, cartilage, and mus-cles. Spinal bending involves the dual ac-tions of tension, compression, and torsion.

The various body motions are not the sole result of muscular action alone; they are also the effect of the structure, balance, and position of the various bones forming the joints acted upon. This cooperative action of muscles and bones is the result of lever-age, and levers operate according to me-chanical laws.

CHAPTER 8

Physiologic Performance and Training Rationale

During human history, the body has adapted to withstand a wide variety of threatening environmental forces. This has resulted in systems designed to work in harmony during ever changing internal and external stimuli. The nervous system provides the necessary intricate coordination. Physiologic measurements offer us data on the essential factors involved in the integrated aspects of organic functions. While voluminous data can be gathered, our major concern involves those aimed at restoring and maintaining homeostasis.

PERFORMANCE PHYSIOLOGY

Human capacity to perform motor activity is determined by three essential aspects: (1) neuromuscular function (strength and skill), (2) energy output (aerobic and anaerobic processes), and (3) psychologic factors (motivation, spirit). These aspects are involved in almost all types of labor, even though of variant emphasis.

Essentially, performance is the result of central and peripheral neuromuscular mechanisms, the energy yield of split elemental compounds, and profound psychologic effects. The cybernetic factor of the central nervous system, complex to measure, relates to an individual's skill or mechanical efficiency, thus directly affects energy requirements.

A wide variety of exercise tests have been utilized in an attempt to measure physical fitness. All offer some, but not complete, data. Such analyses are a step in the right direction in evaluating the factors of human motor performance, but they are only a part of the determining process.

The methods of estimating physical performance capacity of different players can be classified into two major groups: (1) physical fitness tests and (2) physiologic tests. Typical examples of physical fitness tests are sprints, endurance runs, high jumps, long jumps, and throwing. Determination of maximum oxygen intake and determination of muscular strength comprise the common physiologic types of tests, as in (1) determining the mechanical power developed on a bicycle ergometer or staircase; (2) determining the time element necessary to run a specified distance; (3) determining the duration of running on a treadmill at varying degrees of speed and grade; and (4) determining the distance run in a specified time period.

UNDERLYING FACTORS IN PHYSIOLOGIC TESTING

Three basic factors underlie all physiologic tests for physical fitness: (1) metabolic capacity, which determines the amount of activity possible for approximately 2–3 hours through the maximum quantity of energy-yielding substrates available from body reserves during maximum aerobic demands; (2) maximum oxygen intake capacity (aerobic power), which determines the amount of activity possible for approximately 15–30 minutes through coordinated circulatory and respiratory adjustments producing the maximum amount of tissue oxygen; and (3) maximum oxygen debt capacity (anaerobic power), which determines the amount of activity possible with all-out effort for approximately 50 seconds through anaerobic release mechanisms (Fig. 8.1).

Statistics indicate that the day-to-day variability in oxygen consumption in most physical actions is about 5%, and differences of 10% of this percentage among individuals can be expected.

Energy costs vary greatly in different sports (eg, 4.4 kilocalories/minute in archery, 9.1 kilocalories/minute in field hockey, 13.3 kilocalories/minute in judo, and 18.6 kilocalories/minute in squash, for a 150-lb

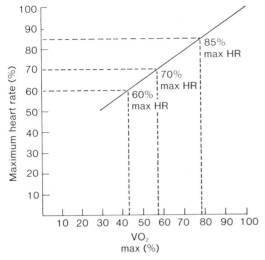

Figure 8.1. Improvement in cardiorespiratory fitness is relative to the level of energy expenditure per min or intensity of training. Because of the linear relationship between heart rate and oxygen intake, intensity can be expressed as either percentage of maximum heart rate or $\dot{V}O_2$ max. As heart rate and oxygen intake have this linear relationship, heart rate is an excellent means for estimating training intensity (with the permission of the Behavioral Research Foundation).

player). Energy output also varies within the same sport depending on such factors as intensity of competition, neuromuscular skill level, position demands, performance level, age, body type, atmospheric conditions, and field conditions. In exercise physiology, however, it has been shown to be valid to measure energy expenditure of muscle tissue in terms of oxygen consumption in liters/minute, but it is not valid to convert such figures into energy units of watts or kilocalories/minute.

When muscular effort must be prolonged longer than a minute, performance becomes increasingly dependent upon the demands of holistic homeostasis and not just that of active tissues. Basically, this involves oxygen supply, carbon dioxide removal, heat balance, and the replenishment of nutrients.

Metabolism

Energy can be neither created nor destroyed. To accomplish work, the body must have energy derived from food which is changed within the body from chemical energy into mechanical energy to produce muscular effort. This fuel is in the form of proteins, carbohydrates, and fats. To maintain health, stored resources (potential energy) must be kept in balance with power expenditures (kinetic energy).

While carbohydrate and fat are normally oxidized quite completely in the human body, protein is not. Protein derivatives of uric acid, urea, and creatinine are excreted in the urine. In addition, not all food ingested is absorbed; that is, only 97% of carbohydrate, 95% of fat, and 92% of protein ingested are absorbed, and these figures do not consider the "coarseness" of foodstuffs such as coarse corn meal or roughly ground whole grains.

Metabolic Rate

Continuous dissimilation and assimilation of energy is characteristic of life. The intensity of energy exchange is lowest during rest and highest during maximum effort. The greater the energy demands, the higher the requirement for oxygen consumption. Total energy is the result of the basal (waking state) metabolic rate (BMR) plus the energy necessary for work, offering a ratio which can be used as an index to measure exercise intensity and performance efficiency. In a given period of time, energy output intensity is directly related to mechanical performance, measured by oxygen consumption in a specified time period. In this sense, oxygen consumption can be considered a reflection of metabolic power.

Metabolic capacity is directly related to performance capacity, reflecting the quantity of energy-yielding nutrients available (2–3 hours) from body reserves under aerobic conditions. Thus, one's maximum aerobic power and metabolic capacity are closely related; yet, there are many individual differences. In addition to metabolic capacity, other indices may be used such as those of glycogen storage, cardiac output, and water balance efficiency.

Metabolic rate has been found to be directly proportional to gross body weight. Such factors as lean body mass, age, diet, sex, height, surface area, and race do not have a significant influence on metabolic rate during muscular performance.

Energy Resources

When metabolized, about 1 g of protein produces 5.5 kilocalories of energy; carbohydrate, 4.5 kilocalories of energy; and fat, 9.5 kilocalories of energy. During strenuous activity, the body prefers fats over carbohydrates as a source of energy; but during submaximum activity, carbohydrates are preferred. Proteins are used as an energy source only when carbohydrate and fat resources fail to meet demands.

During effort, the immediate source of energy is the conversion of adenosine triphosphate (ATP) into adenosine diphosphate (ADP) for continuous muscle contraction, along with the resynthesis of ATP from ADP by utilizing the high energy reserve of creatine phosphate (CP) in muscle tissue. Through the metabolic process, ATP is derived from ingested carbohydrates after they are broken down into simple sugars (especially glucose), with the help of insulin, and transported through the cell membrane and made available as an energy source. When glucose is not used immediately, it is stored in the liver and muscles in the form of glycogen.

The CP and ATP in muscle reservoirs soon become exhausted during prolonged exertion, and ATP resynthesis must be sustained by the oxidation of free fatty acids and carbohydrates. Once oxygen delivery to active muscle tissue becomes inadequate, a portion of energy for muscle function comes from anaerobic metabolism.

Aerobic Power

To produce necessary energy, the body utilizes an aerobic (oxygen) pathway and an anaerobic (nonoxygen) pathway. To maintain life, the primary factor is the continuous and adequate flow of oxygen. Restricted oxygen flow quickly manifests in function deterioration as seen clinically in infarcts and strokes, underscoring why so much emphasis is placed on oxygen demands during physical, psychologic, and environmental stress. Life signs and the degree of life are often evaluated from detectable arterial pulsations; breathing quantity, quality, and rhythm; temperature; and reflexes—all of which are related to oxygen flow.

When oxygen demands exceed supply (oxygen debt) during and following prolonged exertion, lactic acid accumulates within muscle tissue and encourages fatigue. The greater the exercise intensity, the greater the lactic acid accumulation. Following maximum exercise, it may take an hour or longer to attain resting levels. Oxygen debt must be repaid rapidly such as through an increased breathing rate.

Aerobic power is essentially determined by cardiorespiratory function, intrinsic physical fatigue factors, duration and nature of the physical activity, extra demands on temperature regulation, and intrinsic environmental conditions (eg, altitude, temperature, humidity). Maximum aerobic power depends on the efficiency of the total cardiorespiratory system in both oxygen intake and transport. The greater the work accomplished, then the greater the oxygen consumption, the faster the breathing rate, and the faster the heart rate (Fig. 8.2).

Oxygen-dependent aerobic metabolism produces about 50% of the energy utilized in 1 minute of activity; however, this percentage rises to about 80% in 5 minutes and 98% in 60 minutes if necessary cardiorespiratory adjustments are maintained to supply tissue needs.

Maximal oxygen intake variants are seen with (1) body structure, (2) quantity of lean body mass, and (3) various limiting factors. Work requirements increase proportionately with the size of the body. Although fatty tissue may comprise a large amount of body weight, it can be considered quite metabolically inert and thus an important consideration in evaluating the capacity to transport oxygen.

Body Type

Body type is essentially determined by genetic factors. While physical conditioning has been shown to affect maximum oxygen intake, the extent of improvement is controversial: a 3 liter/minute person cannot be trained into a 5 liter/minute person. Habitual physical activities also have a relationship to maximum oxygen intake (ie, physical labor vs sedentary tasks), but it is unclear whether the activities develop high oxygen intake or if people with high oxygen intake are inclined toward such activities.

Weight is the main determination of oxygen consumption; the heavier the person,

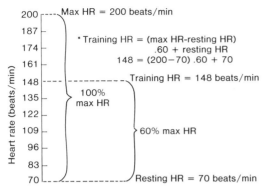

Figure 8.2. Example of calculating percentage of maximum heart rate. To make an accurate estimation of training intensity, it is necessary to know both resting and maximum heart rates. Maximum heart rate can be determined by using the highest heart rate found on a maximum graded exercise test or after a difficult bout of endurance exercise such as a 12-min all-out run (with the permission of the Behavioral Research Foundation).

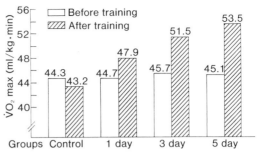

Figure 8.3. Effects of training duration on maximum oxygen intake ($\dot{V}O_2$ max). In one study, men were trained for 15, 30, or 45 min/day, 3 days/week at 85–90% of maximum for 10 weeks. Note that all three exercise groups improved significantly in $\dot{V}O_2$ max with the magnitude of improvement related to duration of exercise. Similar results have been found by others who trained young women on a bicycle ergometer for 10, 20 and 30 min/day, 3 days/week, for 6 weeks (with the permission of the Behavioral Research Foundation).

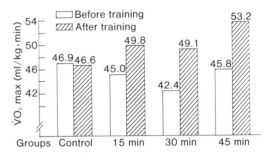

Figure 8.4. Effects of training frequency on maximum oxygen intake ($\dot{V}O_2$ max). Data on 148 previously sedentary males aged 28–64 were trained in random groups 1, 3, or 5 days/week, 30 min/day, for 20 weeks. Significant improvement in $\dot{V}O_2$ max was in direct proportion to frequency of training. Resting heart rate values showed the same relationship (with the permission of the Behavioral Research Foundation).

the higher the oxygen consumption. In contrast, the taller the person, the lower the oxygen consumption. In other words, if two people have the same weight, the shortest one will have the higher oxygen consumption. This is one reason why the tall, lean ectomorph appears to excel in many athletic events requiring endurance. Leg length has been shown to have an influence on energy costs in walking tests, but it is small in comparison to body weight. The obese show high oxygen consumption even at low effort levels.

Limiting Factors

The various limiting factors involved in maximal oxygen intake include the amount of oxygen within inspired air, neuromuscular system status, alveolar space oxygen transfer to hemoglobin, hemoglobin quantity and quality, pulmonary ventilation, nutrients available, blood volume, and cardiac efficiency. Other limiting factors include circulatory distribution, capillary oxygen transfer to cells, muscle tissue receptivity, venous return efficiency, and mitochondrial transfer to adenosine tri- and diphosphate mechanisms (Figs. 8.3–8.5). As strength development does little to develop the heart, the muscularly hypertrophied athlete pre-

sents a lower aerobic power per unit of body weight.

Anaerobic Power

Because the blood, circulation, respiration, and all the other factors contributing to human function during effort cannot be manifested on a moment's notice, nature has provided certain limited anaerobic mechanisms to meet the metabolic demands of active cells. Even with minimal work intensity, there is a period of oxygen defi-

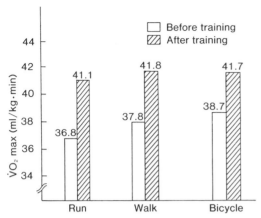

Figure 8.5. Effect of training mode on maximum oxygen intake ($\dot{V}O_2$ max). In a study conducted with middle-aged men, three different modes of training were found to be equally effective in producing a significant cardiorespiratory improvement. Subjects were trained for 30 min, 3 days/week, for 20 weeks, at 85–90% of maximum heart rate (approx. 175 beats/min). Another study comparing jogging, bicycling, and tennis showed jogging and bicycling about equal (14.8%, 13.3%) and both far superior to that of tennis (5.7%) in terms of cardiorespiratory improvement (with the permission of the Behavioral Research Foundation).

ciency which disturbs homeostasis and sets in motion a call for restoration at a higher metabolic level.

Both aerobic and anaerobic mechanisms determine an individual's performance capacity, but anaerobic activity is maintained only for a short time. An anaerobic state exists when oxygen is not used to produce energy and when glucose and glycogen reserves are used. The greater the intensity of the effort, the greater the anaerobic energy contribution. It can be measured by the amount of oxygen intake during the recovery period, usually attaining its peak (maximum oxygen debt) about 50 seconds after intense exercise begins. If performance demands are great enough to exceed maximum oxygen transport capabilities, performance will proceed only until all anaerobic energy stores become exhausted.

Short bursts of effort utilizing primarily explosive strength requiring less than 120 seconds are considered anaerobic activities. An index of work capacity is mechanical power of an anaerobic nature. Common tests are (1) running staircases, as the energy

requirement for maintaining speed in running a specified distance depends on mechanical performance during the time period, and (2) using a bicycle ergometer, where the mechanical work is calculated by recording through a photoelectric circuit the number of wheel revolutions. Activity examples include weight lifting, throwing, 100-yard dash, 100-meter freestyle swim, a basketball fast break, or running bases in baseball.

The Heart and Circulation

The circulatory system provides the physical means for oxygen transport through its tubular arrray of narrowing vascular diameters. Flow on the arterial side is maintained by the pump-like ventricular contraction of the heart, enhanced by the recoil of the aorta. Flow on the venous side is maintained by the "milking" action of muscular contraction and the rhythmically exerted negative pressure of the thorax during inspiration.

Indirect methods of analyzing heart silhouettes on x-ray films or measuring the differences in arterial and venous blood oxygen content offer some cardiac output data. Cardiac output (heart rate and stroke volume) can also be indirectly estimated through the heart rate and pulse pressure ratio. When an electrocardiograph is utilized in evaluating physical fitness, it must be kept in mind that the ECG does not measure cardiac function. It solely detects action potential conduction abnormalities, usually the result of heart disease.

Nutrient Transport

Blood transports oxygen, energy substrates, and metabolic wastes, as well as serves a vital role in temperature regulation. Reduced blood volume, reduced red cells, and reduced hemoglobin lower the body's capacity for aerobic activity. Each tissue has a range of functional response with definite limits of adaptation. In this sense, blood oxygen transport capability is limited by its capacity to carry oxygen (ie, hemoglobin content and oxygen saturation).

An individual's pulmonary blood flow, lung diffusing capacity, rate of oxygen removal, and total hemoglobin all have a close relationship with maximum oxygen intake. Total hemoglobin determines the potential arterial capacity to transport oxygen. For example, low hemoglobin levels in an athlete are often attributed to increased cell destruction, as evidenced by increases in circulating haptoglobins from increased rates in blood flow or extrinsic trauma (eg, runner's feet, boxer's abdomen). Dietary habits are more significant than the minute amounts of iron lost in perspiration.

Cardiac Output

Blood oxygen transport also depends on cardiac output (Fig. 8.6). While evaluation of cardiac output during exertion is helpful in diagnosis, stroke volume is difficult to determine directly. Cardiac output increases with work intensity and is directly related to the quantity of oxygen intake: maximum heart output parallels maximum oxygen intake. Such factors as heat exposure and/or dehydration influence stroke volume and change the relationship between heart rate and stroke volume which alters the relationship between oxygen consumption and heart rate. Cardiac output effectiveness is also determined by relative circulatory distribution among active muscles, viscera, and skin.

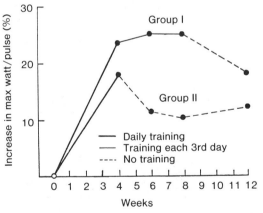

Figure 8.6. Effects of training termination. Two groups of nine subjects each were trained daily for 4 weeks and showed a 20% increase in cardiovascular fitness. Then, group I continued training every third day, and group II ceased training. Note that group I maintained its level of fitness, while group II began to lose its level of working performance within 2 weeks, indicating that training effects are both gained or lost rather quickly. Regular, continual stimulation is necessary to maintain cardiorespiratory efficiency (with the permission of the Behavioral Research Foundation).

The maximum limits of stroke volume are determined by the type of exercise and body posture. For example, in comparison to a runner or swimmer who uses most of the body, a cyclist, in not using his upper extremities for propulsion, often pools a large amount of blood within upper extremity veins. The consequence of this is a reduced stroke volume in the cyclist.

Oxygen Pulse

During exertion, cardiac stroke volume increases and the cells take more oxygen from arterial blood. Both of these factors increase oxygen delivery to cells. The term "oxygen pulse" refers to the quantity of oxygen removed from the blood during each pulse. It is measured in a specified time period by dividing oxygen intake by heart rate. Oxygen pulse increases during exertion, reaching its typical maximum of from 11–17 milliliters at about 135 pulses/minutes and decreasing after further cardiac acceleration.

Heart Rate

Heart rate is closely correlated with maximum oxygen intake. Typically, heart rate is parallel with performance intensity, but maximum cardiac rate decreases with advancing age. There is a linear relationship between heart rate and metabolic rate. Due to the wide variance in individual balance between sympathetic and vagal drives to the cardiac pacemaker, the resting heart rate of the endurance-trained athlete may reach lows of 30/minute. The maximum sustained heart rate during competition is about 185–195/minute or less. In activities of high stress and isometric exertion (eg, skiing), peak heart rates of 250/minute or more may be briefly encountered.

Blood and Pulse Pressures

Blood pressure and pulse pressure also have a close relationship with maximum oxygen intake. To meet oxygen demands during prolonged exertion, the blood quantity in the muscles and the blood flow within the lungs must be increased. By increasing the force of heart muscle contraction, systolic blood pressure is raised as heart rate increases. This increase is minimized in the well-trained athlete and attributed to decreased peripheral resistance because of vasodilation. Pulse pressure, the difference between systolic and diastolic pressures, offers an index to the efficiency of cardiac contraction and stroke volume.

Difficulties in the exchange of oxygen and carbon dioxide in active tissues are rarely anticipated except in specific types of events. For example, an overland cyclist may complain of pain and weakness in leg muscles during hill ascents. This is apparently caused by local circulatory obstruction resulting from vigorous quadricep contractions. However, if activity can be continued in spite of the pain, increased systemic blood pressure tends to overcome the local vascular occlusion. This phenomenon is thought to be a manifestation of the heart failing to develop an immediate and adequate increase in blood pressure.

The Pulmonary Apparatus

The degree of oxygen saturation greatly determines the oxygen-carrying capacity of the blood, and oxygen saturation is dependent on factors which determine the quality and quantity of oxygen diffusion in the lungs. These factors include (1) the quality of pulmonary blood flow and neuromuscular mechanisms, (2) the lung area available for the diffusing process, (3) the time duration in which blood receives alveolar capillary exposure, (4) the thickness of the alveolar capillary membrane, (5) the alveolar air and pulmonary capillaries oxygen pressure differential, and (6) respiratory frequency, which is often linked in the athlete with the rhythm of movement. It therefore becomes apparent that the quality of oxygen transport is dependent upon the blood, the cardiovascular system, and the pulmonary-respiratory system.

Ventilation

Lung function is evaluated by measuring pulmonary residual volume and vital capacity, the components of total lung volume. As an index to breathing capacity, vital capacity is commonly determined by calculating the amount of air maximally exhaled after a maximal inhalation. About 20% of vital capacity is used during rest, while about 70% might be used during prolonged exercise. Up to a quarter of external ventilation is "wasted" in pulmonary "dead space" due to the incomplete mixing of alveolar and airway air, enhanced by the athlete's typically diminished respiratory rate.

Pulmonary ventilation efficiency is assisted as tidal volume increases with decreased respiratory frequency for a given total ventilation. More commonly, ventilation efficiency is judged by the quantity of air inhaled or expired in relation to the amount of oxygen absorbed. Such measurements must take into consideration varying atmospheric conditions and individual, metabolic needs. In that oxygen is essential for life, both oxygen demands and oxygen consumption must be considered.

Lactic Formation and "Choked" Performance

During heavy exercise, lactic acid accumulates within muscle tissue as a result of oxygen demands exceeding oxygen supply. Choking of performance because of excessive competition or poor pacing may lead to early anaerobic demands on metabolism resulting in lactate accumulation (Fig. 8.7). It is witnessed as a premature distressing hyperventilation. Local muscle weakness may also induce premature breathlessness. The hyperventilation from premature lactate ac-

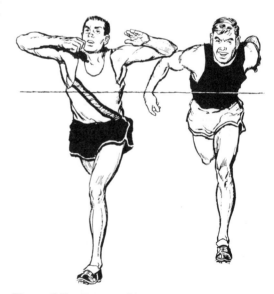

Figure 8.7. Poor pacing or excessive competition may lead to choking of performance as a result of early demands on metabolism leading to excessive lactate accumulation.

cumulation can cause an athlete to exceed normal ventilation adjustments where oxygen delivered to the circulation is less than the corresponding demand for oxygen consumption. It is thus important for an athlete to avoid lactate accumulation until late in activity. If local muscle weakness is the cause, the situation can be corrected by strengthening exercises so the athlete can operate nearer aerobic power before lactate accumulates sufficiently. Marathon runners usually operate just under their lactate threshold until the final sprint.

The "Second Wind"

A second wind is considered the result of an opposite reaction. While early lactate accumulation may be the result of physiologic forces (eg, cardiorespiratory maladjustment), with prolonged activity, systemic blood pressure rises, movement pace is steadied, ventilation diminishes, the respiratory muscles become "warmed-up," which reduces respiratory resistance and the awareness of breathing, and the level of circulating lactate is lowered.

Diffusing Capacity

Many well-conditioned athletes, especially swimmers and other endurance-related participants, exhibit a large pulmonary diffusing capacity (larger pulmonary surface) which enhances oxygen transfer. Such athletes also exhibit an increased ratio of oxygen intake to lung ventilation per min, which decreases as exhaustion approaches. However, even with maximum effort, the equilibrium of pulmonary gases between the blood stream and alveolar spaces is fairly complete. Thus, a gain in diffusing capacity offers little benefit except for swimmers who deliberately hold their breath or for athletes performing in moderate to high altitudes.

Carbon Dioxide Homeostasis

Both low and high levels of carbon dioxide affect normal tissue function. Excessive carbon dioxide elimination may be encountered in high altitudes, witnessed by intermittent ventilation and symptoms of "mountain sickness"; ie, dyspnea, headache, blood pressure and pulse rate changes, and neurologic disorders due to maladjustment to reduced oxygen pressure at high altitudes. Accumulation of carbon dioxide is unusual except for the scuba diver due to the increased rate of carbon dioxide production, the decreased maximum voluntary ventilation, the added external dead weight, and the possible inefficiency of the carbon dioxide-absorbing canisters.

PERFORMANCE ASSESSMENT

The common human performance parameters are those of strength, endurance, flexibility, speed, coordination, balance, and agility. Body type could also be included here, but the subject has been previously discussed. Intelligence, creativity, and motivation are also parameters, and these factors will be left to a later discussion. It would be well to keep in mind that the following factors to be considered do not indicate that highly talented athletes are all endowed with similar traits.

Genetic Influences

Little can be done to modify body type as much as the variables found in body build and its individual physiology, especially in regard to oxygen intake, are genetically determined. While skill has an influence on efficiency, body type places a finite limit on physical achievement goals. It is granted that a great deal of practice time is allotted to the development of skill, but many aspects of skill are inherited (eg, receptor organ sensitivity). The potential "superstar" probably starts life with a peculiar advantage.

Bulk

Body bulk has both its advantages and disadvantages. Muscle bulk, especially in contact sports, provides both force inertia and protection for bones and joints. Body weight is of less consideration in rowing and swimming sports because the weight is supported, it offers some buoyancy advantages, or it provides necessary insulation due to subcutaneous fat (eg, open-water swimming).

In contrast, due to gravitational pull, a heavy bulk is a disadvantage in running sports as it must be raised at each pace. There are also disadvantages in that bulky hypertrophy increases viscous resistance to movement, produces problems from physical apposition, and increases the body mass to be moved. Thus, to avoid mass accumulation in an irrelevant part of the body, muscle training should be specific for the use desired, as indiscriminate muscle hypertrophy is likely to impair performance in endurance events.

Mechanical Advantage

Mechanical advantage and disadvantage has a distinct relationship with performance. For example, pace varies with limb length; thus, long limbs are an advantage in running, especially in long distance events. A higher center of gravity is a disadvantage in that it takes extra postural effort to maintain balance (eg, gymnastics, skating), but it has its advantages in sports (eg, basketball) where increased height places one closer to the goal.

Endurance

Endurance is defined as the capacity to maintain strenuous activity of a large number of muscle groups for a duration sufficient to demand prolonged resistance to fatigue. The term is generally used to denote the ability of skeletal muscle to continue contractions relative to contraction length (time), contraction quantity (per unit of time), and contraction quality (force). During vigorous muscular effort, the endurance factor is determined by the initial glycogen content of muscle fibers (influenced by diet and training).

Endurance, a manifestation of cardiovascular and respiratory function (both aerobic and anaerobic capacity), manifests itself in a variety of ways: eg, gymnastics, crew, cross-country skiing, mountain climbing, wrestling, marathon runs or swims. Both quantity of movements and the time duration involved are reflections of endurance; eg, number of push-ups or pull-ups, time to run a mile.

Strength

The quality of one's strength, power, flexibility, speed, coordination, balance, and agility are determined essentially by neuromuscular functions.

In discussing "strength," terminology is often confusing. The phrase "isometric (equal in length) strength" refers to muscle activity that occurs without shortening of the muscle. "Isotonic (equal in tone) strength" means muscle activity with shortening of the muscle. Both of these general terms of physiologic misnomers in that there is a degree of length change in isometrics due to tendon stretching, and, in isotonics, normal tone is influenced by the altered mechanical advantage and resistance. The word "strength" itself is often a confusing term. For discussion, it can be divided into dynamic (isotonic), explosive, and static (isometric) strength.

1. *Dynamic strength* refers to one's ability to lift, move, and support body weight, calling upon endurance when such functions are strenuously repeated; ie, explosive movements repeated in rapid succession (eg, pullups, sprinting). Limits are imposed by speed-resisting factors and the quantity and quality of energy-exchange factors. If extreme pain, breathlessness, or weakness comes at the end of an athlete's effort, a gain in active muscle strength will do much to improve performance.

2. *Explosive strength* refers to the ability to release maximum power (energy) in the fastest possible time (eg, standing long jump). Single violent efforts are commonly seen in sprinting, jumping, and throwing where speed factors are combined with the force/velocity features of active muscles. Response is determined by mechanical leverage (influenced by body type), immediate energy resources from tissue chemical coupling (influenced by glycogen and mineral ion levels), the quantity of actin and myosin filaments per fiber (influenced by training hypertrophy), and the number of fibers activated (influenced by learning experiences). The performance result of these forces is determined largely by the degree of dynamic viscosity.

3. *Static strength*, a separate factor of physical fitness, means the exertion of a maximum force for a brief period of time against a fairly immovable object (eg, handgrip or arm-pull dynamometer). The importance of static strength is brought out in such activities as weight lifting. Such strength is dependent on the total number of active muscle fibers involved in a specific

activity; ie, the functional (gross muscle less fat and connective tissue) cross-section of the muscle tissue exerting the force, under control of the nervous system, with some assistance from the type of contraction and mechanical advantage in play. Lessening of central inhibition and greater relaxation of antagonists also play a part in the performance effect. Limits are imposed by exhaustion, motivation, Valsalva effects, pain, and quickly diminishing endurance. Muscles required to contract against increasing resistance become progressively stronger and usually, but not inevitably, hypertrophied; ie, women should have no fear that weight lifting with good style will bring gross overdevelopment.

Either progressing central or local fatigue adversely affects skill: diminished skill is commonly associated with approaching exhaustion. As muscle perfusion is greater in a strong muscle as contrasted with that of a weak muscle, fatigue is, to a great extent, due to inadequate perfusion. However, the overt signs of pallor, the energy-wasting poor coordination, confusion, and staggering gait are to be blamed on inadequate blood flow to the posture-regulating center.

Strength also has an effect on recovery in that strength tends to minimize the microtrauma secondary to oxygen lack and local weakness.

Power

Power, the rate of doing work, is determined by the rate at which energy can be released within muscle tissue. While the type of contraction (ie, isometric, eccentric, or concentric), resistance, duration, quantity of repetitions, and number of exercise bouts are important in any exercise program, the most important factor appears to be that the contraction force developed by a muscle must be close to maximum if improved change is to be expected.

It has been well established that low-repetition high-resistance exercises develop power, high-repetition low-resistance exercises develop endurance (Fig. 8.8). Many feel that strength is the only training variable in enhancing the speed of muscle contraction and that tissue viscosity is relatively constant. This is only true, however, when

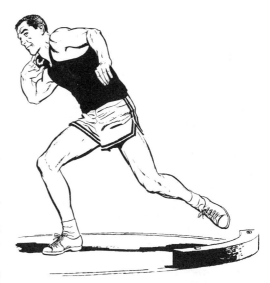

Figure 8.8. Low-repetition, high-resistance exercises develop power; high-repetition, low-resistance exercises develop endurance.

strengthening actions mimic movements used in the sport.

Speed

Speed is highly correlated with muscle power and difficult to isolate. Speed (fastness) can refer to running time or reaction time. It can refer to the legs of a racer, the fists of a boxer, the arms of a goalie, the eyes of a skeet shooter. As inertia is proportional to mass, total speed considers three aspects: time/distance in initiating body movement (explosive force of active muscles); time/distance rate of acceleration to maximum; and time/distance loss of acceleration as the event is prolonged. During the last stage of a run, the reducing metabolic energy must cope with continuing resistances in air flow, tissue viscosity, surface friction, and other energy losses. Good speed is obviously essential in runners, tennis players, and football backs and ends.

Because it is difficult for a bulky frame to accelerate quickly to maximum speed, the ideal physique of a sprinter would be one with powerful legs and little weight elsewhere. In sprinting, performance is enhanced by a preliminary warmup that raises intramuscular temperature because a slight increase in temperature enhances muscle tissue viscosity and utilization of energy resources within the muscles which influence muscle contraction.

Reaction speed is determined by the interval between when stimuli are received by receptor organs (eg, eyes, ears, soles, hands) and when the muscles react. A fast reaction time is necessary for high efficiency in such events as table tennis, dashes, and boxing.

Agility

Agility involves speed with the addition of a sudden change in direction or height such as in a defensive maneuver or a change in attack; it is the ability to change positions in space. The number of positional changes available is obviously almost endless, thus agility is most difficult to evaluate. Good agility is demanded in hockey players, running backs, gymnasts, infielders, divers, boxers, karate enthusiasts, and wrestlers.

TRAINING PHYSIOLOGY

In any type of serious competition, training and practice are essential prerequisites. To keep in top competitive condition, both men and women at younger and younger ages are engaging in weight training programs, interval running schedules, and other developmental activities in addition to their usual practice sessions. This rationale mandates careful health care monitoring.

Training and Practice

The terms "training" and "practice" should be differentiated. Training refers to the improvement or maintenance of physical capacity such as systematic endurance or strength exercises. Normally, these are out of context with a particular sport. Practice means the repeating of specific skill-developing techniques utilized within a specific sport so that they may be executed at a higher level of performance. During practice, a swimmer might practice his pushoff, a tennis player his forehand, a golfer his putting, etc.

What would be called practice in one sport may be called training in another. For example, weight lifting is practice for the weight lifter, training for the tackle. Running is practice for the track athlete, training for the boxer. In addition, as the time available is a concern, the relative degree of emphasis between training and practice varies from sport to sport. Training is minimal in tennis and golf, practice is secondary to training in most explosive strength sports, and most highly skilled team sports require a careful blend of training and practice.

As body type and receptor organ sensitivity is to a greater extent governed genetically, training cannot turn an antelope into an ox or vice versa. Depending upon the genetic foundation, training is an enhancement to potential expression, but many variables are not trainable. Skill is the result of practice, not training. Practice tends to develop timing, accuracy, and conditioned responses so that conscious mental faculties can be concentrating on competitive strategies rather than on physical activities during competition. The term "pressure practice" means practice under highly competitive game conditions (eg, an intersquad scrimmage).

The Development of Endurance

Endurance increases as the result of enhanced muscle hypertrophy, glycogen reserves, myoglobin, and increased vasculature. Local endurance is an effect of muscle strength; we witness this in the power of serves in a long tennis match and in the final paces of the runner. In such instances, repetitions of isotonic overload exercises enhance local endurance. Long-term body endurance, as previously discussed, is related to a high cardiorespiratory circulatory capability and energy reserves.

The Development of Strength

Strength is gained in three ways:

1. *Isotonically* by exercises against resistance in such a manner that body movements are allowed (eg, weights and weight machines, spring or friction devices). Common nonequipment exercise regimens for developing muscular strength and endurance include sit-ups, bar chinning, cross-country jogging, push-ups, spinal extensions, rope climbing, and half-knee bends.

2. *Isometrically* by exercises done against resistance in such a manner that body movements are restricted (eg, pushing against a wall), sometimes offering a short cut to goals of equivalent repetitive drudgery.

3. *Isokinetically* by exercises of a constant velocity against resistance which adapt to the angle of a joint (eg, Orthotron or Cybex II equipment). These exercises are used primarily to rehabilitate up to the point of normal strength, after which other forms of exercise are utilized.

In 1957 and since, Muller has shown that one isometric contraction (slightly more for the well-trained athlete) of 40–60% of maximum held for a few seconds each day would result in the maximum possible increase of muscular strength. From this, while slightly modified, renewed interest in the Charles Atlas type of "dynamic tension" exercises, in addition to isotonic exercises, has become widespread within the sports world.

A 15-year research project in Germany on the subject of muscle building has determined that the maximum contraction of a muscle, held for a matter of seconds, will cause the muscle to grow in strength at an average of 4%/week (*National Health World*, 4/78). These scientists claim that the maximum contraction of a muscle is all that is necessary to strengthen, for example, slackened or weak abdominal muscles. An exercise for these muscles would include pulling in the stomach as far as possible and keeping it there until the muscles quiver, then letting the muscles relax. This exercise, performed once each day to these muscles or other muscles of the body in the sedentary individual will increase the strength of the muscles 50% in 12 weeks according to the research conducted. Thus, evidence of disuse atrophy as seen clinically indicates a severe lack of activity of a muscle group.

One disadvantage of purely isometric exercises is that benefits are confined to a range of motion of only 20° to either side of the training angle at which contraction is performed.

Regardless of the type of exercises and regimens utilized, careful consideration must be made of the total situation of the particular competition involved since there is always the question of how much training is enough, as overtraining can dull an otherwise sharpened performance.

CHAPTER 9

Environmental Influences on Athletic Performance

At one time or another most outdoor sports must be conducted at extreme ranges of temperature and altitude. This is true for both the circuiting professional and the vacationing nonprofessional. This chapter covers the fundamental affects of body temperature, extreme environmental heat, cold, altitude, and water-related activities on athletic performance.

BODY TEMPERATURE

Normal body temperature reflects the balance between heat generation and heat loss, determined by the set point of the temperature-regulating center of the hypothalamus. Temperature is highest at the center of the body, diminishing towards the periphery. When temperatures rise above the set point, the body compensates through peripheral vasodilation, sweating, and hyperventilation to promote heat loss. When temperatures fall below the set point, the body compensates through increasing the metabolic rate, tensing the muscles, and shivering to promote heat generation (Fig. 9.1). In athletics as in clinical practice, with the diagnosis of fever, we must determine if the cause is a dysfunction of heat production, heat loss, or of the hypothalamic thermostat.

Normal Variations

Human body oral temperature is considered to be 98.6°F (37°C) with daily (diurnal) variations from 97°F around 4 a.m. to 99.6°F at about 6 p.m. plus or minus 1°F. The normal average temperature of 98.6°F is an average at rest. It is an arbitrary value, and many people vary somewhat from this. Many healthy people show higher values when active or on a warm day. Subnormal temperatures are also common in many people. Normal functions such as emotional excitement, exercise, digestion, ovulation, pregnancy, or being in a hot room may result in a slight temperature rise. Rectal or vaginal temperature is about 1°F higher than oral, and axillary or groin temperature is about 1°F lower than oral temperature. The pulse rate increases about 10 beats/minute for every 1°F rise in temperature; respiration rate increases 2–3/minute.

False high readings may result from inadequate shaking down of the thermometer, previous ingestion of hot foods, smoking, recent strenuous exercise, or a recently applied hot compress. False low levels may result from incomplete closure of mouth, breathing through the mouth, not leaving the thermometer in place long enough, or the recent ingestion of cold substances. Axillary, groin, and vaginal temperatures are so inaccurate that they are seldom used.

Abnormal Variations

Any form of hypermetabolic condition may create a feverish state through increased heat production, eg, vigorous exercise or hyperthyroidism. Interference with sweating interferes with normal heat loss; eg, dehydration, certain drugs, and primary neurologic defects. Heat stroke is a good example of combined hypermetabolism and diminished sweating from dehydration resulting in high fever.

The most common cause of fever, however, is a change in set point of the hypothalamic thermostat. For an unknown reason, infections and inflammatory processes especially cause the hypothalamic temperature center to become less sensitive to heat.

A temperature between 99°F and 100°F is spoken of as feverishness; a temperature between 100°F and 101°F as a slight fever (hyperthermia); 101°F to 103°F, a moderate fever; and 104°F and 105°F, a high fever. Any temperature below 98°F is said to be

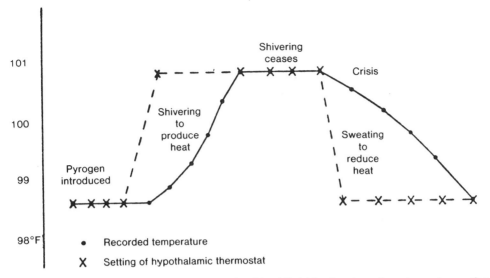

Figure 9.1. Diagram of the mechanisms involved in chills/shivering, hypothermia, and sweating.

subnormal, while a temperature above 106°F (hyperpyrexia) is a grave symptom.

Symptoms of Feverishness

The symptoms of excessive body heat include hot dry skin, flushed face, dry mouth with excessive thirst, malaise, lassitude, languor, anorexia, nausea and vomiting, costiveness of the bowels, scanty highly colored urine, weakness, headache and backache, increased pulse rate, and quickened respiration. In cases of high fever, there may be cerebral symptoms of delirium, stupor, or coma and a suppression of body secretions. All fever or feverish conditions are attended by a preceding sensation of relative chilliness or by a chill with rigors.

With prolonged feverishness, vesicles (fever blisters) of herpes simplex virus often appear around the mouth and nose. While the cause is unknown, it is thought that temperature elevation activates a latent infection that becomes symptomatic or that some visceral reflex is involved.

Local Temperature and Tenderness

In cases of inflammation, the presence of local heat is a valuable sign, noted by passing the outstretched hand rapidly over the affected part to an unaffected part and back again. Any difference in warmth from the affected area to the unaffected area signifies an increase in local temperature. Mild cases of joint involvement invariably present points of warmth and maximum tenderness that correspond to the superficial regions of the endothelium. For example, they are elicited after trauma (1) in the knee on both sides of the patella, (2) in the wrist over the anatomical snuffbox, (3) in the elbow over the radiohumeral joint, and (4) in the ankle at the anterior surface of the joint.

ENVIRONMENTAL HEAT

Heat, even moderate heat, can stress the endurance athlete to extreme. History has shown that many Olympic athletes in top condition have suffered heat exhaustion and heat strokes to the extent of near deaths and fatalities. Summer track and cycling marathons offer many potential hazards. Southern football and even September practices in northern states offer special dangers.

Basic Safeguards

Many fatalities can be prevented when proper precautions are taken to see that safeguards are maintained. The first requirement is a thorough preseason history and examination. Care must be given to see that the use of vasoconstrictor drugs (eg, amphetamines) are restricted, that weight is carefully controlled, and that fluid and salt intake is carefully monitored. Intolerance or maladjustment to environmental heat frequently leads to heat cramps, heat exhaustion, or heat stroke.

In the event that a scheduled endurance event is to occur on a hot/humid day, it is advisable to alert the local hospital emergency room of potential heat problems. Appropriate professional care and ambulance service should be prearranged. Officials must be educated that fluid replacement should never be prohibited by arbitrary rules and that a groggy player should be called to the attention of the coach.

Temperature Maintenance

A person's internal bioclimate possesses unique homeostatic defenses to maintain thermal balance under adverse conditions of both external heat and cold, but even these have their limits (Fig. 9.2). A role of the hypothalamus is to serve as guardian of thermal homeostasis.

The thermoregulatory mechanism (TRM) of the hypothalamus is separated into two divisions which are closely coordinated to act as one unit. When one part is stimulated, the other is inhibited. One section functions to retain and conserve body heat. The other section regulates heat dissipation by affecting cutaneous vasodilation and perspiration.

Hypothalamic heat response is governed by changes in blood temperature and cutaneous reflexes, while its hormonal activity is influenced essentially by electrolytic changes. Normal thermoregulation is upset when work production and the effected heat production becomes so great that the body resources are unable to sufficiently cope.

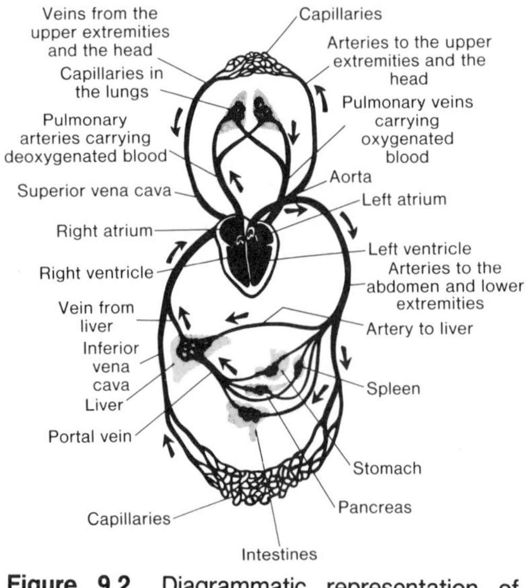

Climate Assessment

Temperature and humidity are crucial factors, but the effects of radiant heat load and windspeed should not be ignored. A sling psychrometer, containing a wet-bulb and a dry-bulb thermometer, is often used on the practice field, at least twice per session, to determine relative humidity (RH). The difference between the two measurements offers an evaluation of the relative wetness-dryness of the environment. The RH, calculated from the difference of the two bulbs, measures moisture percentage relative to the air's capacity to hold water at any given dry-bulb temperature. A RH of 70% indicates that 70 particles of water are being held by a given volume of air capable of holding 100 particles.

A wet-bulb reading of 70°C or slightly higher suggests a rest period after every half hour of activity. Activity should be conducted in light shorts or postponed if the wet bulb records 80°F or higher. Unfortunately, light clothing is almost impossible in football practice where padding is essential protection with sleds, buckers, body contact, and falls. From a health standpoint, athletic activity should never be conducted when humidity is higher than 95%.

Note that temperature and humidity readings make no allowance for air movement. A wind of just 4–5 miles/second can reduce effective temperature by several degrees, although this effect is diminished at high temperatures.

Cooperation among physician, coach, and trainer must assure necessary conditioning, to reduce injuries and increase performance, without health being endangered. While rigid rules and formulae are helpful, any squad deserves reasonable, humanitarian care, and this, more often than not, must be based upon combined experience and instincts rather than on charts and research data. The practical effects of heat are better

Figure 9.2. Diagrammatic representation of blood circulation.

studied on the field rather than in the physiologic laboratory; during training, hot weather persisting through many days of strenuous practice has a cumulative effect.

Fluid and Mineral Requirements

The prolonged cumulative mineral losses through sweat alone may lead to weakness, cramps, spasms, and neurasthenic symptoms. To monitor fluid loss, each player should be weighed before and after each practice session. Data can be recorded on a sheet posted near the scales. During 90 minutes of football practice under adverse conditions, weight losses average 3–5 kilograms. A player exhibiting persistent weight loss should be checked for signs of listlessness, clumsiness, wobbliness, headache, unusual fatigue, slight neuromuscular retardation, and other early signs of dehydration and salt depletion.

Water Deficiency

For some reason, an athlete left to personal inclination will rarely drink enough water during or following an endurance event to compensate for fluid loss. Adjustment can be made for this fact by increasing salt and water intake a few days before competition (preloading). Dehydration usually accompanies poor heat adjustment, making the player more susceptible to fatigue and thus to injury. If an athlete cannot drink enough water to replenish fluid loss, either a decrease in blood volume or an increase in osmotic pressure results in stimulating pituitary secretion of the antidiuretic hormone (ADH) to increase renal reabsorption and reduce excretion of water. Vaporization of moisture from the lungs can exceed a pint of water each day, depending upon the humidity and temperature of inspired air. However, the heat loss from such pulmonary vaporization is insignificant. And, in contrast to kidney action, this moisture loss is without loss of salts.

Sodium/Potassium Balance

Salt imbalance stimulates aldosterone to conserve sodium by encouraging reabsorption of sodium by the kidneys and sweat glands. However, this is at the expense of potassium, which can be excreted to such an extent as to result in a serious deficiency.

To offset this effect, especially during high humidity and hot weather, many trainers increase potassium intake as well as salt intake. If too much salt is utilized, a transient peak of plasma sodium occurs which forces the kidneys to excrete extra water in an attempt to restore electrolytic balance. During severe physical activity, plasma sodium tends to rise, potassium ions "leak" from active muscles as an effect of glycogen depletion, and there is a tendency toward hyperkalemia. At this stage, highly concentrated commercial sodium-potassium supplements are clearly contraindicated.

Heat and Physical Activity Adaptation

Even for the well-trained athlete, the mechanical efficiency of human performance is poor, amounting to about 25% for aerobic activity and 15% for anaerobic activity. Thus, the larger amount of chemical energy used in sports is dispersed as thermal energy. At least 75% of ingested calories is expressed as heat, rather than as mechanical energy, during athletic performance. This heat can be stored in the body for a brief period, exhibited as a rise in body temperature. Heat storage potential is determined essentially by one's weight and initial body temperature prior to exertion.

Heat Storage

The average body can store heat to accommodate full effort for only a limited time. A continuous exchange of heat between the body and its ambient environment is necessary to maintain thermal homeostasis. The skin especially, along with the lungs and excreta, provides the means to accomplish this exchange.

Hyperthermia results if maximum heat storage is not dissipated through a combination of losses from surface conduction, wind convection, and especially perspiration evaporation, along with antiradiation-gain factors such as reflective clothing. During athletic activity, general body temperature increases slightly for about 10–15 minutes, whereafter a plateau (dependent upon dissipation rate) is reached with continued exertion.

The temperature within muscle tissue increases rapidly during the first 5 minutes of work. This tends to improve muscle physiology by dilating intramuscular blood vessels and reducing tissue viscosity.

Core Temperature

Increasing surface temperature reflects the affects of a progressively rising and dangerous core temperature, the increase in subcutaneous circulation, and the amount of perspiration. An increasing core temperature increases oxygen consumption in inactive tissues and diverts a large proportion of the circulation to skin vessels even when optimal cardiac output is maintained. This results in a reduced supply to active muscle tissue.

Because of the demand for heat dissipation, prolonged exertion during hot weather causes a progressive reduction of central blood volume which in turn reduces cardiac stroke volume. As the core temperature increases, peripheral vein capacity increases and the formation of tissue fluid increases during the early minutes of activity. In a hot/dry climate, expired water losses also increase. Sweating contributes greatly to a fall in blood volume and may, under severe conditions, amount to as much as 1–2 liters/hour.

If a player's pulse rate does not reduce during rest periods, it is good evidence that body heat is accumulating. Rectal temperature should be checked for verification.

Note that females sweat less than males, and they cool faster after activity than males. This latter fact is apparently due to a more efficient thermoregulation mechanism.

Perspiration

When the environmental temperature is higher than that of the body, cooling through the evaporation of sweat is the most efficient means to maintain thermal homeostasis. About 0.58 calories of heat are dissipated with every cubic centimeter of water which evaporates. With prolonged athletic endeavor, a player must dissipate 1–2 liters of sweat each hour to maintain heat balance, and this is in addition to conduction-convection losses. One liter of perspiration evaporation dissipates about 580 kilocalories of heat. However, under humid conditions, as much as 50% of evaporation efficiency may be lost. Here, the importance of sweat-absorbing clothing (eg, cotton) to hold moisture until evaporation occurs is underscored.

About a pint of perspiration (3% of body weight) is considered an acceptable perspiratory rate during limited physical activity; however, many marathon runs over 5 hours exceed 5%, decidedly within the danger zone. Up to a 3% loss, the only overt symptom is thirst, and this is probably due to replenishment from catabolism and water liberated from glycogen stores. Once the 3% level is reached, continued exertion exhibits a steady reduction in perspiratory rate. This reduction occurs because the body possesses about 2% of its weight for sweating; once this storage is utilized, additional production becomes increasingly difficult.

The cessation of perspiration is a biologic alert associated with rising core temperature, increasing venous pressure, and a failing of cardiac output. This state may quickly progress into circulatory collapse.

Perspiration must evaporate if sweating is to cause heat loss. Drops of sweat rolling to the ground have no cooling benefit. Because of the capillary action and osmotic pressure involved, the necessary subcutaneous vaporation may become inhibited by equipment pads and inadequate garments. When heat loss is obstructed by improper clothing or hot/humid weather, cardiac output may be reduced to a point where normal cerebral circulation cannot be maintained (ie, heat collapse). If circulatory flow to the skin and kidneys also fails, the resulting hyperpyrexia may be fatal.

In recent years, rubberized or other dehydration apparel are used by some players in an effort to lose "weight." This policy should be prohibited by the physician in charge.

Skin Circulation Flow Distribution

When a player's external environment is hot, subcutaneous arterial vessels dilate to contribute a greater amount of body heat to the surface, and the superficial veins dilate in accommodation. In strenuous exercise, the intensely increased dilatation of subcutaneous vessels offers a potential for flow redistribution because from 16–20% of cardiac output is distributed to the skin. A well-trained athlete with good endurance can tolerate a low skin flow because he or she sweats early, sweats heavily, and adapts well to a high core temperature and because rapid body movements aid convection heat loss. Firm evidence has shown where drugs used in athletics to compromise skin flow have resulted in deaths.

Climate Adaptation

Physical fitness does not constitute environmental fitness. This is frequently seen when a team accustomed to one climate is quickly transported to another climate for competition. When this occurs, gradual acclimatization must be made and substitutions should be made more frequently than normal to benefit team performance.

Heat Syncope

Players who fail to adequately "warm down" after an event or spectators who stand for long periods in the heat may lose consciousness from inadequate cerebral blood flow due to a reduced volume associated with a reduced cardiac stroke output, excessive sweating, relaxed superficial veins, and cutaneous vasodilation which lowers systemic blood pressure. Added to this, players often present an accumulation of fluids within active muscles, standing spectators frequently present extravascular edema in the lower extremities, and either may have a superimposed vasovagal attack featuring general muscular vasodilation and a reduced cardiac rate.

Syncope may also be associated with heat exhaustion or sunstroke. When in doubt, an unconscious or stupored subject with a temperature exceeding 104°F should be treated as a victim of heat stroke until a firm diagnosis can be achieved.

Heat Fatigue and Exhaustion

When physical activity is conducted under highly warm/humid conditions, precautions must be taken to avoid heat cramps, dehydration fatigue, exhaustion, and stroke. *Heat cramps* result from electrolytic depletion and are temporarily disabling. *Heat fatigue* is caused by failure to replenish diminished salt and water lost in perspiration. *Heat exhaustion* is the effect of excessive salt and water depletion. *Heat stroke* results

when the thermoregulatory mechanism fails or is overtaxed.

When early warning signs are ignored, excessive core temperatures rise, and symptoms progress from those of heat fatigue to heat exhaustion and finally to heat stroke. All these stages can be prevented. Keep in mind that both heat exhaustion and heat stroke can occur in the shade. Heat fatigue, the beginning phase of heat exhaustion, is characterized by a dulled alertness, making a player more vulnerable to injury. On a hot day, heat syncope is probably the most common health problem seen.

Dehydration and Heat Exhaustion

There are two types of heat exhaustion syndromes: heat exhaustion and dehydration. During heat problems, nature offers several early-warning signs for the need of fluid and mineral replacement such as thirst and dry skin, lack of sweat, inattentiveness, awkwardness, sluggishness, apathy, headache, undue fatigue, grogginess, unusual nausea, and a marked fall in blood pressure. These are signs of shock as a result of depleted body salt and water.

Poor supervision can lead to chronic maladjustment. During accumulated salt loss, the chronic signs of constipation, scanty urine, and marked weight loss appear. Chronic dehydration exhibits circulatory failure, vomiting that increases salt loss, nausea, sunken eyes, and inelastic skin.

With heat exhaustion, the heart has difficulty in maintaining normal blood pressure and this reduces the circulatory rate and dissipates the core temperature. Exhaustion results. When a player begins to show fatigue and feel warmth, cardiac output and pulse rate increase and sweat moistens the skin. If this state is prolonged, difficult breathing, collapse, and loss of consciousness may occur (Fig. 9.3).

After prolonged sweating and reduced blood volume without fluid replacement, such a dehydration exhaustion also produces cardiac insufficiency. Heart rate increases, physical difficulties occur, and mental disturbances exhibit as dehydration continues. A loss of 5% of fluid body weight results in exhaustion and collapse. Severe heart involvement is exhibited if the lower extremities show extensive edema.

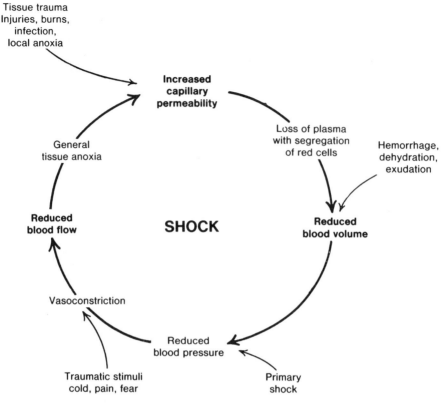

Figure 9.3.   The circulatory picture of shock.

Heat Stroke

Heat stroke is a strict emergency situation; delay can be fatal. There is usually an early hot dry skin (sweat mechanism failure), but profuse sweating is sometimes seen along with a flushed face, frequent and weak-to-full pulse, thirst, fatigue, muscle twitches, heat cramps, and exhaustion. These signs later progress into deep labored respiration, stupor associated with depressed reflexes, or excitement associated with exaggerated reflexes, hallucinations, visual disturbances, loss of sphincter control, and a profound coma.

All these signs and symptoms express a biologic cry for help. If left untreated, irreversible damage to the brain, adrenal cortex (heat shock), liver, and kidneys result because of the reduced cardiac output and rising core temperature. Once organ damage has occurred, massive hematuria, proteinuria, and a rising blood urea may be found.

Predisposing Health Conditions

Many health conditions can be aggravated in hot/humid weather which would not necessarily be unduly affected in cool weather. For example, in the grossly obese, there is difficulty in losing heat because the rate of heat dissipation is influenced by the thickness of subcutaneous fat. In subjects with subclinical heart conditions, the incidence of cardiac deaths is increased. This is probably related to decompensation as a result of increased demands for cutaneous vasodilation. With profound sweating, the electrolytic imbalance tends to increase the possibility of cardiac arrhythmias.

ENVIRONMENTAL COLD

As with heat, health problems rarely arise with a native who is acclimated and experienced, wears proper clothing, and takes necessary precautions. More commonly, they arise with the visitor or sportsperson accustomed to a warmer temperature zone being suddenly exposed to cold (eg, hill walking, sailing, deep diving, cave exploration). Heat loss encourages fatigue and may progress to where the body is unable to compensate without adequate heat production.

When the metabolic rate cannot be increased to prevent chilling, hypothermia may result in collapse and death. Several factors, usually in combination, may lead to a fatal outcome: exhaustion, malnutrition, low physical fitness, poor insulation, moisture-laden clothing, high windspeeds, and psychic confusion and vasodilation from alcohol or other drugs. The windspeed factor is highly important in such events as skiing, bobsledding, snowmobiling, sailing, cycling, and speedskating.

Temperature Homeostasis

Stored body heat helps one to tolerate brief exposures to cold. When the environment begins to cool, heat is conserved by vasoconstriction of the subscutaneous vessels. This is the first physiologic defense, usually taking place from 88°F to 75°F air temperature, and it is greatly impaired by alcohol intake. During exposure to cold, physical efficiency ebbs if core temperature falls only 2°F. This loss must be replaced either by voluntary effort (exertion) or involuntary effort (shivering). Radiant heat loss can be a distinct factor in unheated shelters and after sunset. Conduction heat loss through contact with cold equipment or the ground may contribute to the problem when protective clothing is not adequate.

In prolonged events, subcutaneous arterial vessels further constrict to direct more blood to active muscles, superficial veins constrict to improve venous return, maximum oxygen intake is very slightly increased, tissue viscosity increases, and blood pressure increases (which increases cardiac work).

Heavy clothing, as well as adding to metabolic burden from its weight, may produce excessive sweating during physical activity, which contributes to excessive heat loss through evaporation. Evaporation is also increased with sweat-laden or rain-soaked clothing. Regardless of the cause for the moisture, the body spends 580 kilocalories of heat for the evaporation of each liter of water. In a cold/dry climate, water loss can be considerable even when heavy perspiration and pulmonary vaporization are not noticed, hindering physiologic responses attempting to maintain thermal balance.

Clothing

Clothing provides insulation by trapping still air within its fibers. A larger percentage of the effect of trapped air is lost at high wind speeds. This warmth trapping is highest with animal skins (eg, Eskimo clothing), moderate with natural fibers (eg, wool), and lowest with nylon. Mittens with long cuffs and wrist air seals are more effective than gloves.

Within a cold, dry environment, the best protection during moderate exercise is afforded by loosely woven undergarments covered by windproof outer garments. A fur-trimmed hood helps to shield the face. However, to allow a means for sweat to evaporate during strenuous activity under Arctic conditions such as in downhill skiing, the windproof fabric should be limited to the front only. Here, face masks and extra scrotal insulation are necessary. Within a cold, wet environment, outer garments should be waterproof.

Cold and Physical Activity Adaptation

When muscle tissue is cooled, muscle tone is increased, antagonist muscles relax slower, and contraction speed is slowed, thus power and speed capabilities are hindered. Shivering, active muscle stiffness, and numb hands reduce skill. The risk of muscle tears is increased during physical activity in cold weather because of impaired muscle proprioception, diminished relaxation, impaired cerebral coordination (hypothermic or hypoglycemic), and impaired cutaneous sense organs.

Repetitive exposure to cold temperatures during physical activity, as with hot-temperature acclimation, leads to progressive acclimation to the climate. Studies have shown where it is possible to develop acclimation to both hot and cold environments simultaneously. Once acclimation has been made (7–10 days), an athlete will exhibit less shivering and a reduced general level of cutaneous circulation, present a lower core temperature and increased extremity circulation (increasing dexterity) than the unacclimated, have fewer subjective complaints, show a reduced hypertensive reaction to cold, and acquire normalization of skill.

Frostbite

Frostbite (dermatitis congelationis), a form of localized tissue destruction from freezing, is a danger once skin temperature falls below 30°F. Contributing factors include extremely low air temperatures, contact with cold equipment, severe local vasoconstriction, and extremely high airspeeds.

Etiology

Weak individuals are more susceptible to the injurious effects of cold than are the healthy and fit. Two other important etiologic factors are (a) constriction about the part which interferes with free circulation, and (b) a prolonged constrained position without exercise of the part. The first areas to be affected are the body protuberances such as the ears, nose, fingers, heels, and toes. The genitals, cheeks, chin, and female breasts may also be affected. Moist cold, more than dry cold, is an effective agent in causing this injury. Once clothing becomes soaked with moisture (sweat, snow, rain), the insulation factor is destroyed, encouraging hypothermia and frostbite during rest periods. Frostbite may be classified by three common stages according to the severity (depth of involvement) of the injury: first degree (erythema); second degree (vesication); and third degree (necrosis).

Mild Frostbite and Chilblain

First-degree frostbite features a circumscribed inflammatory skin swelling. The cold initiates a primary contraction of cutaneous blood vessels resulting in pallor. In reaction, the vessels dilate and the area becomes red and swollen, producing a sensation of "burning" pain. White blood cells become disintegrated and liberate a coagulating substance, encouraging thrombosis in peripheral vessels. This impairs circulation along with the spastic ischemia. In mild cases, local signs subside within a few days. In some cases, the erythema may persist for several weeks or may return sharply under the slightest exposure to cold. This hypersensitivity (chilblain or pernio) that develops in a person previously frostbitten presents local areas of congestion which may become inflamed and even ulcerated. This ulceration is often initiated by exercise or exposure to heat, causing itching and stinging sensations.

Severe Frostbite and Gangrene

It is possible for gangrene to develop after exposure even if the temperature is above freezing. Thrombi may remain for weeks or months after exposure and be widespread in the skin and subcutaneous tissues, inducing "late" gangrene. Third-degree frostbite features a blue, marbled, coriaceous skin with vesicle development on the injured area. The area is anesthetic to touch, with pain at the early stage, later progressing to necrosis or mummification and deepening, offering the typical characteristics of dry gangrene. However, if a severely frozen part is suddenly warmed, the resulting hyperemia may produce moist gangrene rather than dry gangrene. If tissue destruction is severe, precautions against dry gangrene, thrombosis, and secondary infection must be taken and professional referral sought.

Hypothermia

When oral temperature falls below 98°F (hypothermia), it signifies a subnormal temperature such as that which commonly occurs immediately after the fall of fever by crisis. It is observed in athletes in cold shock and collapse. In prolonged exposure to cold, the individual may die from exhaustion from shivering rather than from the hypothermia. Shivering, alone, can increase metabolic work as much as 50%. Intrinsic clinical hypothermia results whenever the central nervous system is depressed from drugs, primary brain disease, or toxins that alter the thermostat.

Cold Exhaustion

When rectal temperature falls below 95°F, you can be sure that cerebral and muscular function is being impaired. This is the multiple effect of the decreasing core temperature, exhausted glycogen stores, and reduced blood-sugar level. Cold syncope and collapse are commonly witnessed when an athlete overtaxes heat-sustaining mechanisms, must battle against strong wind factors, or attempts to keep an endurance pace with better conditioned players.

Nature's warning signs prior to syncope are muscle weakness and cramps, followed quickly by locomotor dysfunctions as witnessed by awkwardness, a slowed pace, and poor coordination or stumbling. There is always risk of circulatory, pulmonary, or kidney failure which may require immediate hospitalization. Death is imminent if rectal temperature falls below 90°F.

Predisposing Health Conditions

With many people, cold weather activity presents unusual hazards. Continued exposure to cold has been shown to increase the risk of heart block and pulmonary hypertension in mouth breathers. Infarction may result during exercise, especially isometric, leading from myocardial oxygen deficiency, as seen in an unfit person who shovels heavy snow. People with peripheral vascular problems such as Raynaud's disease or past frostbite are particularly vulnerable to chilblains and frostbite during winter activities. Subjects with subclinical angina or coronary sclerosis tend to have increased symptoms during cold weather. This is partly explained by the oxygen costs from the weight of heavy clothing, the metabolic energy spent in shivering, the hypertensive reactions to cold, and the increased movement difficulty in snow. The inspiration of extremely cold air may so stimulate bronchial nerve endings as to induce a reflex coronary spasm or at least induce bronchiospasm or bronchitis. This is especially true in subjects with an underlying airway or pulmonary disorder.

ALTITUDE AND PHYSICAL ACTIVITY

The typical athlete utilizing maximum effort at sea level has little difficulty in maintaining full arterial oxygenation, but as higher altitudes are attained, unsaturation becomes progressively greater.

Altitude Adaptation

Strict criteria for safe activity are difficult to arrive at, as much is governed by the time alloted for acclimation, the type of activity, the environmental temperature, the intensity of effect, and the individual's state of general health and physical fitness. Diffi-

culties at high altitudes arise more with the aerobic energy-demanding endurance events than the explosive anaerobic activities. In the latter category, performance diminishes because of the accumulated effect of a series of events. At high altitudes, recovery is slowed and fatigue accumulates faster. Once acclimation takes place, lactate utilization is enhanced to speed the rate of recovery after exhaustion.

While impractical for the traveling athlete, full acclimation to a high altitude may take several months. From 3–4 weeks are recommended by Olympic physiologists. Yet, a loss of plasma fluid is seen after about 3 weeks that appears to offer the unacclimated athlete some advantage. During the acclimation period, more frequent and longer rest periods are necessary. After acclimation, an increase in heart rate and ventilation help to compensate for thin air. Other functional adaptations to high altitude include an increased hemoglobin concentration and red cell count to compensate for decreased oxygen saturation, increased myoglobin, increased tissue enzyme activity, reduced tissue bicarbonate levels, and a return to normal blood volume.

Health Concerns

When an athlete enters a new environment, whether it be one of heat, cold, altitude, or underwater, the whole body (structurally, physiologically, emotionally) is affected. The physician's concern must be holistic and not focused entirely on a particular function. For example, ventilation is just as important to the long-distance runner as his leg strength; thermal capability is just as important to a channel swimmer as his stroke.

Predisposing Health Conditions

The effects of a subclinical anemia, angina, or epilepsy may manifest at high altitudes while not apparent at lower altitudes. Any person with an oxygen transport disorder will be stressed at altitudes near or over 8,000 feet. This height may be critical in advanced heart failure, sickle cell anemia (splenic rupture), or chronic lung disease within a weekend athlete. The risk of cerebral hypoxia and cardiac arrhythmias increases greatly with only slight reduction of arterial saturation. Cerebral hypoxia features neuromuscular malcoordination and impaired color vision often associated with central scotoma.

Pulmonary Edema

Potentially fatal pulmonary edema becomes a risk between 8,500–12,000 feet, especially when exertion is prolonged in cold weather. It usually develops within 36 hours of reaching the new altitude. The picture is one of rapid flooding of lungs, usually initiated by severe exertion. Typical clinical signs are those of intense acute dyspnea, loose cough, hemoptysis, nausea and vomiting, x-ray evidence of intense pulmonary congestion, and an ECG indicating right ventricular strain. The lung congestion is encouraged by the increased total blood volume, increased left ventricular pressure resulting from diminished oxygen to the myocardium, peripheral arterial vasoconstriction resulting from carbon dioxide washout, increased pulmonary capillary permeability, pulmonary venous constriction resulting from low alveolar oxygen pressure, and pulmonary hypertension resulting from previous exposure. Hospitalization is often required for bed rest, oxygen, and prevention of secondary infection.

WATER-RELATED ACTIVITIES

The bacterial content of pools and potential safety hazards around swimming areas must be monitored regularly.

Drowning

Even for the experienced swimmer, a life jacket during any boating activity is a necessary precaution. Especially in cold water, swimming is adversely affected by taut muscles, disturbed judgment and orientation, reflex hyperventilation, impaired proprioception, viscous muscle tissue, and inhibited sensory receptors of the skin. Drowning is defined as suffocation due to immersion in water or another liquid. It differs from other types of suffocation in that some water is swallowed and a small amount is aspirated. A victim offers a picture of being pale, limp, livid, cold, with staring and lusterless eyes, dilated pupils, and with water running out of the nose and mouth. Other features include unconsciousness or semiconsciousness, severe dyspnea, rapid and feeble pulse, indistinct or absent heart beat, distended abdomen, and loss of sphincter control.

Scuba Diving

Abnormal accumulation of carbon dioxide is unusual except for the scuba diver (Fig. 9.4). The word scuba is an acronym from Self-Contained Underwater Breathing Apparatus. This sport, requiring highly specialized training, is exceptionally demanding; such activity is a strict contraindication if the individual is suffering even a mild infection or disorder. The equipment contains a large variety of potentially dangerous hazards, thus it must be maintained in excellent condition.

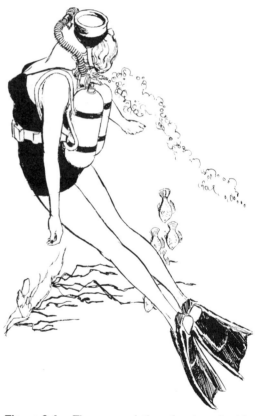

Figure 9.4. The accumulation of carbon dioxide is unusual except for the scuba diver due to the increased rate of carbon dioxide production, the decreased maximum voluntary ventilation, the added external equipment dead weight, and the possible inefficiency of the carbon dioxide-absorbing canisters.

During deep dives, special problems arise from sustaining thermal homeostasis, the physiologic alteration of gases, the changes in renal circulation, the psychosomatic reactions to stress, and the alteration in bacterial characteristics. Two dangers in deep dives are that nitrogen absorption may lead to euphoria resulting in recklessness and that improper ascent will quickly lead to decompression sickness ("the bends").

Skindiving and Snorkel Diving

Skindiving also presents unique hazards. Typically, a deep breath is taken before the person goes underwater. With training, underwater distance and depth can be attained. But this is dangerous in the unexperienced as the initial hyperventilation produces both a hyperoxia of the blood and a hypocapnia of the lungs. The idea is that the exertion will change the state to one of hypoxia aind hypercapnia. Tragedies also occur from hypoxic loss of consciousness as a result of the volitional drive to suppress breathing coupled with a level of hypercapnia which fails to stimulate a respiration urge. During even momentarty unconsciousness, water inhalation is inevitable.

Snorkel tubes provide a short airway from mouth to surface and are used to conserve cylinder air when near the surface and to allow a skindiver to view underwater for long periods. If a youngster uses adult equipment, he may repeatedly inspire and expire the same air until unconsciousness occurs.

Cold Water Hazards

Boating during the cooler months and snowmobiling, ice fishing, or skating across thin ice present common hazards. Convection and conduction heat loss is much more rapid in water than in air. Exposure to water temperature near 40°F can be fatal within an hour; entering near-freezing water can be fatal within 15 minutes. Once exposed, the effects of exertion vary. Activity helps the endomorph, with his or her added layer of fatty insulation, to sustain heat reserves, but effort enhances heat loss for the ectomorph. Keeping the limbs close together as long as possible helps to conserve body heat.

ELECTRICAL INJURIES

Opinions differ as to the physiologic aspects of electrical injury. Some authorities feel that the primary cause of death is due to cardiac fibrillation, others believe respiratory failure is the essential cause, while others consider coagulation and other vascular changes to be effects of the heat itself rather than of electrical phenomena. Autopsy characteristically shows brain and cord hemorrhages along with ganglion cell chromatolysis. Within typical ranges, the higher the voltage, the greater the danger. But, for some reason, extremely high voltages (over 10,000 volts) appear to be less dangerous, if the subject recovers, than the middle levels.

CHAPTER 10

Psychodynamic Aspects of Athletics

Those who care for the athlete soon learn that an appreciation of applied psychology is as important in case management as is specific diagnosis, treatment, and rehabilitative procedures. Performance is the result of total fitness—genetic, structural, functional, and emotional. Psychology bridges the gap between biology and sociology. The mind and body cannot be separated functionally; one sympathizes when the other suffers. Because of this, as D. S. Butt shows, all too often what is found to be "true" in the physiologic laboratory is not true on the playing field.

The role of applied psychology is underscored throughout athletics. There are the psychologic aspects of athletic trauma, mental fatigue (the "burned out" athlete), emotions, acclimation, and will power—all require insight into human behavior. Only through such insight can those responsible provide a suitable environment in which human potential may find a large degree of fulfillment.

PERSONALITY

The interactions in sports between group-and-individual and individual-and-group offer a challenge to social psychologists, as does the mixture of inheritance, environment, goals, early programming, stimulus and response, experience, and role-playing to the behaviorist. Especially under the stress of sports, much can be revealed to the trained eye and ear when the brakes of inhibition are released through physical activity.

The Athletic Personality

Mischel points out that one's habits, attitudes, intelligence, programming, character, temperament, special aptitudes, self-image, perception of reality, basic will power, conditional motivation, stimulus response, and many other factors all combine to form one's unique personality. In general, we think of personality as an individual's most striking traits. Or, as Allport, we can view personality in the manner it calls forth positive or negative reactions from other people. Athletics offers one an opportunity to witness this uniqueness of others. Thus, in viewing the athlete's personality, insight must be gained of how the player views himself and others.

In contrast with much of general society, the athletic situation often presents a setting where one may openly express identification with group goals, gain status, exhibit unusual dedication, define sexuality, trick an opponent and receive applause, gain a release from routine behavior, and manifest a willingness to accept pain and express repressed hostility.

Pressure from fans and sportswriters offers the promise for unusual recognition, attention, and other ego-gratifying needs, as well as the risk of highly irate criticism, contempt, and shame. Unusual stimulation is received from the constant shifting from frustration to achievement, anger to joy, anxiety to hope, and dejection to thrill. Athletic competition demands the highest level of mind-body cooperation and requires this often in the face of potential pain and public humiliation.

Morgan shows that athletes in general, as nonathletes, have different personality structures and different psychic needs and thus require individualized attention and counsel both in human relations and training intensity/duration. However, though there is no conclusive evidence, there appears to be a similarity in psychologic profiles among high-level athletic performers. The danger here is one of insufficient evidence being used to make self-fulfilling prophecies. The tendency in most sports is toward extroversion, with the exception of long-distance runners, who tend to be introverted. Consistent high-level performance requires a high degree of emotional stability. Williams and Sperryn feel that the less successful athlete tends to be more depressed, anxious and confused and has less drive.

Women in Sports

Participation in sports activities, as shown by Pierce and Kuehnie, promotes self-fulfillment, self-confidence, status, a sense of personal limits, goal attainment, self-achievement, and self-esteem—traits that fathers have long encouraged their sons to learn on the playing fields and which liberated women are now expressing. Feelings of helplessness and dependency are lessened as the player learns to cope with problems independently and with personal assertiveness, courage, self-discipline, tenacity, and teamwork. Until recent years, few females have had this opportunity.

In general, female athletes have been shown to be lower in dominance and general anxiety traits. Kane feels this is probably due largely to a lack of opportunities to participate in sports. Traditionally, as shown by J. M. Williams, our culture has conditioned women to be passive, nonaggressive, social, and dependent rather than achievement-oriented. Yet, while environmental forces must be considered, genetic influences also have a profound effect on behavior in that they serve as a blueprint for personality development.

It has been shown that physical activity promotes health and longevity quantitatively and increases the quality of life by promoting better feelings of well-being and self-direction. There are considerable advantages during pregnancy. The body is in better tone, and the expectant mother is accustomed to exercise and the benefits of good conditioning. Exercise helps to maximize physical attractiveness and poise.

As more women are engaging in sports, many false assumptions have been put to rest. Pierce and Kuehnie show that exercise does not encourage a female to become more masculine in appearance or interest, nor does it alter sex drive or sexual preference.

Intelligence and Creativity

Intelligence is an important factor in a number of sports which require planning strategy, game plans, alternative actions, recognition of limitations, and competition data. Hunsicker brings out that the detailed preparation necessary for mountain climbing, scuba expeditions, and deep sea sailing certainly cannot be left to someone with questionable intelligence.

Game playing is not restricted to social human relations. Psychologic "one-upmanship" is an integral part of sports, from the coach's game strategy to the one-on-one player relationship during competition. This later point is just as relevant to heavy-contact sports such as seen with football and judo as it is with highly skilled sports such as the subtle conversational and body-language "psyching" aspects of golf, tennis, pistol shooting, and precision gymnastics. The more physical attributes are equalized, the more emphasis is placed on psychologic "games."

PERSONALITY ASSESSMENT IN ATHLETICS

Because so much emphasis is placed on physical performance, coaches and trainers have often been conditioned to assess player personality strictly through locomotor expression, according to Kenyon. This is but a silhouette-like approach which offers the same dangers as to appraise physiology by examining the superimposed structural shadows portrayed on an x-ray film. One cannot accurately measure the sculptor by examining the statue. On the other hand, the "objective" personality tests and profiles often used require a considerable degree of subjective appraisal. In spite of highly improved methods for analyzing personality, the evaluation of temperament, character, attitude, will power, and motivation is more "art" than "science." Such studies appear to be of interest to everyone concerned except the athlete.

There are three major means for measuring personality: (1) describing the interaction between a person and the environment by evaluating such aspects as needs, drives, ego hungers, instinct, desires, wishes, and the effected roles developed; (2) describing a person relative to the environmental forces acting upon him by measuring the effects of social and physiologic influences; and (3) describing a person relative to his basic traits by assessing those traits which appear to be typical of the human organism.

Profiling Instruments

Our personalities not only affect what type of sports we prefer but in what position we will do best (Fig. 10.1). For example, Straub states that baseball catchers are predominantly extroverted, while outfielders and long-distance runners are introverted.

Many tests are available to help assess maturity, motivation, leadership attributes, and sports preference. For instance, Dolan and Holladay point out that the "Thematic Apperception Test" helps to assess maturity through an index of interpersonal attitudes, self-image, and motivations. The "Athletic Motivation Inventory (AMI)" attempts to reveal latent traits which may influence physical performance. Highly subjective tests such as the Sixteen Personality Factor Test of the "Minnesota Multiphasic Personality Inventory" and the "California Psychological Inventory" attempt to measure personality relative to introversion, extroversion, dominance, etc.

At the secondary level of education, sociometric questionnaires such as "Cowell's Personal Distance Ballot" are sometimes used to determine a player's level of leadership (group standing), but such "popularity" assessment is difficult to equate with reaction to severe stress. The "Edwards Personal Preference Schedule" attempts to relate personal desire with the type of sport selected by evaluating needs for dominance, change, achievement, aggression, etc.

Also popular today are such analytical instruments as (a) the "IPAT 8-Parallel Form Anxiety Battery," which attempts to assess aspects of chronic anxiety; and (b) the "Catell 16 Personality Factor Test (16PF)," which attempts to assess such factors as acute self-assuredness vs apprehension, group dependency vs self-sufficiency, trust vs suspicions, shyness vs courage, etc. These tests offer good data, but not complete data, useful in planning preseason and pregame training.

ENVIRONMENTAL FACTORS

Athletics offer an environment to express or learn self-control, honesty, self-discipline, sociability, teamwork, self-confidence, co-operation, and many more admirable qualities. But to this day, we have not determined whether personality determines sports activity or if sports participation molds personality. Nor, as Ryan and Allman show, do we know whether competition enhances emotional stability or if competition is avoided by the less emotionally stable.

B. F. Skinner, the famous behaviorist, strongly believed that people are shaped by and react differently to varying environmental and situational influences. Thus, an athlete's on-field and at-home behavior may show little resemblance. On the other hand, R. B. Cattell and other trait theorists feel that behavior is stable regardless of environment; ie, nonaggressive people are passive in most everything. Modern training methods, the psychologic factors involved in acclimatization, clothing and protective gear within the environment, and even the behavior of spectators have profound psychologic implications.

The Training Rationale

In any type of serious athletic competition, practice and training are essential prerequisites. To keep in top competitive con-

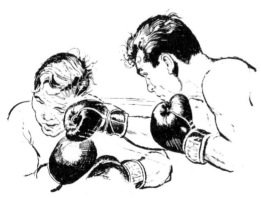

Figure 10.1. One's personality not only affects what type of sports are preferred, but in what position an individual will do best. Many factors, including the behavior of spectators, have profound psychologic implications upon performance.

dition, both boys and girls are engaging today in strenuous and time-consuming programs at younger and younger ages, in demanding interval running or swimming schedules, and in other developmental activities in addition to their usual practice sessions. There are always the questions of how much training is enough, how much training is in the best interests of the team and individual, how much of a young person's life should be devoted to narrow pursuits, and where is the line between adequate training and overtraining. Such questions deserve highly individualized answers.

Basic Training Principles

Four basic principles have been developed by Morehouse and Gross for learning a new skill: (1) The player must have a clear, vivid mental picture of what is to be accomplished. Improvement cannot be made if this image is faulty. (2) The player must come to terms with how far one's present skills will contribute to goal attainment; ie, new skills must be built on old skills previously developed. (3) Skills must be divided into specific components, and the player should start with those components already mastered. In tennis for example, a correct toss should be mastered before the entire service is practiced. (4) The practice speed of a movement component should be gradually made to approach that necessary in competition. The quantity of practice is not as important as its quality. What matters is to practice movements correctly.

Authoritarian Dominance

Many swimmers spend more than 5 hours a day in pool practice alone, and it is not unusual for runners to distance 200 miles/week. The question must be raised as to the effect of such intensive training on immature children and adolescents. A great deal of training favors obedience to authority instead of individual freedom, and youth is not invulnerable to dominance by authority figures (coaches, parents, idols, stopwatch). Intensive training certainly demands obsessional behavior, which replaces time for normal social growth, development, and flexibility.

Proper training should never overlook the need for mental conditioning to overcome the forces of individual self-doubt and apprehension. A peak of mental readiness, based upon eagerness and confidence, is essential for developing the necessary sense of purpose and team cohesion for top performance. Conversely, overtraining can dull an otherwise sharpened performance. Motivation requires a careful understanding of both individual needs and squad morale.

Monotonous Repetition

Stale performance can often be corrected by adequate rest and varying challenges. Many forms of training require many hours of repetitious labor, control by an inhuman stopwatch, and featureless regularity for which many people do not have an inexhaustible appetite. Such conventional training, for many, may degenerate from an initial stimulating experience to profound drudgery, reinforcing feelings of inadequacy and a negative self-image.

Doherty points out that many modern training programs are recognizing the need for a degree of variety, originality, exercise of free will, freshness, personal judgment, and liberty to personally respond to the environment and one's feelings so that a player may benefit from and enjoy the training regimen. One method, "Fartlek," is a speed/play ingredient of training towards such an objective. For example, an athlete is allowed to distance over varying terrain, preferably through beautiful woods and fields, where one may avoid hard surface injuries and respond to the natural challenges of hills and valleys by varying sprints, jogs, walks, strides, and pacing at personal judgment. Fartlek and other free-will training ingredients require a highly self-disciplined, self-motivated person who enjoys setting and achieving personal goals. A degree of self-pressure rather than authoritarian dominance is necessary to sprint up and coast down long inclines.

Socialized Training

School children have been shown by Morgan and Adamson to develop greater fitness during the summer break between semesters than while undergoing school physical education programs. From this fact has developed a form of exercise called "circuit training." In circuit training, a series of from 8–10 exercises, whose variety is limited only by the director's imagination, is done in sequence. During the first session of circuit training, each participant is judged on each exercise for the maximum number of repetitions determined either by time or by the point of exhaustion. This score obtained is divided by three to arrive at the individual's training rate for each exercise. At subsequent sessions, the participant completes three circuits of all prescribed exercises as fast as possible at the training rate. As training progresses, the time necessary to complete the circuits decreases, and adjustments can be made by increasing repetitions.

Circuit training has proved highly effective for teams, clubs, and indoor groups. Because of its competitive and sociable basis, a large number of people presenting wide ranges of fitness and capability are able to train as a group at individual rates. Here, self-competition as well as competition against one another in rate of progress provides a sociable means of motivation during physical and skill development.

Behavioral Modification

Behavior modification has been less applied in sports than in clinical settings. However, Nideffer's Attention-Control Program (ACT) and his "Test of Attentional and Interpersonal Style" have shown benefits in teaching a player to block out external stimuli (eg, the roar of hostile spectators at a road game) which interfere with performance.

Staub feels that data feedback to players has shown to be an effective means to increase performance in athletes. Objective information relative to good or poor aspects of performance via videotape or film help players to review past actions and plan a means to perfect execution. However, while "lessons" are necessary to teach fundamental techniques, Butt shows that only continual practice will develop timing, coordination, and skill.

Psychologic Factors in Acclimatization

Physical fitness does not constitute environmental fitness, nor do either constitute psychologic fitness. This is seen frequently when a team accustomed to one climate is quickly transported to another area and climate for competition. If a player presents an acceptable health status, heat- or cold-related disorders can be prevented by gradual acclimation (7–10 days) to weather conditions and careful monitoring of water and mineral intake. But these dutiful concerns fail to consider the sundry psychologic adjustments necessary.

Arduous training is often associated with sleepless nights, leading to general fatigue. This readily impairs coordination, reaction time, vigilance, and other defense and skill-related mental mechanisms. Williams and Sperryn point out that this physical "down" is frequently coupled with a psychic "up"; that is, a new environment, unfamiliar surroundings, and an unaccustomed climate for the traveling athlete may easily overarouse an already excited player. The brain never rests.

The action of physiologic forces upon psychologic mechanisms, while known to be interrelated, are difficult to differentiate. This is readily brought out in the study of heat exhaustion. During mild heat exhaustion, circulatory inadequacies are exhibited by such physiologic symptoms as hot dry skin, flushed face, dry mouth with excessive thirst, reduced perspiration, muscle cramps, and scanty urine. Associated symptoms of dizziness, momentary blackouts, and fainting spells, along with hallucinations, visual disturbances, headache, nausea, backache, malaise, constipation, weakness, increased pulse rate, and quickened respiration are difficult to relate to specific physiologic or psychologic etiology. In addition, many purely psychologic reactions are witnessed such as loss of initiative, dulled alertness, lassitude, anorexia, inattention, and irritability. If left uncorrected, Syndham and Strydom show that a chronic neurosis may result (heat neurasthenia), characterized by apathy, hysteria, or marked irrational aggression towards other contestants or officials. All these signs and symptoms express a biologic cry for help.

Clothing, Protective Gear, and Equipment

Garments can be considered an environmental factor inasmuch as they are perceived by the senses. The functions of proper athletic clothing and gear are to enhance performance and protect the wearer and opponents, but such attire also has certain psychologic influences. Adrian explains that if an athlete feels safe with certain inferior equipment, he or she will be more apt to move with greater force and speed to accomplish a goal than would be wise. There is also another psychologic effect with attire: if an athlete feels no clothing or equipment binding or restriction, or believes they allow for effective movements, then he or she will perform in a more effective, efficient manner.

It has been shown by Butt to be a misconception that minor changes in equipment alters athletic performance. Once equipment reaches an acceptable level of quality, minor changes such as a steel tennis racket or an expensive pair of sneakers have little effect. Skill is the final determination. However, this would not be the case where, for example, a pair of soccer boots with longer studs than normal for foul weather play may well be the facilitating factor for skillfully carrying out a task.

BEHAVIORAL CHARACTERISTICS

It has been estimated that coaches and trainers spend more than 50% of their professional lives in an attempt to develop or reinforce character qualities which would improve performance in athletic activity. The peculiarities involved are underscored by taking an overview of the human being in an athletic setting that would include the common anxiety-coping mechanism applied and the emotional stability requirements.

Character Traits

The term "character" refers to any consistent and enduring property or quality by means of which a person can be identified. One's character, portrayed in behavior, is deeply embedded within the personality structure. Chaplin believes it to be the effect of one's emotional adjustment; the effect of thoughts and feelings. It taxes a player's fortitude to make continual decisions under stress which affect others as well as self, and these decisions are influenced by sundry needs, attitudes, beliefs, and condi-

tioned responses. For all practical purposes, one's character is exhibited by those choices made which affect the welfare of others.

Due to the nature of sports competition, several personality traits are highly desirable. Ogilvie and Tutko point out that all athletes at one time or another entertain doubts as to self-ability and performance which may interfere with player or team effectiveness. Thus, the influence of assertiveness, fortitude, drive, determination, leadership, and maturity are special concerns (Fig. 10.2).

Will Power

It takes a strong will to train, to practice, to follow rules, to follow the trainer's advice or the doctor's recommendations. Dolan and Holladay state that when an athlete's will is weak, the defect may manifest as irritability, obstinancy, vacillation, and/or precipitation. Irritability is featured in the player with habitual discontentment, pessimism, and frequent signs of hypochondriasis. The obstinate player can be neither persuaded or advised, must have an audience to express his self-assertions, and is a chronic complainer. Vacillation in the athlete is characterized by chronic indecisive-

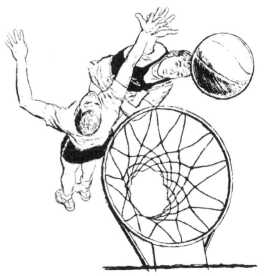

Figure 10.2. An athlete's drive is the goal-directed intensity necessary to be competitive, to comply with strenuous training, to set achievement goals, and to maintain fortitude and trust in teammates and coaches in the face of failure.

ness, hesitant acts, being easily swayed by the actions of others, and by easily falling to temptations to break rules. Aboulia is extreme vacillation where a sympathy-requiring, problem-treating individual offers no resistance to a suggestion, finding it always easier to agree rather than disagree with an impractical idea. Precipitation features impulsive rashness, hasty acts, and impatience with procedures. The greatest physical enemies of will are fatigue and poor health, while the psychologic factors include overstimulation, a lack of knowledge (confidence), immature value judgments, and low drive and determination. Motives must be optimistic and strong enough to produce action, if not for self, then for the squad.

Morale

Rather than being a general personality trait where one athlete has a large quantity and another player has a small quantity, morale is the effect of one's relationship with a particular job or life requirement. If morale is high, a player usually knows his objectives, believes they are worthwhile, thinks they are obtainable, and feels others will consider the goals chosen important. High morale fortifies perserverence and determination to see a job through even if the going is difficult. When morale is high, people are more inclined to want to do what has to be done (eg, pushing on when muscles ache). When morale is low, people have little confidence that they can cope with what the future may bring.

Morale in athletics involves self-satisfaction, zeal, self-confidence, and self-discipline. Self-satisfaction frees one from worry and provides fulfillment in carrying out routine assignments. Zeal is the zest to give more than lip service to policies, rules, and regulations. Self-confidence, based on training and experience, lends a realistic sense of personal worth and the self-esteem necessary to get the job done. Self-discipline is necessary to place personal goals subordinate to team goals and to undertake strenuous training sessions.

Emotional Stability

In addition to the development of a healthy, physically fit body, physical vitality promotes intellectual vitality, and tolerance to frustration promotes emotional stability. The athletic personality offers a challenge to the physician in that the stress involved in the evolving athlete often offers predictable consequences.

Aggressive and Nonaggressive Behavior

The attending doctor should be aware of the numerous social and emotional pressures which direct a player in his or her striving for sacrifice, self-discipline, teamwork, dedication, and the willingness to bear mental and physical pain. The repercussions of stress are frequently recognized as aggressive behavior towards teammates, management, or officials. Some personalities thrive on conflict with authority figures.

Performance "staleness" is a form of depression. The physician often finds himself with the opportunity of offering support to players having difficulty in coping with the stress and emotional demands of competition. The doctor's role as "confidant" can do much to reduce such psychologic stress. The tension generated in young athletes facing competition in front of an audience is tremendous. Carstairs feels that the highly trained athlete is often as delicately tuned as a race horse and can become easily hypochondriac about minor disorders because of preoccupation with physical fitness during training.

Athletic Euphoria Vs Dysthymia

Coaching leadership is constantly trying to promote morale. With good morale, emotional crises can be faced courageously, with zest. High levels of morale are called euphoria, while low levels are called dysthymia, characterized by despair, panic, and feelings of hopelessness where struggle appears futile. Both the athletic coach and the military commander realize the high value of personnel morale and a esprit de corps. A good "team spirit" can make boring practice seem a joyful experience, something that counts and is worthwhile.

Sports euphoria, the "we are number one" syndrome, is characterized by feelings of happiness, thrill, well-being, adventure, hope, excitement, and exceptional skill, as seen in a team's "rally" or spirit to "upset" a favored competitor or to fight on in spite of "bad breaks." The effects of such euphoria are witnessed with an athlete playing beyond his or her usual performance, the baskteball player's "shooting streak," the baseball player's "hitting streak," or a team playing with rare levels of enthusiastic cooperation.

The feelings of euphoria are commonly associated with those situations which promise both joy (potential pleasure) and danger (potential pain); eg, combat with a stronger opponent, parachuting, mountain climbing, high-wire acrobatics, and auto racing. Such relief of surplus energy is often seen in euphoria-seeking drug addiction, postgame fan demonstrations, mob actions, and acts of terrorism. Contrary to popular belief, it has been shown by Goldstein that aggressive sports increase viewer hostility.

A prolonged period of euphoria (winning streak) or performance nearing a record may turn euphoria into a state of athletic dysthymia (slump) because of the increasing pressures of anxiety, along with the knowledge that there is only one way to go from "up." Or, boredom may be the triggering mechanism.

Dysthymia is characterized by feelings of inhibition, painful stress, inadequacy, fear, depression, or "burn out." The effects of dysthymia are witnessed with the professional golfer who misses short putts or the team highly prone to unusual fouls and errors. The shocking upset between supposedly unequal teams is often attributed to the favored team being in a state of dysthymia while the "underdogs" are in a state of euphoria.

The lower an individual's intelligence and the lower the level of maturity, the greater potential for low morale and dysthymia because it takes intelligence and maturity to cope with frustration. It is not uncommon for the child or the childish athlete faced with personal criticism, public humiliation, or defeat to react by projecting blame to others, having temper tantrums, exhibiting sulking self-pity behavior, seeking nurturing personalities, or having a malingering illness or an injury.

Attempts to reduce player tensions and raise the anxiety level by "psyching up" athletes must be used with extreme caution and then only on an individual basis. Highly publicized "pep talks" show no conclusive evidence of improving performance during competition, as little difference has been shown between the anxiety levels of winning or losing teams. Any "psyching up" of athletes before competition will be readily lost because exercise itself reduces anxiety.

EMOTIONAL PROBLEMS IN ATHLETICS

Hanning feels that intellectual grounds for behavior are often overemphasized rather than the psychologic causes rooted in feelings and emotions. We often look for or accept a seemingly healthy athlete's situation at its face or intellectual value and thus eliminate some emotion that is so closely attached to the intellect that it could not function properly without it.

Studies reported by Williams and Sperryn show that emotional "first aid" is just as important following competition as is physical first aid. It is important for a coach to talk to his players after a game to allow for a return to normal psychic function. Naturally, egos must be strengthened in the case of a loss, but insulation must also be extended to average players who have exhibited a high-level performance.

Basic Emotional Processes in Sports

The word "emotion" comes from the Latin term meaning to "stir up." Our "feelings" are reactions to sensations (eg, pleasure, pain) that influence our attitude; ie, feelings and emotions influence the athletic attitude and give one's efforts significance. Pain or displeasure is the result of an individual being out of harmony with his environment.

Emotions cause ductless secretions which can bring about physiologic changes in the body over which the power of reason has little control. Will power rather than reason is the best answer to emotional control. In sports, complex voluntary movements are constantly applied to realize wishes and satisfy desires, and these movements are influenced by emotions built upon past experiences. All emotional reactions are expressed through some physiologic process which results in some type of systemic change (eg, respiratory, cardiovascular, neuromuscular). The mind performs as the emotions dictate.

One generally accepted definition of emotion states that an emotion consists of a mental grasp of a situation as good or bad, pleasant or unpleasant, accompanied by movements of the rational and sense appetites and bodily changes. The basis of an emotion may be an immediate object or situation in an athlete's environment, or it may be something recalled from memory or fantasized. Regardless of its origin, the effects are the same.

In general, emotions are a process of psychic conditioning and displacement. From a psychologic standpoint, a conditioned reflex is one which has been so modified by individual experiences that it may be elicited by a stimulus that ordinarily would not give rise to it. Freud felt that displacement consists of a distortion of emphasis or a means whereby fictitious values are ascribed.

The excitement connected with a "winning" season or adherence to the entire program of training/practice can only be explained on the basis of emotion. During the emotional process, the intellect interprets an object or situation and (a) makes a judgment as to whether the event promises pleasure or pain under the circumstances and (b) evaluates the difficulties to be met with in obtaining what is desired. After this initial interpretation, organic, glandular, and/or locomotor alterations are produced by the thought process and an act of will to create an emotion.

When a player is heavily swayed by emotion, habitual stability for rational judgment is altered. Although intelligence is required to create an emotion, the athlete under emotional sway operates essentially on the sensory plane, becoming a victim of feelings of pleasure and pain, where will and intellect become disassociated from the practicalities which direct the activity. The fading of an emotion is regretted if the associated feeling is pleasurable.

Conflicts and the Unconscious

Petersen relates that emotional disorders due to unresolved conflicts have anxiety as their chief characteristic. In athletics, an individual with an emotional disorder may compete adequately, but performance is shadowed by fears, anxieties, or obsessions.

As Dolan and Holladay point out, many decisions in sports are made at the conscious level, but when a problem becomes complex, the resolution of conflict involves many forces in the unconscious mind. While conflict and frustration are universal, they play an exaggerated role in the life of the neurotic athlete, and this is probably due to the factor of public exposure. Athletic errors are not hidden behind office doors.

Repression, sublimation, projection, and conversion, once unconsiously adopted, are the ego's attempt to resolve conflicts. They show up most clearly in the neurotic individual where the conflicts are greatest. It must be kept in mind that what is vocalized by a player is not necessarily an expression of his conscious or unconscious motives.

Image Development and Body Language

Like most people during stress, an athlete under pressure tends to group images and build concepts which are emotionally tinged ideas and judgments. Such complexes tend to establish fixed patterns in behavior as they influence thinking and actions. Under such conditions, there is an overabundance of feeling and an underabundance of rational thinking. In this manner, emotions beget new combinations of images, generate complexes, and influence the everyday life of the individual. One's mental associations are always a part of an intricate mass (image) of other associations which both influence others and receive influences from others. They do not occur in isolation within the personality.

A good idea of how completely a player has entered the situation can be gained by watching body reactions. The emotional response is a total measurement of mind, will, and body (including the endocrine system and all its ramifications). An athlete's overenthusiastic emotions may alter his psychic approach (perceptions, values) to training, practice, or competition. When under the influence of "hot" emotions, a situation appears different from that which is led by "cold" intelligence.

Emotional tension is almost always manifested as muscle tension and further characterized by anxiety-adrenal reactions such as an increase in pulse and respiratory rates. The palms and plantar surfaces of the feet are cool and moist. Axillary sweat increases. The glance is darting and suspicious, the speech is staccato, the fingers are fidgety, the laugh is nervous, the smile is forced, responses are short, sharp, sarcastic, and frequently angry. A player with high tension usually sits tensely on the edge of the bench with muscles taut, ready to act at a second's notice.

Behavior is rarely fully rational: it is habitually emotional. We may speak wise words as the result of intelligent reasoning, but our entire being reacts to feeling. And for every thought supported by feeling, there is a muscle change. Primary muscle patterns are the biologic heritage of man: man's whole body records his emotional state at the moment. Our entire mental and emotional equipment, temperament, personal experiences and prejudices are utilized in self-expression, influencing and directing the relationship of body parts to the whole. This equipment includes the working unit for motion—the nerve-muscle action on bones. Our osseous structures are much more than nature's coat racks from which to hang muscles and tendons, they play an important role in our sense of control and position in our environment. How we center them determines our degree of self-possession, and they are continually being centered and ex-centered in our rhythm of movement. Mechanically, physiologically, and psychologically, the human body is compelled to struggle for a state of equilibrium.

Emotional Adjustment in the Athlete

Those involved in sports sooner or later must interact with a poorly integrated personality who is easily overwhelmed by the pressures behind internal conflict. Such immaturity is seen in the unstable individual who expresses alternating pendulum-like mood swings of euphoria and dysthymia. Most athletic competition requires constant control of frustration from either or both physical (injuries) or emotional factors (unresolved conflicts).

Maturity Level

The immature athlete cannot realistically appraise his own assets and liabilities, is overly demanding of himself and others, and is easily overcome by frustration. States of sudden, intense feelings can easily drown out rational thoughts. When mental organization is confused by warring impulses, such a dysthymic player can neither participate in a euphoric rally nor react to an opponent's rally with intelligence. This state, called "sports neuroticism," is characterized by overreaction to stimuli, overt hit-or-miss performances, or being overwhelmed by the impasse of seemingly unresolvable choice. What to reasonably do cannot be answered by a player engulfed in and controlled by supervening pressures from ballooning doubts and fears.

In addition to an individual's capacity to tolerate frustration, maturity levels in athletes can be measured by an individual's level of self-set goals relative to ability. It can be readily recognized that moderate ability coupled with high aspirations is conducive to frustration stress. High aspirations to excel in one position may jeopardize a successful career at another position unless the individual has the maturity to adapt desires to abilities or team needs. Immaturity is also seen in the success-avoiding personality who sets goals far beneath his potential and is content with a "lazy" mediocre level of performance. An athlete with a high level of maturity will arrive at a compromise between aspirations (self-demands) and team needs (team/coach demands).

Emotionally Disturbed Behavior

Somatovisceral and viscerosomatic reflexes and their influence upon near or distant visceral or somatic structures are often overlooked. Such reflexes have an effect on both somatic structures and the psyche. It is one thing to determine whether a definite emotional problem exists and another thing to determine the cause of the mental disorder. Psychiatric referral should not be considered until a thorough history and examination has been completed because the mental disorder may be an effect rather than a cause. Treatment and referral will be determined by the severity of functional disturbance and the availability of psychiatric or psychologic consultation.

The overuse of alcohol and drugs is so prevalent in this country today, and at increasingly lower age levels, that these factors cannot be overlooked. Such substances may be at the root of many complaints—physical, functional, or emotional.

The Also-Rans

To achieve championship status, Astrand and others feel that genetic factors account for as much as 94% of the physiologic variance between the "good" player and the "superstar." While skill has an influence on efficiency, body type places a finite limit on achievement goals which may produce emotional disturbances. Every team offers more "bench warmers" than "stars." It is sometimes obvious that a young athlete's ability is clearly limited and realized both within and among peers. Although such an athlete may never attain "first string" status, and without the promise of common motivational reward, self-imposed continual striving and dedication is of the highest order. Hirata reminds us that these players, the vast majority of nonprofessional athletes, deserve profound empathy for what is called "guts."

Suppression, Repression, and Denial

Suppression, states Chaplin, refers to the conscious awareness of inhibiting thoughts from consciousness which are not compatible with one's self-evaluation at the moment. This is the essence of concentration. As the mind can only be conscious of one thought at a time, to be alert to the situation at hand we must suppress thoughts which are not pertinent to the situation. During athletic competition, thoughts of flight, delay, family affairs, social desires, financial yearnings, minor aches and pains, reverie, etc, must be suppressed. Trainers and physicians learn to develop will power to suppress and hide the physical expression of their emotions, and by so doing, feelings become extinguished because passion is nourished and strengthened by gestures. A doctor's picture of calmness is necessary to ease emotional reactions and avoid hysteria on the part of an injured person. It is impossible to reason with a person engulfed in emotion.

Repressed thoughts are those we involuntarily and unconsciously put out of our awareness. Thoughts which may threaten one's security (eg, those of guilt, embarrass-

ment, pain, shame) may be held back from consciousness if they become too unbearable to face. The more highly a thought is distasteful to consciousness, the more tendency there is towards repression (automatic forgetfulness) and towards a higher level of intensity. While a repressed thought is beyond conscious awareness (forgotten), it remains operative within the subconscious. To maintain a state of health, these temporarily repressed thoughts must be expressed at the feeling or action level or they may manifest as symbols psychosomatically or as antisocial behavior. Psychic energy cannot be destroyed, only transferred (conversion). Repression is a valuable tool in athletes. Without it, personal whims and prejudices would be followed rather than game rules. Animal instincts would run rampant. If many unacceptable thoughts were not "buried," the result might lead to penalties, fines, or removal from competition.

Denial is a form of repression where one becomes totally oblivious of an obvious deficiency. In denial, a person fails to see, hear, or touch reality. This is an unhealthy mechanism often witnessed in strong-willed athletes. It is seen in the athlete who plays with such excruciating pain that damage develops to an extent he can never play again. It is seen in the coach who becomes so obsessed with winning that he sees only the hoped-for performance and not that of an injured player. When reality is denied in conditioning, practice, training, competing, treatment, or rehabilitation, appropriate corrective action cannot be taken; and when it is, it is often too late.

Anxiety/Depression States

Anxiety may be defined as a state of apprehension, tension, or uneasiness stemming from an anticipated danger that is largely unknown. Depression manifests subjective feelings of sadness, unhappiness, "sinfulness," and often hopelessness. Little pleases or gives pleasure to the depressed person. In differentiation, anxiety is future-oriented and associated with fear and helplessness. Depression is past-oriented and associated with guilt and hopelessness.

Functional Disturbances

Sympathetic nervous system symptoms

of the fight-or-flight adrenaline reaction are prominent in anxiety. The depressed patient has "given up." Both syndromes may be exhibited by the same athlete at different times. Several features help in differentiation. A player with chronic anxiety is often underweight and has a poor appetite, while obesity and overeating is more common in chronic depression. The anxiety-prone patient usually has trouble getting to sleep, while the depressed patient has trouble staying asleep. Vegetative functional disturbances are also frequently associated, and the intensity of symptoms offers a general clue to the severity of the emotional disturbance involved. In assessing vegetative disturbances, care must be used in ruling out other causes for these problems. An emotional problem may be the major cause for the disturbance, or it might be superimposed upon a functional or organic condition.

Infections

Depression, commonly associated with viral diseases, is especially undermining to an athlete because of his or her constant restlessness to return to heavy training. Williams and Sperryn remind us that the team physician may have a problem with an athlete recovering from mononucleosis, for example. Although the player may feel "ready" and most signs appear normal, frustration often arises with early fatigue. Thus, state Dolan and Holladay, long-term competition should be entered slowly until stamina increases to meet the demands.

An athlete returning to activity after an episode of infection may have an abnormal tendency towards hyperventilation, especially if there is an inclination towards an overly anxious personality. It results from an excessive expiration of carbon dioxide which reduces the normal levels that act upon respiratory centers.

Accident Proneness

A list of athletic injuries in any school during the chosen period of years will reveal that a large percentage of accidents appear among a small percentage of students. Most players prone to accidents present certain basic traits: they tend to live in the immediate present, are shy, and concentrate on immediate pleasures without thought of consequences. There is a relative indifference to potential hazards and a high degree of impulsiveness. Dolan and Holladay report that such students tend to be deeply religious and honest, but rebellious, have poor self-discipline, and present either a low toleration for authority or overconcern about their relationship with authority. Tension is chronic due to preoccupation with health status, exhibited in food fads and unusual "conditioning" programs. They crave excitement and constant stimulation, yet have difficulty in developing warm relationships, and are frequently socially frustrated.

SEXUAL AND MENSTRUAL INFLUENCES

In addition to hormonal abnormalities and medical interference with normal development, the sex of an individual can be disturbed psychologically. While homosexuality appears to have little impact, transvestitism complicates performance. Players who seek athletic competition to prove their sexuality are often those who have not firmly established their sexuality in the first place.

Although sex is usually readily determined by laboratory tests, a few people fall into an intersex zone which requires sympathetic handling. More than one sex test and often several different types of tests are required for the player (male or female) in this intersex zone.

The subject of sexual activity has been enriched through the years by mythical dogmas, social and religious morality concepts, and misled disciplines. There is no evidence to substantiate that a normal level of sexual intercourse, masturbation, or nocturnal emissions has a negative effect upon athletic performance, more so is the effect of associated guilt and anxiety. Deprivation of normal activity, report Williams and Sperryn, may do more harm than good. On the other hand, intensive training and competition have a tendency to temporarily decrease libido in some athletes.

Emotional changes are commonly witnessed with the female athlete during the menstrual cycle wherein there are considerable fluctuations in the level of intellectual and psychologic performance capacity.

INTERPERSONAL RELATIONS

In the middle of the stage—among player stress, coach stress, pressures from conditioning needs, health concerns, training requirements, and the variable frustration tolerances of the fans, the athletic department, the alumni, and the press—are the trainer and team physician who must develop their own method of listening, reacting, and coping (Figs. 10.3 and 10.4). While players and coaches may openly express much of their emotions, those involved in health care are rarely allowed such an outlet.

Physician and Trainer Pressures

The difference between athletes is often slight, but that slight difference may be vital. Games may be won or lost by a slight competitive edge in fractions of inches or seconds, a slight change in attitude or insight, or a last-minute rally in face of tremendous odds. To observe, appreciate, and develop the subtle physical, functional, and

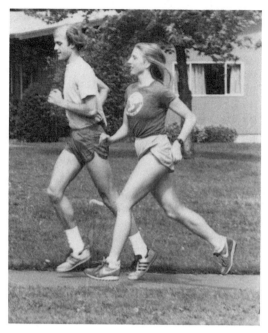

Figure 10.4. *Left*, Dean Clark, a student at Western States Chiropractic College and former track coach at Oregon State and Stanford Universities. *Right*, Dr. Margaret Karg, a competitor in the 1981 Boston Marathon (Photo by Paul M. Everson).

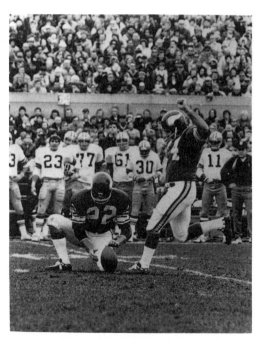

Figure 10.3. Dr. Fred Cox, place-kicker for many years for the Minnesota Vikings, is now a practicing chiropractic physician in Minnesota.

emotional differences of individuals is the mark of effective holistic health care and training. Just as a player with high aspirations and moderate ability can create a situation of chronic frustration, a coach or trainer may become perplexed with a player who sets low goals and is content with performance far below potential.

Coping with Player Frustrations

Athlete anxieties are often expressed in an exaggerated form that would probably not be so bad in a less stressful situation. A player may portray rational, mature behavior at one moment and the temperament of a spoiled child at the next. Such personality switching, states Butt, is often the result of frustrated internal conflicts. This may be the product of critical fans and sportswriters, an overly demanding coach, a postinjury reaction, despair over genetic inabilities, frustrated aspirations, or a number of other factors.

Injury commonly produces player frustrations and anxieties which in turn influence behavior. Postinjury neurotic reactions may exhibit as behavioral changes such as emotional outbursts, feelings of helplessness and despondency, repeated failure or injury, hypersensitivity, and lowered self-esteem. Such frustrations may greatly prolong rehabilitation if left untreated. Chronic hypersensitivity, especially in the body-oriented athlete, may produce functional changes and conversion symptoms (eg, ulcers, hypertension).

Conflicts may arise from a player's desire for adventure and a coach's conservative game plan or between a player's moral values and a "win at any cost" admonition. An athlete's desire for "stardom" may be constantly weighed against a resented role as a cooperative member of a team.

Frustration may also manifest when a player becomes exasperated in competing against another with genetic advantages. For example, Dolan and Holladay relate that Bill Bradley, the superb basketball player, manifested a peripheral vision of 195° when 180° is considered perfect. He could look straight up 70° when 47° is considered perfect and look straight down 70° when 65° is considered perfect.

It has been said that the average person has about seven anomalies, and each may add or subtract from optimal physical performance. About 65% of people have three branches coming off the aorta, 27% have two, and 8% have one branch or as many as four, five, or six branches. Respiratory patterns vary widely, especially in timing and amplitude. Muscles often attach differently in different people, allowing for a mechanical advantage or disadvantage. In one study, only 18% of the athletes checked presented the "normal" temperature of 98.6°F; most were found within a 97–100° range. Dolan and Holladay report that temperature rise during activity can vary as much as 7° among healthy athletes.

Spectator Behavior and Its Influence

There is no doubt that an emotional similarity exists between the modern athletic arena and the men-at-arms events held in ancient coliseums and on jousting fields.

Crowd Effects on Spectator Behavior

The role of the "cheerleader" is twofold: to entertain the crowd and to keep pressure on the players by fanning heated emotions of the spectators. What is generally left unsaid is that aggressive sports stimulate viewer hostility. And there appears to be no difference in the perception of violence among athletic and nonathletic subjects, according to Finn.

Relief of surplus energy is sometimes expressed in society with euphoria-seeking spectator demonstrations, mob actions, and acts of terrorism. Both war and athletics tend to release primitive passions normally held in check by a most thin veneer of civilized restraint. Blood pulsates within the enthusiastic fan in cadence with the blare of the band, the name-calling, the uniforms, the pomp and ceremony, the animated cheering, the potential for supremacy. People tend to act differently when within a crowd. It appears that the crowd offers the vehicle for many repressed individuals to release their tensions by temporarily going crazy together.

Behavior of an unruly crowd is often a progressive ritual: it starts with curiosity about the opposition, turns to amusement, and evolves to crude jokes and ridicule. This progresses to bantered insults and angry shouts. When a highly approved foul is made or a blow is struck which members of the crowd unconsciously wished to strike themselves, a cause is created for individuals most casually related to defend some "principle." Fortunately, most spectators have a greater degree of self-control. When a person intensely identifies with a team, the success of that team gives the person something to brag about. It becomes a symbolic mechanism to enhance self-importance, and that mechanism must be defended.

Crowd Effects on Player Performance

Spectators also have an effect on player performance, and many athletes reflect the lowest denominator of the mob. Some players before spectators and some fans within a crowd lose their sense of reality: play takes on a sense of mysterious importance. The mature athlete develops a personalized mechanism to filter-out much of the reactions of the crowd.

Fickle emotions govern player or coach approval or condemnation. That is, to many fans, an athlete's reputation is never established; it is continually on trial. An injured player is enthusiastically applauded when he returns to combat with suppressed agony, mediocre jokes produce hilarity, a routine goal is widely applauded, and an error is never forgiven during this moment of euphoric escapism.

PSYCHODYNAMIC ASPECTS OF COMMON SKIN DISORDERS

Weiss and English emphasize that the skin, like the eye, is an organ of expression; and the skin, like the eye, is important as a point of contact between the inner and outer worlds. The common phenomena of sweating, blushing, and pallor express anger/excitement, embarrassment, and fear. Yet, beyond these are definite skin manifestations which may express behavioral reactions of an emotional nature.

In dermatology as with most specialities, there is a tendency to seek singular causes. Stokes points out that this sole cause-effect attitude must ultimately give way to a veiwpoint which recognizes multiple causation and interrelations as equally fundamental if not more fundamental than the single, isolated case. Although the psychic rarely appears in dermatoses as a sole cause, this is not reason to believe that it is not a contributing or overlapping cause.

Acne

Acne has multiple causes, but its prevalence in adolescence suggests a factor in retarded emotional and psychosexual development. Sexual conflicts are often associated with profound guilt. In years past, the overly simple recommendation was to suggest marriage. Weiss and English report that acne in the female (rare) is often associated with menstrual disturbances; and the acne often improves as the menstrual disorder is treated. Thus, both endocrine and psychologic factors are probably involved. Severe acne in the athlete often produces a distinct inferiority complex (acne shock) which interferes with competitiveness such as in swimming and basketball. A T-shirt rather than an underwear-type of uniform is better to help hide the lesions in a baskteball player. If leg lesions are present, long socks help to hide as well as to protect both the skin and the ego.

Eczema and Herpes

The term "eczema" comes from the Greek word meaning to "boil over." The cause of eczema may be exogenous or endogenous. The more common causes are external irritants, especially with a person who has inherited sensitive skin. Yet, the skin of most people is potentially sensitive to an irritant after long and repeated exposure. Some researchers have closely related various types of eczema with neurosis. Herpes zoster (shingles) frequently indicates an emotional imbalance from worry added to a general fatigue.

Neurodermatitis

During high periods of anxiety in adult athletics, skin eruptions may be of a psychoneurologic origin. Hostility that cannot be expressed overtly may become self-directed (itching/scratching). Or, as Dolan and Holladay explain, an important game may be "played in the head" to such a degree that a variety of rashes will appear on some athletes before the starting whistle blows. However, many cases of neurodermatitis are misdiagnosed, and careful examination may reveal another previously undetected source for the disorder. Pruritus ani and pruritis vulvae, state Weiss and English, may be associated with guilt over an illicit, fantasied, or duty-bound affair and are often associated with a sexual malfunction.

Erysipelas

While erysipelas is active, the athlete's vision and timing are impaired (up to 3 months) to some degree, some balding may occur, and an associated personality apathy and listlessness are common. These symptoms may produce emotional instability. It usually takes an athlete about 6 weeks to recover his full competition strength, but the physical symptoms begin to ebb after 3 weeks.

Hyperhidrosis

Excessive sweating with a strong odor, as

seen in hyperhidrosis, frequently produces a negative self-image. The fetid odor (bromhidrosis) is the result of perspiration and cellular debris being decomposed by yeasts and bacteria. Berkow feels that hyperhidrois of the palms and soles is psychogenic. Generalized hyperhidrosis may have an endocrine, febrile, or brain basis.

Urticaria

In acute urticaria (hives, nettle rash), allergic factors are frequently clearly recognizable. However, in chronic situations, state Weiss and English, a case may be of multiple causation with important psychic components preceding attacks. Dolan and Holladay report that urticaria is sometimes associated with athletic emotional stress. The theory is that some psychic factor triggers the player's allergic equilibrium; thus it is important to investigate the possibility of anxiety symptoms of anger, excitement, fear, or depression, symptoms of guilt and despondency being related to the onset of the rash.

PSYCHOLOGIC INFLUENCES ON PHYSIOLOGY

While the limits of physical activity may not be set on psychologic effects, there is no doubt that there is a great interaction between psychologic and physiologic factors.

Motivation

There are as many degrees of motivation in athletics as there are players. While intelligence is largely determined genetically as a factor within personality structure, one's motivational level is generally considered an acquired result reflecting how the personality structure functions. Technically, motivation is an intervening attitude variable which is used to account for factors within a person which arouse, maintain, and channel behavior toward a goal. In sports, top-flight performance is paid for by practice time. Thus, Hunsicker feels that one of the most practical gauges of motivation is how much time a player is willing to donate to a long and arduous activity. As athletic participation can be considered a voluntary decision, other conscious options are always available.

While not unique to athletics, there is a distinctly unusual characteristic in sports toward a preparedness to face strong competitive aggression, to persistent determination in the face of pain and discouragement, to sacrifice safety to speed, and to subordinate personal glory to group goals in the team player. Motivation varies from mild to intense and is spurred by a wide number of factors such as love of the sport, social recognition, personal expression, challenge, power and dominance, need for group participation, social contact, a desire to excel, preoccupation with physical condition, financial rewards, or just a need for a break in routine. Regardless of its basis, a degree of motivation is always necessary for any voluntary action. Every movement begins as a thought and a decision to carry it out. Such a thought would be aborted if there were no motivation to carry out the act.

Performance is a function of skill plus motivation, and one's motivation is directly related to one's level of arousal to a point. It has been shown by Staub that performance increases as the level of arousal increases, until a optimal point is exceeded which causes performance to deteriorate. There is an optimal level of arousal for each task depending upon the specific person involved. Each player has an individual level of activation. Naturally, a high-precision task such as golf putting requires a much lower level of excitation than that necessary for football quarterbacking.

The primary source of motivation is believed by Butt to be derived from the id and manifested as assertive, aggressive, neurotic conflict, and competency motives. A secondary source is believed to come from internal (body feelings) or external environmental rewards (crowd approval).

The importance of motivation in strength performance has been clearly shown by Ikai and Steinhaus. By using artificial motivators, strength scores have been increased 7–12% by a shot being fired at the moment of attempt, using intravenous alcohol or using amphetamines. Scores have increased as much as 26% through hypnosis. Increased motivation added to the reassuring accumulation of practice and experience clearly reduces inhibitory restraints. This could be one of the factors involved in nonhypertrophic strength increase.

Cortical Stimulation and Restraints

There is evidence to support the possibility that a large degree of skill and athletic performance differences may be attributable to variations in personality structure. Ogilvie and Tutko feel this link between personality and performance is best explained through the mechanisms of arousal and especially through those factors which influence how stimuli are mediated and modulated through the arousal system. Thus, in this sense, personality may be interpreted as the state of arousal (anxiety).

The discharge pattern of the brain (reticular formation) is increased by environmental stimuli. This is reflected, as shown by Duffy, in the degree of anticipated necessary muscle tone, heart rate, respiratory volume, vigilance, timing, and wakefulness. This degree of "alertness" is readily witnessed in such high-skill actions as long basketball shots, pistol shooting, golf putting, and archery.

Both premature and excessive levels of cortical stimulation have negative effects on performance. When cortical arousal is premature, we see signs of hyperventilation, insomnia, and general fatigue; when it is excessive, poorly coordinated "jerky" movements and "frozen" body segments (eg, fear-inspired) are seen.

The release of extraordinary human potential under hypnosis or the stress of emergency situations shows that a large percentage of the variety of individual capabilities seen in people can be attributed to the quantity and quality of inhibitory impules arising from the cerebral cortex. In the athlete, a great deal of central inhibition is counteracted by the pressures of competition.

Reaction time

The brain can only process one fact at a time. Poulton points out that if cortical arousal is below optimum, the physical response is sluggish. On the other hand, if central stimulation is overaroused, the impulse (eg, a starter's signal) may be delayed by the "computerization" of irrelevant information. Reaction time is also modified by learning. If a response reaction is unfamiliar,

it must be processed through the larger alpha motor fibers. With the trained athlete, when most reactions are the effects of cumulative experience, the data are stored in the cerebellum, via gamma loop settings, and called into play as automatic responses. It has been shown that if a player concentrates on a starting signal (sensory set), a faster reaction time will be attained when he concentrates on the movement (motor set) to be performed.

When faced with threatening stimuli, the experienced athlete will learn to control the physiologic variables to a great extent. Thus, optimal performance varies with the degree of cortical stimulation, skill requirement, and personality. One of the more critical responsibilities of the coach is to manipulate the level of arousal of his players to an optimal level.

Ventilation

Williams and Sperryn report that psychologically limited ventilation has a distinct effect on limiting endurance, although the phenomena involved in "choking" and "second wind" are poorly understood. "Choking" is considered a result of excessive competition or poor pacing leading to early anaerobic demands on metabolism resulting in lactate accumulation, witnessed as a premature distressing hyperventilation. In the absence of lactate accumulation, fear itself may initiate profound ventilation with an associated bronchiospasm which compounds the problem. Whether from anxiety or premature lactate accumulation, hyperventilation can cause an athlete to exceed normal ventilation adjustments where oxygen delivered to the circulation is less than the corresponding demand for oxygen consumption.

A "second wind" is thought to be the result of an opposite reaction to that of "choking." For example, early lactate accumulation may be the result of psychologic forces (eg, jockeying for position, tactical maneuvers) or physiologic forces (eg, cardiorespiratory maladjustment). With prolonged activity, systemic blood pressure rises, movement pace is steadied, ventilation diminishes, the respiratory muscles become "warmed-up," which reduces respiratory resistance and awareness of breathing, and circulating lactate reduces. Even during maximum effort, the blood leaving the lungs is virtually saturated with oxygen, and muscular activity enhances alveolar air pressure. For these reasons, an increase in voluntary ventilation has little benefit, and volitonal control is an insignificant factor in performance.

Familiarity of Movement and Position

Proprioception learning has been shown to be responsible for a large percentage of apparent increases in strength-development programs. The importance of familiarity of movement and position to volitional muscular effort should not be underestimated, warns Rasch and Morehaus. When subjects are evaluated in unfamiliar positions or by unfamiliar methods, isotonic strength increases tend to "disappear." This is true even when the angle of muscle pull is rigorously standardized. When tested in familiar situations, substantial increases in strength of contralateral yet unexercised limbs are also recorded.

EFFECTS OF CHIROPRACTIC ADJUSTMENTS ON THE PSYCHOLOGIC STATE

From the viewpoint of the founder of chiropractic, D. D. Palmer, it made no difference to a nerve what irritated it. Today we consider those irritants to be essentially mechanical, chemical, thermal, or psychic in origin, which cause or contribute to nervous stress, both voluntary and involuntary, resulting in subluxations which in turn result in pathophysiologic processes. This concept encompasses all forms of stress and strain which man encounters, and the irritants may act either singularly or in combination to a degree sufficient to overcome the body's normal resistance and result in structural distortion, subluxations, and disturbed function in somatic and/or visceral structures.

Each athlete has his own breaking point whatever the irritant. For example, mechanical trauma may bruise one person while an equal force may fracture bones in another. Not all people subjected to the same pathogenic microorganisms develop the associated disease syndrome. Likewise, people subjected to the same emotional stress will not always react in the same manner.

A number of conditions are known to have somatopsychic relationships. Thus, it may be assumed that continuous spinal and extraspinal fixations may be effective psychologic irritants after mechanical, chemical, and thermal irritants have been removed. It has been demonstrated that finding and normalizing nerve root lesions and reflex points is an effective method to reduce afferent activity to the psychic centers.

Steward found that adjusted patients as compared to a control group showed: (1) a probable lessening of intensity of patient anxiety and this anxiety would be of a psychologic nature; (2) a lessening of irritation on the sympathetic system, which could be from the removal of the mechanical stimulus (ie, vertebral nerve irritation) or psychologic, where anxieties are lessened, which in turn stops the alarm or stress reaction from taking place within the patient; (3) adjustment does not improve the patient's ability to cope with problems; thus some emotional features are still involved, and the patient needs further psychologic counseling; and (4) once relief is obtained for the stressed parasympathetic and sympathetic systems psychologic stresses remain in a number of cases after adjustment. Therefore, further counseling of a psychologic nature is called for.

CHAPTER 11

Roentgenology in Athletics

Relative to our discussion of examination and evaluation, this chapter offers a general overview of roentgenology in athletics for the examiner well acquainted with the fundamentals of diagnostic roentgenology as applied in general practice. Specific applications will be offered in Part 4 that deal with the case management of particular injuries. Within Part 4, roentgenology is discussed with the objective of bringing forth points of unique pertinence to specific sports injuries, with emphasis upon soft-tissue injury, fractures, subluxations and dislocations, keeping in mind that the significance and scope of any injury vary greatly from athlete to athlete.

INTERPRETATION

Care must be taken so that a film is not used solely to confirm a prior clinical opinion. When this is done, many other facts exhibited on a view which may indicate a different approach may be missed. This often happens when an outstanding feature, visible at a distance, overwhelms a desire to seek other evidence. Whatever is presented on the film must be evaluated; eg, an asymptomatic chronic disease process may be underlying an acute injury. Healthy tissue features and common variances should be recognized at a glance. Once relevant features have been found to classify an abnormality, a search should then be made for those details which enable it to be distinguished from others in the same class. This takes careful evaluation of frequently subtle soft-tissue changes which confirm osseous alterations. The examiner must be well acquainted with the nature of all substances visible on a film.

DIFFERENTIATION

Abnormalities present significant alterations in structure, symmetry, continuity, positional relations, length and breadth, cartilaginous joint space, and density. Calcareous density is much greater than muscle density, fat density is much less than muscle density, and gas density is far less than that of fat density.

Masses, Swellings, and Effusion

Masses are generally soft-tissue enlargements tending to have a spherical outline and a definite limit which differentiates them from healthy tissue. Swellings, on the other hand, tend to be elongated rather than spherical and blend into unswollen tissues without a sharp demarcation.

Inert swelling has features which differentiate it from reactive swelling. Unless its density is extremely close to that of near tissue, inert swelling tends to present a peripheral limit. Poor demarcation of its sides is characteristic of a reactive swelling. This is the result of increased vascularity which fades peripherally in adjacent tissues and the reaction to infectious irritation. The poor demarcation is especially prominent if fat is near the edge of the swollen tissue. The normally invisible deep, abundant, minute vessels become visible and exhibit faint perpendicular striations deep within the tissue.

Effusion is suggested when a joint capsule becomes visibly distended by accumulated material which has the density near that of muscle tissue. If a joint is well supplied with fat pads (eg, knee, ankle), distention is usually quite clear.

Fat Pads

Fat pads help to outline the contour of and view the thickness and smoothness of adjacent articular cartilage. Clear visualization of some tendons (eg, patellar, calcaneal) is made possible on lateral films by adjacent fat pads, helping in the evaluation of stenosing tenosynovitis. Most normal soft-tissue structures show little difference in film shadows except fat which shows as a radiolucency. Warts and sebaceous cysts can produce opacities which can be confusing.

Although calcification of a fat pad is rare,

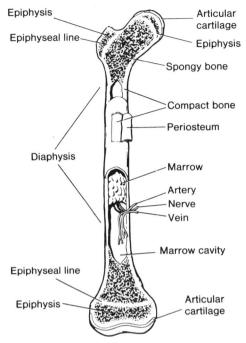

Figure 11.1. A typical long bone, the femur.

it most commonly occurs around a joint after trauma, presenting a picture of minute and multiple amorphous calcifications resembling thin rods in the early stage. Later, they appear more nodular and can sometimes be confused with a tumor.

Joint-Space Alterations

The area between adjacent articular cartilages may be wide, thin, or unbalanced. It is well to keep in mind that function has a considerable effect on joint cartilage thickness. The frequent movements and increased motions of athletes tend to thicken cartilage, while a lack of motion tends to decrease thickness by atrophy or underdevelopment.

In the extremities, an increased joint space is characteristic of a mass or tumor-like development, capsule distention from massive effusion, overdevelopment of cartilage, or a delayed conversion of cartilage into osseous tissue. The area may be reduced by atrophy, cartilage underdevelopment, excessive conversion of cartilage to bone, fibrous degeneration, or destructive disease processes.

Joint imbalance in the extremities is commonly seen in the knee, indicating a de-

rangement of the meniscus on the thin side, especially if there is no other feature except effusion. The medial side may appear thin, while the lateral side will be abnormally wide—or vice versa.

Ossification and Calcification

Care must be taken to differentiate the features of ossification from those of calcification. Ossification is the result of accumulated material of bone density which presents osseous structure when it is laid down. It presents rounded smooth corners, internal reticulation, and a line of continuous calcareous density at the periphery representing the cortex. Common calcareous densities within soft tissues include the ossification seen in sesamoid bones, sesamoidomas, and accessory bones.

On the other hand, calcification is the result of accumulated material of bone density which is initially amorphous. During calcification, bone structure develops slowly and indirectly, thus some areas at the periphery will most likely still be amorphous. Distinction between ossification and calcification is beneficial in identifying many roentgenographic features relevant to sports injuries.

Calcification in soft tissue has a marked relative increased density, usually homogenous in character. Two forms are seen: (1) The most common form is dystrophic calcification. It is associated with local tissue degeneration and reduced blood supply causing low tissue vitality from disease or old age. Dystrophic calcification is usually found in costal and laryngeal cartilages, lymph glands, pericardium, pleura, adrenals, thyroid, uterine fibroid, hypernephroma, dermoid cysts, tuberculous foci, and intracranial calcifications. (2) Less commonly, metabolic calcification occurs in previously normal tissues. It occurs in hyperparathyroidism and some cases of chronic renal insufficiency.

The difference between calcification and ossification is difficult to recognize and is only possible when definite bony trabeculation can be visualized. Bony spurs are often present at tendinous and ligamentous insertions. The most common sites are the os calcis, olecranon, patella, and external occipital protuberance. They are often produced by repeated minor trauma, but are seldom of clinical importance.

Soft-Tissue Calcifications

Most soft-tissue calcareous densities are abnormal, and some of them of significance are mentioned here.

Arteriosclerosis. Calcifications outlining the sides of arterial walls in relatively interrupted lines offer the basis for diagnosis. Calcification in walls of larger arteries of the abdomen and extremities is frequently seen in those over middle age. Two types are seen: (1) One type is characterized by calcific plaques in the medial layers of the vessel wall. These plaques do not narrow the vessel lumen and cause no circulatory interference. (2) Another type is characterized by the formation of atheromatous plaques in the thickened intimal layer. The lumen is narrowed and can lead to clinical signs and symptoms. This type is seen on the radiograph as irregular areas of variable size and shape, distributed irregularly along the course of a vessel.

Phleboliths and Varicose Veins. A phlebolith is a calcified thrombus within a vein. Size varies from most tiny to 0.5 cm in diameter. Oval or rounded calcifications within the walls of veins may tend to offer a degree of central ring-like calcareous density or be homogenous or laminated. They are most common near the pelvic floor, frequently seen in subcutaneous tissue of the lower extremities, and numerous in hemangiomas. Calcification within the wall of the vein proper is rare, but increased width and muscle density surrounded by adjacent fat make tortuous varicose veins quite discernible.

Calcareous Loose Bodies. These are calcifications within a joint, with or without effusion, of such an age as to show advanced signs of ossification. They are normally not free bodies but developments within tissue attached to the joint capsule. Free bodies are demonstrated by a change in position in subsequent examinations. Fragments of a fractured cartilage are rarely visible unless a degree of calcification has taken place.

Chondromatosis. This disorder, characterized by effusion and multiple rounded loose bodies (usually ten or more) in various stages of development, occurs without the typical, osseous features of osteoarthritis.

Posttraumatic Calcifications. Such calcification often occurs after trauma to deep tissues of the extremities. Hemorrhage within a muscle (hematoma) may calcify and, over a period of weeks or months, develop into actual bone. It has a laminated appearance from the hemorrhage following along the muscle planes.

Soft-tissue calcifications occur in posttraumatic states (eg, calcifying fibrositis, myositis, or fat pads); in abnormal tracts (eg, sinus, abscess, wound); and in masses (eg, hematoma, angioma, distended bursa). When a bursa is distended by fluid or granulation, calcification tends to develop as a diffuse amorphous mass or in small clearly defined nodules of varying density, or both.

Posttraumatic calcification in areas of stagnated blood or lymph is limited to involved muscle tissue in calcifying myositis. This type of calcification tends to be initially distributed within muscle(s) axially, fraying outward in the direction of the muscle fibers. As the condition progresses, the calcifying areas become more sharply defined. In differentiation, calcified hematoma presents a relatively round or oval mass in muscle or other tissue. Calcification is confined to the mass, is irregular and amorphous, is diffuse or flocculent, and the nodules are less sharply defined. Fluid stagnation within muscle or fibrous tissue also results in posttraumatic calcifications. These deposits are initially diffuse and amorphous, later tending to become more contracted, dense, and sharply defined. During the final (resorption) stage, the deposits lose density and finally disappear unless stress continues, in which case an osseous texture gradually develops.

Postinfection Calcifications. After inflammation, a reparative-type of calcification may occur in soft tissues during healing. Calcification at the site of a hematoma or calcifying myositis is more regular and less dense than that at the site of a pyogenic infection. While healthy tissue may promote osseous changes during calcification, sclerotic tissue may delay such changes. For example, osseous conversion of the calcification of the patellar tendon following tendinitis may occur promptly and possibly become complete eventually. After being involved by infection, the peripheral lymph nodes may calcify and be seen as nottled areas of calcific density, usually multiple. They are most frequently seen in the cervical chain and next frequently, in the axillary nodes.

Fractures

Hairline fractures, where a true fracture line is not clear, may develop in weight-bearing bones after trauma (Figs. 11.2–11.4). These will usually not be evident in films taken immediately after injury. Often 7–10 days must elapse before they can be visualized. On occasion, they are seen only by overlying periosteal elevation, callus formation, and not by a readily detected fracture line. If symptoms persist without change for 7–10 days after trauma despite negative films taken immediately after the injury, new films should be taken to rule out fracture.

The earlier and the more accurately a fracture is reduced, the sooner function will be restored and the smaller the resulting callus. Calcification begins in a callus in from 1–4 weeks and is usually complete in 6 weeks, depending upon the size of the displacement. The callus may show little early evidence of calcium deposit when

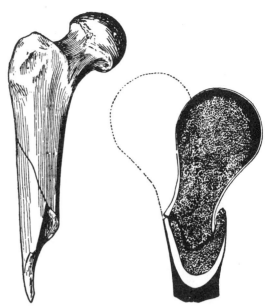

Figure 11.3. *Left*, spiral fracture of the femur. *Right*, impacted fracture of the base of the neck of the femur.

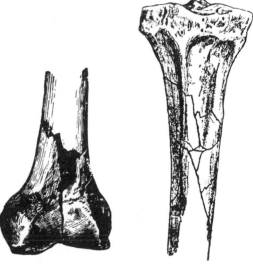

Figure 11.4. *Left*, intercondyloid fracture of the femur. *Right*, comminuted fracture of the tibia.

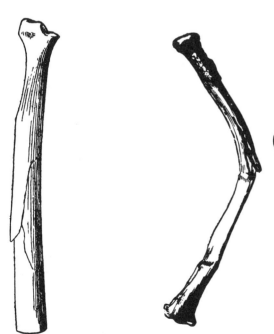

Figure 11.2. *Left*, partial fracture of the ulna. *Right*, partial (greenstick) fracture of the radius.

there is slight or no fragment displacement. However, an extensive comminution or a malposition of fragments should be accompanied by a large and thoroughly calcified callus. In compound fractures, callus formation tends to be slow and irregular. Callus is not seen within joint capsules such as in the neck of the femur, nor is it seen following fractures of the vertebral bodies, skull, or ilia. When fractures involve joints, the prognosis should always be guarded because it is difficult if not impossible to accurately judge the damage to soft tissues or what effect their repair will have on function strictly through roentgenography.

The Fracture Line

An obvious fracture is noted by the lack of normal contour, continuity, organizational structure, and the spiculated surfaces of the fragments; however, difficulty occurs when the division takes place within a cartilage line whether it be a normal or accessory line or one in an unusual, unexpected place. Compression fractures in the spine, whether recent or healed, may be difficult to differentiate from some types of pathologic disorders on the basis of x-ray evaluation alone.

Normally in traumatic cartilage fracture, the line tends to exhibit even width throughout its length with fairly straight and smooth abutting bone surfaces. At the ends of the line, the bone does not tend to be angular, but rounded. In contrast, a bony fracture line tends to be wider at one end than the other with sharply irregular bone surfaces on the line. At the ends of the line, the bone is definitely angular rather than rounded. With reparative change and sclerosis, an old fracture line may be smooth with rounded margins.

Pathologic fractures of bone may accompany a vast list of disorders presenting osteoporotic processes or bone destruction. Such fractures within the spine are usually represented by partial or complete collapse of the vertebral bodies. Hildebrandt points out that partial collapse is invariably seen at the anterior or anterolateral aspects of the vertebral body due to the weight-bearing function of this part along with the lack of support given to the posterior aspect by the articular processes.

Holmes and Robbins state that fracture lines will usually become obliterated in 3–6 months, and, if reposition of the fragments has been accurate, all evidence of the injury may have disappeared in that time. The shadows of linear fracture in the skull, however, may persist for several years after injury. In any fracture, when reduction has been poor or the callus formation extensive, evidence of the deformity may persist for life.

The Fracture Union

Hemorrhage at fragment sites produces posttraumatic calcification (callus) which becomes visible in about 10 days in youth and about 21 days in senior citizens. Rate of development varies greatly with age (faster in youth), apposition of fragments, immobilization, degree of hematoma, quality and quantity of local circulation, and early use after clinical union. When beneath the periosteum, the callus resembles inert subperiosteal calcification. If quite extensive, it appears flocculent and initially amorphous with density following. Resorption begins after several weeks or months until the portion uninvolved in function disappears.

At the surface line of a fracture, calcareous density rapidly diminishes, representing adequate blood flow to wash out the calcium. Under normal conditions, density recovery starts in a few days. Bony union is the result of trabeculae extension from fragment to fragment. Under abnormal conditions, this process fails and a line of calcareous substance forms which joins adjacent trabeculae on each fragment surface until nonunion or pseudoarthrosis develops.

The greater the space between fragments, the longer the time necessary for firm union and the greater the probability of union failure. Fairly firm union normally takes place within 2–3 weeks when fragments are impacted or fully apposed and there is some interlocking between trabeculae. A space of 1 mm may require from 2–3 months for firm union, while a 2–mm space requires several months longer.

The question of union is often difficult to decide. Without evidence of bony union, it is difficult to determine whether an uncalcified callus is present, whether there are soft tissues between the fragments interfering with repair, or whether or not there is fibrous union. Nonunion is prone to occur when the site of fracture involves a nutrient artery or when a bone disease is present. Bony union cannot be said to be complete until trabeculae have been demonstrated across the fracture line. Once clinical union has been determined to have taken place, gradual increased function through direct axial pressure can be started to stimulate strengthening of the union; however, such action prior to clinical union can be quite harmful.

Long Bone Fractures

These fractures present typical evidence, such as a fracture line, a break in outline, and deformity. One exception to this picture is that of the "torus" fracture seen in children where buckling of the cortex occurs and there is no visible fracture line or it is seen as a line of increased density. As healing occurs within a torus fracture, a variable amount of callus formation may be seen. Fractures within long bones may result without direct trauma strictly via muscle exertion if the bone has been previously weakened by the presence of cysts, malignancy, or constitutional disease. With the exception of cancer, it is fortunate that these fractures tend to heal well.

Stress Fractures

Fatigue fractures may be the effect of an improper relation between overstress and adaptability of bone. The most common example of this seen in athletics is similar to the so-called "march foot" of infantry and new track recruits. This is the result of subjects being overstressed in running practice (or forced marching) without adequate preliminary conditioning.

In order of frequency occurrence, the affected bones are the metatarsals with frequent multiple fractures shown as a fine fissure with or without excessive periosteal reaction; the tibia, especially fractures in the upper third of the bone which are often bilateral, the spinous processes of the 7C and T1 vertebrae, especially seen in new players; the fibula, especially above the malleolus; the femoral necks; and the pubic bones.

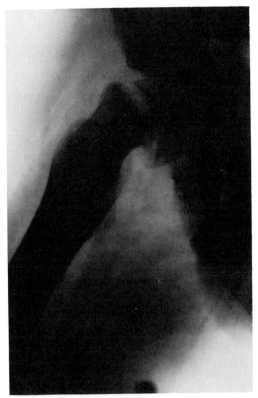

Figure 11.6. Case history: An 11-year-old boy had been involved in Little League football and sustained a blow to the left hip and leg, resulting in some pain. The case was referred to an orthopedic surgeon who x-rayed the knee, found the patient to be essentially normal, and recommended heat and rest for a week before returning to competition. After 2 weeks of rest, pain did not subside and the family brought the boy to a local chiropractor. After appropriate physical examination, the DC questioned the integrity of the left hip and referred the boy to a chiropractic roentgenologist. Radiographs adequately demonstrated evidence of a slipped capital femoral epiphysis. The boy was referred back to the orthopedic surgeon who accepted the diagnosis and continued appropriate care for the case (with the permission of R. B. Phillips, DC).

Dislocations

Dislocations may occur at any joint, but are more common in the shoulder, elbow, wrist, and hips. Except for posterior shoulder dislocations, most are obvious. In posterior shoulder dislocation, a slight widening of space between the anterior margin of the glonoid and the articular surface of the humerus may be noted in the A-P view. The head of the humerus is rotated backward with the lesser tuberosity within the glenoid and the main part of the head behind the scapula. Subcoracoid shoulder dislocations are often associated with a fracture of the greater tuberosity and usually reduced when the humeral head is replaced. Acromioclavicular separations are best seen in A-P views showing both shoulders.

A typical elbow dislocation is backward displacement of the ulna and radius upon the humerus or anterior dislocation of the head of the radius. This latter luxation is frequently related to a fracture of the ulnar shaft. Distally, luxations in the wrist are suspected when there is loss of the normal clear zone of articular cartilage about an individual bone because of the overlapping of adjacent bones. The lunate is the most common bone affected.

Hip dislocation may be congenital or acquired. The latter is rare, but sometimes seen in the young athlete after severe trauma. Displacement may be either anterior or posterior. The congenital form may be double or single. It features a shallow acetabulum, flattening and deformity of the head of the femur which is displaced superior and posterior upon the ilium, external rotation of the head and neck on the femoral shaft, and the development of a false acetabulum.

Athletes frequently present tibiofibular dislocation. The condition is witnessed as a marked widening of the joint space at the knee or ankle.

BONE AND JOINT DISEASES

Active Infection

A wide variety of features determine the characteristics of infection in any one particular case such as the duration and virulence of the disease, the degree of destructive activity, the degree of repair accompanying destruction, the degree and extent of soft-tissue atrophy, the amount of reactive swelling, and the type of decalcification involved. Active infection within a bone or joint means a specific site of active infection. Once activity has subsided, the healed site is referred to as a residual deformity.

Pathologic Features

Edeiken points out that infection in bones and joints is different in infants, children, and adults. In the infant, many vessels penetrate the epiphyseal plate into the epiphysis and vice versa. Thus, in the metaphyseal area, infections are easily spread to the epiphysis and into the soft tissues of the joint since the epiphysis is intra-articular. Fewer vessels penetrate the epiphyseal plate as the child matures; thus there is less chance of epiphyseal infection and joint involvement from metaphyseal infection. Because infants have a loose periosteum, infections readily strip the periosteum and extend to the articular end of the bone.

The metaphyseal vessels in the child loop backward into sinusoids allowing a fertile area for the implantation of infection. Infections easily extend to the joint once the epiphyseal plate closes as there is a direct connection with the epiphyseal vessels.

Infection usually spreads throughout the bone marrow, to a degree depending upon host resistance and the virulence of the microorganism; it may remain localized. If infection reaches the subperiosteal space by breaking through the cortex, the periosteum will be elevated, allowing the infection to spread along the shaft. The cortex becomes necrotic in time, and the periosteum will be stimulated to form successive layers of new bone. Extension into adjacent soft tissues results once the infection breaks through the periosteum. A frequent complication of osteomyelitis is acute pyogenic arthritis as a result of direct extension of the infection into the distal end of the bone and then into the joint space. Reparative changes begin about 10 days after onset.

Destroyed bone is absorbed by the action of granulation tissue which develops about its surface and is fastest at the junction of dead and living bone. Small amounts of dead bone are completely destroyed and leave behind a cavity. In localized osteomyelitis, necrotic cancellous bone is usually entirely absorbed, but large amounts of dead cortex are gradually detached from living tissue to form a jagged, irregular-shaped sequestrum (Fig. 11.5). After complete sequestration, dead bone is less attacked by granulation and is absorbed much slower.

At the site of infection, new bone forms from surviving periosteum (involucrum), endosteum, and cortex, being laid along periosteal and endosteal surfaces. The involucrum gradually increases in density and thickness to create the necessary new shaft, continuous with the new bone formed on

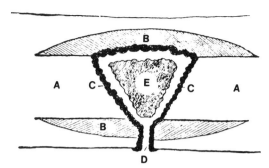

Figure 11.5. Illustration of the formation of a sequestrum: *A*, sound bone; *B*, new bone; *C*, granulations lining involucrum; *D* cloaca; *E*, sequestrum.

the end of the cortex not destroyed by the infection. If infection returns, superimposed layers of involucrum may be formed, and cloacae will be noted at the site of destroyed periosteum. According to the scope and duration of the infection, new bone formation increases in amount and density for several weeks or months. Once the sequestra has been removed or discharged, the cavity left may be filled with new bone, especially in children. The cavity usually persists in adults, especially if the walls are dense. Sometimes the cavity becomes filled with or lined with fibrous tissue and can be associated with a fistula.

During active infections, surviving bone at the site of involvement becomes osteoporotic as the result of disuse atrophy and the amount of inflammation present. When the infection begins to diminish and function begins to return, density increases.

When an infection becomes localized due to either high host resistance or low virulence of the microorganism, the abscess will present a small focus of cancellous or cortical bone destruction. This site becomes limited by adjacent sclerotic bone. During the early stage, the area contains purulent exudate, granulation tissue invades the neighboring bone, and the area destroyed may be completely replaced by fibrous tissue.

Soft-Tissue Reactions

Osseous infection produces the same pathologic changes as infection elsewhere. When a bone or joint becomes infected, hyperemia, edema, effusion, skin warmth,

white cell infiltration, necrosis, and pus are produced. A soft-tissue mass may or may not be present. If it is, it will change shape under pressure and lack roundness. This lack of roundness is the effect of gravity and pressure confined within the fascial planes.

When the capillaries become engorged, the sides of the shadow become indistinct. This is especially clear when the effusion or swelling occurs next to fatty tissue. In active infection, subcutaneous fat, which normally does not show visible minute vessels, presents faint, perpendicular striations within deep tissues.

Effusion offers a wide variety of features. It may present a clearly defined outline or one that is blurred by adjacent swelling. Its shape may be the result of blood clots, tumor, or gout. Its distribution may be limited to a portion of a joint (rare in infection) and tends to collect within areas of least pressure or be widely distributed. The density of effusion is usually that of neighboring muscle or tendon shadows, but it is more dense if hemorrhagic or purulent and less dense if serous.

A reactive area from congestion and fluid stagnation is witnessed in bone as an area of increased soft-tissue density within the bone that is soft, translucent, flat, or hazy, rendering detail indistinct but different from the density of overlying soft-tissue swelling or masses. The cause of this peculiar shadow is from the process involved; ie, resorption of medullary fat under pressure and its replacement by fluid having the density of muscle which diminishes the normal contrast seen in interstices.

As mentioned earlier, initial osseous manifestation of infection on films does not occur until about 10 days after the onset of symptoms. Adjacent soft-tissue swelling commonly appears much earlier than bone destruction, but as Edeiken points out, this swelling may be due to primary cellulitis, thus only presumptive evidence of osteomyelitis.

Subperiosteal Calcification

Subperiosteal calcification is a feature of posttraumatic subperiosteal hemorrhage. In addition, it is seen in stasis, scurvy, cancer, and a benign giant-cell tumor's subperiosteal shell. These inert subperiosteal calcifications must be differentiated from those of active infection.

Inert subperiosteal calcification is limited between healthy periosteum and bone. It conforms to the outline of the periosteum, is fusiform in shape, even in density after the first few days, smooth in outline, and separated from the cortex by a thin dark line. This last point is quite important in distinction.

Infectious subperiosteal calcification develops below diseased periosteum. It presents an uneven outline, density, and depth; and it tends to fuse with the cortex, especially at the ends, rather than being separated from the cortex. Such signs may indicate present or past activity. The degree of subperiosteal calcification may be measured by its density compared with that of the cortex.

As an infection spreads superiosteally, the periosteum is elevated and layers of new bone are laid down parallel to the shaft. This usually takes from 3–6 weeks to appear and is the first evidence of an involucrum forming. Lamellation or a periosteal layer may form and possibly be followed by a mound of bone being deposited on the exterior surface. Rather than being layered, the mound may appear as a relatively thick band of new bone.

The degree of periosteal reaction along the shaft is relative to the extent of the periosteal abscess. Thus, it may involve the entire shaft or be limited to a small area. As new bone continues to be laid down, an involucrum appears around the cortex whose contours become irregular and wavy until a thick bone sleeve is produced. Cloacae defects in the involucrum are the effect of focal periosteal necrosis; ie, channels for the discharge of pus and small sequestra.

Decalcification

Decalcification is the result of a decreased density of calcareous substance as a consequence of diminished calcium salts. In this sense, it differs from absent or diminished substance as a result of atrophy, underdevelopment, congenital fault, surgical removal, or some other like factor.

The three major forms are systemic, local, and general decalcification. Systemic decal-calcification has extensive distribution throughout the body such as seen in some metabolic disorders. Local decalcification features diminished density in a limited and well-circumscribed site, usually the product of a nutritional or circulatory fault in the area affected. Three major types of local decalcification are recognized; cortical, metaphyseal, and superficial. Superficial decalcification on the surface of the cortex is seen as a narrow saucer-shaped area and is the result of vascular disturbance. This fault may be the result of infection-related hypervascularity (especially pyogenic) whose effects are also seen as swelling or effusion. General decalcification is characterized by widespread diminished density about a lesion site or joint which is usually greater distally.

Cortical decalcification is characterized by decreased density of the narrow line of articular cortex which may extend as a thick line of subcortical decalcification of the medullary substance abutting the articular cortex. It is an early feature of pyogenic arthritis and a characteristic of tubercular arthritis. Reduced density from cortical decalcification of the narrow opaque cortex under the articular cartilage should not be confused with subcartilaginous decalcification of adjacent bone where the cortex line holds its normal density. Lack of density from cortical decalcification beneath the articular cartilage is significant in that it points to active joint infection. This point is especially helpful in the spine in evaluating whether a thinned disk is the result of trauma, infection, or degeneration.

Metaphyseal decalcification usually appears as a transverse band of decreased density next to metaphyseal cartilage. It is the result of disturbed circulation in the area of diaphyseal, epiphyseal, or joint infection. Improvement is indicated when density returns to normal after decalcification. Small masses of local decalcification in the wrist bones and epiphyses are often seen in gonorrhea and tuberculosis.

Bone Destruction and Infiltration

In most instances, single or multiple osteolytic areas in the metaphysis denote the first signs of resorption of necrotic bone. When a long bone is infected, thrombosis of the bone's vascular system dictates the extent of the ischemic necrosis and the roentgenologic changes.

A lack of substance indicates an area of destruction, deficient cartilage to bone conversion during development, congenital absence, surgical removal, or some other cause for the absence. The area of substance lack must be examined for details to indicate whether previously present bone is undergoing destruction or has occurred, with reparation yet to take place.

During active destruction, bone will not be resorbed uniformly at the surface. Normal calcareous density will appear to fade from the surface and be seen at deeper levels, and some spicules of bone reticulum will be seen to project at the surface. When healing takes place, the living bone assumes its normal density, and fibrous-filled cavities appear as areas of rarefaction in thickened and sclerosed bone. The site of an old infection will portray dense, sclerotic, irregular, thickened bone for a considerable period.

Infiltrative destruction in active infection is effected by the disease spreading irregularly along bone channels producing several connected areas of active destruction. The area will be somewhat spherical, and adjacent swelling will be present.

Degenerative Disease

In addition to polyosteoarthritis, the most common cause of bone/joint degenerative disease is the result of posttraumatic degenerative arthritis from severe injury or chronic stress. Characteristics include effusion, spurs, and lipping at fibrous tissue attachments, fibrocystic degeneration of articular surfaces, and possibly posttraumatic deformity in bone tissue. In the soft tissues, fibrous and fatty degeneration may be noted.

Deformities

Deformity may be witnessed as abnormal physical changes in angulation, displacement, division or failure of division, loss of continuity, subluxation, or dislocation. A deformity will lack features of other classes of disease and present healthy bone. Inert swelling and calcification after an injury (callus) is sometimes exhibited.

A site of previous disease that is now healthy may present a residual deformity that shows healthy tissue with repair. Other conditions offering deformity are those associated with fracture as seen in osteogenesis imperfecta and osteitis deformans.

Suggested Readings: Part 2
CHAPTERS 7–11

Adrian, MJ: Proper Clothing and Equipment, in Haycock, CE (ed): *Sports Medicine for the Athletic Female,* Oradell, NJ, Medical Economics, 1980.

Aiken, PL: Bilateral Weight Measurement: A Clinical Tool, *ACA Journal of Chiropractic,* April 1980.

Allport, GW: *Pattern and Growth* in Personality, New York, Holt, Rinehart, and Winston, 1961.

A Guide to Medical Evaluation of Candidates for School Sports, Chicago, American Medical Association, 1972.

Anderson, C: *Beyond Freud,* New York, Harper & Row, 1957.

Anderson, LD and D'Alonzo, RT: Fractures of the Odontoid Process of the Axis, *Journal of Bone and Joint Surgery,* 56A: 1663, 1924.

Arends, J: Cardiac Status and Exercise, in Schneider, RC et al (eds): *Sports Injuries: Mechanisms, Prevention, and Treatment,* Baltimore, Williams & Wilkins, 1985, pp 621–626.

Arieti, S (ed): *American Handbook of Psychiatry,* Vol 1–6, ed 2, New York, Basic Books, 1975.

Arnold, LE: *Chiropractic Procedural Examination,* Seminole, FL, Seminole Printing, Inc, 1978.

Astrand, PO: Commentary. Proceedings of International Symposium on Physical Activity and Cardiovascular Health, *Canadian Medical Association Journal,* 96:730, 1967.

Berkow, R (ed): *The Merck Manual,* ed 13, Rahway, NJ, Merck, Sharp & Dohme Research Laboratories, 1977.

Bowerman, JW: *Radiology and Injury in Sport,* Parts I and II, New York Appleton-Century-Crofts, 1977.

Brown, T et al: Psychological Factors in Low Back Pain, *New England Journal of Medicine,* 25:4–22, 1954.

Butt, DS: *Psychology of Sport,* New York, Van Nostrand Reinhold, 1976.

Carstairs, GM: Psychology of Athletic Performance, *British Journal of Sports Medicine,* 2:73, 1970.

Chaplin, JP: *Dictionary of Psychology,* New York, Dell Publishing Company, 1971, p 303.

Combs, AW and Snygg, D: *Individual Behavior: A Perceptual Approach to Behavior,* New York, Harper & Row, 1949.

Craig, TT (ed): *Comments in Sports Medicine,* Chicago, American Medical Association, 1973, p 6.

D'Ambrosia, RD: Roentgenogram Interpretation, in *Musculoskeletal Disorders,* Philadelphia, J. B. Lippincott, 1977.

Doherty, JK: *Modern Track and Field,* London, Bailey Brothers and Swinfen, 1963.

Dolan, JP and Holladay, LJ: *First-Aid Management: Athletics, Physical Education, Recreation,* ed 4, Danville, IL, Interstate Printers & Publishers, Inc., 1974, chapters 1, 2, 14; pp 525, 528–530, 538, 551–557.

Dudley, WN: Preliminary Findings in Thermography of the Back, *ACA Journal of Chiropractic,* November 1978.

Duffy, E: Activation and Behavior, New York, John Wiley and Sons, 1962.

Dunn, JW: A Laboratory Guide for the Orthopedic Practice, *ACA Journal of Chiropractic,* May 1976.

Edeiken, J: Infections of Bones and Joints, in Feldman, F (ed): *Radiology, Pathology, and Immunology of Bones and Joints,* New York, Appleton-Century-Crofts, 1978.

Finn, JA: Perception of Violence Among High-Hostile and Low-Hostile Women Athletes and Nonathletes Before and After Exposure to Sport Films, doctoral dissertation, Springfield, MA, Springfield College, 1976.

Fredenburgh, FA: *The Psychology of Personality and Adjustment,* Menlo Park, CA, Cummings Publishing Company, 1971.

Freedman, AM and Kaplan HI (eds): *Comprehensive Textbook of Psychiatry,* ed 2, Baltimore, Williams & Wilkins, 1975.

Freud, A: *The Ego and the Mechanisms of Defense,* New York, International University, 1946.

Gardner, HH: Low Back Pain—Diagnosis, Psychodynamics and Management, *Industrial Medicine and Surgery,* date unknown.

Goldstein, JH: Associated Press interview, August 23, 1972.

Gonzales, TA: Fatal Injuries in Competitive Sports, *Journal of the American Medical Association,* 146: 1506–11, 1951.

Gottschalk, L: Psychologic Factors in Backache, *General Practitioner,* 33:91–94, 1966.

Hanning, JM: The Role of the Emotions in Clinical Practice, *The Chirogram,* February 1974.

Harper, RA: *Psychoanalysis and Psychotherapy,* Englewood Cliffs, NJ, Prentice-Hall, 1959.

Harris, DV (ed): *Women and Sports: A National Research Congress.* The Pennsylvania State University, H.P.E.R. Series No. 2, University Park, PA, University of Pennsylvania, 1972.

Haugen, GB et al: *A Therapy for Anxiety Tension Reactions,* New York, Macmillan Publishing Company, Inc, 1960.

Haycock, CE: *Sports Medicine for the Athletic Female,* Oradell, NJ, Medical Economics Company, 1980, chapters 2–5.

Hildebrandt, RW: *Chiropractic Spinography,* Des Plaines, IL, Hilmark Publications, 1977.

Hill, AV: The Design of Muscle, *British Medical Bulletin,* 12:165–166, 1956.

Hirata, I, Jr.: *The Doctor and the Athlete,* ed 2, Philadelphia, J. B. Lippincott Company, 1974, chapters 3, 7; p 49.

Hodge, JR: *Practical Psychiatry for the Primary Physician,* Chicago, Nelson-Hall, 1975.

Holmes, GW and Robbins, LL: *Roentgen Interpretation,* ed 7, Philadelphia, Lea & Febiger, 1947.

Holmes, TH and Masuda, M: Psychosomatic Syndrome, *Psychology Today*, April 1972.

Hunsicker, P: Human Performance Factors, in Larsen, LA (ed): *Fitness, Health, and Work Capacity*, New York, Macmillan Publishing Co, 1974.

Ikai, M and Steinhaus, AH: Some Factors Modifying the Expression of Human Strength, *Journal of Applied Physiology*, 16:157, 1961.

Jaquet, P: *An Introduction to Clinical Chiropractic*, Geneva, Switzerland, published by author, 1976.

Jaskoviack, PA and Schafer, RC: *Applied Physiotherapy*, prepublication manuscript, Arlington, VA, American Chiropractic Association, scheduled to be released in 1986.

Johnson, W: *People in Quandries*, New York, Harper & Row, 1946.

Kane, JE: Psychological Aspects of Sport with Special Reference to the Female, Women and Sport: *A National Research Conference*, University Park, PA, College of Health, Physical Education, and Recreation, 1972.

Karpovich, PV and Sinning, WE: *Physiology of Muscular Activity*, Philadelphia, W. B. Saunders Company, 1971.

Kenyon, GS (ed): *Contemporary Psychology of Sport*, Chicago, The Athletic Institute, 1970.

Keesler, HH: *Low Back Pain in Industry*, New York, Commence and Industry Association of New York, Inc, 1953.

Kimber, DC et al: *Textbook of Anatomy and Physiology*, ed 11, New York, Macmillan Publishing Company, Inc, 1942.

Larson, LA: *Fitness, Health, and Work Capacity*, New York, Macmillan Publishing Company, Inc, 1974, chapters 7–20.

LeVeau, B: Dynamics, in Williams and Lissner: *Biomechanics of Human Motion*, Philadelphia, W. B. Saunders Company, 1977, p 199.

MacBryde, CM and Blacklow, RS (eds): *Signs and Symptoms*, ed 5, Philadelphia, J. B. Lippincott Company, 1970, chapter 30.

MacDonald, ML and Stanish, WD: Neuromuscular System, in Scott, WN et al (eds): *Principles of Sports Medicine*, Baltimore, Williams & Wilkins, 1984, pp 15–24.

Marino, N et al: Cardiovascular System, in Scott WN et al (eds): *Principles of Sports Medicine*, Baltimore, Williams & Wilkins, 1984, pp 1–13.

Menninger, WC and Leaf, M: *You and Psychiatry*, New York, Charles Scribner's Sons, 1948.

Miller, TR: *Evaluating Orthopedic Disability*, Oradell, NJ, Medical Economics Company, 1979.

Mischel, W: *Introduction to Personality*, ed 2, New York, Holt, Rinehart, and Winston, 1976.

Morehouse, LE and Gross, L: *Maximum Performance*, New York, Simon and Schuster, 1977.

Morgan, WP: Selected Psychological Considerations, *Research Quarterly*, 45:374, 1974.

Muller, EA: The Regulation of Muscular Strength, *Journal of the Association of Physical Medicine and Rehabilitation*, Vol 112, 1957.

Nideffer, RM: *Test of Attentional and Interpersonal Style*, Rochester, NY, Behavioral Research Applications Group, 1977.

Ogilvie, BC and Tutko, TA: *Problem Athletes and How to Handle Them*, London, Pelham Books, 1966.

Paul, LW and Juhl, JH: *Essentials of Roentgen Interpretation*, New York, Harper and Row, 1965.

Perls, F: *Gerstalt Therapy*, New York, Julian Press, 1951.

Petersen, GJ: Conflicts and the Unconscious, *The Chirogram*, Part I: September 1975, Part II: October 1975.

Phillips, EL: *Psychotherapy: A Modern Theory and Practice*, Englewood Cliffs, NJ, Prentice-Hall, 1956.

Pierce, CM and Kuehnie, KJ: Neuropsychiatric Aspects, in Haycock, CE (ed): *Sports Medicine for the Athletic Female*, Oradell, NJ, Medical Economics, 1980.

Poulton, EC: *Environment and Human Efficiency*, Springfield, IL, Charles C Thomas, 1970.

Rasch, PJ and Morehouse, LE: Effect of Static and Dynamic Exercises on Muscular Strength and Hypertrophy, *Journal of Applied Physiology*, 11:29, 1957.

Risley, WB: *Quick-Reference Laboratory Manual for the Chiropractor*, Phoenix, AZ, published by the author, 1973.

Rothman, RH and Simeone, FA: *The Spine*, Vols I and II, Philadelphia, W. B. Saunders Company, 1975.

Ryan, AJ and Allman, FL (eds): *Sports Medicine*, New York, Academic Press, 1974.

Salter, RB: Injuries of the Ankle in Children, *North American Clinical Orthopaedics*, 5:147, 1974.

Sante, LR: *Principles of Roentgenological Interpretation*, Ann Arbor, MI, Edwards Brothers, Inc, 1961.

Schafer, RC: Inner Forces Which Chain Potential, in *The Magic of Self-Actualization*, Montezuma, Iowa, Behavioral Research Foundation, 1977.

Schafer, RC (ed): *Basic Chiropractic Procedural Manual*, ed 3, Des Moines, IA, American Chiropractic Association, 1980, chapter XIV.

Schafer, RC: *Chiropractic Physical and Spinal Diagnosis*, Oklahoma City, OK, Associated Chiropractic Academic Press, 1980, chapter I.

Schafer, RC: *Symptomatology and Differential Diagnosis*, Arlington, VA, American Chiropractic Association, 1985.

Shanks, SC and Kerley, P: *A Textbook of X-Ray Diagnosis*, Philadelphia, W. B. Saunders Company, 1959.

Smillie, IS: *Injuries of the Knee Joint*, ed 4, Essex, England, Longman, 1971.

Spector, B et al: *Manual of Procedures for Moire Contourography*, Glenhead, NY, New York Chiropractic College, Research Division, 1979.

Steward, SL: An Investigation into the Effect of Chiropractic Adjustments on the Psychological State of the Patient, *Bulletin of the European Chiropractors Union*, date unknown.

Stokes, JH and Beerman, H: *Psychosomatic Medicine*, 2: 438, 1940.

Straub, WF: Psychology of the Athlete, in Haycock, CE (ed): *Sports Medicine for the Athletic Female*, Oradell, NJ, Medical Economics, 1980.

Torrance, EP: *Mental Health and Constructive Behavior*, Belmont, CA, Wadsworth Publishing Company, 1968.

US Army: *Army Medical Department Handbook of Basic Nursing*, Technical Manual 8–230, Washington, US Government Printing Office, 1970.

Weiss, E and English, OS: *Psychosomatic Medicine*, Philadelphia, W. B. Saunders Company, 1957.

White, RW: *The Study of Lives*, New York, Atherton Press, 1963.

Williams, JGP and Sperryn, PN: Sports Medicine, ed 2, Baltimore, Williams & Wilkins Company, 1976, chapter 3.

Williams, JM: Personality Characteristics of the Successful Female Athlete, in *Sports Psychology: An Analysis of Athletic Behavior*, Ithaca, NY, Movement Publications, 1978.

Wyndham, CH and Strydom, NB: Korperliche Arbeit bei Hoher Temperatur, in *Zentrale Themen Des Sportmedizin*, Berlin, Springer, 1972.

Zatzkin, HR: *The Roentgen Diagnosis of Trauma*, Chicago, Year Book Medical Publ, Inc, 1965.

Part 3

GENERAL ASPECTS OF TRAUMA

CHAPTER 12

Basic First Aid and Emergency Care

Before discussing specific injuries by region (Part 4), it is well to review those factors common to all athletic and sports-related injuries to develop a basic rationale of case management which can be used with minor variations throughout this vast and challenging field.

In rendering first aid, the licensed physician is often limited by various ethical and legal restraints not imposed upon the non-professional. Thus, before undertaking emergency care services, the practitioner should be well acquainted with local professional and statutory restrictions.

TENETS OF FIRST AID

First aid has been said to be the first stage in the rehabilitation of the injured person. This is true, and its quality affects the final outcome. The primary concerns must be the preservation of life, protection against further injury or unnecessary distress, and relief of pain, discomfort, and anxiety.

Emergency treatment must be fast. The general priorities for most emergencies are as follows: (1) Clear the airway and restore breathing. (2) Stop any bleeding. (3) Control shock. (4) Dress and bandage wounds if necessary. (5) Prepare for movement (eg, splint fractures). (6) Control swelling. (7) Make the patient as comfortable as possible.

Classification of Injuries

Injuries and wounds are classified by type, location, and causative agent. The extent of injury is described as severe, moderate, slight, superficial (involving surface tissue only), or deep (involving tissues below the subcutaneous layer). See Table 12.1 for classification of injuries by type.

The Acute Injury in Organized Sports

If dealing on-site with organized contact sports (eg, a high school football team), certain precautions must be taken in advance of practice and competition.

Planning Ahead

At the scene, first-aid supplies must be available to well-trained personnel. Good health practices which help to prevent and control the spread of infectious organisms include thorough attendant hand washing, disposal of infectious wastes, and disinfection and sanitization of articles after use. In addition, an athlete should be encouraged to dilute and eliminate toxic materials by increasing fluid intake. Everyone who has a role to play in health care or transportation of the injured should thoroughly understand his or her responsibilities.

Communications

Direct communication should be available for outside assistance if it is necessary for an ambulance to be called. If a player is being transported to emergency-care facilities, the facility should be notified in advance and informed of the player's condition so adequate equipment and staff will be available on arrival. If the player is a minor, the parents should be notified as quickly as possible.

Bleeding and Swelling

In any situation of bleeding or swelling the I-C-E principle should be applied. This acronym refers to ice, compression, and elevation.

The Use of Cold

Many injuries require immediate attention for control of bleeding or the reduction of swelling. In athletics, the use of cold often serves as a substitute hemostat. The effects of cold are local vasoconstriction and a

Table 12.1.
Classification of Injuries by Type

1. **Abrasion.** A wound in which outer layers of the skin have been scraped off. An abrasion results when a rough object is rubbed forcibly along the skin.

2. **Contusion.** A subcutaneous or deeper tissue injury, commonly called a bruise, caused by impact with a blunt object. Swelling and ecchymosis occur as blood leaks internally from injured capillaries; the blood often collects in a pocket of tissues as a hematoma.

3. **Strain.** A tearing or pulling of a muscle-tendon unit from overuse due to a sudden and forceful or chronic stretching or overexertion in lifting, carrying weights, or movement.

4. **Sprain.** An injury caused by overstretching or tearing ligaments around a joint due to a sudden twisting, stretching, or chronic stress of the joint beyond its normal range of motion.

5. **Dislocation.** Displacement of the normal relationship of the bones forming a joint. Displacement of any part, especially a bone where the articulating surfaces have lost contact.

6. **Subluxation.** An incomplete or partial dislocation of any bone; a slight disrelationship existing between two adjacent vertebrae in which their articular processes remain in contact; the alteration of the normal dynamics, anatomic or physiologic relationships of contiguous surfaces, often accompanied by fixation within the normal range of movement.

7. **Fracture.** A break in a bone or part; loss of structural continuity. When there is communication from the broken bone to the outside surface of the skin through a wound channel or by protrusion of a bone fragment, it is an open fracture; with no communication to the overlying skin, it is a closed fracture.

8. **Incision.** A wound made by a sharp-edge object such as knife or razor blade. The wound edges are smooth.

9. **Laceration.** A wound that is irregular and torn, with jagged edges. It is usually caused by objects such as broken glass or splinters.

10. **Penetrating wound.** A wound in which a foreign object enters, but does not go through the body or a part. There will be a wound or entry, but none of exit.

11. **Perforating wound.** A wound that goes all the way through the body, a part, or an organ. There will be wounds of entry and exit.

12. **Puncture.** A stab wound, caused by a sharp, pointed object such as a nail, icepick, needle, or bite. The wounding agent may have been withdrawn from the injured area, but foreign bodies, including bacteria, which have been carried deep into the tissues may remain.

13. **Rupture.** A bursting or breakthrough of a muscle or internal organ through its surrounding membrane. A rupture results from the application of internal or external pressure. With a rupture, there may be no injury to the skin or no external evidence of a wound.

numbing effect to reduce pain. It has the advantage of being easily transported via ice-bags or coldpacks.

It is granted that research shows cold to produce a local vasodilation and an inevitable rebound phenomenon. This is true, as in the case of ethyl chloride where the application is quick. Here, there is an immediate vasoconstriction, followed by a visible rebound capillary flare. However, it takes more than a few seconds of superficial cold

to stop bleeding. The application of cold can often be applied for many hours in injuries prone to recurrent hemorrhage. The danger of frostbite is easily minimized by placing a cloth or piece of clothing between the skin and the cold medium. It also helps to apply a skin lubricant.

Local Pressure

Along with cold, another method used in many injuries is the application of local pressure to control bleeding. Often a loose bandage over a dressing, with or without a pad of sponge rubber, will be adequate. This should never be used tight if later swelling of the part is anticipated, and it usually is. The purpose in applying a sterile dressing with pressure to a hemorrhage wound is three-fold: to facilitate clot formation, to compress open blood vessels, and to protect the wound from further invasion by infectious organisms. More on this subject later.

Immobilization and Elevation

In addition to cold and local pressure, elevation and immobilization of the injured part are often necessary to control swelling and rest the injured part. Elastic tape, adhesive tape, or light casts are commonly used for immobilization. Any type of immobilization must be skillfully applied with consideration to the patient's comfort and apposition of the margins of disrupted tissue (Figs. 12.1 and 12.2).

Elevation of an injured or inflamed extremity permits the force of gravity to drain swollen tissue spaces and blood vessels. The degree of elevation necessary to promote tissue drainage of an extremity is above the level of the heart. To provide this degree of elevation for the arm, the hand and elbow must be higher than the shoulder; for the leg, the foot and knee must be higher than the hip. A patient for whom rest and elevation of an arm or leg are indicated must, therefore, usually be confined to bed with the involved extremity elevated along its

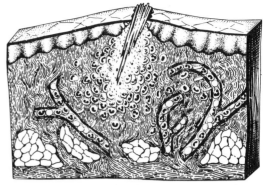

Figure 12.2. Typical tissue changes in inflammation, illustrating phagocytic action of white blood cells.

entire length on properly placed pillow supports.

Rest, inactivity, and immobilization allow the body's defensive efforts to be directed toward healing and combating infection. This can hasten the defensive process of walling off an infected area, thus preventing the body from absorbing a large amount of toxin. Rest also reduces aggravating movement of an inflamed and painful part.

The Healing Injury

Once the acute stage of a sports injury has passed, attention must be given to microscopic considerations. In the typical soft-tissue wound, external healing is complete within 2 weeks but the wound may not be ready for athletic stress. Invariably, the greater the bleeding, the more acute the diffuse the inflammatory stage, and greater induration and fibrous thickening can be anticipated.

The Stages of Healing

Resolution begins after bleeding stops to organize minute thrombi to form the richly vasculated granulation tissue that allows: (1) the *inflammatory stage* where the white blood cells dissolve extravasted blood elements and tissue debris, characterized by swelling and local tenderness; (2) the *reparative stage* where the network of fibrin and the fibroblasts begin the reparative process, characterized by local heat, redness, and diffuse tenderness; (3) the *toughening stage* of fibrous deposition and chronic inflammatory reaction, characterized by palpable thickening and induration in the area of

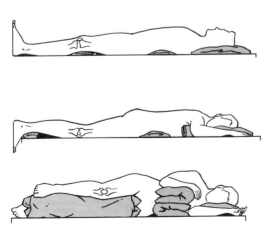

Figure 12.1. Some positions for patient comfort and body alignment.

reaction, with tenderness progressively diminishing.

Care During the Healing Process

Nothing should be done during the complicated healing stage that might disrupt the natural process or restimulate bleeding. The injury itself is all the local stimulation necessary for maximum response. Direct massage, heat, hydrocollators, whirlpool baths, ultrasonics, enzymes, and hormones, etc are usually contraindicated as they only add additional stimulation to an already maximally stimulated part. The best procedure is to anticipate each step in the healing process and provide the opportunity for natural processes to express themselves. If a variation is seen at one of the normal stages of healing, this is not to say that treatment should not be varied accordingly. Increased local swelling and tenderness during a later stage indicate an infectious process.

Good care during healing requires repeated inspection and external support. (1) Periodic and regular appraisal can usually be made, simply through inspection and palpation. When dealing with many athletic injuries, one becomes astute in seeing and feeling the various stages of healing. (2) Continuous support during the resolution stage must be provided by external measures without impairing the natural healing process. The common means are through tapes, bandages, splints, and foam-type braces.

Need for a Holistic Outlook

No injury is static. It continues to produce harmful effects on the injured person until either the injury or the person is defeated. As these effects are systemic as well as local, the response to injury is also both systemic and local. For this reason, injuries and their effects must be evaluated from the standpoint that the whole person is injured and not from the view that an otherwise well-off person is afflicted with a local defect or that only a part of the total system is affected.

Since the effects of injury and the body's efforts to defeat them are constantly changing, the doctor cannot rely on one observation or one major symptom in evaluating the condition of the patient, especially one seriously injured. Repeated observations must be made and indications of the patient's circulatory condition, temperature, blood pressure, pulse, respiration, color, and vitality must all be considered to obtain as clear a picture as possible of the patient's condition and the emergency treatment required at the moment the particular observation is made.

Rehabilitation

Because of the increased vascularity in an athlete's well-conditioned muscles, which is enhanced during exercise, interstitial hemorrhage following tear, sprain, or fracture tends to be quite profuse. This underscores the need for the immediate application of I-C-E.

Once the stage of likely recurrent bleeding has passed, a gradual rehabilitation program can be initiated which encourages the inflammatory reaction of resolution to pass quickly and reduce fibrous thickening of tissues. This program may be accelerated once the stage of fibrous thickening, noted through inspection and palpation, is exhibited. A great deal of atrophy, muscle weakness, and fibrous induration can be eliminated by applying progressive rehabilitation as soon as possible. Naturally, timing must be coordinated with the type of injury; ie, bone injuries require longer support and rehabilitation procedures than do soft-tissue injuries.

The Discomfort Factor

Hirata points out emphatically the "Injections of local anesthetics are not only unnecessary but must be openly condemned." Pain, tenderness, and local swelling are the doctor's primary indices for evaluating the progress of recovery. A numbed joint will never reveal that training was conducted too long or too early. Without the warning signal of pain, the physician has no guidelines for controlling the rehabilitative program. In addition, a local anesthetic injection results in local swelling which complicates the picture of natural injury-related swelling. These factors must be added to the possibility of uncontrolled stress being applied to a numbed, injury-weakened part.

A compromise must be made. Although extensive and prolonged immobilization assures a painless recovery in most instances, it always carries with it related fibrosis and atrophy. On the other hand, quickly initiated and gradual rehabilitation speeds the reduction of swelling and tenderness and minimizes fibrosis and atrophy. Being accustomed to a degree of pain during competition, the typical athlete is far more stoic than the average patient and more interested in how long he or she will be out of competition. While player anxiety to return to the field should not cloud professional judgment, most athletes will choose a treatment regimen that will enable return to competition 7–10 days earlier even if a degree of discomfort is included in the plan.

The Resolution Factor

We recognize that enforced inactivity following major surgery leaves an indurated scar of thick fibrous tissue that remains tight and uncomfortable for a long time after surgery. Likewise, major joint and skeletal injury inevitably results in overabundant scar tissue from necessary immobilization. Even minor disorders treated with long-term immobilization develop large scar masses which permanently restrict function. On the other hand, uncomplicated surgery, wounds, and sprains followed by ambulation in a day or two result in a cicatrix which is not tight, but rather soft and pliable.

Not too long ago the standard treatment for a sprained ankle was 3 days in a plaster boot, followed by 3–4 days of radiant heat and whirlpool baths, and then crutches for another week, all totaling about 2 weeks of therapy. The result was an athlete presenting a distinct limp for 2–4 weeks and an indurated, leather-looking ankle where motion was restricted in all normal arcs. It was not uncommon to take several months before the ankle was considered functionally normal.

Today the procedure and results are much different. For instance, Hirata's experience at Yale is that the same type of injury put on a regimen of straps and cold packs for 1–2 days, supported walking the 2nd day, and jogging to tolerance the 4th day will exhibit a normal-looking ankle on the 5th or 6th day with subsiding tenderness (localized only) and no evidence of edema. With external support, the athlete is able to return to competition. It would appear to be a worthy objective in athletics, if not mandatory, to carefully control rehabilitation towards full return of function with minimal scar tissue.

Postinjury Emotional Trauma

An injured player is often confused and emotionally disturbed, and this should be anticipated. This may be expressed by resisted help and a hostile attitude. Care must be taken to treat such a player with calmness and assuredness.

As some players react with panic or fear while others present denial or withdrawal, only experience can teach one to instantly decide on the right approach for a particular individual. Usually, the physician will be acquainted with the injured player well in advance so that the proper approach is not as difficult to make as it would be with a stranger.

The attending physician must be sympathetic to the injured player's fears and fantasies, while at the same time attempt to gain attention and cooperation. Recognize limitations and avoid impulsiveness by evaluating the situation before taking action. Show sincere personal interest, and use firm, quiet persuasion. Remain close to the injured player at all times, and use mechanical restraints when necessary. If the player is conscious, carefully tell him what you are going to do and why you are going to do it before you do it to reduce the anxiety involved.

The possibility of injury is a contingency in all active sports. In fact, a player may enter a particular sport in an attempt to deny such fears. A secondary factor may also be involved—the excitement of emerging victorious in the face of danger is euphoric, and the associated adrenalin reaction can become just as psychologically habit forming as a drug (ie, an "adrenalin addict").

THE UNCONSCIOUS ATHLETE

The importance of being able to recognize an injury immediately is underscored in the unconscious athlete (Fig. 12.3). In sports, the most common causes are a blow to the abdomen, heat illness, and head or neck injuries. It must always be kept in mind that an athlete is not immune to an epileptic attack or diabetic shock or coma. In undiagnosed coma, a major concern is the need to distinguish anatomic from metabolic causes. Structural causes may require immediate action while metabolic causes, with the exception of anoxia or hypoglycemia, usually allow more time for diagnosis before specific therapy is started.

Salt Loss and Heat Exhaustion

The habit of taking salt tablets during games and vigorous practice sessions to prevent sodium loss is without scientific support; on the other hand, harm can result from such a practice. Plain salt tablets have a tendency to irritate the gastric lining and encourage vomiting, and in most cases, extra salting of foods within logical bounds of taste is sufficient. If too much salt is utilized, a transient peak of plasma sodium occurs which forces the kidneys to excrete extra water in an attempt to restore electrolytic balance. This is the opinion of many research physiologists involved in sports medicine; however, some coaches and team physicians (eg, Dolan and Holladay) feel it advisable to prescribe prophylatic tablets against heat exhaustion, especially during the warm months.

A logical state of hydration should be assured through food/fluid intake. Water intake should be a minimum of eight glasses per day. As salt creates excessive fluid retention, sodium-rich foods such as processed meats, salty snacks, and highly spiced foods should be restricted 24 hours before an event. For vigorous competition, broth or bouillon taken with two or three glasses of water 3 hours before an event provides adequate salt intake.

The classic signs of heat exhaustion are slow-rising excessive sweating, clammy skin, dilated pupils, normal temperature, ashy-gray pallor, dizziness, headache, anorexia, faintness, nausea, muscle weakness, malcoordination, and possibly cramps, vomiting, and blue fingernails. Vital signs are usually normal, but the victim may present a weak rapid pulse, rapid shallow respiration, and a subnormal temperature. Naturally, competitive ability is progressively diminished. These signs, similar to those of shock, are progressive and indicate a serious disturbance of blood flow to the vital organs.

Salt loss through profound sweating has been scaled as follows:

Salt loss	Effect
5%	Lassitude
10%	Loss of will to work
20%	Effort forced
30%	Dizziness
40%	Heat cramps
50%	Prostration

During physical activity, plasma sodium tends to rise, potassium ions "leak" from active muscles as an effect of glycogen depletion, and there is a tendency toward hyperkalemia. At this stage, highly concentrated commercial sodium-potassium supplements are clearly contraindicated. During sodium and potassium loss, blood pressure rises because the blood becomes thicker and more difficult to move. Thus, a weakened artery or vein might rupture as the result of the increased pressure involved.

Long-distance runners often present "heat collapse" as an effect of prolonged muscular effort in a hot humid climate. The active-muscle heat production exceeds the body's compensatory mechanisms causing a rise in core temperature and loss of cerebral function.

First Aid

When symptoms appear, activity must be stopped immediately and emergency measures taken to reduce body temperature as quickly as possible. Treat for shock. The

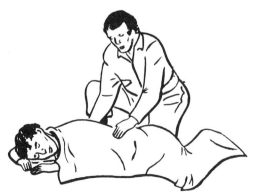

Figure 12.3. Semiprone (coma) position which helps to drain airway.

person should be placed supine, with the head level, in a cool, shady environment; cold wet towels, fanning, cool sprays, or tepid sponging should be applied; clothing should be loosened. Don't allow chilling. The patient will usually recover quickly if allowed to lie flat, rest, and have cooling accelerated by clothing being removed. Keep spectators away that may restrict a breeze. Iced drinks or baths should not be used as they cause vasoconstriction, thus increasing heat retention. Never allow the victim to be pulled to his feet and walked around.

In heat syncope, the lower extremities should be elevated. If the person is conscious, sips of diluted cool salt water (1 tsp/gallon) may be offered. Activity should not be resumed until full recovery is made, exhibited by normal rapid conversation, brightness, and normal rectal temperature. Inadequate treatment in coping with cerebral anoxia can lead to permanent brain damage.

In severe cases, very early medical attention for intravenous fluids and hydrocortisone may be necessary to enhance a reduced systemic blood pressure. Intravenous bicarbonates may be necessary to counteract a metabolic acidosis, and dialysis may be required to compensate for renal failure.

Heat Stroke

Heat stroke or sunstroke is recognized by the state of the weather and the presence of a very high fever (106–115°F). There is no other sure characteristic sign, but low blood pressure, rapid and weak pulse, delirium and convulsions are usually associated and call for immediate attention. This condition is to be differentiated from heat exhaustion in which there is no fever and no coma (Fig. 12.4). Heat stroke is a strict emergency situation where delay can be fatal.

There are three stages of clinical progression:

1. The player's behavior becomes slightly dulled and confused. Early, there is usually a hot, dry skin (sweat mechanism failure), along with a high body temperature, pinpoint pupils, flushed face, frequent and feeble-to-full pulse, thirst, fatigue, headache, nausea, muscle twitching, dizziness, weakness, heat cramps, and exhaustion.

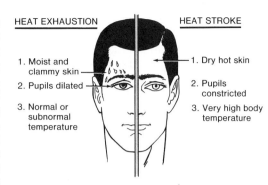

Figure 12.4. Symptoms of heat exhaustion and heat stroke.

2. These signs later progress into deep labored respiration, stupor associated with depressed reflexes or excitement associated with exaggerated reflexes, rising temperature, hallucinations, visual disturbances, and loss of sphincter control.

3. The player enters profound coma from a temperature as high as 113°F, which is often fatal. The skin develops a gray color because of circulatory collapse. The mortality rate is 20%.

All these signs and symptoms express a biologic cry for help. There is a breakdown in the sweating mechanism where the person is unable to eliminate excessive body heat while exercising. If left untreated, irreversible damage to the brain, adrenal cortex (heat shock), liver, and kidneys result because of the reduced cardiac output and rising core temperature. The cause is usually overactivity in an environment of high heat and humidity. For example, players exercising in full football suits often register a temperature 33% higher than those exercising in scrub suits in the same environment. Heat stroke is a better term than sunstroke as exposure to sunlight is not necessary for the condition to develop.

First Aid

In this life-and-death emergency, the longer the victim remains overheated, the more likely he is to suffer irreversible damage or death. Reduce body heat immediately by applying cold wet towels to the whole body, especially under the arms, around the neck, at the ankles, and in the groin. Remove the victim to a cool, well-ventilated place and remove most clothing. Place the patient on his back with his head and shoulders slightly raised. The conscious patient may sip cool water, but never allow hot drinks or stimulants. Transport the victim to an emergency facility as soon as possible, applying cooling measures during transport.

Head and Neck Injuries

Blows to the head or neck may result in unconsciousness. Most blows to the skull do not produce unconsciousness, but rather a "subconcussive" or "punch drunk" effect for a few moments. This state may be the effect of a severe blow to the head or the accumulative effects of many blows. The later is seen in boxers and especially in football centers. The center is defenseless inasmuch as both of his hands are on the football as it is passed.

Both cervical hyperflexion or hyperextension may result in unconsciousness and possible death. Neck hyperflexion injuries, more common in football and gymnastics, result when the head is forced toward the chest. The result may be cervical spine fracture or dislocation, which injures the spinal cord, often fatally if the fracture or dislocation occurs within the upper cervical area. Even mild spinal cord trauma may result in sensory and motor paralysis. Neck hyperextension injuries may cause compression injury to the vertebral arteries causing a temporary oxygen loss to the brain that may result in unconsciousness, if not greater damage, through rupture.

After neck injury, a careful neurologic evaluation must be conducted. Note any signs of impaired consciousness, inequality of pupils, or nystagmus (dancing eyes). Do outstretched arms drift unilaterally when the eyes are closed? Standard coordination tests such as finger-to-nose, heel-to-toe, heel-to-knee, and Romberg's test should be conducted, along with superficial and tendon reflex tests.

First Aid

If there is any doubt, treat the patient as if severe head, neck, or spinal injury exists. If necessary, carefully move the player onto a spine board with the neck aligned with the body for transportation to a neurosurgical facility for observation. It may require seven people involved in the careful lifting process: three on each side and one at the head. If the player attains consciousness within a few moments, continue to recheck symptoms and signs for possible intracranial bleeding. The most common signs are pupil inequality, arm drift with eyes closed, mental disorientation, and headache.

Epilepsy

When their condition is properly controlled, many with epilepsy may enjoy a full athletic career. However, several authorities discourage the epileptic from such activity in fear of the social stigma connected with a seizure in front of an audience. Kennedy points out that youngsters with epilepsy who are engaging in sports have fewer attacks than when they are inactive. Seizure recurrence does not appear to be related to head injury during athletic competition.

Kennedy also shows that there is no increase in seizures during vigorous exercise, although hyperventilation is known to precipitate an attack. Strenuous exercise appears to elevate the seizure threshold. This may be explained by the fact that overbreathing results in an alkalosis which precipitates the small seizures, but long-term breathlessness such as seen in prolonged exercise is associated with a lactate-pyruvate acidosis which inhibits seizures. Seizure susceptibility appears to be greatest during fatigue and sleep. Any sport which might entail a fall from a high spot (eg, skiing, diving, gymnastics) should be discouraged. Swimming requires very close supervision.

First Aid

Rarely will the epileptic not be known to the coach and physician. First aid is only necessary if an injury results from a fall or the thrashing of a grand mal. Such a seizure is not an emergency, but precautions should be taken to prevent the athlete from biting the tongue. The affected player should only be moved if circumstances demand it; eg, occurring on the field of play. Rarely will a seizure last more than 5 minutes.

Diabetic Coma and Insulin Shock

The subject of whether a diabetic should actively compete in athletics is a most controversial question. Levy points out that it has been firmly established that continuous training and exercise are not harmful to the diabetic and can even be a great stabilization factor. However, it has been found that hypoglycemia is a more common occurrence in insulin-dependent diabetics. Kennedy agrees that participation in sports should not be discouraged, and he points out that an exercise-induced increase of glucose uptake by muscle does not occur with marked hyperglycemia. However, most authorities agree that exercise can further aggravate an established state of ketosis in the poorly controlled.

Diabetic coma is the effect of too little insulin producing an accumulation of sugar and acetone in the blood. A player so affected will appear sick and confused, and present a rapid weak pulse and fruity breath odor. Unconsciousness seldom appears until after 24 hours, thus it is gradually progressive. Vomiting is frequent. The skin is dry, the pupils are usually dilated, and reflexes are diminished or lost.

Insulin shock is the result of overexercise, overinsulination, or too little food. The early signs are lightheadedness, weakness, pallor, sweating, and hunger. The affected player later appears intoxicated, sleepy, and uncoordinated and unconsciousness comes rapidly. The onset is rapid (minutes). In contrast to diabetic coma, there is a rapid full pulse and no fruity breath odor. There is usually some muscular twitching and palpitation. The skin is moist, the pupils normal or contracted, and reflexes are normal.

First Aid

The greatest aid is to first know who the diabetic athlete is beforehand. If conscious, ask the player if he/she has eaten and taken his/her insulin. If insulin shock is the cause, and it usually is, seek professional medical aid immediately. A conscious insulin shock victim should be given sips of some form of sugar, orange juice, or honey-flavored drink. Proprietary concentrated sugars (eg, instant glucose) are available. If diabetic coma and insulin shock cannot be differentiated, treat as insulin shock. If it's shock, the sugar will help neutralize the excessive

insulin; if not the sugar will not appreciably alter the comatose situation.

TRANSPORTING THE INJURED PLAYER

This takes extreme care. In moving an injured player, a spine board is better than the customary stretcher because the board helps to prevent further aggravation of a possible vertebral or spinal cord lesion. Craig warns that transporting an injured player should be well-planned, orderly, and conducted in an unhurried manner. Four general steps are involved:

1. The patient should be placed supine with care taken that the head, neck, and spine are in normal alignment. Place the spine board close and parallel to the patient. Place the player's arm adjacent to the board, relaxed at the player's side, and extend the player's other arm over his head.

2. Gently roll the player on his/her side opposite the board toward the extended arm. The athlete should be rolled like a "log" to maintain body alignment. An exception to this would be suspicion of a spinal fracture, whereupon the player should be kept on his/her side and not rolled supine. As mentioned, to move someone with a spinal or cranial injury usually requires seven people; otherwise two people will usually suffice unless the player is extremely large.

3. Next, slip the spine board under the back of the player (not on his/her side), and gently roll him/her onto the spine board. In cases of unconsciousness, facial or mouth fractures, or bleeding from the mouth or nose, keep the player on his/her side to allow drainage and an open airway. Assure that the injured player is in a comfortable position, then snug straps around the board and player to secure the injured player to the spine board during transportation. Remove rings from injured hands, if possible, before swelling occurs.

OXYGEN DEPRIVATION

One of the most critical emergencies is anoxia. The word literally means a lack of oxygen; but physiologically, it refers to an amount of oxygen insufficient to carry on vital processes. The human brain can withstand anoxia for only a few minutes before incurring permanent damage. The heart and other tissues having a high oxygen requirement can withstand anoxia a few minutes longer without damage. The effects of hypoxia, where oxygen is available in amounts less than tissue requirements, will be in proportion to the duration and amount of deprivation. Oxygen deprivation occurs under one or more of three general conditions:

1. *When the atmosphere, or inspired air, contains inadequate oxygen or when impurities inhibit body tissues from carrying or using available oxygen.* Examples are high altitude such as in mountain climbing, traveling in an unpressurized airplane, and poisonous chemical agents that are inhaled, such as carbon monoxide (characterized by cherry-red lips and tongue).

2. *When the respiratory system fails or is so inefficient that inadequate oxygen is inspired.* Head wounds may include damage to the respiratory center of the brain so that respiratory movement is disrupted or halted. The lungs may collapse as a result of chest wounds. Certain drugs (eg, morphine, codeine, barbiturates) may depress the respiratory center so that respiration slows or ceases, or electric shock may paralyze it. Spasm of the chest muscles may result from blast or other compression.

3. *When the cardiovascular system fails to distribute oxygen because of insufficient circulating volume, an insufficient number of red blood cells, or heart failure.* Regional hypoxia occurs when vessels serving a region are occluded by clot or tourniquet or are compressed for an extended period by body weight or tight bandages. Reduced blood volume results from hemorrhage, dehydration, shifts in electrolyte balance, or shifts in volume. Depression of heart action by such forces as oxygen starvation, electrolyte imbalance, electric shock, blows, pressure against the chest, brain injury, drug depression, and emotional upset reduces the overall circulating volume and the number of blood cells passing any given point in the circulatory system and contributes to general oxygen deprivation. If the heart fails, the circulation fails immediately, resulting in absolute anoxia.

The symptoms of oxygen deprivation can be classed as those of hypoxia and anoxia.

The symptoms of hypoxia may include gasping for breath, marked lack of respiratory rhythm, gurgling, croaking, rattling sounds in the respiratory apparatus, or cyanosis of the skin, lips, tongue, and fingernails. In anoxia, the patient is at the point of death. There may be either a marked struggle to breathe or no respiratory movement. The cyanosis gives way to a deathly grey, sometimes mottled or splotchy appearance. Depending on the nature of the underlying cause, the patient may be active or comatose.

Asphyxia

Asphyxia is not common in sports, but it does happen. The usual cause is from the inspiration of foreign bodies (eg, food, chewing gum) or laryngeal edema following a blow to the throat (eg, short-arm tackle). Other rare causes are seen in strangulation (eg, parachute harness) or from the breathing of irrespirable mixtures (eg, gases, swimming pool water).

The classic signs of asphyxia are inactivity of the diaphragm and intercostal muscles, with cyanosed skin in respiratory asphyxia or pale skin in cardiac asphyxia. Partial asphyxia is often difficult to recognize as it is insidiously progressive. This is often seen after traumatic hemothorax, characterized by progressively shallow breathing, a slowly increasing respiratory rate, and possibly slowly developing cyanosis. Difficulty in expanding the patient's chest after airway obstruction has been ruled out suggests pneumothorax or hemothorax. Persistent cyanosis and dyspnea even when the patient can ventilate suggest a flail chest.

Emergency Care

If the patient is not breathing, he requires artificial respiration immediately. If he has no heartbeat, he requires immediate heart massage. If there is both respiratory and cardiac failure, resuscitative measures must be applied to correct both conditions. When possible, one person should perform artificial respiration; another, cardiac massage. If a person is working alone, he must perform both measures alternately.

The most common cause of preventable death in accidents is airway obstruction (tongue, vomitus, blood, dentures, dirt, etc).

After oxygen deprivation, time is of the essence and seconds count in initiating resuscitation. The sooner aid is begun, the more likely it is to succeed. The rescuer's expired air is an efficient air mixture as its 2–3% of carbon dioxide is a respiratory stimulant. When breathing is "not sure," beginning artificial respiration will do no harm; when in doubt, start artificial respiration. Delay may be fatal. An endotracheal tube will prevent aspiration of vomitus and may remain inserted for several days if need be.

Some method based on the operator's expired air technique should be used when possible to inflate the patient's lungs with the operator's breath. Mouth-to-mouth is usually preferred and sometimes mouth-to-nose if the patient's jaws are tightly closed by spasm or when he has a jaw or mouth wound. The Silvester method is used if manipulation of the patient's head or face would cause hemorrhage of or into the airway. These techniques will be discussed later.

Once breathing and heart action normalize, place the subject in the three-quarter prone position for adequate airway drainage, and watch the victim vilgilantly until the ambulance arrives. Make sure the airway is kept clear, that breathing continues, and that there is no restrictive clothing about the neck, chest, or abdomen. Respiratory difficulties often arise after head injury, with froth expelling from the mouth and nose. After brain injury, pulmonary edema can occur insidiously within 30–60 minutes. Continually maintain respiration, and frequently aspirate any froth.

The Heimlich Maneuver

Choking may occur during eating, especially with people who are inebriated or have a partial denture. If the patient is able to stand and several slaps on the back do not help, a foreign body within the airway (eg, food particle) may be expelled using the Heimlich maneuver (Fig. 12.5): Stand in back of the victim and place both your arms around the subject. Make a fist with one hand and grasp it with the other hand. Then, with the thumb toward the patient, press your fist sharply upward against the victim's abdomen, between the naval and the rib cage. Press in and up in quick thrusts.

This causes the diaphragm to elevate, the lungs to compress, and increased air pressure within the thorax and trachea to force out the food particle.

The chest thrust is a variation of the Heimlich abdominal thrust and is equally effective in coping with the choking patient (Fig. 12.6): A tight hand clasp is formed over the patient's midchest. Press in, using several quick thrusts.

Asthma

Asthma can be triggered by exercise as well as by other factors. Kennedy shows where short-term exercise (1–2 minutes)

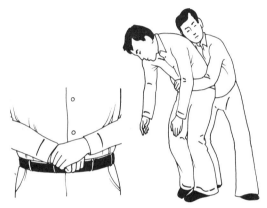

Figure 12.5. *Left*, correct hand position in Heimlich maneuver. *Right*, position for standing abdominal thrust.

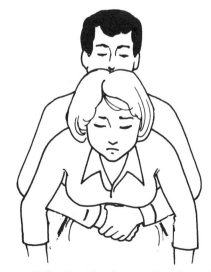

Figure 12.6. Position for standing chest thrust: a Heimlich adaptation.

produces bronchodilation and long-term exercise (4–12 minutes) can result in bronchoconstriction in the asthmatic. Full participation in sports, under proper health-care management, may be enjoyed by the asthmatic, but it is usually best to limit activities to those sports which require energy output of short duration (eg, sprints, softball, skiing, golf). Adequate warmup is often essential to obtain adequate bronchodilation.

Drowning

About 6,500 people die each year from drowning in the United States. A victim offers a picture of being pale, limp, hypoxic, livid, cold, with staring and lusterless eyes, dilated pupils, and with water running out of the nose and mouth. Other features include unconsciousness or semiconsciousness, severe dyspnea, rapid and feeble pulse, ventricular arrhythmias with indistinct or absent heart beat, distended abdomen, and loss of sphincter control.

Immediate cardiopulmonary resuscitation (CPR) and emergency cardiac care (ECC) must be fast, efficient, and unremitting until help arrives. At this vital moment, it is more important to initiate cardiorespiratory function than it is to aspirate water from the lungs of a drowning victim as undoubtedly all lung tissue will not be affected. Many authorities feel that most of the water seen aspirated is from the stomach, not the lungs. The first priority is to restore ventilation to the unaffected lung tissue.

If possible, resuscitation should begin even before the subject is removed from the water. It is usually more efficient if it's conducted in shallow water where the rescuer can touch bottom. A few immediate mouth-to-mouth breaths at this stage may make the difference between life and death. Once circulation and respiration are restored, the victim may require continued support with hospitalization. Precautions against complications such as nephritis, pneumonia, or shock must be taken if possible.

Occasionally, "dry drowning" is seen where a person may die with little or no fluid in the lungs. This is believed to be the result of marked laryngeal spasm with airway occlusion because of a reflex to a slight amount of aspirated fluid. The laryngeal spasm results in asphyxia.

Nitrogen Narcosis and the Bends

During assisted diving, a nitrogen narcosis may result from the effort of nitrogen on the central nervous system. The state is self-limited with adequate oxygen. The symptoms are a mild-to-moderate intoxication encouraging the diver to take abnormal risks or ascend at a higher than optimal rate. Rapid ascent may also produce rupture of the alveoli and tympanic membrane, middle ear problems, and bends.

Bends result from nitrogen bubbles forming within the blood and tissues which block capillary-blood flow. This leads to severe cramps, organic dysfunction, and neurologic symptoms. A thorough examination is required. Symptoms include ear pain, sinus pain, headache, confusion, aching muscles and joints. Signs include shortness of breath, cough, hemoptysis, and air in the subcutaneous tissues.

Management of the bends and barotrauma requires immediate hyperbaric oxygen in a decompression chamber. Until this can be provided, high concentrations of oxygen must be given. If an air embolism within the central nervous system is suspected, the patient should be placed in a head-down position to help dislodge cerebral emboli.

Altitude Sickness

Altitude sickness (eg, mountain sickness) is an acute respiratory failure, often but not always due to pulmonary edema, occurring at high altitudes. Without proper acclimation at altitudes as low as 8,000 feet, symptoms may occur rapidly in hours of over several days and often without warning. The condition occurs in the healthy, but may be predisposed by chronic lung or heart disease. The common complaints are headache, malaise, nausea, and vomiting. Early symptoms include dyspnea on exertion and fatigue with ordinary effort. Signs include rapid respiration, rales, tachycardia, cough, cyanosis, apprehension, distended neck veins, arrhythmia, hypotension, and disturbed consciousness leading to coma. In severe cases, a bloody sputum will be exhibited. The major concern is to get the patient to a lower altitude where supplemental oxygen can be supplied.

Weight Lifter's Syncope

Weight lifters occasionally complain of "blackout" during competition. In subjects studied during activity, the men showed that they lowered their expired carbon dioxide levels through hyperventilation. During the lifts, tachycardia rather than bradycardia and extremely high intrathoracic pressures were recorded. Cardiac size was greatly reduced. Heart, pulmonary artery, and aortic actions were barely perceptible. Immediately after the weight was removed, pulmonary artery pulsations quickly normalized, but a delay was seen in the aortic pulsation (3–4 beats).

It is believed that the fainting is the result of cerebral ischemia produced by a large transient fall in arterial pressure when the elevated thoracic pressure is suddenly released. The condition can be corrected by avoiding hyperventilation and a prolonged squatting position prior to the lift and lifting as rapidly as possible so that normal breathing can be resumed.

CARDIOPULMONARY RESUSCITATION

Cardiac arrest must always be accompanied by an effective means of artificial respiration with closed cardiac massage. Basic life support is an emergency first-aid procedure which consists of recognizing respiratory and cardiac arrest and starting the proper application of cardiopulmonary resuscitation to maintain life until a victim recovers sufficiently to be transported or until advanced life support becomes available. This training and knowledge is essential to all health providers and all are encouraged to enter a certified class of instruction.

There must be a maximum sense of urgency in starting basic life support. The most critical time in such an emergency falls within the first 4–6 minutes after the victim's heart stops or the victim stops breathing. It is within these few minutes that irreversible brain damage begins, thus making recognition of the emergency critical. The indications for basic life support are: (1) respiratory arrest or an airway obstruction; and (2) cardiac arrest from cardiovascular collapse, ventricular fibrillation, or ventricular standstill. Basic life support includes the three basic concerns of CPR: airway, breathing, circulation.

The Mouth-to-Mouth Approach

Butler and others briefly describe the steps and order of priority in assessing and resuscitating an unconscious person in a one-person unwitnessed arrest rescue essentially as follows:

1. The first step is to determine if the victim is conscious by shaking his shoulders and asking questions. If no response, place the victim supine on a firm surface.

2. Kneel at the victim's side and center yourself at shoulder level. Establish an open airway by extending the victim's head back, using your caudal hand under the neck and cephalad hand on the victim's forehead. Once the airway is established, place your ear over the victim's mouth, listen for air movement, and seek moist air cross your cheek. View the chest for respiratory movement.

3. See that an adequate airway is established (Fig. 12.7). Foreign matter (eg, dentures, leaves, dirt), vomitus, or mucus should be removed with a finger. Turn the patient's head to one side and quickly run your fingers behind the patient's lower teeth and over the back of the tongue. Then position the patient's head in the face-up position. If a small rolled blanket or some clothing is immediately available, place it under his shoulders so that his neck will be extended and his chin points upward. In any event, tilt his head back so that the neck is stretched and the head is in a chin-up position.

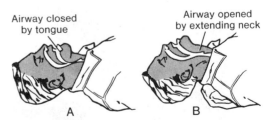

Airway closed by tongue | Airway opened by extending neck

A | B

Figure 12.7. Chin-up position to establish an adequate airway. Note in *A* that the airway is closed by the tongue; in *B*, the airway is opened by extending the neck with a roll under the shoulders.

4. Adjust the patient's lower jaw to a jutting-out position by either the thumb jaw lift (preferred) or the two-hand jaw-lift (Fig. 12.8). This positioning moves the base of the tongue away from the back of the throat, thus clearing or enlarging the air passage to the lungs. In deep unconsciousness, tongue muscle may lose its tone and fall against the back of the throat and mechanically obstruct the pharynx.

5. Once the jaw is supported in a forward position, seal the airway (nose or mouth) that is not to be used, continuing to hold the patient's jaw forward (Fig. 12.9). The seal must be secure to prevent leakage of air during inflation. In the mouth-to-mouth approach, seal the nose by pinching it shut with your free hand or by pressing your cheek firmly against it. In the mouth-to-nose approach, seal the mouth by placing two fingers lengthwise firmly over the patient's lips. If the patient is an infant or small child, cover both his nose and mouth with your mouth, sealing your lips against the skin of his face. Concern must be given that regurgitated gastric contents are not inhaled by the victim. If this does happen,

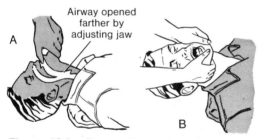

Figure 12.8. Two methods for adjusting the lower jaw to a jutting-out position: *A*, thumb jaw-lift; *B*, two-hand jaw lift.

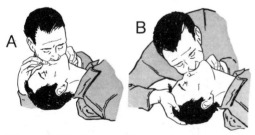

Figure 12.9. Nonused airway closure technique of artificial respiration: *A*, the nose is sealed with thumb and finger; *B*, the nose is sealed with operator's cheek.

quickly aspirate or turn the victim on his side and drain by gravity.

6. If there are no indications of breathing, give four quick, forceful breaths. Focus your eyes on the patient's chest. If the chest rises, it shows that air is reaching his lungs, so continue the procedure. If the chest does not rise, take corrective action. First, hold the jaw up more forcefully and blow harder, making sure that air is not leaking from the mouth or nose. If the chest still does not rise, recheck the mouth for foreign matter and, if necessary turn the patient on his side and strike him between the shoulders with considerable force as often as necessary to dislodge obstruction in the air passage. Then inflate his lungs.

7. Remove your mouth from the patient's airway and listen for return of air from his lungs. If the patient's exhalation is noisy, elevate his jaw further. After each exhalation of air from the patient's lungs, blow another deep breath into his airway. Make the first 5–10 breaths deep (except for infants and small children) and give them at a rapid rate to provide fast reoxygenation. For infants or small children, blow small puffs of air from your cheeks, rather than deep breaths from your lungs. Quickly check the carotid pulse for 5–10 seconds. If breathing alone is absent and you feel a pulse, continue the mouth-to-mouth technique at the rate of one breath every 5 seconds or 12 times a minute (the U.S. Army recommends 12–20 times a minute) until the patient is able to breathe unassisted. Split-second timing is not essential, but smooth rhythm is desired. As the patient attempts to breathe, adjust the timing of your efforts.

If your breathing at first was very deep and rapid, you may become faint, tingle, or even lose consciousness if you persist. But if, after administering the first 5–10 deep rapid breaths, you adjust your breathing to a rate of 12 or more times a minute with only moderate increase in normal volume, you probably will be able to continue to give rescue breathing for a long period without these temporary ill effects. If you become distressed from giving shallow breaths to an infant or small child, interrupt your rhythm occasionally to take a deep breath.

After a period of resuscitation, the patient's abdomen may bulge. This indicates that some air is going into his stomach. Since inflation of the stomach makes it more difficult to inflate his lungs, apply gentle pressure to his abdomen with your hands between inflations. Treat to prevent or lessen shock as soon as the patient is breathing satisfactorily by himself.

Modified Silvester Method

In facial injuries which cause a ventilation problem, the modified Silvester method may be applied. Essentially, this technique requires the operator to hyperextend the subject's neck if not injured, and then alternate arm extension with thoracic compression.

1. Position the patient on this back, and clear his airway as previously described, with jaw jutting forward and neck extended. Position yourself by standing at the patient's head, facing his feet. Kneel near his head on one knee. Place your opposite foot to the other side of the patient's head and against his shoulder to steady it. If you become uncomfortable after a period of time, quickly switch to the other knee.

2. Grasp the patients' hands, and place them over his lower ribs. Rock forward and exert steady, uniform pressure almost directly downward until you meet firm resistance. This pressure should force air out of the patient's lungs. Move the patient's arms slowly outward from his body; then, keeping his arms straight, lift them vertically, past his head. Now stretch them backward as far as possible. This process of lifting and stretching the arms increases the size of the chest and draws air into the lungs.

3. Replace the patient's hands on his chest and repeat the cycle: (a) press, (b) lift, (c) stretch, and (d) replace. Give from 10–12 cycles/minute at a steady, uniform rate. Give longer counts of equal length to the first three steps, making the fourth or "replace" period as short as possible.

If a second person is available, have him relieve you with practically no break in rhythm. Continuing to administer artificial respiration, move to one side while the replacement takes his position from the other side. During the "stretch" step, the replacement grasps the patient's wrists and contin-ues artificial respiration in the same rhythm, shifting his grip to the patient's hands during the "replace" step.

If the patient attempts to breathe, adjust the timing of your efforts so as to assist him. Continue artificial respiration until the patient can breathe without assistance or until he is declared dead by the most competent authority available.

Emergency Cricothyroidotomy

Most airway difficulties are relieved by nonsurgical measures, but persistent obstruction during such a situation requires an emergency surgical airway for relief. In such cases, the procedure of choice for the operator without surgical training is cricothyroidotomy. This consists of an incision made through the skin and cricothyroid membrane covering the cricothyroid space to provide an emergency airway into the larynx because of a supralaryngeal obstruction that cannot be dislodged. However, before attempting this operation, one must have prior training and have tried conservative measures first.

CARDIAC ARREST

A player's left ventricle suddenly starts beating widly. Blood pressure plummets. The other heart chambers lose their steady rhythm and simply flutter and quake ineffectively. These are the signs of a deadly form of a common heart attack: ventricular tachycardia. Without the aid of an electric defibrillator, the victim often dies. Death occurs if not treated within 3–6 minutes.

The etiology is either mechanical or electrical. Cardiac arrest may be caused by blockage of critical blood vessels or by insufficient oxygen to the heart or the brain centers which control its functions such as in massive hemorrhage. Causes include diseases of the heart, pulmonary embolus, aneurysms, sepsis, hypoxia, elevated carbon dioxide, elevated blood potassium especially with concomitant low blood calcium levels, airway obstruction, shock, excessive vagal reflexes, electrocution, malnutrition, anemia, and the effects of drugs, especially those affecting the regulatory brain centers.

The signs of cardiac arrest are unconsciousness, no heart sounds, and no palpable carotid pulse or apex beat. Arrest is quickly followed by cessation of respiration, if that has not previously occurred, and wide dilation of the pupils. The individual is unconscious and limp. Since the diagnosis of cardic arrest must be made with rapidity if the patient is to be resuscitated successfully, the absence of the carotid pulse should be the determining symptom. The pulse of the heart is easily felt with the fingertips by tilting the patient's head to a chin-up position, placing the heel of the hand over the midline of the patient's trachea, and resting the fingers in his throat, parallel to the lower jaw line. If there is doubt, the pulse should be considered absent.

Atherosclerosis begins much earlier in life than was once believed. Leon states that autopsy studies conducted in Korea and Vietnam of war victims frequently showed thickening and narrowing of arterial walls in subjects under 25 years of age who were presumably in good health.

Closed Cardiac Massage

Cardiac massage consists of a rhythmical compression of the patient's heart through the intact chest wall. It is a means of producing circulation artificially, thus keeping blood flowing to the brain and other organs until the heartbeat is established.

Within the thorax, lateral motion of the heart is limited by the pericardium. This loose-fitting, fluid-lubricated, membranous sac surrounding the heart is fastened to structures comprising the boundaries of the thorax. Accordingly, pressure applied on the sternum pushes the heart against the spine, forcing blood from the heart into the arteries. Relaxation of this pressure allows the heart to fill with venous blood. The thoracic cage is normally resistant to pressure but is surprisingly resilient in cardiac arrest.

Cardiac massage must be instituted immediately upon determining the absence of a pulse. Since cardiac arrest is always accompanied by respiratory failure, artificial respiration must be administered simultaneously or alternately with cardiac massage, depending upon whether one or two persons are available to administer these resuscitative measures (Fig. 12.10).

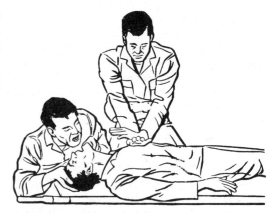

Figure 12.10. Closed-chest heart massage and expired air artificial respiration when two people are available.

Technique

1. Prepare the patient for artificial respiration as previously discussed. Be sure that the surface on which the patient is placed is solid. A litter, floor, or the ground is satisfactory, but a couch or cot is too flexible unless a board has been placed under the mattress.

2. Position yourself by kneeling at a right angle to the patient's chest so that you can use your weight to apply pressure on his sternum (Fig. 12.11). If there is no pulse, position the heel of one hand in the midline lower one-half of the sternum, but be sure to keep 2 or 3 finger widths above the xiphoid process. Spread and raise your fingers so you can apply pressure without pressing the patient's ribs. Place your other hand on top of the first hand, bring your shoulders directly over the center of the victim's chest, and lock your elbows straight.

3. Apply pressure. Lean forward so that your arms are perpendicular to the patient's sternum and press downward with your hands. Exert pressure vertically downward to depress the sternum from 1½–2 inches. Further depression is likely to fracture the patient's ribs and damage underlying soft structures. The compressions must be regular, smooth, and uninterrupted. If the patient is a child, apply relatively light pressure with one hand. For infants, especially the extremely young, the pressure you can apply with your fingers probably will be

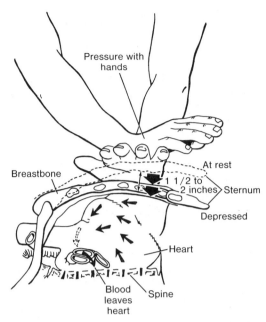

Figure 12.11. Illustration of the mechanics involved in closed-chest heart massage where pressure on the sternum forces blood out of the heart.

more than sufficient to depress the sternum the slight distance necessary to produce blood circulation.

4. Relax your hand contact immediately after compression and for an equal duration to allow for ventricular filling, but do not remove hand contact from the sternum.

The compressions are performed at a rate of 60 compressions/minute, and the compressions and breaths are given in a ratio of 5:1. That is, five compressions followed immediately by a breath. The U.S. Army recommends one cycle of artificial respiration, then four cycles of cardiac massage. Rate does not appear to be as important as duration.

After the first minute of rescue, stop and reassess the presence or absence of breathing or pulse. If no response, return to the compressions and breaths as necessary, stopping to reassess every 2 minutes thereafter. This series is repeated continually until the patient arouses or full life-support help arrives. This may take several hours, long after you feel bodily discomfort and fatigue. However, stopping these measures may be fatal to the arrested player.

If a pulse cannot be detected after several minutes, elevate the patient's legs about 6 inches above the level of his head. Continue cardiac massage and mouth-to-mouth artificial respiration until the patient is able to function without assistance, until you are relieved, or until you are certain the patient is dead.

Defibrillation

Without an ECG, it is almost impossible to differentiate between asystole and fibrillation by palpation and auscultation. An electric defibrillator, as carried by emergency teams, is the best method of defibrillation. In an emergency, however, a firm blow on the sternum over the precordium may halt fibrillation. Such a blow should be quickly followed by external cardiac massage at the rate of a normal pulse. Again, cardiac compressions should be interspersed with lung inflation as described. The chances of restarting a completely asystolic heart are not good, but well worth the effort.

HEMORRHAGE

Acute hemorrhage consists of sudden or rapid loss of blood from the circulatory system within a few minutes or hours as a result of an opening or openings in the system. Life is threatened if blood loss reaches 25–50% of total volume. Concealed bleeding is difficult to estimate. Williams and Sperryn point out that over a quart of blood may be lost into the tissues in a closed fracture of the tibia, yet this is minor compared to be what may be lost within pleural or peritoneal cavities in chest or abdominal injuries.

The body in general and the cardiovascular system in particular react to stress of injury to the circulatory system by shock, which is apparent after sudden loss of 15% or more of the circulating blood volume. The seriousness of hemorrhage lies in both the rate and the quantity of blood volume reduction, which are related to the number, type, and location of the vascular structures opened.

Physiologic Reaction

Whenever an artery or vein is opened, the injured vessel constricts and, if severed, retracts into the tissue, thereby reducing the size of the opening and facilitating clot formation (scalp vessels are an exception). In addition, other blood vessels temporarily constrict as a part of the general reaction to injury. This generalized vasoconstriction helps maintain blood pressure by reducing the capacity of the circulatory system.

At the site of injury, blood tends to clot and plug the opened vessel. If vasconstriction and blood clotting are unsuccessful, the resulting blood volume reduction causes a fall in blood pressure which, among its other affects, facilitates clot formation. If hemorrhage persists, the person dies from lack of oxygen and other nutrients.

Types of Hemorrhage

If a vein and an artery of equal size are severed, blood will escape more rapidly from the artery because it is forced out in spurts under the maximum pressure from each heartbeat. Venous hemorrhage can also be fatal if not controlled.

External Capillary Bleeding

Whole blood lost from capillary damage is of negligible importance in amount. Blood loss from capillaries and small veins is often referred to as "bleeding," as contrasted to large arterial losses that are referred to as "hemorrhage."

Small wounds are often deep and contaminated and require a washing out with fresh blood. Inhibited bleeding can be encouraged either by applying a light venous tourniquet (eg, rubber band, handkerchief, towel) proximal to the lesion or by immerging the limb in warm water. After the wound has been cleaned and the deep anaerobic bacteria have been oxygenated, apply a dressing and cold pack and elevate the limb. Refer for suturing and tetanus prophylaxis if necessary.

External Arterial Hemorrhage

Arterial injuries may be classed as either (1) complete, where the entire vessel wall is disrupted, or (2) incomplete, where only the outer coats or, at most, a portion of the circumference is damaged. These injuries originate from contusions, incised and lacerated wounds, and puncture wounds.

The early manifestations are hemorrhage and possibly the appearance of a hematoma. In the later stages, thrombosis, traumatic aneurysms, and secondary hemorrhage are to be feared.

Control bleeding by grasping the edges of the wound between fingers and thumb, and holding this pressure for 10 minutes or longer if necessary. Once bleeding subsides, cover the site with a large absorbent pad, and cover this with a large firm bandage. Then add more padding and another firm bandage. Nothing more should be done until the patient is in surgery.

Incised and lacerated arterial wounds in the healthy player are usually not serious if they do not penetrate the lumen. Healing progresses without an aneurysm developing. If the lumen is penetrated and divides the artery completely, retraction of the artery's ends tends to inhibit bleeding. The more ragged the tear, the more rapid is the development of the thrombosis. If an injury penetrates the lumen but does not divide the artery, the opening gaps and bleeding is more profuse and prolonged.

Internal Hemorrhage

Seek evidence of "pattern bleeding" where the pattern of clothing texture is imprinted on the skin. This is indicative of severe compression and suggests possible visceral rupture. Note the presence of any blood in vomitus, sputum, or excretions. Hemorrhage within the scalp or lungs may be indicated by bleeding from the nose, mouth, or ears (cranial lesion). Evidence of internal bleeding may also be represented in such signs as restlessness, apprehension, thirst, falling blood pressure, and increasing pulse rate. Swelling and discoloration may be seen in some instances. Treat for shock, and prepare for blood transfusion.

Swelling and pulsation in an arm or leg may indicate arterial hemorrhage within the affected limb. Internal hemorrhage in a thigh may be detected by measuring and comparing the circumferences of the two thighs. Sometimes limb enlargement that cannot otherwise be accounted for indicates internal hemorrhage. If elevation and cold do not relieve the extremity swelling, a tourniquet may be necessary. If the hemorrhage is in the thigh and swelling is severe, a tourniquet is often indicated because the volume of blood lost from general circulation may induce shock and death. This is seldom true of internal hemorrhage in the lower leg or forearm.

Intra-abdominal bleeding is usually the result of a ruptured organ or a branch of the aorta, a mesenteric artery, or a branch of the celiac trunk. In aortic injury, the tear is invariably on the anterior aspect. If such be the case, lying the subject supine should not be done. Rather, curl him up so that his knees compress the abdominal wall, compressing the wall of the artery and reducing the hemorrhage flow. The position may look strange, but it might be life saving. In slight-moderate bleeding from the gastrointestinal tract, sipping ice water or a cold enema may help to slow bleeding and to clear accumulated old blood from the digestive tract.

Hemorrhage within the chest or abdominal cavities may be indicated by signs of shock. First aid can do little directly to control hemorrhage into the patient's thoracic or abdominal cavities. Treating the patient to prevent or lessen shock may help stabilize his condition enough so that he can withstand later surgery. Mortality among such patients may be high, however, despite the best efforts of all concerned.

External Venous Hemorrhage

This can be profuse during competition because of the increased blood flow to active limbs. However, bleeding is often quickly stopped by a pad, firm bandage, and cold pack applied to the elevated limb. Nothing more is usually necessary for the next 24 hours unless surgical cleansing or suturing is required.

Thrombophlebitis and Embolism

Venous stasis and pressure of other injury to vein walls predispose the development of thrombophlebitis. The most common sites are in the veins of the pelvis and legs. This is sometimes seen with severe injuries in remote areas such as during a long hike, mountain climbing, or cross-country skiing, where an individual has remained still for several hours until helps arrives, with relaxed muscles and a resultant slowing of venous circulation in the legs. When inactivity is combined with pressure on the popliteal space and the calf of the leg, the possi-bility of developing thrombophlebitis increases.

The signs and symptoms of thrombophlebitis are cramping pain in the calf; possible redness, warmth, and swelling along the course of the involved vein; and pain which may appear only on dorsiflexion of the foot.

Never rub or massage the affected limb. Keep the affected limb horizontal and at rest, supported by pillows. Cotton elastic bandages may be used if available on each extremity from foot to groin to assist venous circulation. Be alert to any complaint or other evidence of respiratory difficulty or chest pain due to a possible embolism. Sudden dyspnea, violent coughing, hemoptysis, or sharp, severe, stabbing chest pain may be the first sign of a dislodged thrombus. Sudden signs of shock and collapse are common.

Controlling Hemorrhage

Control of external hemorrhage is best accomplished if the wound is first exposed to view. Clothing or other material over the injury should be cut, torn, or lifted away carefully so that additional harm is not inflicted. Unnecessary movement or exposure of the patient to general cold should be avoided if to the extent that it may induce or hasten a lowering of body temperature.

The Pressure Dressing

A sterile dressing applied with pressure to a hemorrhaging wound facilitates clot formation, compresses the open blood vessels and protects the injury from further invasion by infectious organisms:

1. The dressing should be of absorbent material which spreads and slows the blood it absorbs. This spreading and slowing action exposes a relatively large and thin surface of the outflowing blood to the air and thereby facilitates clot formation. Accordingly, one dressing partially filled with the player's blood is more effective in controlling hemorrhage than are a series of others because clot formation is in progress in the bloody dressing. The clot formation tends to spread back toward and into the wound until diminished air exposure, coupled with an adequate circulating speed, brings it to a halt. It is the clot which stops the hemorrhage. If the blood had no ability to clot, the

absorbent dressing applied would merely draw blood out through the wound and do more harm than good. When blood is about to clot, it begins to turn darker in color and becomes progressively darker as the clot takes form. A hard clot is almost black as its iron content oxidizes.

2. Direct pressure on a wound usually is very effective in controlling hemorrhage. Pressure is applied for the purpose of minimizing the size of the vessel opening by compression, temporarily or for an extended period, thereby lessening the amount and the velocity of the escaping blood and aiding clot formation. Considerable pressure may be applied to a wound if there is no broken bone in or near the wound. Hemorrhage does not always stop immediately. At times, hard presssure on the dressing over the wound may be required for several minutes until a clot has formed with sufficient strength to hold with only the help of dressing ties. If a clot does not form, a tourniquet must be considered, if feasible.

3. An external wound becomes contaminated with microorganisms at the moment of occurrence, thus the prompt application of a sterile dressing serves to limit the entrance of infectious organisms. Once a dressing is applied, leave it in place if at all possible. Removal permits entrance of additional microorganisms and may disturb the clot so that hemorrhage recurrs. Also, leaving the original dressing in place helps the surgeon viewing it later to estimate the amount of blood the patient has lost. When a wound is being dressed, care must be taken to avoid either touching the wound or the surface of the dressing that is to be placed directly on the wound, breathing onto the dressing or wound, stirring up dust about the patient area, or allowing other actions which would permit infectious organisms to enter the wound.

Avoid unnecessary prolonged pressure. The dressing should be anchored snugly to prevent slipping, but not tightly. The wounded part, especially if it is an arm or leg, will swell after a time, tightening the bandage still more and impairing or stopping circulation within the part of the detriment of the patient.

Elevation of a Wounded Limb

Frequently hemorrhage, especially of the venous type, can be lessened appreciably by raising the wounded limb to a height above that of the heart. Because elevation tends to drain the elevated limb by gravity, an initial gush of blood downward from open veins may be expected when the limb is first elevated. Elevation helps to lower the blood pressure at the wound site.

Elevation may be used before, during, or after application of a pressure dressing, depending mainly on the type and severity of the wound. The patient may be instructed to elevate a nonserious wound while waiting for a dressing and to maintain the height after the dressing is applied. Serious hemorrhage, especially of the arterial type, may require simultaneous and continuous application of elevation, dressing, pressure, and cold. If there is a broken bone in the wounded limb, elevation must be postponed until after the limb is splinted.

Reactionary Hemorrhage

Realization of the possibility of delayed hemorrhage occurring either externally or internally as a postinjury complication is of utmost importance. Reactionary bleeding may occur within a few hours after injury when blood pressure and circulation return to normal after shock. This increased blood pressure may also cause bleeding by displaced blood clots previously formed. If signs of renewed hemorrhage from the wound appear after a dressing is snugly in place, reapplication of manual pressure may be all that is necessary to assist clot formation with sufficient strength to occlude the vessel(s). Signs of renewed or continued hemorrhage are the appearance or enlargement of a bloodstain on the outer surface of the dressing and the appearance or continuance of blood trickling between the dressing and the skin.

Pressure Points

A pressure point is any site where a main artery supplying the wounded area lies near the skin surface and over a bone or firm tissue (Fig. 12.12). Pressure at these points is applied with the fingers, thumb, or hand. The object of the pressure is to compress

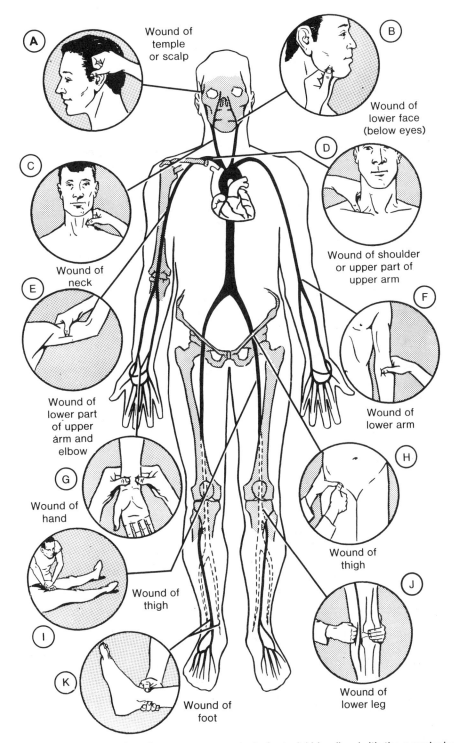

Figure 12.12. Pressure points for temporary control of arterial bleeding (with the permission of the Behavioral Research Foundation).

the artery against a firm substance to occlude the flow of blood from the heart to the wound. Since it is often difficult to maintain occluding pressure manually on a pressure point, the pressure point method is used only until a pressure dressing can be applied. The common pressure points are as follows:

1. *Temple or scalp.* Hemorrhage in the region of the temple or from the scalp may be controlled against the underlying skull just in front of the ear and above the prominent zygomatic arch.

2. *Lower face.* Hemorrhage of the face below the level of the eyes may be controlled by applying digital pressure to the artery in the notch on the under side of the lower jaw. This notch is easily located by running a finger from the angle of the jaw forward until the notch is encountered.

3. *Neck.* Hemorrhage of the neck may be diminished by applying digital pressure below the wound and just in front of the sternocleidomastoideus, pressing inward and slightly backward, thus compressing the carotid artery against the cervical spine. When this pressure point is used, care must be taken not to choke the patient.

4. *Shoulder or upper arm.* If hemorrhage is from either of these areas, digital pressure is applied behind the clavicle. The artery may be compressed against either the clavicle or the underlying first rib. Usually, pressure against the rib produces less pain to the patient.

5. *Midarm or elbow.* Hemorrhage from these areas may be controlled by applying pressure on the medial side of the arm, about halfway between the shoulder and the elbow, compressing the artery against the humerus.

6. *Forearm.* Hemorrhage from the lower arm may be diminished by applying digital pressure at the medial aspect of the cubital fossa of the relaxed elbow.

7. *Hand.* Hemorrhage from the hand may be controlled by applying digital pressure at the inner wrist.

8. *Thigh.* Hemorrhage from the thigh may sometimes be controlled by digital pressure against the midgroin from behind, collapsing the artery against the femur. At other times, pressure against the medial aspect of the midthigh may be more effective.

If midthigh pressure is used, the pressure should be applied with the heel of the hand while the hand is closed into a fist and reinforced by placing the other hand on top. Considerable pressure is necessary at this point to collapse the femoral artery against the femur because both lie deeply imbedded in some of the heaviest musculature of the body.

9. *Leg.* Hemorrhage from the leg between the knee and the foot may be controlled by firm pressure at the posterior knee. Pressure at one or both sides of the knee may be sufficient. If not, hemorrhage may be controlled by holding the front of the knee firmly with one hand and thrusting a fist hard against the vessels within the popliteal space.

10. *Foot.* Pressure by the hand around and just above the ankle is effective in the control of hemorrhage from the foot.

Use of the Tourniquet

A tourniquet is any constricting band placed around the circumference of one of the extremities to stop hemorrhage. In an emergency situation, mature judgment is required in making the decision to apply or withhold a true tourniquet. Both arterial and venous blood flow stop at the tourniquet. Without circulating blood, the part distal to the tourniquet begins to die. Rarely will a tourniquet be required unless a limb is severely mangled.

Professional Judgment

While later surgical amputation of the limb distal to the point of application of the tourniquet does not necessarily always follow, the person who decides to apply a tourniquet must do so with the realization that this distal portion will probably be sacrificed. Thus, a tourniquet applied to a patient must represent a choice between saving a life or saving a limb. It must not represent a choice between the quick results a tourniquet produces and the sometimes tiring application of a pressure dressing.

The decision to apply a tourniquet is irreversible. Once a tourniquet has been applied, it must be left in place until removed by a surgeon as soon as possible. It must not be loosened and retightened in the mistaken belief that the portion of the limb distal to the tourniquet is being kept alive. The patient whose system is stabilized after the tourniquet has reduced the capacity of his circulatory system may not be able to withstand the shock of its sudden enlargement if the tourniquet is loosened.

Guidelines

The use of a tourniquet is minimized when good techniques are used in pressure points, pressure dressings, elevation, local cold, and rest. Nonetheless, hemorrhage from a major artery of the thigh, lower leg, or upper arm, or hemorrhage from multiple arteries that is seen in traumatic amputation may prove beyond control by these methods. There is no set rule as to how long one should continue to try to control hemorrhage by pressure dressing, elevation, etc. However, in the emergency treatment situation, the absorbent capacity of the injured player's first-aid dressing may be used as a guideline:

• If all or nearly all the blood lost by the individual is contained in the dressing, the patient probably has not lost more than 500 ml of blood at most. This is the amount drawn from a donor who gives blood for transfusion. Thus, if the dressing becomes soaked through with blood but signs of clotting are also present, it is probable that continued pressure with elevation and cold, if possible, and perhaps with addition of absorbent material to that already in place, will facilitate clot formation and defeat the hemorrhage.

• If the dressing under hard pressure from the hand becomes soaked through, blood spreads rapidly to dry areas of the dressing and possibly drips or runs off, and no indication of clot formation appears promptly on the dressing, there is little gain from delaying application of a tourniquet.

Application

When a tourniquet is applied, concern must be given to placement, improvisation, tightening, skin protection, dressing, and monitoring until help or transportation arrives (Fig. 12.13).

Placement. When needed, the tourniquet is placed around the limb and between the wound and the body trunk; which is to say, between the wound and the heart. It is

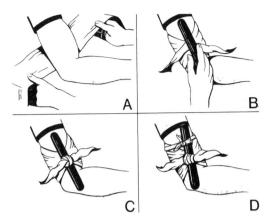

Figure 12.13. Applying a tourniquet.

never placed directly over a wound or fracture. In instances of amputation or partial amputation of the foot, leg, hand, or arm and for bleeding from the upper arm or thigh, place the tourniquet just above the wound or amputation site. For hemorrhage from the hand or forearm with no associated amputation, place the tourniquet immediately above the elbow. For hemorrhage from the foot or lower leg with no associated amputation, place the tourniquet immediately above the knee.

Improvisation. In the absence of a commercial tourniquet, one may be made from strong, soft, pliable material such as gauze or broadcloth bandage, clothing, or hankerchiefs. The material is used with a rigid sticklike object. To minimize skin damage, the improvised tourniquet should be made so that it is at least 1-inch wide *after* tightening. If gauze is used, 3–4-inch widths are preferred.

Pressure During Tightening. The tourniquet is applied with enough pressure to stop blood from passing under it. If a pulse has been detectable in the intact wrist or foot of the affected limb, tourniquet pressure is sufficient when the pulse ceases. If a pulse cannot be used as an indicator, you must rely on your judgment of reduced blood flow from the wound. After a tourniquet is properly tightened, arterial hemorrhage will immediately cease, but bleeding from veins in the distal part of the limb will continue until these vessels are drained. Do not continue to tighten the tourniquet in an attempt to stop this venous drainage.

Skin Protection During Tightening.
The skin beneath the tourniquet should be
protected from pinching, twisting,, and
tourniquet overtightening. Skin is relatively
resistant to oxygen deprivation and may
survive even though the limb beneath it
may require amputation later. Damaging the
skin with the tourniquet may deprive the
surgeon of skin required to cover the stump
properly, thus forcing greater amputation.
Skin may be protected from pinching and
twisting from a tourniquet by placing soft,
smooth material such as a shirt sleeve or
trouser leg around the limb and beneath the
tourniquet before tightening. Protection of
the skin also reduces the amount of pain to
the patient.

Dressing and Covering. After arterial
hemorrhage has ceased and the tourniquet
is securely in place, the wound is dressed to
protect it from further invasion by microorganisms. The condition of both the patient
and the weather may require that the patient be covered. If so, the covering should
be so arranged that the tourniquet remains
in view.

Monitoring. The tourniquet and dressing should be inspected every 15 minutes
until transportation can be made to assure
that arterial hemorrhage has not recurred.
If at any time it is believed that arterial
hemorrhage is continuing, the tourniquet
should be tightened. This judgment should
be made without loosening, lifting, or removing the dressing.

SHOCK

Shock is a body reaction to injury or
disease, a manifestation of the rebellion of
the body against a major insult or injury. It
is, in effect, an alarm reaction. It is a condition in which there is inadequate blood in
circulation to fill the vascular system. As a
result of ineffective circulation, which may
appear suddenly after trauma or develop
insidiously, there is interference with the
basic physiologic process of the blood
stream—delivering oxygen and other essential elements to body tissues and removing
waste products.

The predominant characteristic of shock
is a reduction in volume of circulating blood,
accompanied by vasoconstriction, which is

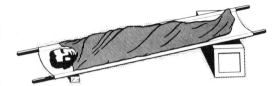

Figure 12.14. Typical position for treatment of
shock.

followed by vasodilation, hypotension,
tachycardia, and prostration. The initial circulatory deficiency is rapidly complicated
by widespread oxygen deprivation and by a
lessening of function of all tissues, especially
the brain, liver, heart, and kidneys.

Types of Shock

Hypovolemic shock is circulatory failure
resulting from loss of blood or other body
fluids from either external or internal
causes. Progressively reducing blood pressure with apathy to coma consciousness are
typical signs. External fluid losses may be
attributed to excessive sweating, burns, severe exudative lesions, renal disorder (eg,
diabetes, diuretics), hemorrhage, severe
vomiting, or diarrhea. Internal fluid loss
causes include fracture, internal rupture, intestinal obstruction, and ascites. When tissue damage occurs from trauma or burns, a
histamine-like substance is liberated which
acts as a peripheral vasodilator. This leads
to capillary stagnation within the splanchnic
area and muscles which results in a progressive circulatory reduction in the vital
organs.

Cardiogenic shock is circulatory failure resulting from cardiac pathology. The patient
presents low blood pressure, tachycardia,
distended neck veins, and pulmonary
edema. The skin is usually moist/pale but
sometimes is dry/warm. The cause is usually arrhythmia, myocardial infarction, severe congestive heart failure, pulmonary
embolism, acute valvular lesions (infection,
trauma), myocardiopathy, acute pericardial
tamponade, or dissecting aortic aneurysm.

Anaphylactic shock is circulatory failure as
the result of an immediate allergic reaction
in 1–60 minutes after exposure to a foreign
substance (antigen). The patient frequently
presents symptoms of dyspnea, wheezing
cough, itching, fainting, apprehension, ab-

dominal cramps, or nausea. Common signs are respiratory distress, bronchospasm, stridor, a red rash, hives, facial swelling, swollen tongue and throat, vomiting, diarrhea, hypotension, and syncope. Typical causes are insect stings or bites, desensitizing extracts of pollen (antigens), drugs (eg, penicillin), diagnostic agents (eg, x-ray contrast media), or foreign serum.

Typical Causes in Sports

Reduction of blood volume in circulation can result from (1) actual loss of blood through internal or external hemorrhage; (2) loss of plasma by seepage into tissues at the site of injury (eg, burns, contusions, crash injuries); (3) excessive loss of fluids and electrolytes from the intestinal tract through severe vomiting or diarrhea; and (4) an abnormally sudden increase in the capacity of the vascular system through vasodilation. In the latter instance, many blood vessels dilate at the same time and, although there is no actual loss in the amount of blood, blood fails to move along in the dilated vessels.

Signs and Symptoms

The signs and symptoms of shock are all related to ineffective circulation and depression of vital body processes (Fig. 12.15). The following signs and symptoms may not be equally prominent or appear in every patient, but they are representative of the picture of a player in shock.

The classical signs of shock reflect the body's attempt to compensate:

1. Early syncope, which is mainly neurogenic and which may be fatal. During this process, the patient will usually present a staring or vacant expression in the eyes. The pupils will be dilated unless morphine has been given.

2. Progressive loss of blood from active circulation, which may lead to failing heart output and insufficient oxygen to cells that are vital for survival. Cold perspiration, pallor, and possibly slight cyanosis reflect the body's attempt to produce peripheral vasoconstriction.

3. Sustained, progressively failing hypotension, which may lead to liver and kidney failure reflected by oliguria, indicative of physiologic-compensation failure.

4. Rapid shallow breathing (air hunger), tachycardia, and rapid weak thready pulse, in compensation for cerebral anoxia. Anxiety, excitement leading to confusion, listlessness, irrelevant phrase repetition, apathy, and coma are also effects of cerebral anoxia.

Preventive Measures

Shock should be anticipated in any player subjected to known causes of shock such as unusual physical and emotional stress, any severe injury, loss of blood, or loss of other body fluids. Shock may develop slowly; in fact, the characteristic signs might not appear for several hours. In incipient or impending shock that has not yet developed, none of the signs may be present, but preventive measures should be taken when shock is considered possible.

The objective of preventive measures is met through the control or relief of factors tending to reduce aeration and circulation of an adequate blood volume. Aside from or even in the absence of hemorrhage, circulatory collapse may be hastened or aggravated by a number of factors including fear, fatigue, and pain; dehydration as the result of vomiting, diarrhea, and excessive sweating; movement of injured parts; a hot environment; and overdoses of morphine.

Keep the patient horizontal so that available circulating blood does not have to move against gravity. If the patient must be moved, move him gently. Cover the player lightly to preserve heat in a cold environment, but with not so many blankets as to increase core temperature. Do whatever is possible to relieve pain. Maintain a quiet, calm attitude to reassure the patient and

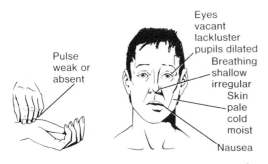

Eyes
vacant
lackluster
pupils dilated
Breathing
shallow
irregular
Skin
pale
cold
moist
Nausea

Pulse
weak or
absent

Figure 12.15. Typical signs and symptoms of a patient in shock.

make him feel secure. Check vital signs frequently to seek signs of irregularities and sudden changes.

Emergency Care

Williams and Sperryn warn that the worst treatment that can be given is overheating as this increases peripheral vascularity which deprives deeper, essential circulation. The only effective treatment of severe shock is transfusion of whole blood. In the meantime, assure that the airway is open, lay the patient supine if conscious or in the three-quarter coma position if unconscious.

The limbs should be raised about 6 inches above the head to let gravity assist venous drainage (see Fig. 12.14). Pillows can be placed beneath the patient's feet (with flexion at the knees) and buttocks. The best manner is to raise the foot end of a cot or litter. This position will create pooling of blood in the abdominal area without pressure on the diaphragm. Placing the head of a sitting victim down is not good as respiration is hindered due to the weight of the viscera causing diaphragm elevation.

The semiprone coma position may be used when the patient is unconscious; when there is a wound of the head, face, neck (except fracture or dislocation), or chest; or when vomiting is likely. When the patient is in this position, drainage from the respiratory tract is assisted. See Figure 12.3.

Loosen tight clothing around the neck, chest, waist, and at any other areas in which clothing tends to bind. Loosen but do not remove shoes. Reassure the patient, if he is conscious, that his best interests are being served. Relieve thirst in the conscious patient who is not vomiting and has no wound in the abdominal cavity or alimentary canal. Warm sweet drinks and oxygen may be offered. Never offer an alcoholic beverage as it dilates the vessels, and never force fluids by mouth. Oxygen must be started immediately at 6 liters/minute if cyanosis of lips, nailbeds, or earlobes is noticed. A critical point for effective kidney function is reached when systolic blood pressure drops below 80 mm Hg. This may be a fatal complication.

Keep the patient comfortable and warm. The patient should not be allowed to become either cooled or overheated. A drop in skin temperature gives rise to constriction of the superficial blood vessels, thereby reducing the volume of the vascular system. In a cool or cold atmosphere, the patient's body and limbs should be covered with blankets. Wet clothing should be removed and blanket coverings tucked close to the patient's skin.

Elevated body temperature places stress on the cardiovascular system. As the superficial vessels dilate in an attempt to cool the blood within them, the system may become too large for the amount of blood it contains. In addition, there is an increased loss of electrolytes, particularly sodium and chloride. In a warm or hot atmosphere, padding used beneath the patient should not be made of wool. The patient should be shaded from the sun. Clothing may be left on and exposed to the atmosphere, provided that a breeze does not evaporate the perspiration in the clothing so rapidly as to chill the patient. He should also be protected against atmospheric temperature changes such as those brought on with nightfall. His temperature should be monitored and perspiration from heat stress differentiated from signs of chilling.

Treatment measures should be discontinued gradually when vital signs return to normal and become stable. One valuable test of return of circulatory control is the ability of the patient to maintain stable vital signs as he changes his position gradually upright. No sudden or abrupt movements should be permitted.

HYPOTHERMIA

In sports, a subnormal temperature is the result of poor heat production, a thermostat abnormality, or exposure to cold, especially when alcohol or barbiturates are in the body. In prolonged exposure to cold, the individual may die from exhaustion from shivering rather than from the hypothermia. Shivering, alone, can increase metabolic work as much as 50%. Intrinsic clinical hypothermia results whenever the central nervous system is depressed from drugs, primary brain disease, or toxins which alter the thermostat.

All cold injuries are similar, varying only in degree of tissue injury. The extent of injury depends on such factors as wind-speed, temperature, type and duration of exposure, and humidity. Tissue freezing is accelerated by wind, humidity, or a combination of the two. Injury caused by cold dry air is less than that caused by cold moist air or exposure to cold air while wearing wet clothing. Fatigue, smoking, drugs, alcohol, emotional stress, dehydration, and severe trauma intensify the harmful effects of cold.

Cold Exhaustion

When rectal temperature falls below 95°F, cerebral and muscular function is being impaired. Oral or axillary temperature give little indication of core temperature. Temperature reduction is the multiple effect of a decreasing core temperature, exhausted glycogen stores, and a reduced blood-sugar level.

Physical findings vary with oral temperature: low 90s, shivering; high 80s, dilated pupils, decreased motor function, bradycardia; low 80s, hypoventilation, areflexia, stupor or coma, arrhythmias.

The warning signs prior to syncope are muscle weakness and cramps, followed quickly by locomotor dysfunctions as witnessed by awkwardness, a slowed pace, and poor coordination or stumbling. The patient becomes talkative, with slurred speech, and excitable. Rapid recovery can be made at this stage if corrective action is taken. If ignored, the state progresses into apathy or anxiety symptoms and finally into collapse within 1–2 hours. During the stage of mental confusion, the subject may become disoriented, subject himself to potential injury, or hallucinate warmth and remove clothing. Intense weakness and paralysis follow. Death is approaching if rectal temperature falls below 90°F.

There appears to be no correlation between chilling and wetness with the common cold. Several studies mentioned by Levy have shown that submerging volunteers in ice baths or hot baths followed by a trip outside in frigid weather failed to show increased incidence. Other studies, however, have shown where cold air blown on the calf of the leg lowered intramuscular temperature between 1–12°F, thus a distinct physiologic alteration is present in drafts.

Nevertheless, in the common cold, fatigue appears to be the most important predisposing factor. Thus, sensible training, diet, and rest should be monitored as much as possible to avoid common colds.

Emergency Care

In an emergency situation of hypothermic cold exhaustion, do whatever is possible to remove moisture from clothing or provide adequate dry clothing, protect the subject from the wind, and provide warm shelter. A well-insulated sleeping bag is helpful. Warm, sweet fluids may be offered if the nondiabetic subject is conscious. Oxygen is helpful, especially if it can be administered prewarmed. Movement by stretcher is extremely slow; escorted walking or another means of transportation (eg, snowmobile) is preferred when possible. If rescue is delayed, the victim can be warmed somewhat by close contact with associates, who also help to screen the wind. Monitor cardiac rhythm frequently; CPR may be necessary.

When returned to safety and shelter, a tepid bath (100–105°F) is helpful in restoring body temperature, but this should not be attempted with the unconscious individual as the risk of convulsions is great. Care must be taken to warm the body somewhat slowly, especially if hypothermia is severe. Never place artificial heat next to the bare skin. A conscious victim can be given warm sips of a nonalcoholic liquid, but do not allow the victim to smoke.

Hypotension is always a danger during rewarming, leading to shock. When the body's heat-regulating mechanisms begin to fail, acid/base balance becomes disturbed, and ventricular fibrillation and cardiac arrest are encouraged. Closely check for signs of respiratory failure or cardiac arrest. There is always risk of circulatory, pulmonary, or kidney failure, which requires immediate hospitalization.

SUDDEN DEATH IN ATHLETICS

Death may be defined as the permanent cessation of the physical and chemical processes upon which the phenomena of life depend. It is necessary, however, to appreciate that there is some difference between the legal and the scientific concept of death.

Thus, each physician should be well-acquainted with statutory definitions.

Sudden death occasionally occurs in an athlete where even standard autopsy fails to show clear evidence of cause. In extensive examination, some cases of sudden and unexpected deaths have been attributed to fibrosis within the cardiac conduction system associated with a narrowed coronary artery. Other cases have shown signs of myocarditis related to old trauma.

Conditions Simulating Death. As death is accompanied by cessation of circulation and respiration, the conditions which may simulate death are those accompanied by temporary respiratory and circulatory inhibition such as syncope, partial asphyxia, and trance. When death occurs, the surface of the body takes on an ashy-white color which is quite characteristic and serves as evidence of cessation of circulation. However, there are many exceptions to the rule that such pallor indicates actual death. The same is true of tests for respiration and muscle tone applied too soon after death. Immediately after death, the eyes begin to lose their luster and become dull and glazed; but in rare cases, this may not occur for some time.

Death Signs. Death in sports may come suddenly or in minutes before transportation to an emergency facility can be made. Healthcare personnel need to be aware of signs commonly associated with approachiong death and need to recognize how these physiologic changes modify management of the individual. In such cases, anticipate the need for privacy, and attempt to meet all physical needs for hygiene and comfort.

FIRST-AID SUPPLIES

Half of good health care is good planning. Table 12.2 includes those basic items that are typically available in the training room during games and practice sessions. While certain basic equipment should be available when needed, the doctor and first-aid assistant must be able to improvise on a moment's notice, sometimes under the most difficult circumstances. Knowing the "why"

of any procedure differentiates the professional from the amateur who has only been taught "what" and "how."

**Table 12.2.
First-Aid Supplies**

Absorbents	Hydrocolator packs
Adhesive bandages	Ice
Adhesive felt	Jaw wedge
Adhesive tape	Lubricating ointment
(various sizes)	Magnifying glass
Analgesics	Massage oil
Anhidrotics	Mouthwash
Antiglare ointment	Nail cutters
Antiphlogistics	Ophthalmoscope
Antiseptics	Otoscope-nasoscope
Artificial airway	Penlight
Aspiration sucker	Percussion hammer
pump (hand	Pinwheel
operated)	Protective pads (assorted sizes)
Astringents	
Bandage scissors	Razor blades
Bandages (sterile)	Resin
Benzoin tincture	Rubefacients
Blackboard	Safety pins
Blankets	Salt tablets and dispenser
Bulletin board	
Cervical collars	Scalpel
Chafing powder	Scissors
Cleat wrenches	Sink with hot and cold water
Clock	
Cold packs	Skin pencils
Contact lens suction	Slings
cup	Sphygmomanometer
Cotton balls	Spine boards
Counterirritants	Splints
Deodorants	Sterile gauze pads
Disinfectants	Stethoscope
Drinking cups	Sting-relief lotion
(paper)	Stockinetts
Elastic tape (various	Styptics
sizes)	Swabs
Emollients	Tape cutters
Endotrachial tube	Taping tables
Eye chart	Thermometer
Eye patches	Timer
Felt	Tongue blades
Fire extinguisher	Tongue forceps
Finger cots	Towels
Foam rubber	Tracheotomy tube
padding	Tuning forks
Gauze rolls	Two-way artificial airway (various sizes)
Hair clippers	
Heel cups	Weight/height scales
Hemostatics	Wool felt

CHAPTER 13

Physiologic Therapeutics in Sports

Chiropractic physiologic therapeutics is defined by the ACA Council on Physiotherapy as the application of forces and substances that induce a physiologic response and use and/or allow the body's natural processes to return to a more normal state of health.

This section is not intended to be instructional in specific modality application, but rather to bring to attention commonly utilized procedures and their rationale within the management of sports injuries. For this reason, emphasis will be on application-rationale within athletics, indications, and contraindications, rather than technique.

PHYSIOLOGIC THERAPEUTICS

Physiologic therapeutics make use of the therapeutic effects of mechanotherapy, hydrotherapy, electrotherapy, light, heat, cold, air, soft-tissue manipulation, and massage. The rational application of these natural forces requires a knowledge of the actions and effects on pathophysiologic processes.

The use of physiotherapy to facilitate basic chiropractic care has been popular within the profession since the turn of the century. However, any therapeutic agent possesses a potential for effectiveness and a potential for danger. Each modality has its indications and contraindications, and certain precautions must be observed if the modality is to be applied safely and effectively in line with the biophysics and physiologic responses involved.

When properly applied, benefits are gained in normalizing function, preventing and minimizing pain and deformities, and maintaining what has been gained in treatment. The physician-operator must be well acquainted with the physics involved and the underlying application fundamentals to properly prescribe or utilize an appropriate modality—as well as be skilled in the technique of application, its intensity and duration—and to effectively analyze the anticipated effects.

Effects of Common Physical Agents

Each of the common physical agents utilized has more or less specific primary effects and secondary effects. Heat from any source, for example, has a primary thermal effect with secondary effects in hyperemia, sedation, and attentuation of microorganisms. Cold from any source offers a hypothermal primary effect with secondary effects of decongestion, ischemia, and sedation.

Photochemical and electrochemical effects are seen with some physical agents. For example, sunlight, heated metals, and carbon or mercury-vapor arcs present primary photochemical effects and secondary effects of erythema, pigmentation, and activation of ergosterol. Galvanic current offers a primary electrochemical effect and secondary polarization and vasomotor effects.

Kinetic and electrokinetic effects are seen with other physical agents. For example, vibration, massage, traction, and therapeutic exercise offer primary kinetic effects with secondary actions of muscle stimulation, increased venous and lymph flow, tissue stretching, and reflex stimulation. Electric currents (eg, low-frequency, alternating, interrupted, sinusoidal) present primary electrokinetic effects with secondary effects of muscle stimulation, increased venous and lymph flow, tissue stretching, and reflex stimulation.

Ultrasound therapy is unique in that it offers primary mechanothermochemical effects with secondary effects of intracellular massage and thermal sedation.

Reflex Considerations

The efficiency of physical therapy in the treatment of injury and disease depends to a great deal on (1) the direct reflex effects of the stimulating agent employed and (2) the influence of these agents exerted through the autonomic centers.

The relief of visceral pain by means of any stimulating agent applied to the skin which elicits localized peripheral vasodilation probably depends mainly on the associated visceral hyperemia. Traumatic and visceral pains are not uncommonly associated with ischemia of the organ or tissues involved. The pain receptors involved are stimulated by a chemical substance which accumulates in the tissues because the circulation is insufficient to remove it. The function of the vasomotor nerve consequently plays a major role in both the cause of pain and its alleviation.

Procedure Applications Relative to Pathogenesis

As disease is a dynamic process rather than a static entity, the primary intent of chiropractic physiotherapeutics is to assist the body in adapting to and/or normalizing the aberrant processes within an abnormal state. The abnormal process existing at the time of therapy determines the particular type of therapy applicable. Any injury or disease state comprises a number of abnormal physiologic reactions depending on its state of healing or adaptation. Thus, therapy *must* be varied according to the process at hand to assist the body in normalizing or adapting to the condition. The therapeutic goal is often to stop or reverse a noxious reaction which is preventing or delaying normal healing processes. (See Fig. 13.1.)

Brandstetter points out that whether a tissue becomes primarily injured through frank trauma or microtrauma or is undergoing a change such as a secondary reaction to a neuropathic process initiated elsewhere, four stages usually occur (see Table 13.1). While these stages and their processes usually exist in varying degrees within tissues simultaneously, one process usually dominates. Treatment should be directed primarily at the dominant process and altered as the dominant feature changes. In this regard, as Brandstetter states, the presence of a coexisting neuropathy must be realized and the area of therapy should be considered as not only at the site of local symptoms but also at the neuromere or spinal segment directly or indirectly involved.

In any particular stage of physiologic activity, a misapplied or too vigorous appli-

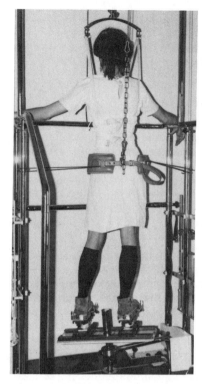

Figure 13.1. A tortion locomotion apparatus designed to facilitate antigravitational dorsolumbar adjustive procedures.

cation may be an insult to the lesion as well as to healthy tissue, causing a return to active inflammation. Any overtreatment, whether it be of time or intensity, may counteract the beneficial effects desired.

A professional treatment table can be an important adjunct in providing relaxation, stretching, or gravitational assistance during the application of various types of physiologic therapeutics. Some examples are shown in Figure 13.2.

THERAPEUTIC COLD

Winning or losing a game often depends upon getting an injured athlete back into competitive form as soon as possible. The application of cold to an acute injury is probably the fastest and safest therapy available. In traumatic sprains, strains, contusions, and abrasions, ice or other types of cold applications with appropriate support (eg, tape, padding) often offer dramatic relief.

Table 13.1.
Modalities and the Physiologic Stages Involved in Healing

I. **Stage of hyperemia or active congestion**
1. *Ice packs*: vasoconstrictive effects.
2. *Positive galvanism*: vasoconstrictive, hardening of tissues effects.
3. *Ultrasound*: dispersing effects; increased membrane permeability effects.
4. *Rest*, with possible support: prevents irritation and further injury.

II. **Stage of passive congestion**
1. *Alternating hot and cold applications*, preferably in 3:1 ratio every few hours: revulsive effects.
2. *Light massage*, particularly effleurage: revulsive effects.
3. *Passive manipulation*: effects of revulsion, maintenance of muscle tone, freeing of coagulate and possibly early adhesions.
4. *Mild range of motion exercise*: effects same as 3.
5. *Sinusoidal stimulation*, of a surging nature: effects same as 3.
6. *Ultrasound*: increase in gaseous exchange, dispersion of fluids, liquefaction of gels, and increased membrane permeability effects.

III. **Stage of consolidation and/or formation of fibrinous coagulant**
1. *Local moderate heat*, preferably of a moist nature: mild vasodilation, increased membrane permeability effect.
2. *Moderate active exercise*: revulsive effects, freeing of coagulant and early adhesions, maintenance of tone, and ligamentous and muscular integrity effects.
3. *Motorized alternating traction*: effects same as 2.
4. *Moderate range of motion manipulation*: effects same as 2.
5. *Ultrasound*: hyperemia, liquefaction of gels, dispersion of gases and fluids, increased membrane permeability, and tissue-softening effects.
6. *Sinusoidal current*, surging or pulsating: effects same as 2.

IV. **Stage of fibroblastic activity and fibrosis**
1. *Deep heat*, prolonged (eg, diathermy): prolonged vasodilation, increased membrane permeability, increased chemical activity effects.
2. *Deep massage* (eg, petrissage or other soft-tissue manipulation: tends to break down fibrotic tissue and create more elasticity.
3. *Vigorous active exercise*, preferably with slight traction or at least without weight bearing: maintains muscle and ligamentous integrity, stretches fibrotic tissues, breaks adhesions, and creates greater elasticity.
4. *Motorized alternating traction*: effects same as 3.
5. *Negative galvanism*, particularly with an antisclerotic (eg, potassium iodine): vasodilation, softening, liquefaction, and antisclerotic activity effects.
6. *Ultrasound*: effects causing softening of tissues as previously mentioned.
7. *Active joint manipulation*: reduction of muscular spasm, breaking of adhesions and fibrotic tissue, and restoration of physiologic motion effects.

Adapted from 1975 report of the ACA Council on Physiotherapy

Cold may be applied by numerous methods such as plastic bag packs, vapor coolant sprays, ice massages, immersion baths and whirlpools, or coldpacks. Cryokinetics (cooling a part, followed by active exercise) and contrast baths are often used in stimulating peripheral circulation.

Physiologic Effects of Cold

When applied locally, cold produces vasoconstriction, which reduces secretions and exudation. Thus, as Andrews shows, it has a reverse effect on inflammation by decreasing capillary pressure and diminishing the amount of hemorrhage into tissue spaces that facilitates lymphatic drainage to reduce swelling (Fig. 13.3).

Prolonged cold also produces sedation and numbness and increases muscle tone. A reflex vasoconstriction effect occurs in internal organs. If cold is prolonged, the vasoconstrictive effects are fatigued and the opposite effects develop, such as local vasodilation, reflex internal vasodilation, increased blood pressure, and decreased respiratory rate. The initial decreased capillary

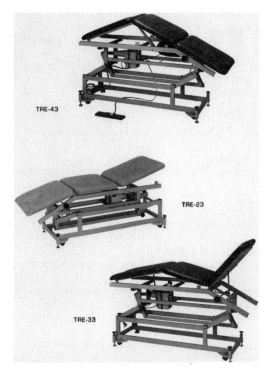

Figure 13.2. Some Triton treatment tables (with the permission of the Chattanooga Corp.).

blood pressure is followed in 5–8 minutes by increased blood pressure and a slowed pulse.

As cold is a counterirritant and as the speed with which a nerve transmits an impulse is reduced in decreased temperatures, the pain threshold is increased. This is one reason why cold applications allow a painful joint to be placed through greater angles of passive and active ranges of motion without discomfort.

The general physiologic effects of cold include increased heart and respiratory rates, leucocytosis, and decreased fatigue. The color change occurring as blanched skin changes to red or blue-red in prolonged cold is the result of a histamine release associated paradoxically with an increase in utilization of oxygen by local tissue. When cold is removed, the demand for tissue oxygen is increased and the vessels dilate in compensation to produce a hyperemia.

Cold is much more penetrating than heat. Studies in ice massage show that temperature drops 18°F at a depth of 1 cm with effects lasting up to 3 hours. Ice massage can reduce surface skin temperature to 60–

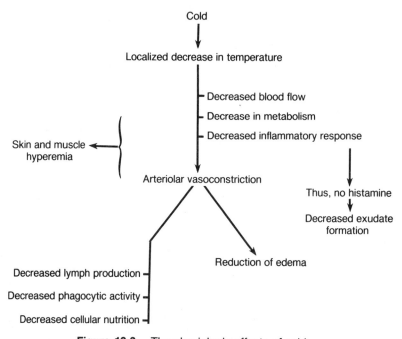

Figure 13.3. The physiologic effects of cold.

58°F, and no ill effects to normal skin are seen until skin temperature is reduced below 50°F. But it takes time for cold to penetrate. For example, when icebags whose water temperature is 32°F are continually placed on an extremity, the outside of the towel covering the bag will be about 40°F. It takes 15 minutes for the skin temperature to drop from 84–43°F, about 60 minutes for subcutaneous tissue to drop from 94–70°F, and about 2 hours for intramuscular temperature to drop from 98–79°F.

Indications and Contraindications

Cold is indicated whenever the physiologic effects are desired, thus readily appropriate in musculoskeletal strains, sprains, bursitis, arthritis, tendinitis, fibrositis, myositis and splinting. Muscle "pulls" and cervical strains respond well to cold. Many trainers report excellent results with cold therapy in the management of ligamentous irritations of the ankle, knee, hips, ribs, shoulder, elbow, and wrist.

While cryotherapy has been used for centuries, its exact physiologic effects are not completely understood, but current research is showing its profound effects. For example, in cases of advanced multiple sclerosis, poliomyelitis, arthritis, and periarthritis, cold applications applied both proximal and distal to a joint tested have shown to offer a marked but often unsustained decrease in resistance to passive stretch and thus a marked increase in joint mobility, whether or not pain and tenderness are present. Such a decrease in resistance to passive stretch lasts from a few minutes up to 24 hours. It is also unexplained why patients with rheumatic afflictions who have decreased joint mobility on cold damp days are benefited by ice massage.

There are few contraindications to cold in sports as compared to clinical practice with the weak, very old or young, or advanced cardiovascular or peripheral vascular conditions. Obviously, cold is contraindicated when blood flow is impeded or the thermal sense is diminished. Cold should not be applied in an area previously affected by frostbite. Even when frostbite is not within the history, some people are hypersensitive and intolerant to cold.

THERAPEUTIC HEAT

Heat is applied in a number of fashions such as hot water, whirlpools, steam baths, sauna-like hot air, sand and mud, paraffin dips, hydrocollator packs, hot moist packs, electric pads, ultrasound, shortwave diathermy, microwave, radiant heaters, sunlight, infrared rays, and incandescent lamps. Regardless of the mechanism used, the surface effects of heat on tissues are essentially the same, but deeper effects vary according to intensity, concentration of application, duration, wave-length, and the vascularity of the area (Fig. 13.4).

Physiologic Effects of Heat

The rule of thumb is that heat should never be applied to a body part until 48 hours after injury, or even longer if recurrent bleeding is a danger. When tissue is injured, the body establishes a defensive inflammatory mechanism that temporarily blocks circulation and white and red cells

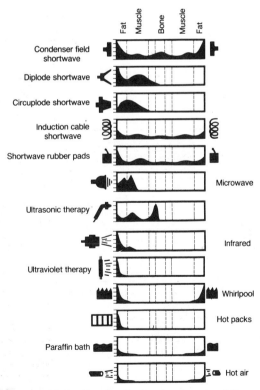

Figure 13.4. Depth effects of various heat-therapy modalities (after Hill).

hasten to the affected part. After the acute stage has passed, fresh blood must be brought to the injured part to carry on the battle to enhance healing processes. Because lesion waste products are difficult to move through the small venous vessels, heat is an aid. See Figure 13.5.

It takes time for heat to penetrate. For example, when hot water bags whose temperature is 133°F are continually placed on an extremity, the outside of the towel covering the bag will be about 122°F. It takes about 30 minutes for the skin temperature to rise from 90°F to 110°F, about 40 minutes for subcutaneous tissue to rise from 91.2°F to 105.5°F, and about 50 minutes for intramuscular temperature to rise from 94.2°F to 99.6°F.

As with cold, the exact physiologic mechanisms by which heat achieves its effects are not completely understood. For example, paradoxical decreases in intra-articular temperatures have been recorded, and increases have been recorded with surface cold.

Indications and Contraindications

Local heat relieves muscle spasm, dilates superficial blood and lymph vessels, increases phagocytosis and perspiration, and sedates the nervous system. It also reflexly dilates blood and lymph vessels in deeper tissues in various degrees depending upon the application site.

General heat applied to the body increases circulation, heart rise, perspiration, respiration, and urine formation. The blood tends to become more alkaline while the tissues become more acidic.

Some authorities have shown that variations of temperature applications to various parts of the body will produce vascular shifts and also have a toning effect upon the blood vessels, thus explaining the benefits of alternate hot and cold applications.

Local heat is contraindicated in acute inflammations, suppuration, hemorrhagic tendencies, impaired or hypersensitive thermal sense, or over encapsulated swellings where vasodilation may result in rupture or dispersion. Heat should never be applied to an acute injury where extravasated blood

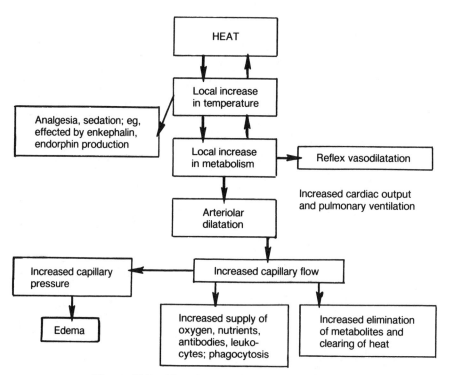

Figure 13.5. The physiologic effects of local heating.

and fluids occur because great damage can be done by increasing localized edema and bleeding from ruptured capillaries. Great care must be used in applying local heat to the diabetic.

Physiologic Effects of Shortwave Diathermy

Different wave lengths have different effects; ie, the shorter the wave length, the deeper the penetration. As the name implies, this modality utilizes high-frequency alternated currents of short wavelengths.

Shortwave diathermy produces local hyperlymphemia and sedation. Histamine production is increased, which causes vasodilation. Enlargement of the venous capillary system hastens resorption and removal of bacteria and waste products at the site of the lesion. Because defensive mechanisms (phagocytosis) are assisted by the effect on serum and leukocytes, a bactericidal effect is present. Both locally and generally, phagocytosis and leukocytosis are increased through increased circulation rate. Osmosis of serum proteins is reestablished from increased capillary pressure, and metabolism is influenced from the increased oxidation rate of blood. There is a general rise in body temperature, associated with increased heart, BMR, perspiration, and respiratory rates.

Indications and Contraindications

The deep heat from diathermy relieves muscle cramps, spasms, and associated pain and increases glandular secretions. Because of a lowered concentration of pain-producing substances below the irritation level of nerve receptors, a general sedative effect and relief of pain occurs.

Shortwave diathermy uses high-frequency current (27 megacycles) to heat body tissues, the result of tissue resistance to the current. It is probably the most common modality used when deep heat is desired. Subacute and chronic strains, sprains, tenosynovitis, and myositis respond well. It should be kept in mind, however, that the deeper tissues affected by diathermy do not have the heat sensitivity enjoyed by the superficial tissues. Thus, thermal devitalization can occur in deep tissues without

pain or other warning signs. For this reason, it is best to apply deep heat cautiously.

The common contraindications seen in athletics are acute injury and inflammations, deficient thermal sensation, menstruation, large or inflamed varicosities, over epiphyses, through the brain, or whenever systemic fever would be contraindicated. As seen in general practice, states of tuberculosis, malignancy, pregnancy, cardiovascular or renal disease, metallic implants, ulcerative disorders, advanced osteoporosis, and severe weakness are certainly contraindications. Even in the healthy, only one-half of the normal rate should be applied over encapsulated organs.

Physiologic Effects of Ultrasonic Diathermy

Ultrasound therapy is produced by a frequency about 1 million cycles/second far above that perceptible to the human ear. The depth of penetration is 4 cm or more, and its primary effect is the result of the vibrations passing into tissue causing an internal friction which results in heat. Unlike light, ultrasound passes through all tissue liquids and solids which inhibit the passage of light.

Mechanical, thermal, chemical, and neural effects are seen with the use of ultrasound. Mechanically, there is a dispersion of fluids, an increase in molecular movement (cellular micromassage), and increased membrane permeability. Thermally, hyperemia (thus increased leukocytosis and alkalosis) and increased glandular activity are produced. Chemically, ionization through membranes, chemical oxidation, and gaseous exchange are increased. Thixotrophic gels may be converted into liquid forms.

Phonophoresis is presently being investigated, wherein certain substances are incorporated into the coupling medium to enhance the therapeutic effect. Adequate data on this noninvasive innovation are not as yet available.

Pathophysiologic Neural Effects

Whether they be mechanical, chemical, or psychic, irritations cause the nervous system to alter its normal physiologic response, and it is such altered responses that are exhibited as signs and symptoms of a given disorder. A paper by the ACA Council on Physiotherapy brings out that, "This neurotrophic response may also be sensitized and result in an aberration of normal irritability with the subsequent maintenance, facilitation, and/or production of disease processes occurring as the nervous system responds to the average extrinsic and intrinsic stresses of normal life processes. Ultrasound affects the nervous system in such a way as to reduce its conductivity and, therefore, tends to abort the maintenance of a neural pattern of disease."

Because of this latter effect, ultrasound is wisely applied to several areas which parallel the pathogenic process. For example: (1) The local area, to scatter or dissolve the pathologic process before neuropathy is firmly established and to provide symptomatic relief. (2) Known areas of referred or reflex activity, to halt or dissolve areas of neuropathy. (3) Over the synaptic areas of specific neuromeres when "sensitization" of the neurotrophic process may have occurred.

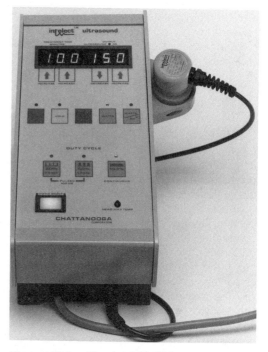

Figure 13.6. The Intelect 205 ultrasound unit (with the permission of the Chattanooga Corp.).

Therapy over a neurologic area (eg, nerve root) should be conducted at half duration and at a lower intensity as compared to that utilized over the primary site. Ultrasound can also be used as a diagnostic probe in locating paravertebral and peripheral trigger points and deep-seated areas of sensitivity (Fig. 13.6).

Contraindications

Ultrasound is generally contraindicated over sites of potential hemorrhage, the stellate ganglion, gonads, eyes, growing or unfused epiphyses, implants, infections, and bony protuberances. In general practice, advanced heart disease, malignancies, pregnancy, pulmonary tuberculosis, and sensory paralysis are also contraindications.

Microwave Diathermy

Microwave diathermy is rarely used because its depth of heat is limited to the most superficial tissues, eliminating deep joint therapy, and the treatment area is limited to a small field. However, it is easy to apply and sometimes the treatment of choice when mild heating is desired. Greater research into application is necessary.

Microwave therapy is contraindicated whenever heat is inadvisable. It should never be applied in high dosages over edematous tissues or wet dressings, near metallic implants, or over adhesive tape. Extreme caution must be used when applications are made over bony prominences.

GALVANIC CURRENT

Ever since Guillaume Duchenne published *Physiologic des Mouvements* in 1867, galvanism has been used in the treatment of injuries and disease. Galvanic current is the only current that is applied in regard to polarity. Its physiologic effects are those of heat and chemical processes and as a cellular excitant. The chemical effect is derived from the dislocation of sodium from tissue salt.

Most galvanic current is of a direct current of low voltage usually not exceeding 100 volts and of low amperage usually not greater than 50 milliamperes. The current is unidirectional, consisting of a stream of ions which flow at low tension. No muscle contraction results unless the current is interrupted.

Polar Effects of Galvanism

The negative pole tends to attract alkalies and repel acids, to increase circulation via vasodilation (thus relieving chronic pain), to decrease nerve sensitivity at high intensities, to increase irritability at low intensities, and to soften tissue. The positive pole tends to attract acids and repel alkalies, to decongest tissues via vasoconstriction (thus relieving acute pain), to inhibit nerve irritability, and to toughen tissue.

Contraindications

High-intensity current should never be applied through the heart or brain, or on an individual with impaired sensory response. Galvanism is contraindicated in any condition where its effects would be inadvisable for the state of a disorder at the time or in any disease process where stimulation might produce harmful results (eg, possible tumor).

Iontophoresis

Iontophoresis consists of transferring ions into the body by an electromotive force. The greatest concentration is moved into the skin where the skin is broken or along sweat glands and hair follicles. Because the depth is minimal, the ions transferred into the skin are taken up by the circulation and do not proceed through the tissues to the other electrode.

The caustic ions of heavy metals such as copper and zinc have been found useful in the management of septic surfaces and in chronic infections of cavities (eg, sinuses). Copper salts (2%), for example, are 12 times more microbicidal when taken into tissues through iontophoresis. Iodine and chlorine ions are often used for softening fibrotic tissue and loosening adhesions and superficial scars after joint injuries.

HIGH-VOLT MODALITIES

During the past few years, relatively high-voltage units have been employed with outstanding results. The physiologic effects apparently are produced by the increased capability to move bound and unbound tissue fluids.

Kaesberg, who has studied various models, lists the primary advantages as circulation stimulation, elimination of muscle spasms in minutes, immediate pain control, and ability to locate and break trigger points in seconds. This rapid removal of pain fills a long need within chiropractic in highly acute disorders. Another interesting point is that following shortwave or ultrasonic diathermy, high-voltage therapy greatly reduces the adverse and hidden deep-tissue edematous effects created by deep heat without interfering with the therapeutic value of these modalities. (Fig. 13.7).

High-volt units are neither galvanic in action, nor similar in most ways to low-voltage units. High-volt units generate an electromotive force of up to 500 volts. They use a unidirectional, monophasic, interrupted (noncontinuous) current that consists of twin spikes. The total pulses per second can be manually varied by the operator. In comparison to pulsed low-volt units, the pulses of high-volt units are on for an extremely short time and this interval may be controlled to some extent in some units. High-volt units have a relatively low current amperage, averaging between 1.0 and 1.5 milliamperes.

Jaskoviak points out that high-volt stimulators have a distinct advantage over low-

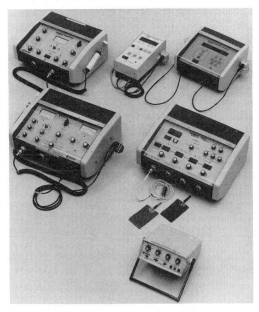

Figure 13.7. An array of Intelect high-volt, ultrasound, and muscle stimulator units (with the permission of the Chattanooga Corp.).

volt units in that the former have the ability to reach much higher wave peaks. The ability to achieve this without burning the patient is possible in high-volt units because the *pulse duration* is extremely short; ie, a low average current is produced. In other words, high-volt units generate a relatively high-peak wave with a low–average current amperage.

Physiologic Effects

High-volt therapy generally affects body tissues in certain ways to modulate pain, muscle spasm, inflammation, tissue healing and repair, based on the way that the control settings on the unit are adjusted. The major effects may be summarized as: (1) pain reduction, (2) muscle spasm reduction, (3) muscular exercise and reeducation, (4) circulation enhancement, (5) edema reduction, and (6) insignificant chemical changes without appreciable iontophoresis.

Contraindications

High-volt modalities are one of the safest electrotherapies in use today. The worst effects possible appear to be caused by increasing the intensity too fast, thereby pushing the current at such a rapid rate that tissue accommodation cannot occur. If this happens, considerable discomfort is suffered by the patient even though a burn does not occur.

The three standard contraindications to applying high-volt therapy are: (1) applications over the low back or abdomen during pregnancy, (2) applications over neoplastic areas, and (3) use of the therapy on patients wearing a pacemaker. It should also be noted that extreme caution must be used if the application is made near the heart or carotid sinus, and any possible clinical value of applying high-volt transcerebrally is highly questionable.

MUSCLE STIMULATORS

To be effective, a muscle must have a certain intensity and duration. In addition, its final intensity must rise with adequate speed.

Any procedure used to stimulate muscle tissue by electricity falls under the general category of *electrical muscle stimulation*.

Various types of modalities, frequencies, and wave forms can be utilized to stimulate muscle fibers electrically. Common objectives of electrical muscle stimulation include the reduction of spasticity, the exercise of weak muscles, and diagnostic evaluations to determine the state of a possible degree of degeneration. The therapy may be applied to normally innervated muscles or to muscles that are abnormally innervated or denervated.

Muscle stimulators are typically low frequency modalities. Low frequency currents are those electrical currents that can stimulate a patient at a frequency of under 1000 pulses/second. Such currents are primarily used to exercise muscles after injury, develop muscular strength and tone, trigger chemical changes, alleviate pain, and break muscle spasm. The primary reasons for applying electrical stimulation to muscle tissue are weakness of innervated muscle, muscle spasm, and dysfunction of denervated muscle.

The basic effect on the body is muscle contraction if an alternating current of 1 Hz is applied to normal innervated muscle; ie, a single twitch-like contraction will occur. As the pulse rate is gradually increased, the rate of twitching correspondingly increases. As the frequency nears 20 Hz, the contractions merge until a tetanic contracture (persistent tonic spasm) results.

TENS UNITS

The acronym TENS refers to *transcutaneous electrical nerve stimulation*, a procedure where an electric current is passed across the skin. In its broadest sense, TENS refers to many types of therapeutic devices, including high-volt modalities. However, the term is generally reserved for those small portable electrical units that the patient wears to control pain.

TENS units are designed to provide sensory and not motor stimulation. This fact is important because motor stimulation will produce contractions in many cases of severe pain that result in aggravation of the patient's complaint.

Application

TENS is intended for the symptomatic relief of a large number of painful syndromes until the cause can be found, the relief of chronic intractable pain syndromes, or cases where analgesic drugs would be contraindicated. The pain modulation usually lasts only while the current is turned on; ie, it has no residual posttherapy effects.

Many excellent types of stimulators are available for home and professional use; the following features are common to most pain control TENS devices:

1. Because afferent nerve fibers differ greatly from efferent nerve fibers in (a) length of refractory period, (b) accommodation to stimuli, (c) threshold of firing, and (d) response to different wave forms, TENS wave form widths are 40–500 milliseconds or less (usually under 130 milliseconds), while pulse widths for triggering millisecond motor responses are 500 milliseconds or better, and frequencies can usually be set in the 70–150 pulses/second range for effective pain control.

2. The wave forms are usually spiked; ie, they are not smooth symmetrical waves. Most units have a wave that alternates and is a variation on the faradic or square wave.

3. Electrode placement should be on the same dermatome(s) as is the patient's perception of pain, preferably over or proximal to the site of pain. In radiating pain, electrodes may additionally be placed over the major nerve pathways (eg, in sciatica). In cases of nerve damage, electrodes should be placed proximal (never distal) to the site of pain. If the site of pain is so sensitive that the slightest stimulation is excruciating, the stimulation of the contralateral area will initially provide partial relief that tends to become more effective after a few days. Acupuncture points far distant from the site of pain have also proved to be successful sites of stimulation. In fact, some authorities have suggested that TENS and acupuncture have a similar mode of action.

A great deal has been written about TENS, and there are many fine charts available as a guide for the placement of electrodes. Some examples are shown in Figure 13.8. Studies have shown that TENS provides significant short-term relief for 65–80% of patients and long-term relief for 30–35%.

Contraindications

Electrical stimulation of any type should

obviously be used with caution in undiagnosed pain syndromes where the etiology has been firmly established. The only contraindication known, when used with a physician's prescription, is in a patient's use of a demand-type pacemaker. However, stimulation over the carotid sinus, the heart in patients with known arrhythmias or myocardial disease, the pregnant uterus, open wounds, or the pharyngeal/laryngeal muscles would undoubtedly be hazardous.

INTERFERENTIAL CURRENT

Interferential current is totally different from the other modalities that have been described. It consists of two medium frequency currents that cross deep within a body part, and, in so doing, trigger the formation of a third current that radiates from the *inside to the outside* of a body part, thus creating an *endogenous* physiotherapeutic approach.

The Physiological Basis

To fully appreciate this type of therapy, it should be remembered that one of the major effects of high-frequency stimulation is that the frequency or rapidity with which the stimulus bombards the skin is so rapid that skin resistance is immediately overcome, allowing for deep penetration of the therapy. Low-frequency currents, in contrast, have frequencies of under 1,000 Hz and do not produce such deep penetration, but they do have a profound effect on electroexcitable tissues (eg, muscles, nerves).

The medium frequencies that are applied with interferential current are generally 4,000 cps sine wave currents that are crossed simultaneously (triggered by two generators). However, they cross at slightly different frequencies. One of the sine waves has a fixed frequency (generally, 4000 Hz), and the frequency of the other current can be set at a variable amount that is usually between 4000 and 4250 Hz.

The linear superimposition of the second wave on the first wave is called *interference*. In Figure 13.9, it can be seen that the placement of four electrodes on the skin, as shown, will establish the specific location where current intersection takes place. By placing the two currents close to one another, the depth of penetration is kept su-

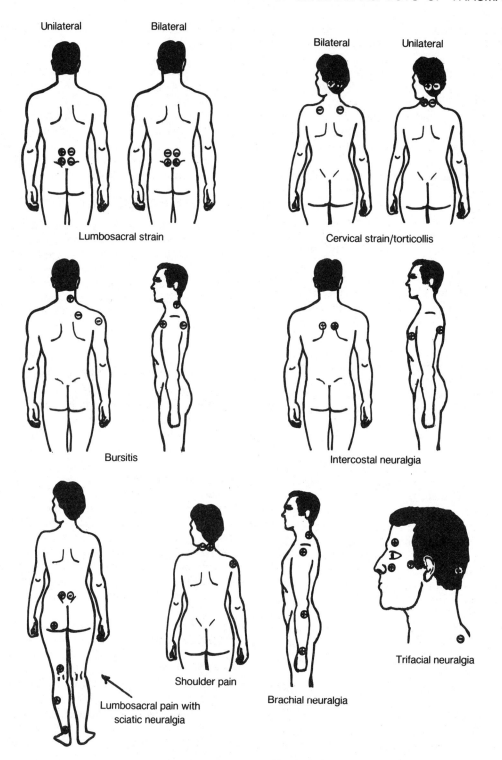

Figure 13.8. Some examples of TENS electrode pad placement. Refer to manufacturer's guidelines for detailed instructions.

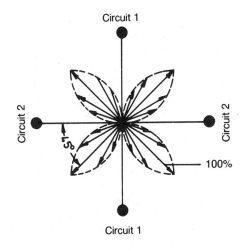

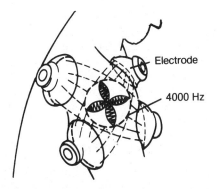

Figure 13.9. *Top*, schematic of an interferential current pattern. *Bottom*, two-circuit application to the right shoulder.

perficial, while placing the electrodes farther apart will increase the depth of penetration. The density of the body tissues involved will also alter the depth of penetration and the locale of intersection. At the area of intersection, a low-frequency endogenous current will be generated. This endogenous current, for all practical purposes, has a frequency that is the difference of the two frequencies which were originally applied.

Because interference current therapy is a by-product of a superimposition of two altering sine wave currents, there will be no direct current effects within the involved tissues. Chemical alterations and polar changes do not occur as they do with direct current. Because of this factor, an operator need not be especially concerned about burning the patient with interferential ther-

apy. As explained, the placement of electrodes predetermines the exact site and degree of interference.

Application

The following points are considered to be some of the major advantages of interferential therapy: (1) endogenous stimulation, (2) slight or no danger of burns from therapy, (3) use over areas with nonelectronic metallic implants, (4) great depth of penetration, (5) minimal resistance of the skin between 3000 and 4000 Hz, thus higher intensities can be provided without patient discomfort, and (6) hypesthesia is not a contraindication.

Contraindications and Special Precautions

The following special concerns and contraindications should always be taken into account prior to treatment with interferential current: (1) metastatic carcinoma, (2) implanted pacemaker, (3) pregnant uterus, (4) over carotid sinus, (5) transcerebrally, and (6) through the chest or over the heart.

Special care and consideration should likewise be given before interferential therapy is administered in the following cases: (1) localized inflammatory processes; (2) thrombosis, decreased vascularity, poor circulation, varicosities; (3) tendency to hemorrhage; (4) tuberculosis; (5) over pelvic organs during menstruation; and (6) hyperpyrexia.

Interferential vs High-Volt Therapy

Interferential current has its effect by an intersection (superimposition) that occurs within the tissues, the depth of which is determined by where the electrodes are applied. Although intersection may occur in muscles, tendons, and ligaments, its effect is not dramatic. High-volt therapy is preferred when a dramatic effect would be desirable. On the other hand, high-volt currents do not penetrate as deeply. Thus, interferential is preferred in the treatment of deep joints such as the shoulder, hip, knee, or spine.

The general rules to apply are: (1) if it's a deep or large joint problem, interferential is the modality of choice; (2) if it's a soft-tissue injury of muscles, tendons, ligaments, and/

or other pariarticular tissues, then high-volt therapy is the preferred modality.

High-volt therapy is quite effective in triggering endorphin production with the small-diameter electrode, and apparently more so than interferential therapy. However, interferential therapy has been found to be more beneficial in blocking deep-seated pain or pain arising from visceral dysfunction.

Interferential therapy is quite useful for building strength in muscles, tendons, and ligaments, especially during postinjury rehabilitation. It is not, however, the modality of choice to use for passive exercise when denervation is present. Interferential therapy may also prove to be of value in many other clinical entities. Future research may establish more specific parameters.

ULTRAVIOLET RAYS

Inasmuch as human skin sensitivity varies within a wide normal range due to variations in skin thickness and pigmentation, a "minimal erythema dose" must be conducted on each patient prior to therapy to determine an "average" dose. Application is generally utilized in acne, psoriasis, indolent ulcers, and certain fungal disorders.

Physiologic Effects

The physiologic effects of ultraviolet light include local erythema, pigmentation, metabolic effects, bactericidal effects, and counterirritation effects.

Degrees of Erythema

First Degree: slight reddening appears in a few hours and disappears in 1–2 days.
Second Degree: visible reddening followed by slight desquamation and pigmentation such as seen in common sunburn.
Third Degree: intense redness, slight edema, marked desquamation and pigmentation. This degree is often called the counterirritant dose.
Fourth Degree: increased third-degree signs with painful blistering. Often called the destructive or bactericidal dose.

Metabolic Effects

Several metabolic effects are noted from ultraviolet rays. Skin sterols are activated to vitamin D, thus aiding in calcium absorption and calcium-phosphorus metabolism (ie, an antirachitic effect). Ultraviolet improves skin tone, elasticity, and secretory functions, and increases both red blood cells and reticulocytes. It also raises the BMR and general physiologic activity of the body.

Bactericidal and Counterirritation Effects

Ultraviolet has a lethal effect on some bacteria, viruses, fungi, and other pathognomonic organisms if exposed to the proper spectrum. The counterirritation effects are produced by absorption of destroyed albumin of the irradiated area and the reflex stimulation of the irradiated zone.

Contraindications

Few contraindications are seen in sports such as are seen in general practice in cases of diabetes mellitus, severe weakness, advanced cardiovascular or renal disease, hyperthyroidism, tuberculosis, hemorrhagic tendencies, suppurative dermatitis, and skin cancer.

HYDROTHERAPY

Water is an excellent medium for therapy because of its high specific heat. This property allows for (1) slow absorption of heat by the body through the process of conduction and (2) slow cooling of the body or any of its exposed parts. Water is quite versatile to use because it permits full or partial immersion of a part or it can be specifically directed by spraying onto an isolated area of the skin.

The most common technique for hydrotherapy involves the use of the small whirlpool tank, which permits immersion of one or more extremities within agitated water or the patient may sit in the tub. Larger therapy units (eg, a Hubbard tank), incorporating larger whirlpools, can accommodate both a patient and a therapist. This latter type of therapy is beneficial when passive exercise is indicated during the treatment.

Several different types of hydrotherapy are in common use. Examples are whirlpools, sitz baths, hot and cold sprays and douches, and colonic irrigation. Some authorities include several other modalities of care under the general classification of hydrotherapy, including applications of ice; hot or cold moist packs, compresses, and dressings; and paraffin.

The Physiologic Basis

Water as a therapeutic agent allows for several remarkable possibilities. There are many reasons why water can be utilized successfully as a method of therapy for a patient in distress. The major properties that serve as the basis for intelligent application are water's buoyancy, the cohesion and viscosity factor, hydrostatic pressure, mechanical stimulation, conductivity, versatility, temperature, and the chemical effects involved. The application of heat or cold in any form to one area of the body has an effect on circulation in other areas.

Several factors determine the extent of the effects of water as a therapeutic agent that should be taken into consideration prior to the use of water as a modality: (1) the degree of temperature change desired; (2) the water temperature itself; (3) the suddenness with which the water therapy is applied; (4) the duration and pressure of application; (5) the extent of body surface treated; (6) the frequency of application; and (7) the age, weight, and general condition of the patient.

Indications

The major physiologic effects of hydrotherapy and the corresponding indications for care may be summarized as follows: (1) thermal or hypothermal effects; (2) increase in circulation; (3) increase in mobility, especially when exercise is performed underwater; (4) relaxation; (5) analgesia or sedation, especially during cold water therapy; (6) debridement (eg, open wounds); (7) promotion of tissue healing and repair; and (8) relief of muscle spasm. Water also has variable cleansing, diaphoretic, and hypnotic effects.

TRACTION

Traction is the act of drawing or pulling a body part or parts by any means. It was crudely practiced therapeutically even prior to Hippocrates for the reduction of structural compression, alterations, and deform-

ity. Skin traction is both a definitive treatment method as well as a first-aid measure. The traction force applied to the skin is transmitted to bone by way of underlying fascia and muscle. (See Figs. 13.10–13.13.)

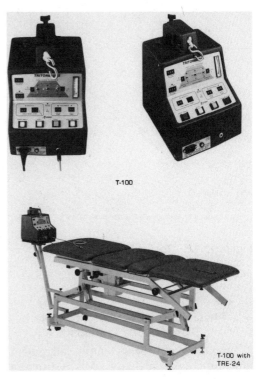

T-100

T-100 with
TRE-24

Figure 13.10. The Triton T-100 traction unit (with the permission of the Chattanooga Corp.).

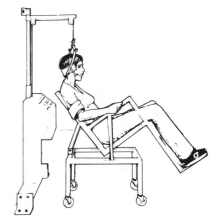

Figure 13.11. Some mobile traction units offer four modes of treatment: progressive intermittent, intermittent, static, or progressive static (with the permission of STC, Inc).

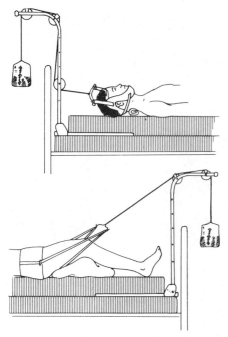

Figure 13.12. *Top*, portable continuous cervical traction unit. *Bottom*, pelvic continuous traction unit (with the permission of STC, Inc).

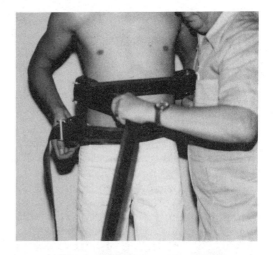

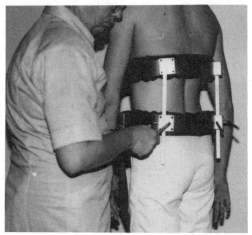

Figure 13.13. Tracto-O-Belt, an ambulatory traction unit. *Top*, adjusting tension on straps. *Bottom*, cranking belt up until skin is tight (with the permission of VRB, Inc).

Physiologic Effects of Moderate Continuous Traction

Traction encourages length, alignment, and functional stability. Mild structural compression results in ischemia and pain sited either locally and/or distally, resulting in muscle spasm producing functional contraction. The associated nerve irritation, which may be sensory or motor or both, may exhibit signs of pain, flaccidity, and diminished reflexes.

Continuous moderate traction tends to immobilize and "splint" strained musculoskeletal tissue, to relieve spasms by placing them in "physiologic rest," and to stimulate proprioceptive reflexes, thus relieving associated pain and tenderness. It stretches fibrotic tissues and adhesions (anticontracture factor) and relieves compression effects on articular tissues (eg, cartilage, discs) due to muscular spasm, gravity, or other compression forces (commonly seen in chronic subluxations) to restore connective tissue resiliency and contour. Traction can reduce edema in an extremity if the traction unit elevates the affected part above the heart.

In the spine, traction reduces the circumference of the intervertebral disc, thus helping to restore its normal positioning (eg, suction, molding, axial pull), and relieves compression effects of foraminal distortion and/or narrowing; ie, increases the intervertebral foramen's diameter. A by-product of these effects is the dissipation of congestion, stasis, edema, and dural-sleeve adhesions in associated tissues.

Physiologic Effects of Intermittent Traction

Intermittent or alternating traction effects include increased vascular and lymphatic flow (suction aspiration effect) which tends to reduce stasis, edema, and coagulates in chronic congestions. It tends to stretch and free periarticular and articular adhesions and fibrotic infiltrations and is an efficient supplement to manual adjustments. Traction stimulates proprioceptive reflexes and helps to tone muscles that tends to reduce fatigue, restore elasticity, and restore resiliency. In the spine, it encourages the expansion and contraction of disc tissues, thus improving their nutrition.

Indications and Contraindications of Traction

Traction is indicated whenever the physiologic effects are desired and structure is in such a state as to withstand the stress. It has been found helpful in brachial neuritis, occipital neuralgia, osteoarthritis, scalenus anticus syndrome, spinal curvatures, vertebral disc thinning, spinal neuralgia, Steinbrocker's syndrome, and subacute torticollis, vertebral subluxation, and whiplash syndrome.

Traction is contraindicated in localized and vascular disease, acute trauma syndromes, hemorrhagic states and for healing fractures and dislocations. Few other contraindications are seen in sports as are seen in clinical practice in cases of bone disease, spinal cord afflictions, severe cardiovascular disease, pregnancy, and hypertensive disorders. In addition to these factors, intermittent or alternating traction is contraindicated in inflammatory joint conditions, severe muscle spasms, chronic musculoskeletal inflammations (eg, bursitis, tendinitis), and an acute intervertebral disc syndrome. Excessive traction will easily result in skin damage, thus careful monitoring must be done on proper padding, strapping, and angulation.

STRETCHING

Therapeutic stretching may involve any manual or mechanical force that is designed to lengthen abnormally shortened soft tissues to produce an increase in joint range of motion. It may or may not involve pure traction forces. The tissues affected may be skin, fascia, ligaments, and/or muscles and tendons, and the cause of the exhibited tissue shortening may be (1) trauma, (2) any infection or degenerative pathology that results in fibrosis, adhesions, or contractures, (3) a connective-tissue disorder, or (4) restricted mobility of physiologic (eg, spasticity), postural, neuromyogenic (eg, scoliosis), or disuse (eg, immobilization) etiologies.

General Considerations

The physiologic effects of stretching therapy are similar to those of soft-tissue traction. Besides manual application, various devices are available for this purpose (Figs. 13.14 and 13.15).

Stretching therapy may be applied (1) passively with or without mechanical advantage such as a pulley or lever apparatus, (2) actively by the patient (with or without mechanical assistance), or (3) actively assisted. The therapy is invariably indicated in such situations as profound weakness or paralysis.

Heat is helpful during stretching therapy, but cold and vapocoolant sprays have been shown to be more effective in acute cases. Combined mild isotonic exercises are also useful for improving circulation and inducing the stretch reflex, especially in the cervical extensors. These exercises should be done supine to reduce exteroceptive influences on the central nervous system. In chronic cases, relaxation training with biofeedback is helpful.

Indications and Contraindications

Therapeutic stretching is usually recommended for any state of abnormal soft-tissue shortening that interferes with normal

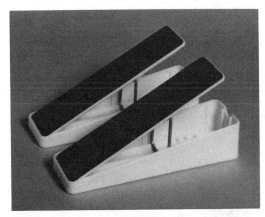

Figure 13.14. Flex-Wedge apparatus, for actively stretching lower extremity muscles and tendons in the standing position by body weight (with the permission of the Flex-Wedge Company).

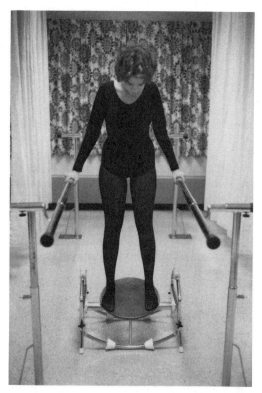

Figure 13.15. Adapto-Disc, for controlled angle of motion in the development and rehabilitation of ankle joints and leg muscles (with the permission of Widen Tool & Stamping, Inc).

function (eg, adhesions, contractures, spasticity, myogenic or ligamentous articular fixation, IVD thinning, paralytic, or immobilization atrophy, lack of exercise, etc). The reduction of spasm and/or the easing of contractures are often necessary prior to structural correction and to maintain a corrected position after adjustment. Mild passive stretch is an excellent method of reducing spasm in the long muscles. Heavy passive stretch, however, destroys the beneficial reflexes.

The contraindications of therapeutic stretching are similar to those of traction.

VIBRATORY AND RELATED THERAPIES

Mechanical vibration to stimulate preprioceptive functions has gained increasing interest in recent years. It may be applied manually or mechanically, superficially with relatively horizontal oscillations, or to deeper tissues via percussion strokes.

Physiologic Effects

The primary action of vibration, under whose general classification one can include forms of percussion and concussion, is kinetic, which effects an increase in circulation and lymphatic flow and a decrease in systemic nervous tension and general or local muscle spasm.

Deep, rapid, short-duration percussion, applied either by hand or by a percussion-type vibrator, upon spinous processes at a rate of 1–2 impulses/second for about 20 seconds with 30-second rest intervals can be used to stimulate a spinal center. Prolonged stimulation such as for 3 minutes or longer appears to fatigue excitability and produces an inhibitory effect.

Associated Therapies

Sinusoidal current has shown to be an excellent method to contract involuntary muscle without irritation. Pulsating ultrasound is also effective in stimulating spinal centers. Therapeutic heat in almost any form increases nerve conductivity; thus, it may benefit vibratory, percussion, sinusoidal, and ultrasound therapies to spinal centers. Interspaced heat and cold can also be used in conjunction with vibratory therapy, depending upon the effect to be achieved.

Voss reports that the tonic vibration reflex is stronger under isotonic conditions and that the reflex response induced is sustained contraction of the vibrated muscle with simultaneous relaxation of the prime antagonist. An active vibrator placed over a muscle belly appears to serve as a further stretch stimulus, producing an increased response and further range of motion of the involved joint.

Indications and Contraindications

A large number of musculoskeletal ailments can be effectively treated with vibratory therapy. The most common complaints include edema, hypomyotonia, myalgia, spasticity, and stasis. In addition, several practitioners report excellent results with high-speed vibratory therapy in treating palpable trigger points. A fairly firm cone-shaped attachment with a small diameter is used for this purpose, which can be specifically directed and rolled beneath a congested or taut muscle or ligament if necessary.

Because of the deep penetration produced by the typical unit, there is no need to apply heavy pressure while moving the applicator. Excessive pressure or moving the unit too rapidly may cause patient discomfort and/or bruise the patient's skin. Use of a dry towel at the applicator-skin interface prevents body oils and perspiration from contaminating the attachment and prolongs the life of the attachment. It also contributes a dispersive cushioning factor. The operator should also avoid sliding the applicator back and forth over the spinal column or bony prominences or moving the applicator too fast. When the extremities are being treated, treatment should always be applied toward the heart; ie, in the direction of venous and lymph flow.

MECHANICAL SUPPORTS

Mechanical supports include such items as strapping, taping, braces, casts, corsets, canes, collars, crutches, slings, shoelifts, and certain bandages. (See Figs. 13.16–13.19.)

Physiologic Effects

Most mechanical supports are designed to relieve weight bearing or motion stress on bones and joints and to immobilize structures in a sustained position so as to assist healing. A by-product of these features is to relieve muscle spasm and pain. Shoelifts

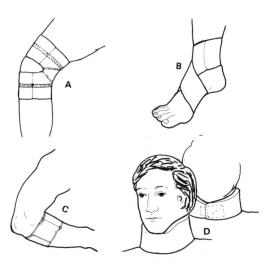

Figure 13.17. Various types of supports: *A*, knee support; *B*, ankle wrap support; *C*, tennis elbow support; *D*, foam cervical wrap (with the permission of STC, Inc).

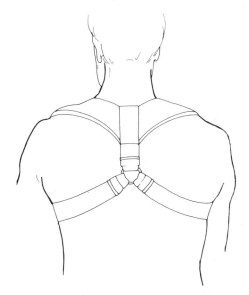

Figure 13.18. Stretch type, adjustable, clavicle splint with padded shoulder straps (with the permission of STC, Inc).

and some other supports allow for contracture and/or stretching of musculoskeletal tissues to encourage structural change. In acquired or congenital malformations, such supports help to relieve poorly compensated structural and functional inadequacies.

Indications and Contraindications

The use of supportive appliances is a matter of clinical judgment. When used wisely

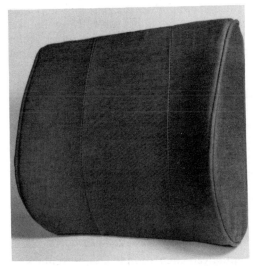

Figure 13.16. Back-Hugger cushion, for relief of resistant or recurring back pain (with the permission of the Controus Comfort Company).

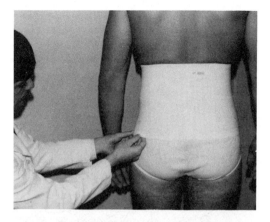

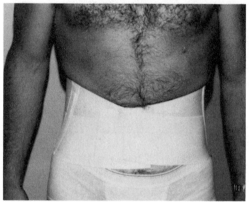

Figure 13.19.   Simple lumbrosacral support.

with a thorough knowledge of the biomechanics involved and corrective chiropractic care, recovery can be greatly enhanced. Mechanical support is usually indicated in situations of pain, weakness, deformity, function assistance, or paralysis of a part of the body.

Mechanical supports are contraindicated whenever immobilization tends to promote muscular atrophy and weakness or when immobilization tends to promote the organization of inflammatory coagulant and consequent adhesions and/or fibrotic infiltration, depending upon the nature and stage of the condition. Support is also contraindicated whenever immobilization may produce congestion, ischemia, or vascular stasis or when immobilization or a fixed position may induce unsatisfactory stretching and/or contracture changes. These contraindications depend greatly upon the nature and stage of the condition.

Bandaging

Bandaging is used to secure dressings and splints, to limit motion of a part, and to apply compression to a wound to control hemorrhage. Cotton cloth is commonly used over a dressing or to secure splints. Rolled gauze secures dressings and serves as a protective support beneath strappings. Elastic bandages provide compression.

Adhesive Strapping

Adhesive taping or strapping is used in athletics for both injury prevention and treatment to limit joint motion, to secure protective devices and padding, to support and stabilize a part, and to hold dressings secure. Tape should be stored on end, never on its side, in a cool dry location.

The rule of thumb is, the larger the part, the wider the tape; eg, 2–3-inch tape is best for thighs or shoulders, and half-inch tape for fingers and toes. In athletics, heavy backed (85 longitudinal fibers/sq inch) with a rubber-base adhesive is usually preferred for greater backing strength and superior adhesion as opposed to the acrylic adhesives and lighter backing used in surgery. Before tape is positioned, clean and dry the skin, treat cuts, shave hair, and apply a nonallergenic skin adherent.

Strips of adhesive tape are used, rather than one continuous winding, to avoid constriction. After one turn of the tape, the tape is torn. Further strips are overlapped 1 inch at the ends and at least a half inch above or below. Tape must be carefully smoothed and molded to fit the natural contour of the part as it is laid on the skin with equal tension.

Most irritation is seen in the mechanical irritation caused by tape removal, but the reddened area disappears quickly. Allergic reactions are rarely seen and are characterized by erythema, papules, vesicles, and edema. A patch test will indicate a positive reaction within 48 hours if a sensitivity exists. The irritative effects of inhibited sweating beneath tape may be relieved by using a porous nonocclusive-type tape.

Extremity Pressure Supports

Enhanced circulation in any musculoskeletal injury is almost always a benefit, and this is especially true if immobilization is required. The use of hot packs, ultrasound, massage, and sometimes whirlpools have been of some, but not excellent, benefit in this regard. There also has been a problem obtaining lightweight but strong supports that restrict motion in some ranges but still allow some type of activity (eg, locomotion). Some technical advances, as described below, appear to have solved some of these problems.

The Aircast/Airstirrup System

Aircasts and Airstirrups have proved themselves excellent innovations in the treatment of extremity injuries and have overcome many of the disadvantages of conventional plaster casting or adhesive strapping. An Aircast consists of two plastic half shells that are connected by Velcro straps, and two or more self-inflated/self-sealing air bags are attached to the inner surface of the shells (Fig. 13.20). Airstirrups are similar U-shaped appliances for the lower extremity.

An athlete with a mildly sprained ankle, for example, can continue running almost immediately in many instances when the appliance has been applied. Such appliances also allow normal, gradual recuperative functions to take place, prevent recurrence of injury during rehabilitation, and eliminate motion pain while still allowing motion in nonpainful directions. They appear to efficiently bridge the gap between immovable plaster casts and inefficient flexible supports.

Hydropulse and Pression Units

To meet the need for immobilization and support without some venous and lymphatic circulatory deficit, new approaches have been introduced in recent years that pulsate warm water or air within specially designed cuffs. Two examples are the Hydropulse and Pression units. Such appliances, which optimally offer a unidirectional action towards the heart, are efficient in treating sprains, strains, spasticity, cramps, decreased circulation, local edema, and other types of pain or discomfort arising from a degree of anoxia and/or circulatory stasis.

Mobilization After Support

To minimize strength loss, improve nutrition of the part, and reduce atrophy, exercise of adjacent joints should be advised when support is provided as well as thereafter. Both progressive passive manipulation and active exercise are the keys to fast recovery. However, joint movement should not be made whenever it increases pain, muscle spasm, or involuntary splinting.

Postinjury edema soon becomes filled with fibroblasts (joint glue), and excessive collagen formation produces stiffness, especially when collateral ligaments are immobilized in a position shorter than that for the functional position. However, a normal joint can tolerate a long session of immobilization without ill effects, such as that seen in fracture healing. Degenerative changes, in intra-articular adhesions, and periarticular stiffness are more of a concern in the

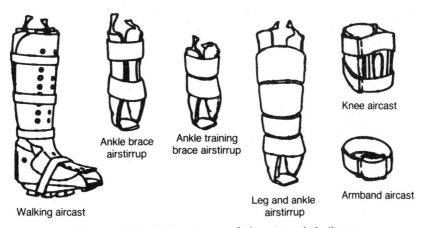

Figure 13.20. Various types of aircasts and airstirrups.

Walking aircast

Ankle brace airstirrup

Ankle training brace airstirrup

Knee aircast

Leg and ankle airstirrup

Armband aircast

elderly patient in short-term immobilization than the young athlete in long-term immobilization. It is not abnormal to have some swelling after removal of a lower-extremity support, but this may be minimized by elastic stockings and contrast baths followed by elevation.

TREATMENT FREQUENCY

Athletes typically demand immediate relief of pain; however, this should be no excuse for overutilization. The specific modality used; the patient's age, sex, and physical condition; and the severity and duration of each complaint—all should play a part in determining the number and frequency of treatments that will be required.

General Guidelines

The following general guidelines for musculoskeletal complaints were developed by Jaskoviak. They may be used in developing a treatment program for a patient. However, each practitioner must remain responsible for basing every therapeutic program on an individual patient's current physical condition.

Phases of Therapy

1. *Acute stage.* Following an acute musculoskeletal injury, especially during the first 24–48 hours, it may be necessary to treat the patient once or several times each day until the pain subsides. In some patients with severe IVD injuries, multiple treatments or concentrated care combined with bed rest is often the regimen of choice.

2. *Postacute healing stage.* Treatments for musculoskeletal complaints after the acute pain has subsided need not be spaced as close together as during the acute stage. Treatment is usually administered on a daily basis, then every other day, and eventually to about once per week. If pain persists after 10–15 visits, it is probably advisable to completely re-examine the patient and re-evaluate the initial diagnosis, seek consultation, or refer the patient for further specialized evaluation before therapy is continued.

3. *Strengthening stage.* As healing becomes more complete, treatment should be directed to developing strength and tone in the injured muscles, tendons, and ligaments. Therapy during this stage is frequently scheduled once (possibly twice) a week and is usually combined with a specific exercise program that is given to the patient (by demonstration/explanation and writing) to apply at home.

Response to Therapy

Results should not be expected with just one or two applications of a modality. Changing therapies after each one or two visits when a patient is not responding is not practical and serves no useful purpose. If 8–10 treatments with one specific modality have been given with no apparent results, re-examination, an alternative therapy, or referral should be seriously considered. Modalities such as ultrasound or shortwave diathermy typically have a cumulative effect, and the results are usually minimal until after 2–4 visits.

Prognosis

If denervation occurs in patients with motor disturbances, therapy should be instituted as soon as possible. The process of atrophy begins immediately and will be apparent within 7–14 days without care. With peripheral nerve injuries, low-volt galvanic is the *only* effective wave form because of its long pulse duration. Treatment time in the acute stage should be about 3–5 minutes. Frequent therapy (5–6 times a day) or a supplemented vigorous exercise regimen to prevent atrophy is often necessary. If regeneration occurs within the first year, the outlook is good. The prognosis after 2–3 years without results is dismal. The objective is always to retard the process of atrophy somehow so that the degree of recovery can be increased as far as possible.

BASIC CONCEPTS UNDERLYING PAIN CONTROL

Pain reflects the body's alarm system. It is helpful and immobilizing, yet agonizing. When prolonged, it can lead to anxiety, depression, anorexia, dyspnea, fatigue, insomnia, and countless other adverse signs and symptoms.

Pain can be controlled through either drug or nondrug means. The use of opium as an analgesic was known to the Egyptians as early as the 16th century B.C. It was also known that repeated applications of chili pepper, oil of cloves, and ginger cause sensory nerves to become numb. But one of the most effective means to relieve acute pain without the use of drugs has been the use of counterirritation. The age-old practices of acupuncture, cupping, deep massage, heat, ice rubs, manipulation, moxa, plasters, and poultices are well known. In more recent times, articular adjustments, needle sprays, percussion, trigger-point therapy, deep heat, galvanism, TENS, ultrasound, and other forms of electrotherapy undoubtedly have a counterirritative effect.

While the exact mechanisms of how counterirritation relieves pain is not fully explained, its effects are readily demonstrable. Rubbing an injured area, for example, is almost an instinctive reaction. It has only been during the last 2 decades, however, that several theories have been advanced that have improved the professional management of painful syndromes.

Receptor-Pathway Mechanisms

Hirschy describes five types of sensory receptors: (1) *mechanoreceptors*, which detect mechanical deformation of the receptors or cells adjacent to the receptors; (2) *chemoreceptors*, which detect tastes, odors, arterial oxygen levels, osmolarity of body fluids, CO_2 concentrations, and other factors that make up body chemistry; (3) *thermoreceptors*, which detect changes in temperature, with some receptors detecting cold and others warmth; (4) *electromagnetic receptors*, which detect light on the retina; and last but not least, the (5) *nociceptors*, which detect damage in the tissues, whether it be of a physical or chemical nature. These sensory receptors initiate impulses from their sites to the spinal cord via Type A, B, and C afferent fibers.

Pain signals are essentially transmitted centrally by Type A fibers at velocities between 3 and 10 meters/second and by Type C fibers at velocities between 0.5 and 2 meters/second. Guyton states that these latter fibers constitute over two-thirds of all fibers within the peripheral nervous system.

Upon entering the spinal cord at the dorsal roots, pain and temperature impulses enter the tract of Lissauer where they are transmitted up or down 1–3 segments and then terminate with second-order neurons in the gray matter of the posterior horns of the cord. From here, fibers pass through the anterior commissure to the opposite side of the cord where they form the lateral spinothalamic tract, whose impulses eventually terminate in the intralaminar nuclei of the thalamus, medulla, pons, and mescencephalon. Communication with the cerebral cortex is made via third-order neurons from the thalamus and intralaminar nuclei.

Specificity Theories

Von Frey proposed the most famous specificity theory. It suggested that there are specific receptors or fibers that respond to different stimuli and transmit specific signals of pain, pressure, temperature, and position to higher centers in the brain. This theory, which serves as the anatomical basis of surgical intervention and "nerve blocks" to control intractable pain, has brought attention to the fact that there are extremely specific subcutaneous receptors and pathways.

Pattern Theories

Livingston's "summation" theory is the most famous pattern theory. It proposes that abnormal volleys of patterned nerve impulses are conveyed to the brain via the dorsal horns where the neurons undergo intense stimulation. Once these circuits are established, a chain of self-exciting neuronal circuits are believed to be produced to create a continuous self-generating mechanism that is unrelated to the initial trauma, thus explaining the phantom limb pain of an amputated limb. Other pattern theories include those of (1) Noordenbos, whose "sensory interaction" theory proposed that the large afferent fibers had an inhibitory effect upon on central transmission, while the small afferents had an excitatory effect; and (2) Goldscheider, who suggested that stimulus intensity and central summation are the two critical determinants of pain. However, as Siegele points out, it has been Melzack and Wall's "Gate" theory that has encouraged the most practical applications in the field of pain management. Yet even this theory does not answer all the questions posed.

The Gate Control Theory of Pain

The original gate theory suggested a mutual presynaptic inhibition between receptors that register pain (nociceptors) and those that do not (eg, mechanoreceptors) (Fig. 13.21). The nociceptor path is comprised principally of unmyelinated Type C and small Type A fibers, and the mechanoreceptor path represents the Type A fibers that mediate sensations of touch and pressure. Once these fibers have entered the dorsal gray horn of the spinal cord (probably within the substantia gelatinosa of Rolando), both the mechanoreceptor and nociceptor fibers send projections to second-order neurons. These second-order neurons synapse with what is called a trigger cell (T cell), which has access to the higher somesthetic centers involved in the perception of pain via the paleospinothalamic tract. A higher central decoding mechanism located somewhere in the brain is hypothesized, which subsequently monitors spinothalamic activity and exerts descending control on the system. Prior to communicating with the T cell, however, the mechanoreceptor and nociceptor fibers give off collateral axons that terminate with interneurons in the dorsal horn. Impulses of the mechanoreceptor collateral axons impose presynaptic inhibition, which produces primary afferent depolarization of the mechanoreceptor and nociceptor terminals ending on the T cell and thus inhibit the mechanoreceptor and nociceptors impulses reaching the T cell. In contrast to the mechanoreceptor collateral, the collateral circuit from the nociceptor has a second interneuron interposed in its pathway. This is an inhibitory interneuron that silences the presynaptic inhibitory interneuron whenever the nociceptor is stimulated. The effect of this is to remove the presynaptic inhibitory effect from the system.

Thus, according to the gate theory, mechanoreceptor stimulation (eg, counterirritation) tends to "close" the gate, inhibiting mechanoreceptor and nociceptor input to the T cell, while nociceptor stimulation tends to "open" the gate, allowing both mechanoreceptor and nociceptor input to reach the T cell.

The original gate theory, however, did not support further findings. For example, several studies have shown that (1) nociceptor stimulation does not appear to open the gate and (2) the hypothetical T cell has never been found. Nevertheless, most authorities agree that there is presynaptic inhibition in both the mechanoreceptor and nociceptor pathways. In recent years, a revised concept has been proposed that is based on the fact that "like impulses presynaptically inhibit like impulses." For example, nociceptors presynaptically inhibit other tonic nociceptors, phasic mechanoreceptors presynaptically inhibit other phasic mechanoreceptors, and tonic mechanoreceptors presynaptically inhibit other tonic mechanoreceptors.

In Figure 13.22 the dotted lines joining the interneurons communicating with the mechanoreceptor and nociceptor collaterals represent some spillover from one receptor type to the other, but the dominant presynaptic effect is reflected back upon the input involved. Thus, there must be a functional spillover of the presynaptic inhibitory effect from mechanoreceptor to nociceptor, or vice versa, to induce the gating phenomenon.

Neither the original nor the revised gate theory have been firmly established anatomically and physiologically. Other factors must be involved because even the revised gate theory does not adequately account for the various nonsegmental, psychologic, social, and cultural factors that influence an individual's pain threshold and/or perception. However, even if the gate phenome-

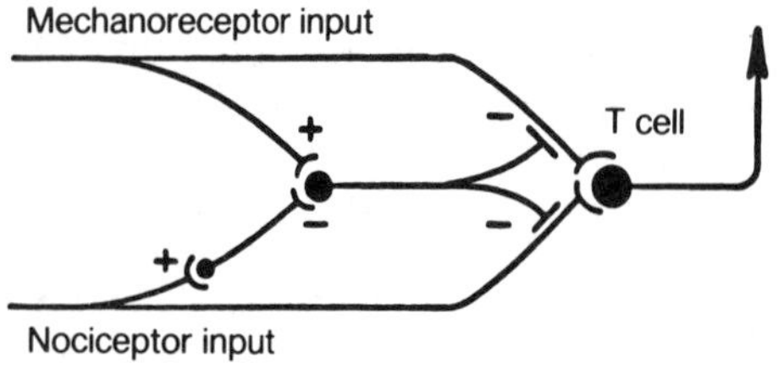

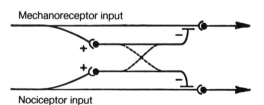

Figure 13.21. Schematic of the original gate theory.

Figure 13.22. Schematic of the revised gate theory. Compare this concept with that of Figure 13.21.

non is not exact as described, many of its clinical predictions have proven useful empirically (eg, TENS). Fortunately, some answers have been found in studies involving the production of endogenous opiate-like substances.

Selective Neural Mechanisms

It has been known for several years that central stimulation can produce pain, but only within the last decade or so has it been found that the stimulation of specific intracranial sites is capable of inhibiting pain.

Analgesia from Central Stimulation

Mayer and Price have shown that intracranial stimulation-produced analgesia is an extremely *specific* antinociceptive effect, rather than a generalized sensory, motor, or psychologic deficit (ie, subjects will respond to mild temperature and light touch stimuli within the area of analgesia). At times, this stimulation-produced analgesia may last for many minutes or hours following stimulation, but the key to purposefully prolonging this effect has yet to be found. It appears that such stimulation does not result from a temporary disruption of pain afferents but exerts its effects caudally through active, selective inhibition of afferent volleys elsewhere in the nervous system such as in the spinal cord or the nucleus of the 5th cranial nerve.

The sites, mechanisms, and effects of intracranial stimulation-produced analgesia are closely parallel with those of morphine. These extremely specific sites are broadly and unevenly distributed throughout the brain. Optimal sites appear to be located in the periaqueductal gray matter of the midbrain.

The Opiate Receptors

Opiates such as morphine, which have extreme chemical specificity, appear to produce their effects by interacting with specific postsynaptic receptors. This fact suggests that if morphine can effect the CNS, there must be an anatomical receptor site or sites present to elicit its effects. As it is doubtful that the body would evolve receptors just for the extracts of poppy seeds, it was theorized that the nervous system must produce some substances that are similar or equivalent to morphine. Some of these substances have recently been isolated, and they are collectively called *endorphins*—naturally occurring endogenous substances whose analgesic effect can be 200 times stronger than that of morphine.

It has been found that naloxone, a specific narcotic antagonist, blocks morphine analgesia, simulation analgesia, and acupuncture analgesia; thus all three must involve an opiate-like receptor. Such receptors have been found in the marginal cell zone and substantia gelatinosa of the dorsal horn of the spinal cord, the trigeminal nucleus, various components of the vagal system, and the area postrema.

The Endorphins

To date, many endogenous substances that possess opioid properties pharmacologically have been found. The first two endorphins to be isolated turned out to be pentapeptides, and they were called *enkephalins*. Endorphins and enkephalins are the body's own natural opiates, and they are produced in certain tissues (eg, pituitary gland) in response to pain, high stress, acupuncture, electrical stimulation, and other stimuli, either centrally or peripherally. Hundreds of types have been discovered, and each affects pain in a *different* region or regions of the body.

Stimulating the Production of Endorphins. Stimulations of the skin with a needle or an electric impulse triggers the brainstem to increase endorphin levels in the blood stream, cerebrospinal fluid, and the gastrointestinal tract. The levels build up within 30 seconds; however, clinical results are often not appreciated by the patient until 12–24 hours later. It should be carefully noted that the site of stimulation determines the type of endorphin that is released and the area of the body that it will affect. Thus, endorphins are *site specific* in their effect. Since an active endorphin is a circulating hormone, the side of the body (when bilateral points exist) stimulated makes little or no difference (other than psychological). When electrotherapy is utilized, a small diameter electrode, no larger than a dime, should be used. Most research indicates that from 1 to 10 pulses/second (Hertz) for the frequency of stimulation is appropriate.

However, recent evidence seems to indicate that the best results occur at 4–6 Hz.

Stimulating the Production of Enkephalins. Stimulating the production of enkephalins clinically is primarily by means of electrical stimulation to the skin. Dampened sponge electrodes, 3 or 4 square inches in size, are commonly used. Firm skin contact is essential. Stiff electrodes that do not readily conform to the shape of the surface make poor conductors and greatly limit the depth of impulse penetration. Research appears to indicate that pulse rates of 70–130 Hz when using high-volt modalities and 90–100 Hz when using interferential units are most valuable. Some studies with interferential therapy tend to indicate that modulation of frequency is valuable because it limits accommodation. Although almost all modalities produce some analgesic properties, low frequency spiked-wave therapies (eg, TENS) are preferred. Note that careful placement at the segmental level of involvement is essential. With patients in acute pain (eg, an IVD syndrome), it should be made certain that the intensity of the stimulation is just to the level where the patient barely perceives the current. In this manner, the physician is able to achieve effective sensory stimulation without aggravating the patient's complaint by producing muscle contractions.

Closing Remarks

Adjustive therapy, electrotherapy, cryotherapy, acupuncture, TENS, hypnosis, autosuggestion, biofeedback, certain drugs, and neurosurgery have all earned respectable places in the arsenal of pain control. As the understanding of pain pathways and mechanisms improve, researchers have great hopes of discovering even better methods of analgesia. The search is on for better methods of producing nonadditive endogenous analgesics.

CHAPTER 14

Skin and Related Injuries

A wide variety of dermatologic conditions come to the attention of the sports-related physician. Acne, boils, infestations, infections, heat rashes, contact dermatitis, toxic eruptions, and other contagious and infectious skin diseases have been discussed previously. In this section, we shall limit our concern to the recognition and management of problems related to skin and soft-tissue environment injuries.

THE SKIN AND SUBCUTANEOUS TISSUES

The skin has unique functions and characteristics in that it provides an interface between internal and external environments, it is selectively permeable, it serves as a homeostatic mechanism, and it attempts to regulate temperature despite external extremes (Fig. 14.1). It contains the same basic elements as do the major organs: connective tissue, blood and lymph vessels, nerves and glands. It has excretory, secretory, absorptive, synthetic, and sensory functions. Just 1 square inch of surface area contains over 3,000,000 cells, 4 yards of nerves, and at least a yard of capillaries.

Skin Trauma

In most injuries, the skin is the first to suffer. The top layer of the skin is usually quite tough. The true skin just under the epidermis is abundant with connective tissue which readily serves as a nest for infection that is easily transported throughout the body via the circulation. Any abrasion, laceration, or puncture wound offers a potential site for secondary infection. It is also important to be mindful that many skin conditions and associated complications are directly or indirectly associated with poor hygiene practices during management or aggravated by poor management and prevention techniques.

The two most common skin injuries seen in sports are contusions and friction injuries. Depending on the degree of pressure, friction injuries produce calluses and painful, tender blisters, erosions or fissures. Most friction injuries occur early in the season before the player's skin has had a chance to accommodate to stress. Later in the season, subcallus blisters are a concern.

Examination

Examination of the skin includes skin color, texture, moistness, and lesions, along with mucous membranes, hair, and nails. Cutaneous temperature, texture, and moisture have a kinship which is determined by hormones, nutrition, and environmental exposure and contact. While the skin is the largest body organ in terms of surface area and the most visible, it is often the most overlooked. This is probably because the skin manifests a complicated array of both meaningful and unimportant information. Thus, it is necessary to acquire a definite understanding of the various lesions encountered in skin injuries and diseases as it is the aggregate of these that constitutes clinical change and establishes the basis for recognition and management.

CLEANLINESS

It has long been recognized that a thorough showering is a necessity after physical activity to remove accumulated sweat residue, bacteria, dirt, and debris. Because of the postactivity shower routine in athletics, players practice far better habits of cleanliness (are more thoroughly and frequently washed) than those of the general population.

Soap and Water

Usually, a 4–5 minute shower in water of 80–90°F is sufficient. There is no scientific basis in the habit of following a hot shower with a blast of cold water to "close the

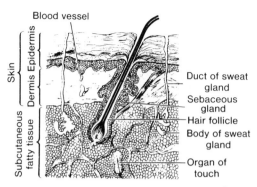

Figure 14.1. Structure of the skin.

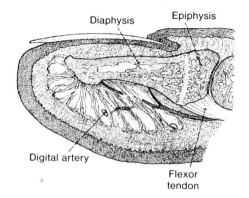

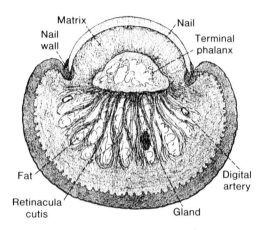

pores," but there is in drying off quickly to prevent chill. The conditioned skin of most athletes adapts well to common bath soaps. On rare occasions, an athlete may be found who is susceptible to alkali irritation and will require a mild nonallergenic-type of pH controlled soap. For dry sensitive skin, Oilatum soap has been found to be beneficial.

Skin Residues

Taping is common in athletics, and the residue left from adhesive tape is rarely completely removed by the after-game shower. Usually more is needed besides soap and water. Commercial solutions are available which are very effective, but many contain carbon tetrachloride that requires extreme caution against breathing the fumes. Gasoline or other explosive mixtures should never be used. Two football players at Purdue were killed several years ago in a shower-room blast while using gasoline to remove tape residue.

Other residues are often a problem. Dried calamine lotion, flakes, and powders may be removed with a light oil. Nonexplosive cleaning fluids, or effective detergents can be used in removing greases, ointments, and rubefacients. A cheesecloth bandage saturated with a light oil (eg, mineral, cottonseed, olive) is often helpful in removing skin scales and crusts. A solution of sodium thiosulfate tends to dissolve iodine stains, while spirits of ammonia and alcohol help in removing gentian violet stains.

BLISTERS

Blisters, common nuisances in sports, are produced by localized pressure and friction.

Figure 14.2. *Top*, longitudinal section of a terminal phalanx of the finger. The anterior closed space (eg, where a felon develops) corresponds to the portion of the pad which overlies the diaphysis of the bone. The epiphysis and termination of the flexor tendon lie outside this space. Small branches of the digital artery supplying the diaphysis pass through dense confines of space and are quickly compressed by an inflammatory swelling. *Bottom*, cross–section of terminal phalanx of a finger. Dense fibrous columns (retinacula cutis) pass from the lower layer of skin to attach to the bone's periosteum. Between these columns is fatty tissue containing sweat glands, nerve fibers, and blood vessels.

They are common on the hands and fingers in bowling, rowing, racket, stick, club, and fencing sports; and on the feet in all running sports.

Background

Blisters can often be traced to new or poorly fitted shoes, quick stops and turns, sock seams, and wrinkled socks. New ath-

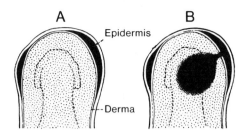

Figure 14.3. Subepithelial abscess. *A*, abscesses located at tip of finger lie between dense epidermis and derma. *B*, subepithelial abscess developing from a felon which perforates derma and spreads beneath epidermis, which is lifted up in a manner analogous to a blister.

letic shoes should be worn for several weeks prior to use during athletic activity. In addition, taping, protective equipment, heat, and constant sweat within athletics contribute to blister formation.

In blister development, an accumulation of serum occurs between intradermal layers after friction has separated the layers. Prior to development, a "hot spot" will be noted at the site of irritation. Without proper care, infection can develop a mild irritation into a distinct disability with serious complications. The associated pain varies with intensity, often inhibiting performance in a given activity by producing a "favoring" away from the irritation which easily predisposes sprains and strains through changes in normal biomechanics.

Management

Whether to puncture a blister or not depends on the blister's size, location, and degree of inflammation involved. Most trainers advocate sterile aspiration or puncturing the blister at its base with the point of a sterile scalpel or needle parallel to the skin surface, after the area has been thoroughly sterilized. The area is then greased with petroleum jelly and covered with a light pressure pad that won't "mat" during activity. Aspiration is initially effective, but fluid accumulation returns quite rapidly in most cases.

Several trainers recommend covering foot blisters with a soft sterile dressing over a Telfa sheet dressing. The use of Neosporin powder is advised for foot blisters by many team doctors.

Some authorities such as Williams and Sperryn feel that the quickest way to handle frank blisters within athletics is to thoroughly clean the area, immediately deroof the blister in a sterile manner, and let it dry in the open air with frequent alcohol washes. While this method is more painful, it does assure the most rapid return to competition as it avoids the irritating layers of lint and friction between equipment-dressing-lesion. Hirata, on the other hand, points out that this method removes the blister's outer layer and exposes the easily abraded thin inner layer, the site being the equivalent to a third degree burn, predisposing secondary infection. He prefers that the blister be opened widely but with the outer skin hinged so that it may be used as a natural inner dressing for protection against abrasion. When the inner layer thickens in 2–4 days, the flap drops off. During this process, the site should be greased with an appropriate ointment or jelly and covered by a pressure pad to maintain drainage and inhibit infection. Subcallus blisters can be treated in the same manner.

Prevention

Sensitivity to blister development can be reduced by painting weight-bearing portions of the soles with oil, silicones, or powder. Athletes who wear wool socks should be advised to wear cotton or silk stockings next to the skin to reduce blister development. It is also helpful to have the player reverse sweat socks so that the seams are away from the skin.

Tincture of benzoin should rarely be used as a "protective pad" because it makes the foot "sticky" and increases friction. Greasing the entire foot with a lanolin ointment is both a preventive practice and an aid to healing, but it quickly destroys athletic socks.

CALLOSITIES

Callosities are localized areas of hyperplasia of the horny layer of the epidermis as a result of pressure and friction.

Background

Plantar callosities, probably more than any other type, can become disabling in track when they produce a subcallus blister. Divers also present a special problem from

A

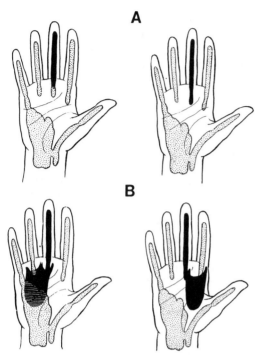

B

Figure 14.4. Illustration of the progressive extension (*A* and *B*) of tenosynovitis of the middle finger. Either the middle palmar or thenar space may be invaded by spread of infection following rupture of the tendon sheath.

board friction. The problem occurs because the constant immersion in pool water and showers leaches natural skin oils from the keratinized plaque. This causes the area to dry, crack, and split, often to the degree of bleeding and secondary infection.

Management

Regular use of a callus file and frequent greasing with a lanolin-base ointment is recommended as a palliative measure. Pool work must be restricted until all signs of infection have subsided.

Subcallus Blisters

Callus formation is nature's response to chronic irritation. Once a callus becomes thick, it in itself can become a chronic irritant as a keratinized plaque and produce a subcallus blister in the deeper tissues. Once developed, treatment is the same as for a superficial blister, but prevention can be accomplished by having the player periodically use a fine emery board (ie, callus file) to prevent undue callus buildup.

CORNS

Corns are round or cone-shaped localized callosities of skin which possess a horny core.

Background

The picture is one of a circumscribed area of hypertrophied skin resembling a small shell containing a harder core which presses on nerves of the foot in the weight-bearing position. The cause of corns can usually be attributed to atypical bone formation or position (often requiring adjustment), to undue external pressure, or to repeated trauma. There are two types, soft and hard corns.

Management

Soft corns form in areas where skin touches skin (eg, between the toes) in an area where heat is poorly released, perspiration has difficulty in evaporating, and an adjacent bone puts pressure on the skin. Prevention is aided by keeping the feet clean and dry, wearing round-toed shoes with metatarsal crescents, wearing silk or nylon undersocks, adjusting subluxated-fixated bones of the feet, and performing exercises to strengthen the metatarsal arch.

First aid consists of the above preventive measures plus using an alcohol foot wash frequently, drying thoroughly, and applying a foot powder. Another method used by many trainers is to dust between the toes with a powder such as sulfomerthiolate or bismuth formic iodide. Lamb's wool placed

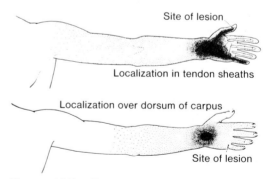

Figure 14.5. *Top*, acute spreading infection starting from a lesion on the volar surface of the hand with eventual localization in the radial and ulnar bursae. *Bottom*, acute spreading infection, starting from a lesion on the dorsal surface with eventual localization on the dorsum of the wrist.

between the toes will help keep the area dry.

Hard corns are firm, rigid, and dense. They arise over prominent protuberances on parts of the foot where sport shoes exert considerable pressure such as the lateral side of the small toe and the top of the middle toes. Many trainers use a first-aid measure to eliminate pressure on the area with pads and rings and frequently cover the corn with an effective "corn paint." Stubborn cases should be referred to a chiropodist.

CONTUSIONS

A contusion represents an area of subcutaneous extravasated blood wherein tissue has been crushed and devitalized but not thoroughly killed. Inevitably, there is some degree of tissue disorganization or cellular death. The extravasated blood either diffuses into an ecchymosis or encapsulates into a hematoma.

Background

Even minor bruises can cause considerable problems (eg, bleeding, swelling) if not offered quality initial treatment. Pain, discoloration, and swelling are common to all forms of contusions, but these signs vary according to the nature of the violence, the site of trauma, and the susceptibility of the individual. Athletic function is impaired to the degree of associated pain, swelling, tissue disorganization, and psychic factors.

Hirata refers to the closed soft-tissue swelling associated with contusions to be one of the most frequent problems seen in contact sports. The greater the vascularity of the tissue involved, the greater the swelling. Thus, the degree of injury cannot be determined by the quality of swelling alone. Swelling varies in degree from a slight puffiness to the size of a large hematoma.

Management

Treatment is directed toward relief of pain, restoration of function, and prevention of residual defects. Stop bleeding by cold, moderate compression, elevation, and rest of the part. After 48–72 hours, local heat and massage may be used to alleviate any associated local tenderness, but it is usually not necessary. Activity can be slowly

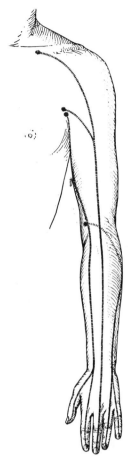

Figure 14.6. Diagram of the routes of lymphatic drainage from the hand. The lymphatics from the little and ring fingers drain through epitrochlear nodes. Vessels from the thumb and index finger pass through axillary nodes. Those from the middle finger pass through axillary glands in 85% of cases; in the remainder, they pass directly into subclavian glands and into venous circulation.

increased to tolerance, then increased gradually to the demand of the sport. The site should be protected with padding during healing to prevent further injury.

ABRASIONS

The word "abrasion" means a rubbing, planing, or scrapping off of skin or mucous membrane. Abrasions are often referred to in baseball as "strawberries" and in basketball as "floor burns." Turf sports and track events often present abrasions highly contaminated with debris.

Background

Friction abrasions are common in most all sports. The skin is removed, leaving a weeping, extremely tender base which is readily subject to infection.

Management

Most trainers gently but thoroughly clean the site with a detergent surgical soap and follow this with a topical ointment with a local antibiotic effect (eg, polymyxin B). Penicillin or tetracycline ointments are best avoided because of the possibility of producing sensitization or hindering future needs.

Slightly implanted foreign bodies should be sought and gently removed under local anesthesia if necessary. Most can be "teased out" with the point of a sterile needle until they can be grasped with a tweezers.

Warm local compresses are routine for mildly infected abrasions. Dressings should be changed at least daily after showering. After healing, the site should be protected for 1–2 weeks until it reaches its normal degree of "toughness." Except in the most severe cases, return to activity can be immediate with adequate protection.

LACERATIONS

A laceration refers to any torn, ragged, or mangled wound. Puncture wounds may be minor or serious; the chief danger in minor wounds is the formation of thrombosis and possible release of emboli.

Background

A clot protruding beyond the surface of the skin is presumptive evidence of arterial damage. The circulation of the part distal to the injury may be jeopardized because of marked damage to vital vessels or may be merely a result of pressure resulting from a hematoma.

If subcutaneous fat is exposed in a laceration, the rule of thumb is that the wound should be sutured. The emergency attendant is rarely directly involved in the handling of wound closure materials such as suture needles or thread. However, it may be necessary to apply specially prepared adhesive strips for a sutureless wound closure prior to transportation.

Temporary Small Wound Closure Technique

The following technique is used for closure of a small, shallow incision when gaping is minimal and skin edges can be apposed with no difficulty. Two types of sutureless closures may be used—a commercially packaged sterile strip or an improvised butterfly adhesive closure.

1. Sterile skin-closure strip (Fig. 14.7). These strips are made of porous, nonirritating material. The adhesive surface is applied directly to the wound surface. Usually, ½-inch-wide, 4-inch-long strips are packaged in a peel-back plastic or paper enclosure. The strips are handled with sterile gloves to bring the skin edges together. One or more strips are used for closure. A sterile dry dressing is applied over the strips and then bandaged.

2. Butterfly adhesive closure (Fig. 14.8). A butterfly adhesive closure can be made from an ordinary 1-inch wide, 4-inch long adhesive strip. It provides less exact

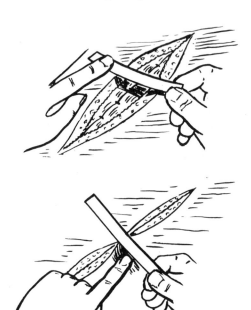

Figure 14.7. Sutureless skin closure, sterile-strip technique. *Top*, apply one-half of adhesive strip to one side of skin at midpoint of wound, press firmly into place, and apply strip at right angles to the wound. *Bottom*, hold other end of strip for traction, appose skin edges using gloved fingers, and press free half of strip into place.

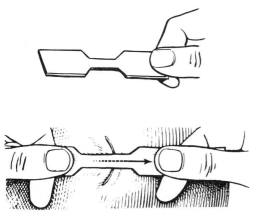

Figure 14.8. Sutureless skin closure, butterfly tape technique. *Top*, cut two diagonal slashes on top and bottom toward center of strip and fold under edges to make a nonadherent bridge; flame the underside of the bridge, holding a match or lighter just close enough to scorch the fabric; do not touch the flamed portion as this will lie over the edges of the wound; allow heated portion to cool. *Bottom*, attach adhesive portion at right angle to one side of laceration, press firmly to anchor it to the skin, apply traction to other end of strip to appose skin edges, and anchor the free end.

skin closure than a commercially prepared sterile strip, but it often is useful as an improvised measure. A sterile dry dressing may be applied over the butterfly strip for protection, but the surface of the strip is not sterile.

ACUTE TRAUMATIC GANGRENE

This is a form of direct gangrene in a limb where the blood supply has been restricted by traumatic obliteration. The hand or foot is usually affected.

Background

The condition usually results from extensive laceration or a crushing contusion wherein most soft tissues and often the bones of the part are involved. When dirt or debris are ground into the wound, tetanus and gas gangrene are always potential complications.

Management

First aid consists of cold and compression and what other means are available to control pain and hemorrhage. If available, dust-

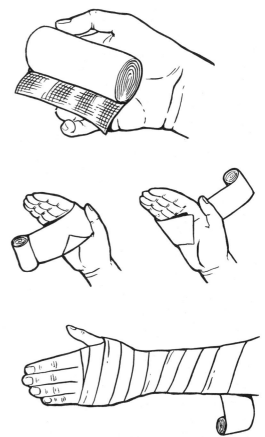

Figure 14.9. Basic methods of applying roller bandage to hand and arm. *Top*, start by holding roller bandage with loose end at the bottom, external surface to be applied to the part. *Middle* diagrams, anchor by placing the loose end of the bandage on the part; then anchor with a few circular turns. *Bottom*, spiral anchor by using succeeding diagonal turns, overlapping each turn by one-third of the bandage.

ing with a sulfa powder or equivalent is recommended, but avoid strong antiseptics which tend to further devitalize tissues. Immediate referral is necessary for probable amputation, tetanus antitoxin and antibiotics.

HEMATOMAS

A hematoma represents a rapid extravasation of blood and tissue fluid which pools into a singular large fluctuant mass. It may localize within a tissue, space, or organ at any depth at most any site in the body after injury.

Background

After a hematoma develops, the body's reaction is to make an inflammatory response, enabling it to cope with the blood pool. This reaction increases local tenderness and heat similar to that seen in cellulitis for 2–3 days until the stage of reactionary inflammation subsides. A large hematoma is never absorbed: it undergoes organization, fibrosis, and scar.

Carefully note the extent of a palpable hematoma, the tension of the tissues, and the presence of a bruit. If the hematoma pulsates, it may be due to transmitted arterial impulses or to the development of an aneurysm. In case of an aneurysm, a bruit will usually be present on auscultation. The hematoma itself is not tender, but adjacent soft tissues are frequently so. As the hematoma begins to age, the initial pool firms. If palpable, it will feel from doughy to fluctuant depending upon its stage.

Management

Typical hemorrhage first aid is indicated, such as I-C-E and rest. While even a distinctly large extremity hematoma may become obliterated in 1–2 days with such treatment, local compression and padding should be continued from 1–2 weeks to assure complete resolution.

In severe cases or when fluctuation is firmly in evidence, referral for aspiration may be necessary. If so, it must be early as a clot cannot be aspirated; open drainage must be used for evacuation. Aspiration should be followed by continued compression. If a semifirm clot resists aspiration, continued compression and padding are applied to encourage clot liquefaction. This should occur within 2–5 days. Open surgery is rarely necessary; when it is, the probability of secondary infection is always a problem. A dozen or more needle aspirations are safer than one incision. Certain enzymes tend to help dispersement of a hematoma but are less effective than evacuation.

Uniqueness of Athletic Injury

The well-conditioned athlete has not only increased work capacity but also has altered typical metabolism at the microscopic level. Injury not only interrupts training, which causes a diminished level of physical fitness, it also produces a different type of lesion than that seen in general practice. This is due to the effects of training which increase muscle-fiber bulk and interstitial tissue vascularity.

The uniqueness of the athletic lesion is clearly brought out in hematoma. Because of the increased muscle bulk, vascularity, and conditioning to high demands, bleeding is more marked than in the unconditioned individual. In addition, the trained muscle offers more efficient physiologic mechanisms to remove extravasated blood from muscle with the result that absorption is much more rapid. Thus, in the treatment of hematoma or any athletic injury, treatment must be modified in dealing with the rigorously trained or the sedentary person.

Danders of Coagulants

The use of "blood-stoppers" in sports, especially by unqualified "cut men," has been a nasty part of athletics for many years. In boxing especially, as the cut man has just 45 seconds to stop bleeding during a large-purse bout, dangerous drugs and chemicals are often applied:

- Monsel's solution quickly sears torn blood vessels shut when swabbed or powdered into a wound. A thick, black, hard mass of scar tissue results which must be removed surgically. If the solution accidently enters a fighter's eye, permanent blindness can occur.
- Adrenalin is sometimes used to restrict bleeding blood vessels. Side effects include increased heart rate and blood pressure, which can later cause the vessel to rupture.
- Negatan is a cauterizing drug containing formaldehyde which turns to the skin into leather within seconds. Many boxing cuts appear in the temporal and supraorbital area of the head, and if negatan enters a fighter's eye or an opponent's eye, the cornea may become permanently scarred.

MOIST DRESSINGS

Although usually contraindicated in the elderly because of circulatory insufficiencies, wet dressings, as commonly used in the athletic aid station, are helpful in maintaining constant lesion drainage, cleansing

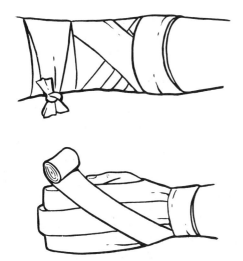

Figure 14.10. *Top*, figure-eight bandage for knee or elbow is anchored below the joint, spiraled upward for circular turn above the joint, then spiraled down to form an X with upward turn; repeat, overlapping each turn. *Bottom*, for recurrent bandage of hand or foot, anchor distal to part to be covered, then fold bandage back at right angle and carry over surfaces, reversing right-angle turn to carry back to origin; repeat, alternating to left and right of centerline; secure recurrent turns with spiral turns. Padding between skin surfaces is not shown.

skin injuries, maintaining a constant site temperature, softening and removing crusts, opening blisters without lancing, and allowing medications to penetrate deeper into infected areas. Room-temperature wet packs tend to produce a soothing anesthetic effect.

Application

The best wet dressing is made from cheese-cloth, as absorbent cotton hardens when wet, dries quickly, and becomes an irritant. The dressing is dipped in water, wrung, and then applied to the skin when still wet but not dripping. Any water used in a wet dressing should be first boiled or distilled. The wet dressing is covered with plastic sheeting to retard evaporation and then covered with a light elastic bandage for security. Warm clothing should be worn over the bandage to prevent chilling.

Petroleum jelly should be applied to the skin near the area being treated to prevent maceration of allied tissues. The dressing should never be allowed to become dry. Trying to add water to the ends of the pack will never suffice; periodically, the dressing must be completely reapplied. If topical medications have been prescribed, the site must be watched very carefully the first 24 hours to note reaction. This may require a wet pack without a protective covering. Ointments should be applied abundantly.

Contraindications

Cleanse irritated skin by washing with a cleansing spray, but avoid vigorous applications of green soap. Wet dressings are contraindicated in any condition where circulation is seriously impaired or where the skin becomes drawn or begins to crack.

Adhesive tape should never be applied near a moist lesion, area of infection, or suppurative lesion as later removal will insult the lesion. Care must be taken when the dressing is secured that no "tourniquet" effect results. A penicillin ointment should never be applied unless it is known before hand that the player is nonallergic. Tar preparations (eg, ichthtol, pragmatar) are contraindicated in skin areas exhibiting heavy hair growth as they tend to produce pustules.

BITES AND STINGS

Animal and severe insect bites are not common in sports, but they occasionally occur to a degree greater than an annoyance. The athletic physician should be prepared to handle such a situation.

Dog Bites

Dog bites are a special hazard to cross-country runners and cyclists, and occasionally a dog will run onto the field of an outdoor arena. Such bites are usually contaminated and present torn edges. Bleeding should be encouraged to clean the wound and a dressing is applied and strapped securely for adequate closure of the wound. Unless the patient has received a recent antitetanus vaccine or booster shot, referral is the typical recommendation. Rabies is always a concern.

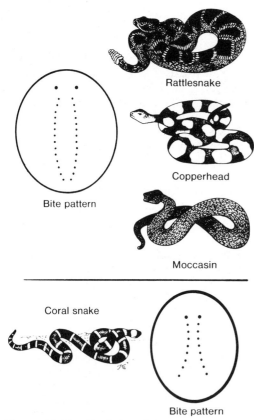

Figure 14.11. North American snakes and their bite pattern.

Snake Bites

Snake bites are a special hazard to cross-country runners. Neurogenic shock is the first concern. Other cases can occur at almost any outdoor event. The lesion should be encouraged to bleed for cleansing purposes, suction applied, then a constricting band applied proximal to the lesion and released at 15–20 minute intervals.

Background

The two poisonous types of snakes in America are coral snakes and pit vipers (cottonmouth moccasins, rattlesnakes, copperheads) (Fig. 14.11). Coral snake venom has a great effect on nerves, causing respiratory paralysis, while that of pit vipers causes local tissue destruction. Only some foreign sea snakes have venom that is both neurotoxic and hemotoxic. Thus, it is important to differentiate for proper treatment.

Coral snakes have a black nose and red, yellow, and black bands on the body. Pit vipers have triangular heads that are wider than their necks, slit-like pupils, pits between their eyes and nostrils that look like extra nostrils, long needle-like hollow fangs that fold against the roof of their mouth when not in use, and a distinctive bit pattern. If feasible, kill the biting reptile without damage to its head. Save the entire snake for positive identification later. Immediate referral to an antivenom facility must be made, taking the dead snake with the patient if possible.

The symptomatic pictures differ. Little local pain and swelling result from a coral snake bite for several hours. Early symptoms include difficult speaking and swallowing, dizziness, shortness of breath, confusion, nausea, vomiting, and general weakness. These progress into flaccidness, respiratory failure, coma, and death. Pit viper bites are immediately painful (local burning). Local swelling progresses centrally, and ecchymosis may spread throughout the extremity. This reaction is followed by blisters and numbness of the limb. Systemic reactions include early sweating, rapid pulse, nausea, vomiting, weakness, facial tingling, progressing to tachycardia, shock, and death. If only minimal swelling occurs within 30 minutes, the bite will almost certainly have been from a nonpoisonous variety or possibly from a poisonous snake which did not inject venom.

Emergency Procedures

Within practical limits, achieve immediate, absolute immobilization of the affected part in a position that is lower than the level of the heart. Immediate attention must be given to reduce toxic absorption at the injection site.

If the bite is on an extremity, place a lightly constricting band such as a rubber band 2–4 inches closer to the heart than to the site of the bite (Fig. 14.12). It should be tight enough to halt the flow of blood in superficial vessels but not tight enough to stop the pulse. You should be able to easily insert a finger between the constricting band and the limb. Relax the band 1 minute every 10 minutes and periodically move it slightly ahead of any advancing edema. There is no benefit from a band applied 30 minutes or

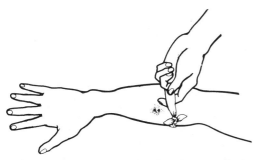

Figure 14.12. Constricting band, properly applied.

more after the bite. Never use ice or cold packs. Reassure the victim if he is conscious, but do not give alcohol or stimulants. Monitor vital signs, low blood pressure, and arrhythmias; apply CPR measures as necessary. Transport to a hospital as soon as possible.

Incision and Suction

If less than 30 minutes have elapsed since a pit snake bite, make a linear incision no more than ½ inch in length through each puncture wound parallel to the involved limb. The incisions should extend about ½ inch beyond the fang marks. Do not make such incisions or suction on finger bites. Avoid injury to nerves, tendons, and blood vessels, and do not use cross-like or multiple incisions. Apply suction by a suction device or by mouth (spit it out). Any venom accidently swallowed during suction will be quickly neutralized by stomach acids. Once flow has begun, let it continue for 30 minutes. Never delay transportation to a health facility, however, just to continue suction. Splint the affected extremity for transportation.

In cases of a neurotoxic coral snake bite, the treatment is the same except that incision and suction are not recommended. There is little local effect from the bite. The danger is to the nervous system.

Insect Bites

Insect bites are rarely disabling, but often annoying with their itchy hive-like lesions. The exception to this are stings on mucous membrane and in those allergic to the par-

ticular injection. When the environment warrants it, an insect repellent may be recommended as a preventive procedure, but sweating and wiping washes off much of its effect. Ant stings may cause redness, itching, and swelling at the site or more serious effects if there is an allergic reaction.

Background

The common type of strings requiring attention are hymenopteran stings from hornets, bees, yellow jackets, and wasps. The reaction is immediate pain and a reaction that may vary from local to fulminant anaphylaxis. Insects are infrequently the cause of tick paralysis and Rocky Mountain spotted fever in this country.

Certain American spider bites are also serious, but rarely fatal:

1. Black widow spiders are common in the southern states. They are recognized as being jet black with orange markings in the shape of an hourglass on the underside. Pain is immediate, often subsiding and then recurring. Reactions may be painful muscle cramps within 30–120 minutes, spinal and abdominal pain, weakness, respiratory paralysis, and convulsions.

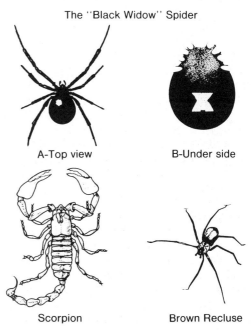

The "Black Widow" Spider

A-Top view   B-Under side

Scorpion   Brown Recluse

Figure 14.13. Black widow spider, scorpion, and brown recluse spider.

2. Brown recluse spiders have a yellow to dusty-brown color and present a brownish violin-shaped design on their back. Pain is rarely immediate, usually localizing within an hour, with blisters developing at the bite site. Reactions may be nausea, vomiting, weakness, arrhythmias, fever, shock, red blood cell breakdown, and kidney failure.

3. Scorpion stings in the United States are usually not serious with the exception of a variety found in the Southwest, especially Arizona. Most scorpion stings produce a burning sensation at the site of the bite followed by pain that spreads to the entire limb. Skin discoloration may be present. Stings from the dangerous species produce nausea, vomiting, convulsions, abdominal pain, excessive salivation, and shock. The victim may develop respiratory failure, cardiac arrest, coma, and die.

Emergency Care

After stinging, bees leave their stinger within the lesion. This lance should be removed by using a magnifying glass and fine tweezers or gently scraping it off with the edge of a knife blade. Do not try to grasp the sac or stinger since this simply forces the remaining venom into the skin. Wasps retract their stingers.

First aid for hymenopteran stings may be provided by cold and a commercial sting-relief lotion or cream. Temporary relief can be achieved with a topical freezing anesthetic such as Fluori-Methane (Gebauer Chemical Co.), ethyl chloride, or ice. Non-prescription antihistamine preparations have little benefit. However, if a mouth sting shows signs of edema with possible consequences of obstruction, referral should be made for antihistamine and/or corticosteroid therapy.

As black widow spider bites may lead to serious consequences, hospitalization is required to manage convulsive and respiratory difficulties. Antivenom may be necessary. With brown recluse bites, quick hospitalization is necessary for excision of the bite area.

In major reactions from any type of insect bite, make the patient lie down and immobilize the area immediately. Remove all jewelry from an affected limb. Apply a con-

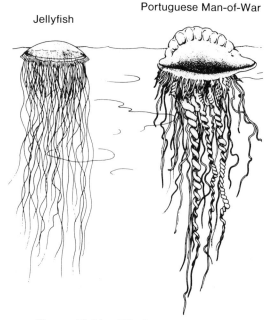

Jellyfish   Portuguese Man-of-War

Figure 14.14. Stinging sea animals.

stricting band to the affected limb which is placed lower than the heart. Apply cold to the part while the victim is being transported.

Marine Bites

These usually arise from stings, bites, puncturing, or sticking with poisonous tentacles such as from jellyfish, Portuguese man-of-war, corals, hydras, and anemones—all of which release venom into the individual's skin. Reactions range from local burning pain and irritation to anaphylactic shock and death (rarely). Muscle cramps, nausea, vomiting, and respiratory distress may be associated. Gently remove clinging tentacles with a towel. Diluted ammonia or rubbing alcohol poured over the site and left for 10 minutes helps to inactivate any stingers that have not as yet fired. After this, the acidic venom can be neutralized at the site with a sodium bicarbonate solution. A restricting band above the site helps to delay systemic absorption of the venom. Anaphylactic shock is always a danger.

Spiny fish, stingrays, urchins, and cone shells inject their venom by puncturing with spines. General signs and symptoms include swelling, nausea, vomiting, generalized cramps, diarrhea, muscular paralysis, and shock. Deaths are rare. Emergency care consists of soaking the wounds in hot water for 30–60 minutes, controlling bleeding, applying a dressing, and obtaining medical assistance.

BURNS AND SCALDS

Burns constitute any injury caused by contact with heat, flame, chemicals, electricity, or radiation. First- and second-degree burns are referred to as partial-thickness burns, and third-degree burns as full-thickness burns.

Background

Sunburn is the most common type of burn seen in sports, but other types of burns are occasionally seen in land and water vehicle-driven sports such as automobile racing, motorcycle events, and power boating. For the most part, burns caused by agents other than heat are treated as heat burns.

Actinic injury may be acute or chronic, and the acute form is usually that from sunburn which can produce varying degrees of pain, tenderness, erythema, blisters, and crusts. Sunburn is usually of greatest concern early in the season before the skin has had a chance to accommodate by thickening and tanning.

Chronic actinic injury produces premature skin wrinkling and lentigines and, more seriously, predisposes actinic keratoses, basal-cell carcinomas, and squamous-cell carcinomas. Basal-cell carcinomas do not metastasize, but they can deeply invade adjacent tissues. The result is often severe disfigurement, especially about the face and ears. Early signs are a small sore or mass which heals slowly and bleeds readily. Squamous-cell carcinomas are commonly sited on the face, lips, or back of the hands. They tend to grow slower than basal-cell carcinomas, do not bleed as readily, aggressively metastasize, disfigure, and lead to disability and death.

Management

First aid in burns requires immediate removal from the source of heat. This should be immediately followed by cool washings, cold applications for at least 30 minutes to reduce blisters and pain, protection from

infection, and management of the accompanying shock. Topical vitamin E and "special waters" have proved helpful. Prevention for sunburn is provided by hats, clothing, and sunscreens; however, sunscreens are quickly washed away by the sweating athlete.

Fluori-Methane or ethyl chloride may be used to alleviate the pain of first- and second-degree burns. The Spra-Pak nozzle should be used which offers a mist-like spray to lessen the impact of the vapocoolant on the affected area. Spray lightly until the skin just begins to frost, but never frost the skin.

Severity

The severity of burns is measured by the degree or depth to which tissues are injured and by the extent or percentage of body surface burned (Fig. 14.15).

First-Degree Burns

A first-degree burn is superficial; it involves only the outer layers of the epidermis. A typical example is sunburn, in which the skin is red and painful but with no blisters or fluid loss. It is not an open wound and, for this reason, does not become infected.

Second-Degree Burns

A second-degree burn extends into but not completely through the dermis, destroying or damaging skin cells, glands, blood vessels, and other structures. This burn is

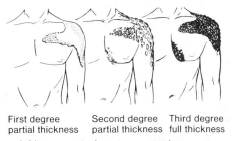

First degree   Second degree   Third degree
partial thickness   partial thickness full thickness

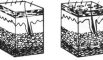

Epidermis
Dermis
Fat
Muscle

Skin reddened   Blisters   Charring

Figure 14.15. Major characteristics of first-, second-, and third-degree burns.

characterized by redness, pain, vesication, and blisters, and sometimes it exudes matter. Body fluids are lost through the damaged skin. A second-degree burn is an open wound susceptible to infection.

Third-Degree Burns

A third-degree burn destroys all layers of the dermis and may extend through the subcutaneous tissue into skeletal musle and underlying bone. There may be amputation of a part. This burn is characterized by insensitivity to pain since nerve branches are destroyed and by a hard dry surface which is either charred or pearly white. The surface is usually depressed below that of surrounding, painful, second-degree burned tissue. Enormous amounts of body fluids are lost into the damaged tissues and through the nonviable skin. A third-degree burn is an open necrotic wound highly susceptible to infection.

Pathology in Second- and Third-Degree Burns

Phase 1

In the first phase of a burn, there is always some destruction of the skin that results in a loss of plasma. In second-degree burns, there is a temporary loss of plasma in the form of edema fluid and a permanent loss through blister fluid or through weeping burned surfaces. Because of the plasma loss, the local vascular mechanism is affected in the burned area. Excessive permeability and blood stagnation in the involved and adjacent capillaries occur immediately after the injury and cause plasma to seep into surrounding tissues. This exudate rapidly infiltrates these tissues and gives rise to widespread edema. The edema begins to develop at the time of burning and is evident within a few hours. It continues for 2–3 days. Excessive capillary permeability is also responsible for the large amount of plasma lost through damage of the skin. In second- and third-degree burns, particularly the latter, there is an appreciable destruction of red blood cells.

Phase 2

The second phase of burn begins, as a rule, on the third day after injury, with a reversal of the phenomena just described. The coagulum which forms on the surface of second-degree burns reduces further surface losses. Edema fluid is now absorbed from the injured site into the blood stream. Finally, the arteriocapillary circulation, which was first distributed by vasodilation and then by vasoconstriction, returns to normal. The source of the exudation therefore dries up spontaneously. The eschar which forms on second- and third-degree burns reduces surface losses.

Phase 3

In the third phase of a burn, infection develops. Second- and third-degree burns are wounds subject to contamination from the moment of their occurrence. The existence of any wound exposes tissues to infection from bacteria because of the contact of the wound with the environment. The injury is contaminated almost immediately, sometimes as the patient falls to the ground. Improper emergency rescue measures, makeshift first-aid dressings, careless handling, and personnel breathing on a patient's burns are factors which lead to infection.

FROSTBITE

Frostbite (dermatitis congelationis), a form of localized tissue destruction from freezing where ice crystals form in the skin or deeper tissues, is a danger once skin temperature falls below 32°F. Contributing factors include fairly low air temperatures, contact with cold equipment, severe local vasoconstriction, and high airspeeds and altitude.

Background

Weak individuals are most susceptible to the injurious affects of cold than the healthy and fit. Two other important etiologic factors are (1) constriction about the part which interferes with free circulation, and (2) a prolonged constrained position or posture without exercise of the part. The first areas to be affected are the body protuberances such as the ears, nose, fingers, heels, and toes. The genitals, cheeks, chin, and female breasts may also be affected. Moist cold, more than dry cold, is an effective agent in causing this injury. Once clothing becomes soaked with moisture (sweat, snow, rain), the insulation factor is destroyed, encouraging hypothermia and frostbite during rest periods.

Mild Frostbite and Chilblain

Frostbite may be classified by three common stages according to the severity (depth of involvement) of the injury: first degree (erythema); second degree (vesication); and third degree (necrosis).

First-degree frostbite features a circumscribed inflammatory skin swelling. The cold initiates a primary contraction of cutaneous blood vessels resulting in pallor. In reaction, the vessels dilate and the area becomes red and swollen, producing a "burning" pain. White blood cells become disintegrated and liberate a coagulating substance, encouraging thrombosis in peripheral vessels. This impairs circulation along with the spastic ischemia. Symptoms progress with continued exposure to numbness of the part which appears white, yellow-white, or mottled bluish-white, and the part is cold, hard, and insensitive to touch or pressure.

In mild cases, local signs subside within a few days. In some cases, the erythema may persist for several weeks or may return sharply under the slightest exposure to cold. This hypersensitivity (chilblain or pernio), which develops in a person previously frostbitten, presents local areas of congestion which may become inflammed and even ulcerate. The ulceration is often initiated by exercise or exposure to heat, causing itching and stinging sensations.

Management

The prevention of frostbite is more important than its cure: feet must be kept dry, moist socks must be changed frequently, and shoes must not be so tight as to restrict slight toe and heel movement.

If the skin is livid and obviously not gangrenous, first aid for frostbite consists of brief rewarming of the affected part(s) with body heat, warm air, or tepid water. Heat should never be applied immediately. Never rub a frostbite area. Before wrapping the part(s) in cotton wool, gauze should be placed between affected digits. Once the tissue destruction process has been halted, the part should be kept cool to reduce secondary edema and ease the metabolic demands called for by the injured tissues.

In cases of deep frostbite, the skin appears hard and will not move over bony ridges. Never attempt to thaw the frostbitten area if there is a chance of refreezing. It is better to leave the part frozen until transportation can be made because refreezing of a thawed extremity causes severe and disabling damage. Much of what appears to be devitalized tissue may return to normal with proper care; ie, frostbite often appears worse on first examination than it really is.

CHAPTER 15

Bone and Joint Injuries

The relationship between structure and function, and the interrelationship between all body systems, cannot be denied. Muscles, bones, and connective tissues are involved in both local and systemic pathology and in a wide assortment of functional and referred disturbances. Thus, great care must be taken in eliciting the details of a complaint when any musculoskeletal disorder is suspected. This section reviews the basis of alert management of bone and joint injuries within the health care of athletic and recreational injuries.

BONE INJURIES

Correlation of the history of the present complaint with musculoskeletal dysfunction must be done in detail and with care. Maintain accurate initial and progress records with repeated monitoring.

Background

Musculoskeletal symptoms may be the first clues toward poor structural adaptation or stress adaptation. The most common musculoskeletal symptoms are joint stiffness, joint swelling, and joint pain. The nature of the damage depends on the direction of the applied force on the bones and the manner in which these bones are attached to other structures. The principal acute skeletal injuries are sprains, strains, subluxations, fractures, and dislocations.

Normal bone has an excellent blood supply with some exception in the metaphyseal area; but tendons, ligaments, discs, and cartilage are poorly vascularized. Yet both bone and joints challenge the host's defensive mechanisms. The pressure of pus under hard bone blocks circulation, and emboli and thrombosis can cause additional devascularization. When circulation is deficient, local phagocytic function and nutrition are deficient, and cure is stymied.

The most accurate diagnosis can be made immediately after injury, before swelling clouds the picture. Many fracture and dislocation complications such as nerve and vessel injury occur not from the trauma itself but from poor first aid which does not provide adequate splinting prior to movement. Traumatic bone injury rarely occurs without significant soft-tissue damage. The physical examination must be gentle but thorough because soft-tissue trauma is poorly visible on roentgenograms for several days after injury. For example, a working diagnosis of stress fracture may have to be made in the absence of classic symptoms by bony tenderness alone as the fracture may not be demonstrable on x-ray films for 10–14 days or longer.

Probing the History

Whether pain is present or not, the history must be probed to determine if the dysfunction is the result of bone, the joint, or the motor apparatus involved in the joint motion.

When subjected to weight-bearing, traumatic, or occupational stress, bone demineralizes and undergoes degenerative changes, resulting in deformity of the articulating surfaces. Concurrently, the attending excoriation of the articular periosteal margins results in proliferative changes in the form of lipping and spur formations or eburnation.

Bones break from either direct blows or indirect blows such as a fall on an outstretched hand resulting in a fracture of the forearm, elbow, shoulder, or clavicle. It is thus imperative that the injured person be examined as a whole. For example, even if a fall on the outstretched hand does not result in fracture, a rib or spinal subluxation may result. The inexperienced doctor may overlook a slipped femoral capital epiphysis in a young player whose complaints are restricted to the knee. The list can go on and on.

Bone Bruises

Certain simple contusions which involve subcutaneous tissues overlying bone and the periosteum are often referred to in sports as "bone bruises." Because the periosteum is richly endowed with nerves and vessels, severe bruises and fractures are quite painful despite a lack of roentgenographic evidence. When the periosteum is affected, tenderness will be present long after true soft-tissue tenderness has eased, sometimes for several months. Wherever the site, the athlete is disabled or considerably hampered as long as tenderness exists.

Initial treatment must be quick to minimize bleeding and swelling through ice, compression, elevation, and rest. Padding, often specially designed, must be worn as long as tenderness persists. During recovery, corrective manipulation, local heat, ultrasound, and massage may be applied to relieve related soreness.

FRACTURES

Fractures are classified as open or closed. An open fracture is one in which there is a break in the skin that is contiguous with the fracture. The bone is either protruding from the wound or exposed through a wound channel such as one produced by an arrow, javelin, bullet, or other missile. A closed fracture is not complicated by a break in the skin, but there is usually soft-tissue damage beneath the intact skin.

Intra-articular fractures are not uncommon in sports. They involve the articular surfaces of joints and the associated articular cartilage. Osteoarthrosis results if reduction is not accurate. However, a displaced fragment need not be removed if it does not interfere with function by impingement. Fracture dislocations often involve joint impaction and fragmentation. They usually present great instability and require operative repair.

Symptoms of Fracture

A working diagnosis of fracture may be based on any one of several symptoms. Additional assistance in diagnosis may be obtained from the history and roentgenography. A history of falling, receiving a blow, or of having felt or heard a bone snap may help in the discovery of more evidence such as:

1. Tenderness over the site of injury. Tenderness or pain upon slight pressure on the injured part may indicate a fracture.

2. Swelling and discoloration. These signs at the site of injury increase with time and may indicate fracture. The swelling is due to the accumulation of tissue fluid and blood. When blood collects near the surface of the skin, a bluish discoloration may be seen.

3. Abnormalities with movements. Deep, sharp pain upon an attempt to move the bone is presumptive evidence of fracture. Grating of bone ends against each other indicates fracture. Movement, however, should rarely be attempted to see if crepitation is present as it causes further damage to the surrounding tissues and promotes shock.

4. Deformity of the part. Protrusion of a bone segment through the skin, unnatural depression, or abnormal flexion may indicate fracture.

Some diagnostic pitfalls in orthopedics, as pointed out by Iversen and Clawson, include: (1) considering accessory ossicles as fractures; (2) overlooking an osteochondral, a tibial-spine, or a stress fracture; (3) forgetting that an upper-tibial fracture might progress into valgus; (4) failing to realize the instability of an apparently undisplaced lateral condyle fracture of the humerus; and (5) not appreciating the frequency of distal forearm fractures that slip.

The Repair Process in Fractures

Although bone is noted for its hardness and supportive characteristics, bone is similar to soft tissue in that it is resilient, highly vascular, and constantly changing. It adapts to disease and heals itself when fractured. Both bone growth and repair are most efficient during youth and adolescence, as witnessed in rapid fracture healing. Abnormally slow healing can almost always be contributed to a deficiency in minerals and vitamins, rarely to endocrine or metabolic etiologies. However, too much site motion, joint distraction, infection and other compound-fracture complications can cause delayed union or nonunion.

After fracture, a hematoma develops between the split ends. This space becomes invaded within a few days by granulation tissue, which in time becomes converted into fibrocartilage. This fibrocartilage is an osteoid tissue where new bone is laid down for union. After this stage, resorption and remodelling occur to reduce the initial callus formation in an attempt to restore the bone to its original size and shape.

While normal bone is highly vascular, readily repairs itself, and resists infection, avascular bone is defenseless in participating in the reparative process. Thus, after injury, treatment must be directed to prevent further devascularization and to encourage improved vascularity. Intra-articular and metaphyseal fractures enjoy an abundant blood supply; thus, early and active movement of the joint should be encouraged. However, proper stabilization of distal and proximal joints must be maintained in diaphyseal fractures because of the relatively poor blood supply. Thus, special concern must be given to increasing circulation and preventing stiffness.

General Emergency Treatment

The first step is to make a brief but thorough examination to determine the extent of injuries. Treatment of any life-endangering condition such as respiratory failure, cardiac arrest, or hemorrhage takes precedence over that for fracture. The care applied directly to the fracture is a part of the prevention or lessening of shock because pain is lessened and the likelihood of further trauma is reduced.

In the treatment for fractures, the rule, "splint them where they lie," applies. Open fractures are dressed before splints are applied. Care must be taken to avoid moving the fractured part as the razor-sharp ends of fractured bone can easily cut through vessels, nerves, muscles, and skin. Such additional damage would, of course, increase the possibility of hemorrhage, shock, or loss of limb or life. If movement of the patient is unavoidable or is essential in treatment, the fractured part must be supported if further damage is to be avoided. Slight traction-adjustment of the fractured part may be necessary to restore circulation, the lack of which is evidenced by absence of the pulse distal to the fracture. This is especially common in elbow fracture.

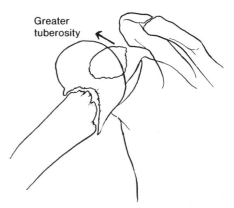

Figure 15.1. X-ray film tracing of fracture-subluxation of the surgical neck of the humerus where the greater tuberosity is displaced upward between the rotated head and glenoid.

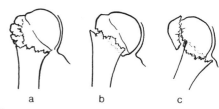

Figure 15.2. Diagrams of the three common types of fractures of the surgical neck of the humerous: *a*, crack without displacement with comminuted fracture of the greater tuberosity; *b*, adduction fracture; *c*, abduction fracture with separation of the greater tuberosity.

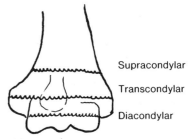

Figure 15.3. Diagram indicating the various levels of transverse fractures of the lower end of the humerus. The supracondylar type is by far the most common variety.

In the individual suffering multiple injuries, the most commonly overlooked injuries are fractures of the basilar skull, C7 vertebra, femoral neck, orbit, pelvis, radial head, talus, tibial plateau, T12 and L1 vertebrae, and zygomatic arch; and dislocations of the lunate, perilunate, posterior femoral head, posterior shoulder, and scaphoid.

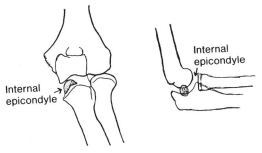

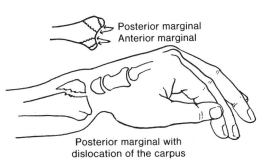

Figure 15.4. Internal epicondyle of elbow separated and lying in the ulnohumeral compartment of the joint. This injury often passes unnoticed in cursory analysis of roentgenograms.

Figure 15.6. Typical marginal fractures of distal radius. If separated, fragment is large. There may be an accompanying carpal dislocation.

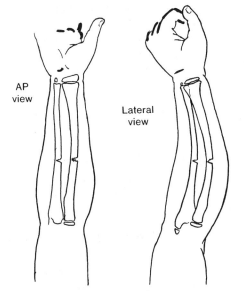

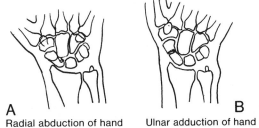

Figure 15.5. Greenstick fractures of the midshaft radius and ulna.

Figure 15.7. Illustrations of how a scaphoid fracture may be (*A*) hidden by overlapping bone due to faulty position of the hand during roentgenology; (*B*) revealed when the hand is adducted toward the ulnar side.

Emergency Immobilization (Splints)

To prevent further damage, a fractured bone must be immobilized by splinting the joints above and below the fracture, as movement of these joints would move the bone segments. All splints should be well padded to protect the skin from injury, loss of circulation, inflammation, and infection. Bandages used to secure a splint must not be applied so tightly that they impair circulation even for a few minutes. A bluish discoloration of the nailbeds or skin of the affected limb indicates that one or more bandages are too taut. Security bandages should never be tied directly across a wound.

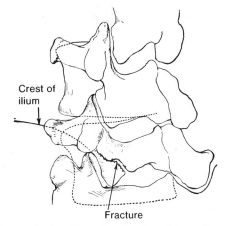

Figure 15.8. X-ray film tracing of irregular unilateral fracture of inferior articular facet and inferior margin of lamina; result of torsion injury.

Splints commonly used to immobilize fractures of the extremities are the wire ladder, cage, and Thomas leg splint. If this equipment is not available or training has not been provided for correct application, splints may be improvised by using such items as boards, stiff tree limbs, rolled news-papers, belts, etc.

In limb fracture, the pneumatic inflatable splint is especially useful as it offers both immobilization and compression to mini-mize hemorrhage. It must be applied only tight enough to support the fragments with-out inhibiting circulation.

To immobilize a fractured bone in the thigh or hip, an improvised splint must ex-tend from the groin and the armpit to sev-eral inches below the foot. Padding should extend over the ends of the splint at the groin and the armpit.

Fatigue Fractures

Fatigue (stress) fractures can be the result of any severe repetitive stress (eg, dancing, jumping, marching, running, throwing).

Etiology and Incidence in Sports

The causative factor appears to involve tensile forces from severe musculature con-tractions rather than the compressive forces of external trauma. Fatigue fractures of the leg and foot are most commonly seen in runners, and fatigue hip fractures are often seen in jumpers. Other patterns of incidence appear to be the pars interarticularis in foot-ball linemen and gymnasts; the patella, soc-cer players; ischiopubic area, hurdlers; ul-nar, tennis players and pitchers; and the pisiform, volleyball players.

The vast majority (95%) of fatigue frac-tures occur in the lower extremities, and most are associated with competitive run-ning. The three most common sites of fa-tigue fractures associated with sports in-volve the femoral neck, tibia (especially the distal third), metatarsals (especially the 2nd and 3rd metatarsals), and tarsals (os calcis, talus, or cuneiform). Less frequently, a site may be found in the pelvis, especially in-volving the ischiopubic arch of female ath-letes.

Symptomatology and Physical Findings

Vague pain may be the only early symp-tom. The typical case history will reveal the onset of insidious local soreness during a stressful activity. With repeated activity, progressively severe discomfort occurs both during and following the activity and often during the night while resting.

Physical findings typically include an-talgic postures and maneuvers, increased pain on percussion, localized swelling, point tenderness, referred pain, and a restricted range of motion (soft-tissue related). If sig-nificant stress is superimposed on a fatigue fracture (eg, fall, blow), a displaced frag-ment may be produced.

Roentgenographic and Ultrasonic Findings

Roentgenographic evidence rarely ap-pears until 10 days after the precipitating trauma, and it may not appear until 40 days after the incident. The first signs are endos-teal or medullary sclerosis and a break or nick in the cortex that is followed by the development of a periosteal callus.

Bone scans have been found to be more sensitive in detecting fatigue fractures than conventional x-ray procedures. This is an important consideration because if a fatigue fracture is found in one area, nonsympto-matic contralateral or remote fatigue frac-tures may be associated that could lead to serious complications.

EPIPHYSEAL DISORDERS

The growth plates in the young are highly susceptible to severe stress because of their vascularity.

Osteochondritis

Traumatic changes as the result of stress (osteochondritis) are featured by displace-ment, bony fragments, distortion or col-lapse, and irregular ossification during late stages. Osteochondritis may occur at almost any epiphyseal plate, and it is often named after a descriptive author. For example, fem-oral head, Perthe's disease; heel, Sever's apophysitis; metatarsal heads, Freiberg's disease; tarsal navicular, Kohler's disease; tibial tubercle, Osgood-Schlatter's disease; and the vertebral plates, Scheuermann's disease. Such terminology is confusing as the condition is not a disease, and this should be stressed to the afflicted.

Epiphyseal Displacements

These are seen in the young and are al-most always associated with severe trauma. They may occur spontaneously such as in the hip when associated with unexplained knee pain. The growth plate is weakest at the site of cell degeneration and provisional calcification, especially in children who are undergoing a rapid spurt in growth or who are overweight in proportion to their skeletal maturity. A common pitfall in orthopedics is to confuse an epiphyseal slip for a ligament injury; eg, at the knee joint. Epiphyseal slips should be treated as fractures, for fractures are what they are rather than a disease process.

Osteochondritis Dissecans

This disorder features inflammation of subchondral bone and articular cartilage which results in split pieces of cartilage within an affected joint. The cause is not completely understood, but the damage is inevitably at a point where compression occurs in a jarring injury. The clinical picture is one of avascular necrosis, where flakes or loose bodies of bone and/or cartilage are extruded into the joint. The knee, ankle, and elbow are most often affected.

BONE INFLAMMATIONS AND INFECTIONS

The earliest symptoms and signs of acute bone or joint infection are local pain and tenderness in the periarticular region. The patient has extreme difficulty or refuses to move the joint. The cardinal signs of infection (heat, redness, swelling) may appear much later than pain and tenderness, and sometimes never appear. Rotentgenograms are of little help in arriving at an early diagnosis; when evidence is obvious, the disease is chronic. Sometimes comparative bilateral films exhibit slight soft-tissue evidence.

Traumatic Arthritis

Traumatic arthritis presents signs of pain, possible ecchymosis, and soft-tissue swelling of periarticular tissue that may be limited to effusion within the capsule or obliterate bony prominences depending upon the severity of trauma, tenderness on pressure, and loss of function. Motion is usually limited because of pain, and there will be joint instability if the injury is sufficient to tear a tendon or joint capsule. Intra-articular fractures and fragments may be associated. The prognosis is excellent in those receiving efficient treatment; however, a subacute arthritis may, at times, persist indefinitely.

Periostitis

Periostitis is commonly associated with joint injury, especially that of the knee. It is the result of violent muscle strain which damages the periosteum. If severe enough to detach the periosteum, a degree of hematoma develops. The bruised joint is swollen, extremely tender, and movements are restricted. Physical examination makes one suspicious of fracture, but early roentgenographic findings are negative. Later, ossification of the hematoma is exhibited by induration of the swelling and new bone formation.

If severe hematoma is associated, aspiration may be necessary. In milder cases, firm support and physical therapy are appropriate. The condition is slow to heal and usually requires at least seasonal restriction from further athletic activity.

Osteomyelitis

With the exception of compound fractures, repeated injuries, and piercing wounds, osteomyelitis is rare in sports. When diagnosed, antibiotics are invariably required for control. Staphylococcus aureus is the common agent in all ages, and over 50% of the strains are penicillin resistant. Blacks are prone to develop a subacute form of osteomyelitis, especially if there is any indication of sickle cell anemia.

The time between initial infection and circulatory troubles is often rather short. If effective treatment is delayed and partial circulatory embarrassment is allowed for more than just 72 hours after the infection begins, surgery may be the only alternative and loss of joint function may be the result.

Posttraumatic Painful Osteoporosis (Sudeck's Atrophy)

Following extremity trauma, bone (being reactive tissue as other tissues) undergoes rapid and extensive physiochemical changes under the influence of the circulatory and trophic disturbances which frequently follow injury.

Background

It is common for immobilized bones to lose considerable mineral salts and show osteoporotic areas on x-ray examination. This type of disuse atrophy has little clinical importance as normal bone density and strength return quickly when function is resumed. It is essentially asymptomatic. Osteoporosis can be differentiated from such disuse atrophy in that true osteoporosis is characterized by a patchy decalcification of extremity bone in which there are coexisting signs of pain, vasomotor changes, and trophic disturbances.

A *neurogenic* type of bone atrophy may show its effects long after the effects of the original trauma have subsided or after fractured bones have united in good position. Not infrequently, it manifests 3–6 weeks after some apparently trivial injury to a polyarticular joint and is confused with malingering when insurance or compensation cases are involved.

Clinical Picture

In the early stages, it is characterized by constant aching pain, hyperesthesia, local swelling and hypervascularization, local heat, redness, marked joint stiffness, and abnormal sudomotor response of the previously injured part. These indications progress to vasoconstriction and edema, with a moist, cold, cyanotic part. In late stages, the skin becomes atrophic, thin, and shiny, and there is attrition of the nails, excessive hair growth on the part, and diffuse osteoporosis is demonstrated on x-ray films.

Any neural or circulatory interference to the part must be normalized. Vigorous physiotherapeutic measures are necessary to reduce edema, maintain joint motion, and increase deteriorating muscle activity. Minimal immobilization should be followed by active movement, heat, and massage.

Related Inflammatory Processes

Tendinitis, tenosynovitis, peritendinitis, and bursitis directly in a joint region are noninfectious inflammatory processes involving a tendon, a tendon sheath, or a bursa. They may be related to a specific single severe trauma or a series of microtraumas from joint stress and fatigue as often seen in weightlifters, tennis players, and even piano players and typists. Nelson states that they may be the result of reduced microcirculation caused by reflex mechanisms. The symptoms are a gradual onset of pain radiating along the involved tendon upon active contraction or passive stretching. The swelling is localized and soft, and the area may present heat and redness.

JOINT INJURIES

Most joints permit movement in the joint itself and/or fix a limb portion while another joint is in motion. They also function in transmitting stress when stabilized by musculature. This stabilization is necessary so that muscles can achieve their maximum leverage for joint motion (eg, angular, gliding, rotational).

The stability of synovial joints is primarily established by action of surrounding musculature. Excessive joint stress results in strained muscles and sprained or ruptured ligaments. When stress is chronic, degenerative changes occur. Joints are usually stressed from a direct blow leading to connective-tissue contusion and possible intra-articular fracture or a slipped growth plate in the young. The blow is often an unexpected one where protective mechanisms have not been put in force, or it may be so excessive that protective mechanisms fail.

The synovial lining is slightly phagocytic, is regenerative if damaged, and secretes synovial fluid which is a nutritive lubricant that has bacteriostatic and anticoagulant characteristics. This anticoagulant effect may result in poor callus formation in a situation of intra-articular fracture where the fracture line is exposed to synovial fluid.

Examination generally includes inspection, bony palpation, soft-tissue palpation, determination of the passive and active range of motion, muscle integrity and strength test, superficial and deep reflex tests, and investigation of associated areas.

Inspection

First seek gross abnormalities. Observe gait, and note any awkwardness in rhythm, weight shifting, or imbalance. Note any bone distortion, angulation, or limp. When a specific joint is involved, observe any gross deformity or swelling from either (1) fluid, where a wave can be demonstrated, or (2) thickened synovial tissue, where there is no wave but boggy tissue can be palpated. Inflammation associated with a red and swollen area suggests an acute synovitis. Inspect muscles for hypertrophy and atrophy, and note areas of old ecchymoses which point to previous trauma. Sinus formation is rarely seen. When present, the sinus leads to necrosed bone, to gouty tophi, or to abscess in or near the joint.

Irregularities of contour may be the result of osteophytes or lipping (attached to the bone); gouty tophi (not attached to the bone); constriction line opposite the articulation; or protrusion of joint-pockets in large effusions filling natural depressions. Irregularities of contour are easily recognized provided the normal contour of different body types is familiar. Note distortion or malposition due to muscle contractures near the joint, to necrosis, to exudation, or to subluxation.

Palpation and Percussion

Note any trophic lesions over or near a joint (cold, sweaty, mottled, cyanosed, white, or glossy skin; muscle atrophy). Palpate the joint for masses and points of tenderness which may indicate osteoarthritis, synovitis, a torn ligament or meniscus.

Palpate for muscle tone, fasciculations, and spasms. Fasciculations are small, isolated, involuntary contractions of a portion of muscle fibers, representing spontaneous discharge of a number of fibers innervated by a single motor nerve filament. Spasms are readily palpable, tender, and frequently accentuated during passive joint movement.

Palpate bone for tenderness and masses. Bone tenderness suggests inflammation, tumor, fracture, or complications from trauma. A suggestion of bone inflammation is enhanced when the bone is percussed at a site distant from the point of tenderness and pain is felt at the site of tenderness rather than at the site of percussion.

A hard enlargement is probably of bony origin. If boggy, it is probably infiltration or thickening of the capsule and periarticular structures. If fluctuating, it is probably from fluid in the joint. Enlargement is generally unmistakable; but when there is considerable muscular atrophy between the joints of a mature weekend athlete, the joints may seem enlarged by contrast when in fact they are not.

Fluid or semifluid exudates in joints may fill up and smooth out the natural depressions around the joint, or, if the exudate is large, may bulge the joint pockets. In the knee joint, four eminences may take the place of the natural depressions, two above and two below the patella.

Motion Evaluation

Functional limitation may be the result of (1) pain associated with movement, (2) bone or joint instability (eg, muscle weakness, fracture, torn ligament), or (3) restricted joint movement by effusion, muscular spasm, ankylosis, thickening or adhesion in the capsule and periarticular structures, obstruction by bony overgrowths or gouty tophi.

Determine active and passive ranges of motion bilaterally, and palpate the joint simultaneously to determine the presence of crepitation. Crepitus and creaking are detected simply by resting one hand on the suspected joint, with the other hand putting the joint through its normal range of motion while the patient remains passive. Note bone integrity by its abilitiy to resist a deforming force.

The examination of the musculoskeletal system must be greatly adapted in examining an acutely injured patient from that of a patient presenting nontraumatic complaints. For instance, active and passive range of spinal motion should not be conducted until after roentgenograms have demonstrated the mechanical integrity of the joint.

Excessive motion such as in joint tears is recognized simply by contrast with the limits furnished us by our knowledge of anatomy and physiology of joint motion at different ages. When bone and cartilage appear normal or are not grossly injured, we call the excessive motility of the joint a nonfixated subluxation, but excessive motility may also be due to destruction of bone and other essentials of the joint.

Measurements and Reflexes

Take circumference and limb length measurements at equal points above and below involved joints bilaterally and compare. Swelling enlargement or telescoping of the joint with shortening may be found, evidenced by careful limb measurements.

Test deep tendon reflexes. Upper limb

muscles are supplied essentially by C2-T1; lower limb muscles by L1-S2.

Indirect Methods

Indirectly we may gain information about joint disorders by noting: (1) general constitutional symptoms, their presence or absence, including fever, chills, leukocytosis, glandular enlargement, albuminuria, and emaciation; (2) blood analyses such as tuberculin and Wassermann reactions, bacterial presence or absence; (3) disease of other organs, their presence or absence; and (4), the course of the disease and the results of treatment.

PERTINENT SIGNS AND SYMPTOMS

Typical abnormalities that may be discovered in disorders of the musculoskeletal system include: (1) color changes such as ecchymoses and redness; (2) local heat; (3) soft-tissue swelling from synovial thickening, periarticular swelling, or nodules; (4) swelling from bony enlargement; (5) deformity from abnormal bone angulation, subluxation, scoliosis, kyphosis, lordosis; (6) wasting from atrophy or distrophy; (7) tenderness on palpation; (8) pain on motion; (9) limitation of motion; (10) joint instability; and (11) carriage and gait abnormalities.

If the history indicates recent travel abroad, the symptomatic picture may represent problems not usually seen in this country. For example, joint pain may be the result of hydatid disease, amebiasis, fungal infections, or some tropical diseases that may express themselves in joints during their acute or chronic course.

Joint Pain

Probing into the character, origin, timing, onset, and absence of pain offers important clues. Referred pain is often associated with musculoskeletal disorders, as are somato-somatic, somatovisceral, and other reflexes.

Unusual causes may be found. A history of childhood heart disease, St. Vitus dance, or chorea suggests joint pain resulting from acute rheumatic fever. Allergic conditions (eg, hay fever, asthma, migraine) point to a diagnosis of nonspecific intermittent hydrarthosis. Joint pain associated with a history of joint aspiration or intra-articular medication injections suggests pyarthosis. Or, joint pain may be associated with a venereal disease.

Character

Fracture pain is severe, throbbing, and aggravated by movement of the part. A sharp, severe pain (associated with muscle changes and sensory disturbances) radiating along the distribution of a nerve is characteristic of acute nerve compression. Severe throbbing pain is characteristic of gout and septic arthritis. Pain from degenerative arthritis and muscular disorders is an aching type which is relieved by rest, aggravated by certain motions, and often accompanied by splinting and paresthesias. Bone pain resulting from tumor or aneurysm is usually deep, constant, boring, more intense at night, and rarely relieved by rest or a change in position. Severe and persistent pain in one joint that begins to spread to adjacent joints is characteristic of inflammatory arthritis that is chronic and nonspecific in nature.

Origin

Although bone proper is insensitive to pain, orthopedic pain originates from the periosteum, joint capsules, surrounding connective tissues, irritated or inflamed bursa. A fractured bone produces pain from the periosteal rupture and soft-tissue hemorrhage pressure. Arthritis is painful because of the joint capsule irritation. A bone tumor yields pain due to the pressure upon and/or stretching of the periosteum. A history of a recent injection of antitoxin or the administration of a new drug may suggest joint symptoms have an allergic basis.

Timing

Joint pain worse in the morning after rest that is relieved after mild exercise but worse in the evening points to joint disease. Deep, aching, throbbing, dull or sharp pain that may be either constant or spasmodic is typical of joint disease. Pain from a herniated disc is relieved by rest and gets progressively worse as the day goes on. A dull ache during rest that's aggravated by motion suggests inflammatory arthritis. Pain lasting for several weeks or longer is common in chronic arthritis. In acute rheumatic fever and often in gonococcal arthritis, pain lasts for several hours, disappears, then reappears in other joints.

Onset

Sharp pain occurring only when the joint is moved a certain way and which is usually relieved by rest or immobilization points to joint dysfunction. In degenerative joint disease of the weekend athlete, the pain which occurs on motion and is relieved by rest is the result of joint dysfunction rather than the arthrosis itself.

Both primary joint dysfunction and joint disease may present sudden pain following trauma or an episode of stress; however, joint swelling is uncharacteristic of joint dysfunction but characteristic of joint disease. Joint disease may also have an insidious onset that is unusual in joint dysfunction. An exception to this would be intrinsic trauma causing joint dysfunction occurring during sleep or unconsciousness.

The onset of pain in several joints simultaneously points to joint disease unless several joints have been immobilized such as in multiple fractures or involved in severe trauma with multiple bruises. Gradually developing pain is often associated with chronic nonspecific arthritis. A rapid onset is seen in acute rheumatic conditions and gout.

Absence of Pain

Neuropathy is suspect when there is no pain but obvious joint disease. In such cases, diabetes mellitus is the usual fault. When pain fibers are destroyed or deadened in joint disease, injury is not safeguarded against properly and traumatic osteoarthritis advances rapidly. In the history of a non-medicated painless limp, muscle disease is the first suspect, but a metabolic bone disease or an endocrine dysfunction may be involved in children.

Joint Swelling

Periarticular swellings are classified as (1) swellings arising in the joint proper, (2) swellings derived from the bones adjoining the joint, or (3) swellings originating in the extra-articular tissues around the joint.

Joint swelling is the result of thickening of the synovial membrane or of excess fluid in the joint cavity. Such swelling is often obscured by bones, muscles, and tendons which overlie the joint cavity or its pouches; however, it is noticeable over thinly covered areas of the joint. For instance, swelling in the hip joint is almost impossible to detect. Swelling in the elbow is observed only at the posterior aspect on the sides of the olecranon process because the anterior surface of the elbow joint is thickly covered with muscles and the lateral aspects by strong collateral ligaments which prevent protrusion. For the same reasons, a wrist swelling is least noticeable when viewed from the front and radial side, and a knee swelling is least noticeable when viewed from the medial or posterior aspect.

Character

Joint trauma is profiled by a cool periarticular swelling that's very tender. Trauma or inflammation may result in hemorrhage or effusion. Painless bony lumps and asymptomatic joint swelling can often be traced back to forgotten trauma, especially when associated with sports injuries. For example, surf-board enthusiasts will often present bony lumps slightly inferior to the tibial prominence.

Swelling around a joint can be caused by edema from fluid overload or venous insufficiency. If this is the situation, pain and tenderness will be absent. Swelling around a joint that is warm and painful is characteristic of gout and rheumatic arthritis. Synovial inflammation is characteristic of nonspecific arthritides, rheumatic fever, septic arthritis, gout, and various collagen-vascular diseases.

In degenerative joint diseases, the trauma may be only normal activity to elicit effusion. A gonococcal wrist or ankle joint will usually be associated with nearby tenosynovitis. Infiltration, effusion, or inflammation can cause direct joint swelling. Localized infiltration is seen in leukemia, myeloma, and amyloid disorders.

Positioning

Because of the relative position of various bones and associated relaxation of the muscles around joints, every joint has one position in which the synovial cavity attains the greatest dimensions. When tension increases in the synovial cavity because of effusion, the patient will adopt a position that affords the greatest relief. For instance, the following positions of the larger joints offer the greatest ease: (1) hip: slight flexion, eversion, abduction, (2) knee: slight flexion, (3) elbow: flexion and midposition, (4) wrist: slight flexion, and (5) ankle: plantar flexion and eversion.

Shape

Shape of the swelling corresponds to that of the synovial membrane distended in toto. For instance, when a subcrureal pouch becomes dilated, the knee joint swelling may extend as much as 7 inches above the joint line. Distention of the tabular process of endothelium about the long head of the biceps in the shoulder may present enlargement over the surgical neck of the humerus.

Motion Restriction

In general, joint motion becomes restricted from either pain or mechanical disability. Intra-articular swellings inpair both active and passive movements, while extra-articular swellings impair one type of movement or none. Foreign bodies or fragments within a joint that result in effusion are associated with intermittent motion restriction.

Fluctuation

All swellings should be tested for fluctuation if they are more than an inch in diameter. Testing for fluctuation is made in two planes at right angles to each other. If a mass fluctuates in one plane but not another, it is negative for swelling because a swelling fluctuates in both planes. In testing for fluctuation, fat or muscle also transmit an impulse, but less perfectly than fluid.

Moderate swellings are tested for fluctuation by pressure exerted with the tip of a finger midway between the center and outer border of the swelling while the tip of the other finger is placed at an equal distance on the opposite side but remains stationary. The stationary finger moves passively from the pressure exerted by the action finger on the other side. Then reverse the procedure with the originally passive finger becoming the active finger and vice versa. If displacement takes place in two planes at right angles to each other, there is little doubt that the swelling contains fluid. When examining small swellings, it is often best to use two fingers of each hand.

A swelling of less than an inch is difficult to test for fluctuation. In such a case, use Paget's test, which consists of pressing the mass with a fingertip. A solid swelling is hardest in the center, while a cyst is softest in its center.

In the knee, the examiner tests for "floating" of the patella over an effusion by surrounding the joint with both hands, pressed slightly toward each other to limit the escape of fluid in either direction, and then suddenly making quick pressure on the patella with one finger. If the examiner feels or hears the patella knock against the bone below and rebound as the pressure is released, fluid in abnormal quantity is present.

Crepitus

There are several types of crepitus which characterize a specific type of lesion: bone crepitus, traumatic pulmonary emphysematous crepitus, joint crepitus, and tendosynovitis crepitations.

Bone fractures elicit an audible grating when the ends of the broken fragments rub against each other during movement. The crepitation from an epiphyseal separation resembles that of a broken bone but is softer in character than bone crepitus from a fracture.

A fractured rib in which a fragment of bone has pierced a lung allows air from the lung to escape into the subcutaneous tissues. Crepitus may be felt when the fingers are placed with mild pressure over the affected area.

Joint crepitus may be tested by placing a hand over the joint while passively moving the joint with the other hand. When coarse crepitations are transmitted to the palm of the palpating hand, osteoarthritis is usually involved. Other acute or chronic lesions present fine crepitations. To amplify the crepitations involved, it is often helpful to apply a stethoscope to the joint during the passive motions.

Crepitus may be felt over an effused joint following inflammation of the tendon sheath. In traumatic tendosynovitis of the extensor tendon sheaths of the forearm, for example, test by grasping the arm above the wrist while instructing the patient to clench his fist and open his hand with rapid motion several times. The presence of effusion will result in a transmittable or audible crepitation.

Pitting on Pressure

Pitting is a sign of liquid infiltration into the underlying tissues. Tenderness associated with pitting is indicative of inflammatory edema. While edema gives rise to a soft pitting, a degree of induration can be felt if pus is present.

A suspicion of edema may be confirmed by applying thumb pressure over the area in cases of massive infiltrations and index-finger pressure in cases of localized swelling. This pressure should be maintained for about 15 seconds. A positive sign of edema is indicated by a depression in the area after the action thumb or finger is removed. The depression is often palpable with the fingertips even if it is not visible.

Local Temperature and Tenderness

In cases of inflammation, the presence of local heat is a valuable sign. This may be noted by passing the outstretched hand rapidly over the affected part to an unaffected part and back again. Any difference in warmth from the affected area to the unaffected area signifies an increase in local temperature.

Mild cases of joint involvement invariably present points of maximum tenderness which correspond to those regions of the endothelium most superficial. For example, they are elicited (1) in the knee on both sides of the patella, (2) in the wrist over the anatomical snuffbox, (3) in the elbow over the radiohumeral joint, and (4) in the ankle at the anterior surface of the joint.

Turgor Test

This is a screening test to judge tissue hydration/collagen content. First, the examiner lightly pinches and lifts the skin on the back of the patient's hand with the thumb and forefinger. Hold the suspended skin taut for 30 seconds, release, and observe the area. It should quickly flatten and be complete within 3–5 seconds (a negative sign). If the area that has been pinched gradually creeps back to its normal state, the test is considered positive for probable collagen deficiency and/or an associated sign of osteoporosis.

Joint Stiffness

Joint stiffness is often the result of an overly stressed muscle in a young player or a sign of degenerative changes in an older athlete. The history of joint stiffness should be recorded as to distribution, duration, and associated circumstances. The stiffness may be in one joint or several. It may last only a few moments or for several hours or days. Inquire about the related circumstances: what aggravates and what relieves the stiffness?

Joint stiffness is often caused by edema or structural changes. Edema around the joint capsule is found in inflammatory disorders. Edema in the joint capsule secondary to inflammation is characterized by being worse after rest; eg, in the morning or arising after sitting for a long period. Stiffness that lasts for more than a half hour points toward the inflammatory arthritides, wherein it may last for several hours.

Stiffness resulting from structural changes is usually traced to cartilage degeneration or capsule tears. Previous trauma or inflammation of a capsule or associated tendons and sheaths may have resulted in adhesion formation. Stiffness resulting from degenerative disease becomes pronounced when area muscle compensation fails to protect thinning cartilage. Here also the stiffness is more pronounced after rest; however, it is quickly relieved by mild exercise.

Joint Restrictions

To distinguish muscular spasm from bony outgrowth in the weekend athlete as a cause of limited joint motion, notice that bony outgrowths (eg, in the hip) allow perfectly free motion up to a certain point, then motion is arrested suddenly completely, and without great pain. Muscular spasm, on the contrary, checks motion a little from the onset. The resistance and pain gradually increase until the examiner's efforts are arrested at some point, vaguely determined by the examiner's strength and hard-heartedness and by the patient's ability to bear the pain. Bony outgrowths within the joint are sometimes only recognized by the sudden arrest of an otherwise free joint motion at a certain point. In most cases, roentgenography is necessary. In true ankylosis, there is no mobility whatever.

Motions limited by capsular thickening and adhesions are not, as a rule, so painful after the first limbering-up process is over. There is no sudden arrest after a range of free mobility, but motion is limited from the first and usually in all directions, although the muscles around the joint are not rigid. The possibility of more or less limbering-out after active exercise (or passive motion) distinguishes this type of limitation.

Loose Bodies

Free bodies in the joint are not palpable externally and are recognized only by their symptoms, by roentgenography, and by operation. These loose bodies in a joint are the result of trauma, degeneration, or an inflammatory process. They may be singular or multiple, free or attached, and of bony, cartilaginous, or synovial origin. Loose-body formation is the outstanding symptom of osteochondritis dissecans and osteochondromatosis. They rarely present a problem; but if persistent joint "locking" occurs, surgery is usually advised.

There are certain other conditions in which loose bodies occur as a complication of a pathologic process: (1) breaking loose of new bone processes and cartilage in certain degenerative joint disorders (eg, osteoarthritis); (2) the organization of clots of fibrin forming rice bodies and melon-seed bodies; and (3) intra-articular fractures, especially compression fractures.

JOINT DYSFUNCTION VS JOINT DISEASE

Joint dysfunction implies the loss of one or more movements within the normal range of motion and associated pain. Joint dysfunction is only one possible problem that must be differentiated from other causes of joint pain. In a history of joint pain, there may be many clues pointing to the diagnosis of joint disease and many strongly suggesting joint dysfunction. This may represent separate problems overlapping on one another or be one complex problem. Thus, joint and periarticular pain and discomfort must be fully understood to arrive at a correct diagnosis because they appear in such a large variety of dysfunctions and diseases which may underlie an apparently acute athletic injury.

Joint Dysfunction

Primary joint dysfunction is usually the effect of intrinsic joint stress occurring at an unguarded moment when the joint is active within its normal range of motion. Another cause is that of extrinsic joint stress following a definite but minor trauma, often classified as a sprain and/or strain.

Secondary joint dysfunction is often overlooked in traditional medicine. Yet joint dysfunction is, according to Mennell, "the commonest cause of residual symptoms after severe bone and joint injury and after almost every joint disease when the primary pathologic condition has been eradicated, has healed, or is quiescent." Immobilization after surgery, immobilization from a fracture case even if the fracture is far from a joint, and immobilization from a taped sprain all cause residual symptoms of joint dysfunction.

Symptoms also follow joint inflammation or resolution of systemic joint disease with or without internal adhesions. When joint dysfunction causes residual symptoms after so-called joint disease recovery, the symptoms change from those of joint disease to joint dysfunction. That is, during the active process, rest increases joint pain and stiffness; during the residual dysfunction, rest relieves and action aggravates the pain. These points should be brought out during the case history.

To review the key history points of primary joint dysfunction: (1) the pain has a sudden onset and is sharp, (2) it usually follows stress at some unguarded joint motion, (3) pain is limited to one or adjacent joints, (4) pain is aggravated by movement and usually at some particular area of motion, (5) rest relieves the pain and doesn't produce stiffness, and (6) marked swelling or warmth is not associated.

Joint Disease

Peculiar features elicited in the history point directly to certain diseases. For instance, hemarthosis has a history of trauma and is characterized by slight but rapid swelling from blood; the joint is hot and acutely painful. Synovitis also has a history of trauma, but the swelling due to excess synovial fluid may not occur for many hours, the joint may feel warm rather than hot, and aching rather than acutely painful. The athlete, young or old, is not immune to rheumatic or degenerative joint conditions. It is all too easy to think of every joint injury of a sportsman as solely traumatic. Gout, osteoarthrosis, and infection are sometimes underlying factors. Gout may occur in any limb joint and is occasionally found in the spine, and it is not always associated with tophi or limited to the feet and hands.

Infection

Infection may be the result of a penetrating wound or be blood borne. A hematoma or hemarthrosis is an invitation to a subclinical blood-borne condition to manifest. Persistent pain following adequate treatment may indicate the presence of a secondary low-grade and unsymptomatic infection or irritation in spite of blood reports to the contrary. In such cases, suspicion should be directed toward a distant focus of infection. But, it need not be infection. It could be irritation from malfunction in a part of the gastrointestinal tract that reflexly produces vasospasm in the joint and hence pain. We must be aware that irritation produced by malfunction of a viscus can produce many difficult–to–diagnose symptoms.

Secondary Causes

Painless swelling of the feet or ankles is a common sign in heart failure, in certain kidney conditions, and in the use of estrogens, and it is the result of several idiopathic origins. However, the musculoskeletal system is often overlooked, and the swelling may be the result of venous and/or lymphatic congestion due to pelvic, thoracolumbar, diaphragm, or rib-cage dysfunction.

Periarthritis is another ill-defined disorder associated with an active process originating elsewhere. The clinical picture is one of infiltration, generalized tenderness, pain on movement, and joint heat. Management consists of seeking the causative factor, normalizing neural or vascular interference, regulating diet and rest, and applying moist heat.

SOFT-TISSUE JOINT INJURIES

Sprains

A sprain is a joint injury in which the ligaments, capsule, and surrounding tissues are partially torn or severely stretched without dislocation being present. There may have been a partial dislocation that spontaneously reduced itself. The cause is primarily from forcing a range of motion beyond the power of a ligament to withstand the stress, such as from overstretching or overexertion. The extent of damage depends upon the amount and duration of the force.

Background

Sprains are classified by severity as acute, subacute, or chronic, or by the area of involvement such as cervical, thoracic, thoracocervical, brachiocervical, thoracocostal, thoracolumbar, lumbar, lumbosacral, sacroiliac, or iliofemoral. Although the terms subacute and chronic may be diagnostic entities, these terms are confusing and an explanation of the subacute or chronic joint instability is more descriptive and desirable.

In differentiating sprain from strain, keep in mind that sprain involves the ligaments of a joint and strain involves the muscular and tendinous structures. Sprain usually elicits pain on movement of the affected joint even without muscular effort; strain elicits pain on muscular effort even without movement as in resisted contraction. However, any tissue may be strained in injury if the word "strain" is being used as a verb. When used as a noun or state of being, however, sprain refers to ligamentous injury and strain to muscular or tendinous injury.

When ligamentous tissue is subjected to continuous stress, it will become chronically inflamed and invaded by collagen substance and mineral salts. This results in sclerosing and even varying degrees of calcification. In addition, when ligamentous tissues are sub-

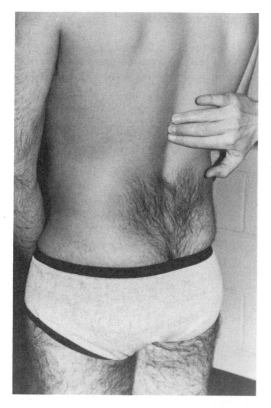

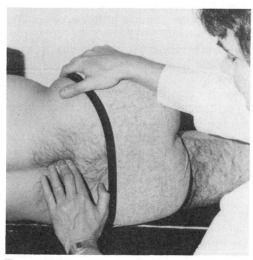

Figure 15.9. Palpation of lumbar spinous processes.

jected to acute traumatic stress, they will experience rupture of some of the comprising fasciculi that is attended by minute hemorrhages. If the involved ligament possesses elastic fibers, there will be a definite shortening.

Classification

Sprains, as strains, are divided into three degrees of injury:

1. First-Degree Sprain. In a mild sprain, there is a small amount of internal bleeding in a localized area of the ligament with only a few fibers separated. No actual loss of function or reduced strength is present. Generally, the ligament requires no protection and is not weakened. It is characterized by tenderness over the ligament that is not marked at the bony insertion by swelling and other symptoms of mild local inflammation. Joint instability is negligible.

2. Second-Degree Sprain. This is a moderate sprain with a partial ligamentous tear, characterized by increased severity of first-degree symptoms. A tendency toward recurrence is a complication, as is the possibility of traumatic arthritis and permanent instability. A moderate sprain results from severe tearing of the ligaments, although at least half of the fibers remain undamaged. This type of sprain shows some loss of function in the injured area even if the torn ligaments are not widely separated. They will join together again during the natural healing process unless the damage is great. If so, considerable scar tissue may form, and a permanent weakness of this section of the ligament may result. Moderate sprain is characterized by a greater degree of symptoms than presented by a mild sprain, lack of normal ligamentous resistance on digital pressure, and increased joint movement on tension as seen with movement or manipulation.

3. Third-Degree Sprain. This is a severe sprain with a complete ligamentous tear, characterized by severe swelling, hemorrhage, tenderness, complete loss of function, abnormal motion, and possible deformity. When a sprain is termed severe, it denotes a complete loss of function of the ligament caused by a force sufficient to pull it completely apart or tear it loose from the surrounding tissues. A severe sprain is characterized by a greater degree of symptoms than presented by a moderate sprain plus marked excessive joint motion indicating definite separation on tension or motion. Severe pain may or may not be present. Abnormal motion may be exhibited on bilateral stress roentgenograms. Persistent instability and traumatic arthritis are common complications. If seen soon after injury before swelling occurs, a palpable gap may be felt at the site of tear.

Management

If only a few fibers are stretched or torn, the part should be elevated and treated with cold packs to minimize swelling and relieve pain. Joint stability must be maintained until strength returns; a sprain should be supported (eg, ankle hitch) to prevent further stretching. If there is any doubt as to the severity of the injury, it should be treated as a fracture.

The same regimen is advised if several fibers are torn but the joint remains quite stable. The only change is that movement is delayed and initiated slowly with gentle non-weight-bearing passive movements only. This can be followed by swimming and carefully monitored flexion-extension active movements. Lateral and rotational movements should not be allowed until 2–3 weeks. When such injuries are numbered by an anesthetic so a player may return to competition, the results can be disastrous.

Torn large ligaments may require from 8–16 weeks for the scar to mature enough for protection. In severe sprain, a decision must be made whether motion or stability is the most important consideration. Early mobilization is necessary if motion is the priority; immobilization until solid healing occurs is necessary if stability is the priority. Surgical repair is usually required if the ends of the ligament cannot be approximated, the joint cannot be reduced, or there is complete lack of stability.

Fibrocartilage Damage

These are usually associated with the spine and knee but are occasionally related to the temporomandibular, sternoclavicular, and distal radioulnar joints. Moderate cases can usually be managed by manipulation, rest, physical therapy, and muscle reeducation, but crippling cases may require surgery.

Cartilaginous and disc substance when traumatized will progressively undergo degenerative change with possible dehydration and fragmentation. Disc damage results from repeated vertebral subluxations and the strain of mechanical and postural incompetence that tend to weaken the anulus, and, in the cervical and lumbar spine areas especially, at the posterolateral aspects with possible bulging into the intervertebral foramen. There may also be a visceral reflex causing a slight vasospasm that leads to degeneration.

Capsular Tears

A capsule tear usually results from an unexpected joint force, often occurring in an abnormal plane of motion. The torn tissues produce hemorrhage and local tenderness. Damage to the synovial membrane is commonly associated, resulting in effusion and possible hemarthrosis. Unless joint stability is severely disrupted, these disorders improve well with conservative care. Early treatment should consider cold, pressure, rest, and a graduated muscle education and exercise regimen. On the third or fourth day, contrast baths, deep heat, and more active movement can begin. Associated contusions are treated the same as the sprain.

Intracapsular Pinches

A sudden, usually rotational, joint stress may cause some soft tissue to be pinched within articular structures. This is most frequently seen in the knee where infrapatellar fat is nipped, resulting in effusion and possibly hemorrhage. Management is the same as that for sprain, but movement is slightly delayed because injured fat is slow to heal.

DISLOCATIONS

An osseous dislocation is the displacement of the normal relationship of the articular surfaces of the bones that make up a movable joint.

Background

Dislocation places considerable strain on ligaments which normally maintain joint position. There may be injury to these ligaments, the capsule they form around some joints, articular cartilage, synovial membrane, and other soft tissues, as well as hemorrhage into or around the joint. A dislocation may result in a complete luxation or a subluxation. In the extremities, a presented subluxation may be the effect of a spontaneously reduced dislocation and be associated with considerable capsule and ligament damage. Pain, swelling, and deformity are centered about the joint. Usually, there is also loss of motion.

Emergency Treatment

A dislocation is immobilized in the same way as a fracture: close to the joint. Cold compresses may be applied to the joint to relieve pain and reduce swelling, but the patient's temperature must not be lowered so as to invite shock. Related ligaments are frequently torn and require surgical repair. Postreduction immobilization usually requires 6 weeks in the lower extremity, 3 weeks in the upper extremity. Inadequate care, especially in ankle and shoulder dislocations, leads to chronic weakness, movement restrictions, instability, and recurrent dislocation wherein subsequent surgery has a poor prognosis for restoration to the preinjury status. Most all dislocations require x-ray analysis prior to reduction.

OBJECTIVES OF JOINT INJURY MANAGEMENT

Prevention is better than cure. A large percentage of traumatic joint injuries can be avoided with proper conditioning, training, and practice. After injury, the following points are the aims of good case management.

Reduce and Reabsorb Swelling. Early cold, compression, elevation, and rest will do much to avoid the hazards of excessive swelling. Heat, massage, and exercise are contraindicated in the early stages, but beneficial in the later stages. Aspiration is contraindicated unless necessary for diagnosis or relief of severe pressure. To prevent capsular stretch from chronic effusion, local compression, elevation, contrast baths, and muscular activity are beneficial after 48 hours. Normal joint movement and tendon function cannot be achieved until periarticular swelling has been absorbed.

Minimize Deformity and Wasting. An attempt must be made to normalize existing deformity, mechanical obstruction, and articular irregularities so that normal joint motion and configuration can be achieved. Joint stability must be achieved by conservative measures (eg, manipulation, physiotherapy, proprioceptive neuromuscular reeducation) or surgical and postoperative rehabilitative methods. Progressively increased exercises are necessary to minimize the muscle wasting that rapidly follows joint trauma. A protective reflex muscle spasm may interfere with early rehabilitation. It is best treated with cold and cryokinetics.

Normalize Joint Movements and Function. Progressively increased remedial exercises of a well-supported joint help to restore normal joint motion. Support should not restrict motion in an unaffected plane. Once the joint's full range of normal motion is obtained painlessly, strength-developing and skill exercises can be carefully incorporated with emphasis upon rhythm to avoid tissue breakdown.

CHAPTER 16

Muscle, Fascia, and Tendon Injuries

Muscles are often injured in sports by strain, contusion, laceration, indirect trauma, rupture, hernia and, occasionally, disease. This chapter offers the practicalities behind alert management of muscle-tendon unit trauma and related disorders.

INTRODUCTION

The body is composed of over 600 muscles that move over 200 bones, and each is somewhat unique to an individual. When working in a synchronous manner, bones, nerves, muscles, and ligaments give the body the ability to perform all motor functions, whether they be gross movements or artistic functions.

The typical muscle contains 75% water and 20% protein, and the remaining 5% is composed of carbohydrates, lipids, inorganic salts and extractions. It has been estimated that 42% of a male's total body weight is made up of muscle tissue, as compared to 39% of a female's weight.

MUSCLE INJURY

The degree of vascularity of the capillary network between skeletal muscle fibers and in associated tissues depends greatly upon the type of training. The quantity of interstitial fat, most marked in atrophied muscle, is also determined by the degree of training. Lymph vessels are not found within voluntary muscle. A muscle caused to be in traumatic or reflex spasm will become modestly inflamed. Some transudation precipitation of fibrin, collagen, and mineral salt deposition may result, and, if extended, a chronic myositis and myofibrosis may manifest. In addition, the myofascial planes of the erectors will become inflamed at the points of major strain. Transudation and fibrin formation may produce myofascial plane adhesions.

Muscle Soreness and Stiffness

Muscle soreness may occur shortly after activity and pass quickly, or it may not appear until up to 48 hours after exercise and persist for several days. Stiffness, a sign of poor physical fitness in the weekend athlete or unusual stress in the trained athlete, may be confused with minor strain as both stiffness and strain produce pain due to increased intramuscular pressure. The stiffness syndrome features gradually increasing pain, swelling, and restricted motion.

Most authorities today feel that the disorder is not involved with the local accumulation of lactic acid: stiffness results from the accumulation of extracellular muscle fluid due to increased capillary-filtration pressure in an unconditioned muscle where the vascular bed is unable to keep up with the necessary vascular return. The disperal of the accumulating extracellular fluid is also delayed because of the lack of lymphatics within voluntary muscle.

Muscle Cramps and Spasms

Cramps are characterized by spontaneous, prolonged, painful muscle contraction, usually occurring in the voluntary weight-bearing muscles. They often develop during sleep or soon after violent exertion and may vary from slight contractions to violent spasms. Cramps frequently follow drinking ice water or other cold drinks too quickly or in too large a quantity after exercise. Normally, many motor units rest while others are firing; but in the cramp phenomenon, all motor units fire and cause the spasm. Why this happens is not clear, but impaired electrolytic balance and blood flow are often involved.

Background

Heat cramps are often caused by excessive salt loss. However, the other factors may be involved such as muscle anoxia, cold, a blow or strain, or for some yet undetermined other reason. Cramps are differentiated from heat stroke and heat exhaustion in that the mental state is clear, the temperature is normal, and blood pressure and ECG are normal. Swimming too soon after a meal increases the danger of active-extremity cramps because much of the general circulation is diverted to the abdomen for absorption purposes. Hormonal factors may be involved in the female athlete, especially during the menstrual period.

Muscle spasm is an involuntary and aberrant contraction of a muscle part or whole as a result of some excessive motor fiber stimulation such as irritation of: (1) the anterior horn cells by the toxic elements of catabolic debris, accumulations consequent to faulty elimination, and circulatory disturbances; (2) an encroached nerve root from subluxation, paraforaminal congestion, herniated disc, and/or ligamentous thickening; (3) a nerve trunk or plexus (eg, piriformis psoas major, scalenus anticus contraction); or (4) peripheral nerve branches (eg, common peroneus by contracted tensor fascia lata or occipital nerve by suboccipital spasm). Spasm may also occur as splinting secondary to injury as in sprain, avulsion fracture, and compression within a muscle as the result of direct injury or irritation, often resulting from toxic accumulations (eg, toxic lumbago); or consequent to emotional or mental stress.

Management

Relief can be provided by stretching the affected muscle within its normal range after intermittent cold applications, then applying firm pressure kneading. Relaxation and warmth of the affected muscles usually offers further relief, and it sometimes helps to massage the spastic area toward the periphery.

In severe muscle tightness, cold is often effective when combined with exercise. Have the patient flex or extend the limb against manual resistance in the direction of tightness and in the range where limitation occurs, followed by voluntary relaxation. This should be done while cold applications are being applied. As the part begins to

relax, the joint should be passively put through its normal range of motion. Probably one of the most effective techniques is that of "spray and stretch," which is discussed later in this chapter with trigger areas.

The incidence of cramps can be reduced by adequate warmup, salt, water, and protective equipment to prevent contusion. Muscle fatigue is frequently averted by sympathetic stimulation effecting an adrenalin reaction, as well as correcting postural faults, endocrine imbalances, neural and circulatory impairment, and actions which enhance respiratory efficiency. If salt loss is the cause, therapy consists of salt tablets (1 gram every 1–3 hours) until symptoms subside.

Muscle Contusion

Muscular contusion is a disturbance of muscle tissue in the nature of a bruise re-

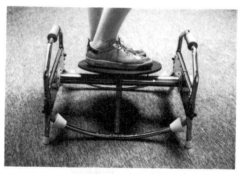

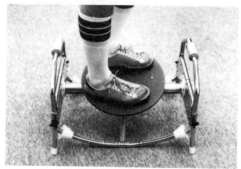

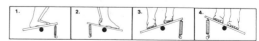

Figure 16.1. Adapto-Disc, for controlled ankle motion in the prevention and rehabilitation of ankle, shin, and leg problems (with the permission of Widen Tool & Stamping, Inc.).

sulting from a direct force over the muscle. Usually, there is no or little accompanying disturbance to the skin or subcutaneous tissues. However, muscles may be lacerated by sharp or pointed objects. A compound wound has the added problem of infection and must be treated by surgical methods.

Background

After contusion, there is local swelling, tenderness, pain on motion, and mild function impairment. Following repeated intermittent trauma to a muscle, the normal resolution is interrupted and fibrous scarring occurs in the hemorrhagic area. This is frequently followed by calcification (myositis ossificans).

Management

Ice, compression, elevation, and rest of the part is necessary in the acute stage to minimize bleeding. Heat and exercise are indicated after 72 hours. The initial pain of traumatic bruises, contusions, abrasions, swelling, and minor strains may be controlled with a vapocoolant such as ethyl chloride. The affected area is sprayed until the tissue just begins to frost and turn white. Further spraying is contraindicated because excessive spraying is likely to intensify pain from muscle spasm and increase motion limitation. Rapid evaporation of the coolant absorbs heat and causes cooling depending on the dosage. The smallest dosage needed to produce the desired effect should be used because the anesthetic time interval (10–60 seconds) is often sufficient to help relieve the initial pain from trauma.

Muscle Ruptures

A muscle action not balanced by reciprocal inhibition of the antagonistic muscle (eg, blow, unexpected force) may result in the rupture by sudden contraction or a less common injury to its antagonist by overstretching. Muscles previously weakened by fatigue or disease are more apt to rupture.

Rupture is characterized by knife-like pain, followed by a sensation of extreme local weakness. If a complete tear occurs, the lesion is usually at the tendinous attachment to the muscle belly. Normal continuity is broken and quite obvious on palpation until obliterated by hemorrhage and swelling. Function is lost in proportion to the degree of tear. Direct evidence is gained by testing function with gravity eliminated. The asymptomatic ripple-pattern (ladder muscle) seen in some athletes on passive stretch is not of traumatic origin but considered an effect of banding of the overlying fascia.

Muscle ruptures associated with nonpenetrating wounds are seen in both the young and old. In youth, they occur when a muscle is suddenly stressed beyond its tensile strength and the muscle fails at the musculotendinous junction. Such rupture is characterized by painful voluntary contraction, ecchymosis at an area of local tenderness, swelling, edema, and hemorrhage. Palpation will often reveal the defect. After the acute stage, persistent weakness remains and there is an increase in muscle bulk proximal to the rupture site upon contraction.

In the elderly, muscle rupture occurs under minimal loads as a result of degeneration within the muscle's tendon. These ruptures feature considerably less pain, swelling, tenderness, and ecchymosis; however, they do present the later persistent weakness and increased bulk upon contraction.

Management

Treatment for hemorrhage must be provided in the early stage. Support, progressive exercises, heat, ultrasound, and massage are indicated in the later stage. In severe lacerations, surgical approximation of the torn ends is necessary.

Muscle Hernia and Dislocation

Complete muscle rupture is rare, but a split in a muscle sheath due to weakness or a break may allow the muscle tissue to herniate during contraction. It may follow injury or be a surgical complication. The sheath opening may be large or small. A soft mass is noted at the site of the opening during palpation which disappears when the muscle is contracted and reappears on relaxation. Weakness may be a complaint. Permanent correction can only be made by surgery.

Muscle Weakness

With the possible exception of spinal dysarthrias, disuse atrophy is the most common cause of muscle weakness. It may be the result of immobilization, an occupational lack of use of a particular muscle group, or disuse as a result of painful injury, nerve disease, or primary muscle disease. Atrophy is demonstrated in evaluations of muscle strength as well as a decrease in bulk. Because of this decrease in mass, bilaterally compared circumferential measurements of limbs are helpful in evaluation when practical. Muscle rupture and prolonged spasm are also causes of muscle weakness witnessed in athletics. Other causes of muscle weakness and spasm such as spastic paralysis, flaccid paralysis, myopathy, myasthenia gravis, periodic paralysis, root or nerve disease, upper and lower motor neuron syndromes, parkinsonism, and cerebellar disease are rarely encountered in athletic care, but their possibility should be considered.

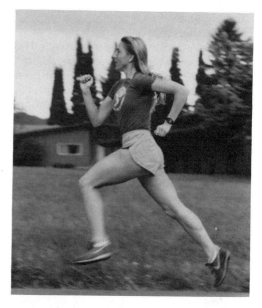

Figure 16.2. Dr. Margaret Karg demonstrates good running form (photo by Paul M. Everson, with the permission of the ACA Council of Women Chiropractors).

MUSCLE AND TENDON STRAINS

Soft-tissue damage is usually more painful and can be more serious than bone injury. Bone heals with calcium, whereas soft tissue heals with fibrous or scar tissue. The latter is different from the original soft tissue and lacks the elasticity or viability of the original tissue. Soft tissue also takes longer to heal than bone tissue. Bone tissue may actually be stronger after the healing process has taken effect, whereas soft tissue is usually weaker after repair.

The most common muscle injury is strain of a few muscle fibers and associated connective tissue. Players refer to it as a muscle pull or tear. In strain, both intrinsic or extrinsic muscle stress can produce torn muscle fibers, connective tissues, and vessels within a muscle belly or at its points of origin or insertion. A strain cannot affect a muscle and not the tendon or vice versa; if it affects one part of the unit, it affects the other. Thus, the musculotendinous unit must be considered as a whole in cases of strain.

Chronic strain is the result of prolonged overuse which produces an inflammation at the tendinous attachment, musculotendinous junction, or within the tendon itself. As activity continues, the inflammatory reaction progresses to calcification at the muscle origin or tendon insertion with possible spur development. Intramuscular hemorrhage is not uncommon in conditions of chronic strain. Tendons with sheaths are more likely to become inflamed, with the inflammation spreading between the tendon proper and the sheath.

Background

The incidence in upper extremities is highest in the biceps and triceps (eg, glass arm), and in the elbow, wrist, and fingers in tennis players. Incidence is highest in lower extremities in the quadriceps, hamstrings (eg, sprinting), anterior tibial, adductors (eg, horseback riding), triceps surae (eg, tennis), and Achilles tendon (eg, older runners). Pulled spinal muscles are often seen in weight lifting, gymnastics, and rowing. Pectonius and psoas muscle strain is often seen in ballet dancers and athletes who do considerable kicking.

The exact cause of muscle tears is unknown. Some feel they are the result of technical error, some unknown circulating toxin, or a postural fault where an activator muscle is jerked into action before the prime fixers are ready. Regardless, the mechanism appears to be a breakdown in coordination of the reflex inhibition necessary for synchronous contraction of antagonistic muscle groups; eg, fatigue, weakness, and straining are known to cause a cortical bombardment of the spinal centers, manifested in overstriding.

Hematoma Formation

Interstitial hematomas are usually the result of contusion, while intramuscular hematomas are the result of intrinsic tears. Both contractile and noncontractile elements are damaged during muscle strain, but the greatest injury is suffered by the capillary network between skeletal muscle fibers. The effect is seepage of blood and tissue fluid into interstitial and extracellular muscle spaces which are already engored by activity hyperemia. A degree of hematoma is the result, and it may protude within the potential space between muscles. When extrinsic stress is severe, bleeding may also result within the deep and subcutaneous connective tissues to compound the problem.

Hematoma development is smaller and localized in open wounds because the open surface relieves pressure, restricting tracking into deeper tissues. When intramuscular tension returns after injury, intramuscular bleeding points tend to become compressed. Clotting occurs within a few hours, but slight trauma (eg, massage) may cause further hemorrhage even after 2–3 days. Resolution follows with a degree of absorption and fibrosis as previously described.

Symptoms

The onset is acute with searing pain which rapidly fades into a full ache. Pain is increased on movement, especially against gravity. Weakness is not commonly associated. Examination presents a locally spastic and tender muscle with swelling. If rupture is severe, a gap may be palpated. A bulge in the long axis (eg, thigh) on vigorous contraction points to hernia. Contraction against resistance and passive stretching produces pain relative to the degree of hematoma. In the late stage, extensive skin discoloration is common and often appears some distance from the site of injury. Subacute and/or chronic strains may result in a myofascitis and/or myofibrositis.

Classes of Muscle and Tendon Strains

Strains are classified by either severity or by area. When classified by severity, the terms mild, moderate, and severe are generally applied. When classified by area, specific musculature are used such as gluteal, cervical paravertebral, intercostal, abdominal. If the muscles involved are of a nonspecific multiple nature surrounding a joint, the general area may be used as a descriptor such as a right iliofemoral strain, left knee strain, thoracocostal strain of T7-T9.

Muscle strains can be classified into three degrees of injury:

1. First-Degree Strain. This is a mild muscle pull caused by trauma to a part of the musculoskeletal unit from forceful stretch that results in a low-grade inflammation and some muscle-tendon disruption. Hemorrhage, disability, and strength or function loss are mild. It is characterized by local pain aggravated by movement or muscle tension. Physical signs include local tenderness, swelling, mild spasm, ecchymosis, and minor strength and function loss. The common complication is recurring strain; tendinitis and periostitis at the site of attachment may develop.

2. Second-Degree Strain. This is a moderately pulled muscle caused by trauma to the musculoskeletal unit from excessive stretch or violent contraction that results in torn fibers without complete disruption. It is characterized by increased first-degree strain symptoms. There is moderate hemorrhage and swelling. Muscle spasm and function loss are especially greater. The complications are similar to those seen in first-degree strain.

3. Third-Degree Strain. This is a severely strained muscle. The trauma results in a ruptured muscle or torn tendon which may be represented as a muscle-muscle, muscle-tendon, or tendon-bone separation. A palpable defect is often present. It is characterized by severe pain, tenderness, swelling, spasm, disability, ecchymosis, hematoma, and muscle function loss. Prolonged disability is the major complication. After the acute stage, roentgenograms exhibit soft-tissue swelling and an avulsion fracture at the tendinous attachment.

Tendons repair slowly and handle infection poorly because of their relative avascularity. Sheath trauma or infection can block nutrition, especially in those tendons which extend via long tunnels and are served with a long-axis blood supply.

GENERAL TREATMENT OF MUSCLE INJURIES

It is typical of muscle injuries that the pain is out of proportion to the extent of damage. This pain is the result of hematoma pressure which stretches adjacent muscle fibers and connective tissues, as well as the result of irritation from extravasated blood. As complete muscle rupture is rare, loss of functional ability is usually a secondary concern.

Emergency Care

Immediately after injury, a cold pressure pad should be applied to inhibit bleeding. If occurring on a limb, elevation should also be applied to the limb which has been elastic bandaged (distal to proximal) up the limb. In minor tears, gentle active movement should be encouraged to reduce the pain, in spite of the discomfort, but this is inadvisable when swelling is rapid.

Case Management

Treatment should be designed to inhibit hematoma development and promote rapid resolution. Such care reduces pain (the chief complaint) and inhibits excessive adhesions and scar tissue (the disability factor). In cases of intrinsic injury, the cause of injury must be determined and preventive measures instigated.

The pressure pad should remain in place 2–3 days, with tightening when necessary. Gentle, active unresisted exercise should be encouraged. Bed rest may be required if bruising is severe, but rest has no place in treatment after the first 48–72 hours unless complete rupture or myositis ossificans is knowingly in progress. Rest after the acute stage promotes atrophy, adhesion formation, and scarring.

Appropriate physiotherapeutic measures (eg, diathermy) may be started in 2–3 days after injury to promote vasodilation and reduce spasm. Later, ultrasound, massage, and progressive resistance exercises may be instigated to encourage dispersal. As improvement continues, exercises are increased in variety and vigor to tolerance until they meet activity needs. Local anesthetic injections to diminish pain are dangerous because they deaden natural protective mechanisms and increase the size of the space-occupying lesion. Jaskoviak has found acupuncture to be an effective adjunct.

Rehabilitation

During strain recovery, full exercise of the unaffected parts, depending upon the site and scope of injury, may be carried out to maintain general fitness. Faradism has been found useful in stimulating inhibited muscles, but it is contraindicated if there is any suspicion of myositis ossificans. When a case is first presented long after injury, a program of progressive mobilization is necessary due to the probable marked fibrosis. Rehabilitation is not complete until the player is physically capable of returning to competition, knows one's capability, and demonstrates full muscle extensibility.

Determining the Anatomical Movers of Human Movement

Training a person to properly analyze the anatomical movers at the point of performance has been a difficult task until recently. Chun has developed a method that depends on the principle that a body moves along the direction of the resultant of the applied separate forces. A body segment must move along the direction of the resultant of muscular tension, tissue passive resistances, and external forces applied on the segment such as gravity, elasticity of the equipment used, friction, muscular tension of opponents, etc. Generally, the direction of the segmental motion and the external forces would be known. The direction of the muscular tension as well as the principle muscles responsible for the movement could therefore be determined.

To develop analytical capabilities, Chun states that the examiner should be aware that there are usually three types of situations in which the determination of the principle movers of human motion are possible.

1. First, the direction of segmental motion would be classified as opposite to the direction of the external forces (ie, gravity, etc). This would indicate that the movers are located on the same anatomical side as that of the segmental motion.

2. Second, slow moving segmental actions would occur in the same direction as that of the external forces. As a consequence, the movers would be located on the opposite side of the segmental motion.

3. Third, rapid segmental movements would also occur in the same direction as that of the external forces. The movers would now represent muscles lying on the same side of the segmental motion.

Muscle Training via Resistance Exercise Equipment

Ariel and associates emphasize that the ultimate objective in weight training for sports activities or rehabilitation is to exercise the muscle at maximum efficiency throughout its range of movement. This goal necessitates proper assignment of force, displacement, velocity, and when desired, time, acceleration, and the amount of work and power. To accomplish this, it is necessary to assess the individual's biomechanical changes and then to develop a resistance and velocity intensity that will accommodate those changes in a functional manner. This means that the variations in resistance intensity and velocity must be precisely and wisely incorporated into a resistive mechanism. It is also essential that the operation of such a mechanism is not adversely affected by improper machine design. To prevent design failure, the relative effects of inertia must be understood. Inertial forces affect the motion and magnitude of the muscle's movement. The smaller the inertial forces produced by the machine's moving parts, the greater the muscular involvement.

All gravity-dependent exercise machines are subject to inertial forces and also apply the resistance in only one direction. Thus, only the agonist muscle group is exercised and the training is not followed by a correspondingly balanced antagonist muscle activity.

Exercise equipment that employs springs, torsion bars, etc, are able to overcome the inertia problem to some extent and can partially overcome the unidirectional force restriction. However, the problems of safety, nonlinear resistance, and the nonadaptability of the machine to an individual's force characteristics are still serious drawbacks. For this reason, most trainers consider them unacceptable.

Another type of machine in common use operates on a constant velocity principle where the resistance is changed in direct relationship to the forces acting on the moving bar. This equipment, however, operates on an open loop mechanism that does not allow feedback control of the exercise while it is in progress and the velocities cannot be changed in a manner that will simulate ballistic human motion.

Hydraulic mechanisms can overcome the inertial problem as well as the unidirectional problem. However, applications of such a mechanism are limited by a fixed flow rate that restricts the user to move at a limited number of preset velocities and, at any given moment, the user is unsure of just what his performing force or velocity actually is.

Fortunately for professional use, a computerized closed-loop feedback control exercise mechanism has recently been developed that can overcome these problems and provide the user with the flexibility and the adaptability to exercise at any resistance or velocity pattern throughout the range of movement.

COMPLICATIONS TO STRAIN

Infection, myositis ossificans, and cyst formation are typical complications of muscle strain. Other complications such as aneurysm, arteriovascular fistulae, phlebitis, and phlebothrombosis will be discussed in Part 4 on a regional basis.

The spine and extremity joints commonly suffer strains and sprains, which may be uncomplicated or complicated. For example, an uncomplicated spinal strain is a simple subluxation involving the muscular component primarily and does not contain a serious neurologic deficit. A complicated strain is accompanied by mild autonomic disturbances and may be associated with preexisting arthropathy or discopathy, congenital deformities (osseous or muscular), systemic diseases (eg, diabetes mellitus), myofascitis, or age. An uncomplicated sprain is a ligamentous injury unaccompanied by an preexisting pathology or injury to the spinal column contents. A complicated sprain is accompanied by preexisting pathology or injury to the spinal column contents. In general, complications result in strain/sprain when the tissues are abnormal or the general system is physiologically deficient at the time of injury because the lowered vitality of the damaged cells and the accumulation of exudate may provide fertile soil for the invasion of inflammatory processes and delayed repair.

Acute and Chronic Spasticity

When muscles become acutely spastic or chronically indurated, normal movement is impaired and foci for referred pain are established. Even with proper conditioning and warmup procedures, myalgic syndromes are commonly seen when treating athletes because they habitually ignore the warning signals of pain. The degree of impairment is essentially determined by the severity of spasm, the amount of induration, and the extent of functional disability.

Both spastic and indurated muscles are characterized by circulatory stasis, which is essentially the effect of compressed vessels. This leads to poor nutrition and the accumulation of metabolic debris. Palpation will often reveal tender areas that feel taut, gristly, ropy, or nodular.

An area of chronically indurated muscle tissue is often adjacent to an area of muscle that has entered into a state of fatty degeneration. When found through palpation, this area should not be confused with that of a lipoma (adipoma). These soft benign fatty tumors are frequently multiple but not metastatic, varying in size from a pea to a large egg. While most lipomata are located subcutaneously, those embedded deep within skeletal muscle tend to rise to the surface when the involved muscle is exercised and to recede during rest.

Management

Treatment should be directed to normalize the continuous motor firing, dislodge

collections of metabolic debris, and improve circulation and drainage. Regardless of the modality used, intensity should be maintained below the threshold of pain to prevent a protective contraction of the involved musculature. Heat (superficial or deep), sine-wave muscle stimulation, negative galvanism, and massage have all proved themselves effective. When deep mechanical vibration is used, several clinicians believe that pressure across muscle fibers tends to release accumulated metabolic by-products while pressure parallel to muscle fibers (directed to the heart) enhances drainage.

Lowe points out that when spastic areas do not release adequately or conventional methods only offer temporary relief, a nutritional evaluation should be made. A calcium, Vitamin D, and/or magnesium deficiency may be a contributing cause.

Infection

Infection is rare except in open wounds or aspirated hematomas. Especially if a bacteriemia exists, a hematoma may become infected and produce suppuration. This is a greater possibility if the hematoma is sited in a relatively poorly vasculated area. Rest and referral for antibiotics and surgical drainage is usually indicated. Progressive exercises may begin as soon as drainage stops, with normal training after healing is complete.

Traumatic Myositis

Myositis is an inflammation of muscle tissue, usually involving only the skeletal muscles. Contusion and trauma may cause an inflammation of muscles wherein the involved muscles become red, swollen, tender, painful, and almost of wooden hardness. This type of myositis usually subsides without any suppuration.

Background

Disease of muscle tissue is often mistaken for disease of the adjacent joint, tendon sheath, or some type of neuralgia. Muscle pain is not localized subjectively with the same accuracy as is pain in the more superficial structures, thus such vague localization requires a most careful examination. Functional use of a muscle is painless if the inflammatory process lies entirely within the muscle sheath, but perimyositis may cause pain during function. Myositis causes pain only when the muscle is palpated or stretched. Whenever stretching a muscle causes pain, that muscle should be carefully palpated for sensitive areas and palpable swelling or induration. Points of sharply defined tenderness can usually be found. In testing muscle tenderness, portions of the muscle should be pressed between two fingers rather than pressing the muscle upon underlying bone to avoid mistaking a periostitis for a myositis.

Management

Rest, local heat, and acupuncture may be helpful. Massage is beneficial if applied in the later stages.

Traumatic Myositis Ossificans

Myositis ossificans is a condition of heterotopic bone formation which can occur in collagenous supportive tissues such as skeletal muscles, ligaments, tendons, and fascia following hematoma. It is commonly the effect of direct muscle bruising, especially repeated contusions, as seen in contact sports, on the anterior aspects of thighs and arms.

Background

Connective tissue which surrounds the muscle rapidly invades the traumatized area, and connective tissue retains its embryonal ability to be transformed into more differentiated tissue. Following the primary interstitial myositis, there is a transformation of the connective tissue into bone. A fluffy calcification shows on roentgenography in 2–4 weeks after injury. The calcification matures in 3 months, and in 5 months ossification appears. The lesion is characterized by an indurated, tender, indistinct mass of a single muscle group that presents local heat. It is common in teenagers and young adult males, and it occurs 80% of the time in the biceps brachialis after dislocations and is frequently seen in the thigh (quadriceps). Periosteal tears undoubtedly encourage ossification.

Management

Early cold, rest, and compression to the injured muscle helps to reduce potential ossification. Immobilization is usually required for about 2 weeks after injury, followed by progressive active range-of-motion exercises. Exercise should not be begun early as it provokes extension of the calcareous deposits. Heat is helpful in the later stages. Extremely large and painful lesions may require surgery after ossification is mature and when the site is near a joint disturbing function. Protection of the part is the best preventive measure.

Cyst Development

Absorption is inhibited if bleeding is excessive or if a hematoma forms within lax tissues. When the clot retracts, a serum-filled cavity (presenting a fluctuant swelling) is left which is lined with organizing fibrin deposits. Aspiration is seldom successful, thus surgical drainage is indicated. Progressive exercises may be begun gently even when the pressure bandage is still applied as an inserted drain is rarely necessary.

MYALGIA (FIBROSITIS)

Myalgia or muscular rheumatism is a generalized term referring to aching muscles associated with stiffness, tenderness, and varying degrees of disability increased by active motion. Rare is the person who has not suffered some form of stiff neck, pleurodynia, scapulodynia, dorsodynia, lumbago, or sore leg muscles after unusual exertion or chilling. It appears to be the commonest form of persistently recurring pain, other than headaches.

Background

Fibrositis is a better term than myalgia since the changes occur chiefly in the white fibrous connective tissue of tendons, muscles, nerve sheaths, fascia, periosteum, joint capsule, and ligaments. These changes are a hypothermic edema and proliferation of white fibrous connective tissue as a result of chilling, toxic influences, acute trauma, chronic strain, or physical fatigue.

Thermal and barometric changes, vitamin B deficiency, chemical intoxication, metabolic imbalances, as well as dampness and respiratory infection, are important precipitating factors. Focal infection is often an important factor, as is a malfunctioning co-

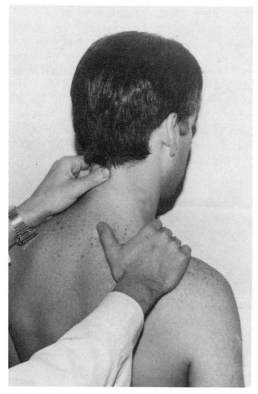

Figure 16.3. Palpation of the superior nuchial ligament.

lon. Regardless, the mode factor is via the capillary circulation and the nervous system.

The early state is one of effusion with a localized inflammatory serofibrinous exudate causing puffy swelling. The exudate may be absorbed or organized by fibroblast invasion and proliferation of fibrous tissue. In the latter stage of fibrous thickening, fibrous bands and nodules sometimes form in the muscles and fascia as adhesions and press on arterioles and nerve filaments producing contracture and atrophy.

Common Causes of Myalgia

While any disease that primarily affects joints may cause an associated poorly localized aching in a muscle or muscles, the following conditions are those which usually present muscle pain with minimal or no articular involvement.

Infection. The patient reports an acute onset associated with fever and other signs of infection.

Psychogenic Rheumatism. The history presents poorly localized muscle pain, more commonly reported by females. The course is chronic, nonprogressive, and nondeforming. There is diffuse or localized areas of muscle tenderness.

Tendinitis, Peritendinitis, and Capsulitis. The history commonly presents an acute or insidious onset associated with trauma to or excessive strain of the involved area. Some investigators, however, dispute this, feeling that many times there is no overt trauma involved. Bennett contends visceral irritation produces local skeletal vasoconstriction which sets up spasm, joint irritation, etc. Thus, a joint or tendon may become painful without trauma, either overt or covert. The course is self-limiting, but joint deformity may result (eg, shoulder). There is local tenderness over the tendon insertion and around the joint. Motion limitation is common.

Drug-induced Myalgia. There is a history of administration of steroids, diuretics, clofibrate, chloroquin, anticonvulsants, procainamide, etc, often where remissions can be associated with not taking the drug. Physical findings are usually negative, but there may be some pulmonary involvement.

Other causes rarely seen in athletics include rheumatoid arthritis, polymyalgia rheumatica, dermatomyositis, scleroderma, systemic lupus erythematosus, and various connective-tissue diseases.

Management

Whenever possible, the underlying cause must be found and eliminated. Treatment is a challenge. The first concern should be to remove neural and circulatory interference. Relaxation, heat, dietary supplementation, low-salt intake, support of the affected part, contrast baths, exercise, counterirritation, acupuncture, and massage all help somewhat but seldom completely.

COMPARTMENT SYNDROMES

Muscles are enclosed and supported by strong fascial compartments. A compartment syndrome is any condition that increases pressure within an anatomic space which results in circulatory embarrassment to the contents of the space. Any muscle crush or interference with circulation may result in muscle swelling restricted by the fascial sheath, which leads to extreme pressure and cellular death.

Background

The syndromes are seen in both the upper and lower extremities, especially in the forearm and leg. Typical locations in the upper extremities include the volar and dorsal compartments of the forearm and the intrinsic compartments of the hand. Lower extremity locations are found at the anterior, lateral, and posterior superficial and deep compartments of the leg. The disorder is often seen in football where a limb is stepped on by a studded shoe.

Increased pressure within a compartment may effect vascular closure, a reflex vasospasm, and/or decreased perfusion pressure. The cause for the increased pressure may be traced to either an increase in compartment content or a decrease in compartment size by some factor(s). Hemorrhage, increased capillary permeability or capillary pressure, infusion, and hypertrophy are common causes of an increased compartment content. A decrease in compartment size is usually the effect of localized external pressure (eg, a tight dressing).

Examination

During the neurologic examination, be sure to test light touch and two-point discrimination. Laboratory data are of little help. Grade muscle strength of potentially involved muscles, and palpate for tenseness. Passive muscle stretch will increase pain in ischemic muscles. Each syndrome has its individual clinical picture of pain, tenseness, weakened muscles, and sensory changes (see Table 16.1).

A diminished peripheral pulse may point to either a compartment syndrome or arterial occlusion. Hot red skin overlying an affected compartment suggests a complication of thrombophlebitis or cellulitis. Kidney failure or myoglobinuria may add to and complicate the picture. A poorly responding case of shin splints with pain even on rest suggests a compartment syndrome.

Management

As certain players appear to have a predisposition toward compartment syndromes, they should be identified as early as possible and examined frequently because the syndrome is usually progressive. Maintain careful records of examination findings. In severe cases, referral for early decompression may be indicated.

TENDON DISORDERS

Tendons are contiguous with periosteum, with some fibers entering the bony cortex. Tendons have great intrinsic strength capable of withstanding the action of strong

Table 16.1.
Lower Extremity Compartment Syndromes

Sign	Anterior	Lateral	Posterior — Superficial	Posterior — Deep
Pain on passive movement	Toe flexion	Foot inversion	Foot dorsiflexion	Toe extension
Site of tissue tenseness	Between fibula and tibia, anteriorly	Lateral fibula area	Bulk of calf	Between tibia and Achilles in posterior-medial lower leg
Weakened muscles	Tibialis anterior, toe extensors	Peronei	Gastrocnemius, soleus	Tibialis anterior, toe flexors
Sensory change distribution	First web space (deep peroneal)	Dorsum of foot (deep and superficial peroneal)	No signs	Plantar surface (posterior tibial)

muscle contraction yet are often incapable of withstanding an unexpected stretching force (eg, misstep). For protection, the Golgi tendon-stretch receptors have an inhibitory effect on muscle contraction. This tends to counterbalance the stretch receptors within muscle which excite contraction upon stretch.

Tenosynovitis

Tendon sheaths are lined with specialized connective tissue cells similar to cells lining bursae and the synovial membrane of joints. Thus, reactions within tendon sheaths to external influences are akin to those seen in bursae and joint cavity affections. The term tenosynovitis generally includes all affections of the tendons and their enveloping sheaths.

Background

Continual pain at a tendinous insertion can usually be traced to a sudden unexpected strain, to chronic stress, and rarely to contusion. Nerve entrapment, epicondylitis, soft-tissue nipping, and osteoarthritis may be confused or superimposed within the clinical picture. The two most common sites are at the origin of the extensor tendon at the lateral epicondyle (tennis elbow) and

the origin of the adductor longus at the pubis.

Tenosynovitis is usually the result of overuse or compression of a tendon possessing a synovial sheath or secondary to systemic infection. The disorder is usually acute and relieved by rest but may become chronic and resemble rheumatoid arthritis. Chronic inflammation of the sheath always holds the danger of stenosis, especially at sites where tendons cross (eg, De Quervain's disease, snap finger).

Types

Traumatic tenosynovitis (peritendinitis crepitans) is divided into two types. The common form is due to repeated overuse of a musculotendinous unit to a point of fatigue where the tissues cannot functionally adapt. Vigorous exercise in a sedentary weekend athlete is an example of overactivity which may bring on the characteristic symptoms. Within a few hours after a hard session of unaccustomed effort, and the involved tendon sheath becomes edematous. Pathologic changes are particularly evident at the musculotendinous junction and in the peritendinous areolar tissue. Thrombosis of the venules occurs, and fibrin is thrown out into the aveolar tissue and between muscle fibers. A sticky fibronous exudate is thus produced which may be accompanied by a serous effusion within the tendon sheath. The adjacent muscle fibers show degenerative changes, lose glycogen content, and accumulate lactic acid, which spreads over the tendon. This acidity causes the edematous swelling. The second form is an acute hemorrhagic type resulting from direct contusion or a puncture wound which does not introduce infection. A sterile outpouring of bloody and serous fluid occurs within the tendon sheath.

Symptoms develop in 24–28 hours after injury. There is a gradual onset of pain radiating along the involved tendon upon active contractive or passive stretching. There is a soft, hot, frequently red, localized swelling at the musculotendinous junction which usually renders an audible silky or leathery crepitus whenever the tendon is moved. In the hemorrhagic type, the pain is dull and aching, a feeling of fullness is perceived at the site of the affected tendon

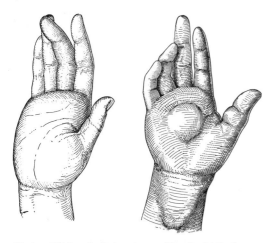

Figure 16.4. *Left*, tenosynovitis of middle finger with rupture of sheath and invasion of middle palmar space. Finger symmetrically swollen, flexed, and the concavity of the palm is lost. *Right*, tenosynovitis of radial and ulnar bursae with rupture into the palm.

sheath, and crepitation is not usually prominent.

Inflammation of the areolar tissue around a tendon (peritendonitis) is a common result of sudden training increases. It features swelling, pain which is relieved by activity, tenderness, and palpable crepitus.

Management

Rest and support are necesary from 1–2 weeks, followed by massage, progressive exercises, and therapeutic heat.

Tendon Rupture

Rupture is exceedingly rare in players under the age of 40 years. Both complete and partial ruptures are most commonly seen of the Achilles tendon of middle-aged athletes. Tendinitis with healing and repair might precede an episode of complete rupture requiring prolonged casting or surgical repair. The cause is usually traced to overuse, direct violence during stretch, or a poorly placed injection. Its site is commonly found just away from the point of insertion into bone. The rare event of spontaneous tendon rupture occurs only when the tendon is weakened by degenerative processes.

Rupture Near Insertion. Rupture here is characterized by sharp pain, often accompanied by perception of an abrupt "thud" at the site. The sharp pain soon subsides, but joint weakness does not. Partial rupture is characterized by acute pain during activity which persists until stress can be avoided. When activity is resumed, severe pain returns. A tender swelling is inevitably noted on palpation. Surgery presents the risks of complications but usually leads to a quicker return to activity (within 3–4 months) than conservative measures.

Rupture at the Musculotendinous Junction. This features a sudden stabbing pain followed by swelling and sometimes hematoma. Pain is increased when the affected muscle is contracted. A gap may be noted when swelling subsides to indicate a degree of muscle tear, but surgery is rarely necessary.

Ganglion. The localized cystic swelling to which the term "weeping sinew" is applied is the result of a mucinous degeneration of connective tissue occurring near a

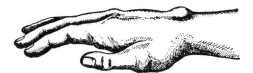

Figure 16.5. Ganglion of the wrist.

tendon sheath or joint capsule. The cause is unclear, but trauma is thought to be a factor.

Background

One large cyst may be felt, or several small cysts may coalesce to form a multilocular cyst. The walls are composed of dense fibrous tissue. Bundles of nerve fibers are often seen in the areas of mucinous degeneration. Ganglions are usually seen on the dorsum of the wrist or foot. They give rise to a localized swelling, gradual or sudden in onset, which may vary in size from time to time. Weakness and mild neuralgia may be perceived. If connected to a tendon sheath, the ganglion becomes prominent when the tendon is stretched.

Management

Small ganglia may be ruptured by pressure or a sudden blow. After disruption of the gelatinous material into the tissues, the area should be firmly compressed for a few days. However, this method is not successful if the ganglion is attached to the joint capsule; surgical incision may be necessary.

Calcific Tendinitis

The tendons of the rotator cuff and the origin of the elbow extensors are the common sites of deposits of calcium. Deposition is usually abrupt and associated with an acute inflammation of the joint capsule and its lining, characterized by pain and muscle spasm which limits movement. Relief may occur suddenly as a deposit is spontaneously ruptured into a bursa or joint cavity. Occasionally, deposition is a slow asymptomatic manifestation of tendinous degeneration.

Ossification of Tendons

Due to stress at points of tendinous insertion, cracks may appear in the cortex which cause the area to become invaded by osseous tissue. In late stages, compact bone may be found on roentgenography to extend well over an inch in the tendon. Such extensions are subject to fracture, but without undue stress they are asymptomatic.

TRIGGER POINTS (MYODYSNEURIAS)

Sola believes that myofascial pain may be the most common pain problem faced by most physicians. It may present as a primary complaint or as a crippling adjunct to any number of other problems (eg, unequal leg lengths, disuse, immobilization, chronic strains, poor posture, gait disturbances, connective-tissue diseases, arthritides). Trigger point syndromes often appear related to a lack of appropriate exercise; thus, they are less common (but not absent) in athletes and laborers than they are in sedentary workers.

A trigger point can be demonstrated much easier than it can be defined. Clinicians for many years have found highly localized, exquisitely sensitive areas within or near a painful region. When pressure is placed on the sensitive spot (trigger point), local pain, referred pain, or both may be initiated. Besides deep pressure, an application of heat, cold, electrical stimulation, needling, or some other stimulus may evoke a painful trigger-point reaction. The power of such a reaction appears to be moderated by a number of general factors (eg, conditioning, genetic predisposition, hormonal balance, personality, previous injury (scar tissue), and emotions).

Trigger points are foci of stress inflammation which result in binding cobweb adhesions that incarcerate sensory nerve endings to produce sharp demarcation of referred pain especially upon pressure. A trigger point itself, or myodysneuria, is a small, deep, hypersensitive area in a myofascial structure from which high-intensity impulses bombard the central nervous system and give rise to deep-aching referred pain—as contrasted with the ischemic-compression nerve pain of prickling, tingling, and numbing which follows the segmental distribution of an entrapped peripheral nerve.

An irritable trigger point in or near a muscle is often a little-recognized cause of spasm and myofascial pain. Many cases of torticollis, shoulder pain, tennis elbow, substernal aches, lumbago, sciatica, hip pain, knee pain, and ankle pain can be traced to trigger-point mechanisms. Such conditions are frequently misdiagnosed as myalgia, myofascitis, nonarticular rheumatism, and sometimes as muscle strain or joint sprain. This is especially true when symptoms persist long after precipitating events.

Etiology

Myofascial trigger areas, as pointed out by Johnson and others, may be produced by direct trauma to muscle or joint, chronic muscular stress, chilling of fatigued muscles, acute myositis, nerve root trauma, visceral ischemia or dyskinesia, arthritis, and hysteria. Long-term myofascial pain following activation of a trigger area is believed to be a reflex pain cycle sustained by the trigger area. Predisposing influences may be any factor which leads to chronic stress (physical or emotional) and fatigue. Nerve root compression, chronic visceral dysfunction, remote joint lesions, chronic infection, heavy alcohol consumption, a low metaboic rate with creatinuria, diminished serum potassium or calcium levels, diminished vitamin C or B levels, estrogen deficiency, and hypothyroidism are frequent factors in contributing to noxious feedback which perpetuate trigger points. The opposite is also true; ie, somatovisceral reflexes from trigger points may reinforce and perpetuate a visceral disorder such as ectopic cardiac rhythm, for one example.

Impulse discharges from a trigger area may be related to vasoconstriction and other autonomic effects which are limited to a more or less predictable reference zone of pain. This is true for both visceral disease and the myofascial structures. One must distinguish between the site of pain (the reference zone) and the source of pain (the trigger area). Thus, it is important to differentiate true somatic pain from the somatic pain component of visceral pain. Although the somatic component of such pain syndromes may be relieved and indicated for this use, the visceral cause of the pain complex must never be overlooked by casual therapy for temporary relief of a trigger area.

Causes of Trigger Point Pain

Trigger points are generally considered to be "weak" points within myofascial tissue that are particularly sensitive to stress-induced change. That is, they may remain quiescent until a certain stress triggers a syndrome that involves a number of positive feedback cycles such as sensory and motor reflexes, sympathicotonia, vascular responses, and, possibly, extracellular fluid changes, which eventually lead to hypertonia, fatigue, and endogenous pain or the intensification of traumatic pain.

Although the exact physiological mechanisms of trigger point pain are unknown, Sola offers a rational neurophysiologic explanation. He feels that, because of physiologic defense mechanisms such as splinting and bracing of muscles, vasomotor changes, increased sympathetic discharge, and hormonal and other humoral changes in plasma and extracellular fluids, the spastic muscle or fascia (which is probably more sensitive than surrounding tissue due to previous injury or a genetic weakness) fatigues and signals its distress to the central nervous system. A number of responses may result. For example, various muscles associated with the trigger point may become more tense and begin to fatigue because of motor reflexes. Sympathetic responses lead to vasomotor changes within and around the trigger point. Zimmerman reports that local ischemia following vasoconstriction or increased vascular permeability following vasodilation may lead to changes in the extracellular environment of the cells involved, release of algesic agents (eg, bradykinins, prostaglandins), osmotic changes, and pH changes—all of which may increase the sensitivity or activity of nociceptors in the area. The sympathetic hyperactivity may also cause smooth muscle contraction in the vicinity of nociceptors, thus increasing their activity. This increased nociceptor input may then contribute to the cycle by increasing motor and sympathetic activity, which, in turn, leads to increased pain. This pain may be shadowed by growing fatigue that adds an overall mood of distress to the patient's status and feeds back to the cycle. Sola believes that, as tense muscles in the affected area begin to fatigue in an environment of sympathicotonia and local biochemical change, latent trigger points within the involved muscles may also begin to fire, thus adding to the positive feedback cycle and spreading the pain to these muscles or muscle groups. Finally, the stress of pain and fatigue, coupled with both increased muscle tension and sympathicotonia throughout the body (conceivably with ipsilateral emphasis through the sympathetic chain), may lead to focal exacerbations or trigger points in other muscles that are far remote from the initial area of pain.

On the other hand, Simons offers a neurochemical explanation of trigger point development that deserves consideration. He feels that a traumatically induced tear in the sarcoplasmic reticulum initially causes the release of calcium that acts in conjunction with adenosine triphosphate (ATP) to continuously stimulate local contractile activity. This uncontrolled contraction shortens and tenses fibers within the involved muscle bundle(s). Such increased physiologic activity can initiate a subsequent increase in sustained, uncontrolled, localized metabolic activity by the muscles that is capable of producing substances which cause a hypersensitivity of involved sensory nerve fibers and, possibly, stimulate localized reflex vasoconstriction to help control what otherwise might be a rapidly increasing metabolic activity. The result is local tenderness, referred pain, and decreased blood flow within the involved muscle area. Once the local energy and nutrient supply becomes restricted in this manner, ATP stores become depleted. When this occurs, the local physiologic contracture of muscle fibers is converted to an energy-deficient contraction. Thus, the sarcoplasmic reticulum of the muscle must be repaired. If sufficient energy is not available, the calcium pump (which is the most energy-sensitive step in the contractile mechanism) will respond with continued muscle contraction, creating an even greater energy depletion. It is hypothesized that normal function may be restored by stretching the locked actin and myosin filaments far enough apart to eliminate contraction. Simons believes that enough ATP will then accumulate to restore a normal sarcoplasmic reticulum, which would allow the inhibited circulation to slowly remove the accumulation of metabolic by-products. In this context, Sandman feels that the amount of degeneration or pathologic alteration created may relate directly to the length of time these conditions are allowed to exist within a muscle.

Reference Zones

Muscle pain exists in recognizable patterns in correspondence to a trigger point, but these pain patterns are often obscure or distant from the trigger point itself. That is, the site where the patient feels pain and the place where the pain originates are not usually the same. Not all trigger areas, however, are widely removed from their reference zones; the reference of pain may at times even circumscribe the trigger area. They may or may not follow the distribution of dermatomes, sclerotomes, peripheral nerves, or acupuncture meridians. Common trigger points are illustrated in future chapters.

The referred pain is initiated or the site is found whenever the trigger site is stimulated by deep pressure, a small-blunt probe, ultrasound, needling, extreme heat or cold, or stretching motions of the structure containing the trigger area. The resistance to stretching produces shortening of the affected muscle which limits motion and causes some weakness without atrophy. Trigger areas in myofascial structures can maintain pain cycles indefinitely; ie, the pain cycle may continue long after the precipitating cause has vanished because the mechanism that set the pain in motion initially is not necessarily the same as that which keeps it going.

Common Sites

Although one or more trigger points may occur in any muscle, they usually form in clusters and certain muscles and muscle groups (eg, antigravity muscles) appear to be more liable than others. Common trigger point syndromes are described in Table 16.2. It should be noted that reference patterns vary considerably according to the severity and chronicity of the trigger point phenomenon involved.

Trigger points are primarily found in the "stress sites" of the myofascial planes of the erector muscles of the back, pelvis, neck, and shoulder girdle. A trigger area at a

Table 16.2.
Common Trigger Point Syndromes*

Upper Body Location	Primary Reference Zone or Symptoms
Infraspinatus	Posterior and lateral aspects of the shoulder.
Intercostal muscles	Thoracodynia, especially during inspiration.
Levator scapulae	Posterior neck, scalp, around the ear.
Pectoralis major	Anteromedial shoulder, arm.
Pectoralis minor	Muscle origin or insertion.
Quadratus lumborum	Anterior abdominal wall, 12th rib, iliac crest.
Rectus abdominus	Anterior abdominal wall.
Semispinalis capitis	Headache, facial pain, dizziness.
Splenius cervicis	Headache, facial pain, dizziness.
Sternocleidomastoideus	Headache, dizziness, neck pain, ipsilateral ptosis, lacrimation, conjunctival reddening, earache, facial and forehead pain.
Trapezius	Lower neck and upper thoracic pain, headache.

Lower Body Location	Primary Reference Zone or Symptoms
Anterior tibialis	Anterior leg and posterior ankle.
Gastrocnemius/soleus	Posterior leg, from popliteal space to heel. These trigger points may be involved in intermittent claudication.
Gluteus medius	Quadratus lumborum, tensor fasciae latae, gluteus maximus and minimus, sacroiliac joints, hip, groin, posterior thigh and calf, cervical extensors, upper thoracic muscles.
Tensor fasciae latae	Lateral aspect of the thigh, from ilium to the knee.

* Adapted from Sola.

particular site gives rise to a consistent distribution of referred pain which varies only slightly from person to person, indicating that the impulses follow fixed pathways. These pathways are similar to those of visceral pain which is referred in predictable patterns that do not follow a simple segmental distribution. Once the pain reference pattern of a trigger point is known, it can be used to locate the muscle that is the source of the pain.

In time, a chain reaction is often seen where satellite trigger points eventually develop. Travell gives the example that trigger points in the sternal division of the sternocleidomastoid muscle which refer pain to the sternum are often associated with satellites in the sternalis muscle on the anterior sternum which refer pain deep under the sternum, across the upper pectoral region, and sometimes down the arm—often leading to a misdiagnosis of angina or mastalgia.

Secondary Sites

Trigger point pain may be localized in one muscle or group, or it may also involve remote muscles or groups. Primary trigger points in the gluteus medius, for example, are commonly related to secondary trigger points in the neck and shoulder girdle. Thus, while trigger points in the neck and upper thoracic muscles may be found to be responsible for tension headaches, a group of "mother" trigger points should be sought on the dorsal aspect of the ilia.

Diagnosis and Management

Cycles of physiologic responses arising from trigger points typically involve (1) well-defined pathways (eg, motor reflexes, sensory changes), (2) anticipated autonomic feedback reflexes, and (3) hypothesized microscopic tissue changes. Motor and sensory reactions are usually exhibited in local and general muscle fatigue, hypertonia, weakness, possibly a fine tremor, hyperirritability, pain, and hypoesthesia. The autonomic concomitants are similar to those seen with Meridian acupoints. Travell believes that these are frequently expressed as decreased skin resistance, increased pilomotor reaction in the reference area, vasodilation (possibly with dermatographia), and skin temperature changes (coolness).

In the typical myofascial syndrome, standard physical diagnostic procedures, laboratory analyses, and roentgenography fail to show significant bone, joint, or metabolic changes. According to Sandman and others, the focus of pain appears to be from exercise of an ischemic muscle and/or chemoreceptor and mechanoreceptor stimulation from pressure by accumulated metabolic debris or irritation by released acetylcholine, blood serum, bradykinin, histamine, inflammatory exudates, substance P, and 5-hydroxytryptamine.

Primary points can be localized through electric stimulation, blunt mechanical probing, or ultrasonic searches. With practice, digital pressure may localize a deep tender point of taut or ropy muscle tissue. At this point, a positive "jump sign," with referred pain, is often associated. This sign is the result of a visible shortening of the msucle which contains the trigger point by placing the muscle in a relaxed position, applying moderate passive stretch, and snapping the trigger site briskly with a finger or probe. Chronic trigger points are often "latent," ie, they are less apt to produce pain (except on needling) and are less irritable on deep palpation. But, they frequently produce a reflex jerk of the part (jump sign) as do active trigger points.

Deep direct digital pressure for 5–10 seconds, pulsating ultrasound, nonsurging sinusoidal currents to tolerance, ice massage, acupuncture, acupressure, intermittent traction, therapeutic exercise, saline or procaine injections, and nonfrosting sweeping sprays of a surface coolant across the site and zone with passive stretching of the affected muscle have been reported to be beneficial. Of the noninvasive techniques, the intermittent application of intense cold by the "spray and stretch" method is considered the most simple and most effective. Keep in mind, however, that trigger points themselves are frequently secondary to another condition (eg, strain, subluxation, stasis, visceral disorder) which must be diagnosed and treated.

Any trigger point therapy is generally considered more effective if the involved area is placed in a position of relaxed passive stretch during treatment. In addition, regardless of the type of procedure utilized to treate trigger points, the intensity of the therapy must be kept just below the threshold of pain because pain will initiate a defensive reflex contraction that would aggravate the disorder rather than alleviate it. Most authorities feel that, regardless of the therapy utilized, it should be concluded with some form of therapeutic heat that is followed by passive stretching movements in all ranges of motion that are conducted within patient tolerance.

Spray and Stretch Technique

Fluori-methane and ethyl chloride may be used as a counterirritant in the management of myofascial pain, restricted motion, and muscle spasm with or without related trigger points. Fluori-methane is preferred to ethyl chloride in that it is less cold to the patient, noninflammable, not explosive, not a general anesthetic, and nontoxic when used correctly.

The vapoccoolant is applied in one direction, never back and forth, at a distance of 18–24 inches and at the rate of 4 inches/second. A fine stream is used, not a mist. The rhythm should be a few seconds on and a few seconds off. If spraying near the face, take precautions to cover the patient's eyes, nose, and mouth. The degree of cooling with from two to four unhurried, even parallel, nonoverlapping sweeps with the spray, about ¼-inch apart, does not result in local anesthesia, but it is often enough to cause immediate and sometimes lasting disappearance of pain in acute joint sprain or muscle spasm precipitated by trauma.

If an irritative trigger point is involved, spray from the active trigger point to the referred pain zone. Continue the therapy until all trigger points found (several are common) have been sprayed.

To be effective, passive movement must be used while spraying to gently stretch the muscle containing the trigger area. Spray and stretch until the muscle reaches its maximum or normal resting length. The stretch of the muscle should begin as you start spraying the affected area. It should be gentle but firmly applied by a sustaining passive stretch to the muscle while the patient remains relaxed. Overchilling muscle tissue or overstretching will set up painful spasms which defeat the purpose of the therapy. During stretching, you should feel a gradual increase in range of motion of the affected muscle. Active motion in the direction of restriction should be tested after every one or two sweeps. The spraying and stretching may require from two to four applications to achieve the results desired. Stop the treatment if there is no positive effect in 5 minutes. A few sweeps are usually sufficient to cover the skin representation of the affected muscle and extinguish the pain. Avoid skin frosting. The benefits may last several hours, days, or be permanent.

It takes about 5 minutes for skin and subcutaneous tissues to rewarm. During this time, moist hot packs can be applied to the area while the procedure is being conducted in another region. Following treatment, the patient should be given some simple exercises to be carried out a few times each day. It is not uncommon to find on a follow-up visit that the original trigger points have vanished and the remaining discomfort can be traced to secondary trigger points missed on the first treatment.

The relief of pain facilitates early mobilization in restoration of muscle function. The benefits are apparently derived from the spray-producing nociceptive impulses that propel faster from skin receptors along afferent nerves to higher centers than do noxious impulses from the muscle spindles which travel along smaller afferents. The nociceptive impulses seem to set up a refractory state that blocks the slower muscle-pain impulses. Thus, the muscle is allowed to relax and be stretched to its normal resting length and pain-free state.

While vapocoolant sprays are quite beneficial in acute cases, chronic cases sometimes show better results with acupuncture. This is probably due to an acute case being a purely neurophysiologic disorder at the onset which in time develops organic changes that are benefited by the mechanical effects of the needling of the trigger areas but not by the cooling effect. Nevertheless, dramatic relief of painful motion of many years standing without structural deformity has been reported with only a few sprayings.

Acupuncture

In some cases, trigger sites are more associated with acupunture points than they are with established trigger-point pathways. It appears that the introduction of impulses by any means at a rate more rapid than pain overloads the dorsal horn of the spinal cord to such an extent that the transmission of pain impulses is not perceived by the patient (gate theory).

CHAPTER 17

Peripheral Nerve Injuries

The diagnosis of neurologic injuries and diseases can be frustrating because of the transient nature of many symptoms and signs. In addition to frequent symptomatic peaks and valleys, neurologic symptoms may mimic a large variety of organic and functional disturbances. The various aspects of general nerve injury which do not lend themselves to a regional basis are discussed in this section. Some of the topics discussed will be infrequently seen in the active athlete, but they often arise with the weekend athlete who seeks attention long after the condition has manifested.

EXAMINATION

The neurologic examination should incorporate testing muscle tone, strength, reflexes, coordination, and sensation, along with evaluating structural and functional abnormalities. No objective neurologic examination is complete without a thorough patient history and physical examination of the whole body.

History

All symptoms of pain, neurologic episodes, malcoordination, and behavioral changes should be investigated thoroughly. Symptoms of headache, weakness, sensory perversions, seizures, tics, syncope, and vertigo lend suspicion to a neurologic disorder. One should assess the nervous system in relation to its influence on other systems and the manner in which its functions are influenced by all the other systems of the body. If a problem is somatic, for example: (1) consider the autonomic, motor, and sensory nerve supply to the area, (2) consider the visceral and somatic structures that receive innervation from those same areas, and (3) consider the influence each may have on the others. Thus, if a problem concerns a visceral area, consider the somatic structures and other viscera that share the same autonomic, motor, and sensory innervation as the organ involved. It is for this reason that reflexes are labeled somatosomatic, somatovisceral, viscerovisceral, or viscerosomatic.

Spinal Reflexes and Muscle Tone

Healthy muscle possesses a small amount of tension even at complete rest. It feels resilient rather than flabby. During passive manipulation of a joint, a slight degree of resistance is encountered in the muscle that is not a conscious effort on the part of the patient. Thus, the chief characteristics of normal muscle tone are subdued activity during relaxation and an involuntary reaction opposing mechanical stretch. If the function of the ventral roots are impaired, a muscle loses its tone immediately; and the same is true if the dorsal roots containing sensory fibers from the muscle are damaged. Thus, tone must be considered not a property of muscle itself, but of reflex activity.

The basic neural mechanism for maintaining muscle tone is the stretch reflex. In addition to this function of tone maintenance, the stretch reflex is responsible for regulating tension within various muscle groups that provides the basis of postural muscle tone on which voluntary movements are superimposed. Stretch (myotatic) reflexes are tested via the tendon reflexes.

While a diagnosis of a neurologic disorder cannot be determined by reflexes alone, they are important aids in establishing the type and location of a lesion. Deep reflexes vary in direct proportion to muscle tone. Superficial reflexes apply to any reflex phenomenon which may be induced by a light stimulus such as stroking the skin with a wisp of cotton, resulting in horripilation (gooseflesh) or muscle contraction. Note that: (1) in upper motor neuron or pyramidal fiber lesions, the deep tendon reflexes are exaggerated, but the superficial skin reflexes are decreased or absent; (2) in lesions of a lower motor neuron or the motor fibers from the anterior horn cells of the cord, both the deep and the superficial reflexes are decreased or absent.

Evaluating the Sensory System

Localize areas of diminished or absent tactile sensation, increased pain sensation, and abnormal sensations. Seek temperature, vibratory, and proprioceptive impairments. Once sensory perceptions are found to be abnormal and the areas can be localized, the spinal nerves or higher centers affected can then be identifed. Sensory deficits are usually found in areas of pain, muscle weakness and atrophy, and excessive sweating, when found in conjunction with sympathetic nervous system involvement.

General Patterns of Sensory Loss. The pattern of sensory loss is helpful in differentiating lower and upper motor lesions. Sensory loss in one half of the body usually points toward impairment in the cerebral or thalamic area and above the pons, wherein the deficit is almost to the midline of the body. In hysteria, the deficit is to the midline or greater. Sensory loss in the saddle area, associated with absent anal sphincter and anal skin reflexes, points toward a tumor in the conus medullaris of the spinal cord or a malignancy in the cord, probably from the prostate. A lower motor neuron lesion is usually at the upper lumbar area. If the lower lumbar and sacral nerves are involved, it usually means a lesion in the cauda equina. An upper motor lesion results in loss of bladder and bowel control and a loss of potency. Sensory loss in the lower trunk and legs is indicative of spinal cord lesions. Sensory loss in the distal half of the extremities (stocking-glove deficit) is a common finding in peripheral neuropathy and sometimes in hysteria.

Diagnostic Sensory Areas. Most skin areas are innervated by an overlapping nerve supply from adjacent nerve branches, thus making it difficult in testing cutaneous sensations to isolate a specific spinal nerve that may be affected. However, in certain parts of the body, there are isolated areas of cutaneous innervation by a specific nerve (diagnostic sensory areas). Skully lists the more important areas as follows:

• The radial sensory area, located on the back of the hand toward the thumb.

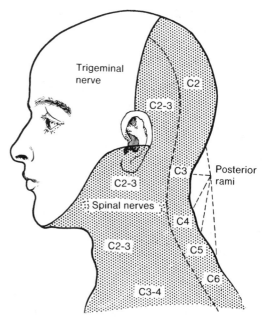

Figure 17.1. Sensory innervation of the head and neck.

• The median areas, occupying the tips of the index and middle fingers.
• The ulnar area, limited to the small finger.
• The musculocutaneous area, located on the medial aspect of the forearm.
• The axillary area, located over the point of the shoulder.
• The femoral area, situated on the anterior medial aspect of the thigh.
• The femoral lateral-cutaneous area, located over the distal part of the lateral surface of the thigh.
• The common peroneal area, presented as a vertical strip on the front of the ankle.
• The sciatic sensory area, occupying the entire foot and ankle except the medial aspect.

Peripheral vs Central Lesions. By evaluating the sensory bed, it is often possible to determine if a lesion is in the peripheral nerves or whether it is in the central system. Peripheral lesions give a segmental loss picture, and the loss will be on the same side as the lesion (eg, nerve root compression). Central lesions cause a sensory loss from the level of the lesion caudally in the following manner: (a) the loss will be on the side opposite the lesion for exteroceptive sensations; or (b) the loss will be on the same side as the lesion for proprioceptive sensations, because exteroceptive fibers cross in the cord while proprioceptive fibers do not.

Evaluating the Motor System

Any sign of muscle weakness, atrophy, paralysis, and incoordination is significant. The muscular aspect of the motor system is checked for tone, strength, and muscle volume (mass), while nerve integrity is judged by the deep and superficial reflexes Motor disorders may be caused by the same processes as sensory disturbances such as from direct nerve injury, pathology, reflexes from visceral organs, and particularly nerve root involvement or upper motor neuron lesions.

Motor nerve root involvement is characterized by deep muscular pain in the muscles innervated. Early hypertonicity or muscular spasm is evident. Later on in chronic conditions, loss of tendon reflexes, muscular weakness, atrophy, and even trophic changes in the overlying skin may be present. Motor disturbances from upper motor lesions may also be a factor (hyperreflexia). Remember that abnormal reflexes, particularly if bilateral or similar in other reflexes, may be normal for a particular person. All signs must be correlated.

Muscle Strength. Have the patient perform various muscular actions against resistance, and always test bilaterally. Be mindful that the nervous system is concerned with patterns of movement and not with contraction of isolated muscles.

Muscle Mass. Palpation and mensuration are used to determine muscle volume. Upon palpation, there should be a mass that

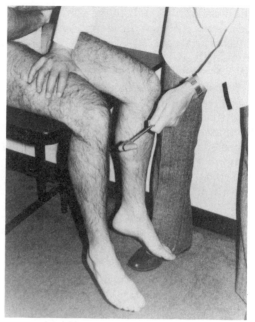

Figure 17.3. Testing the knee jerk in the sitting position while the extremity is relaxed.

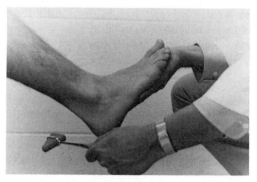

Figure 17.4. Testing the Achilles reflex.

is symmetrical bilaterally. A decrease in size (eg, midcalf or thigh) is indicative of atrophy and usually associated with some degree of hypotonicity. Atrophy is difficult to evaluate in the aged or malnourished individual. The affected muscle becomes shrunken, poor in tone, and weak in strength. Take age, sex, occupation, righthandedness and lefthandedness into consideration.

Muscle Tone. The typical feeling of a normal muscle upon palpation is one of resilience. An increased perception of tone by the examiner denotes a hypertonic muscle; decreased tone, a hypotonic muscle. In

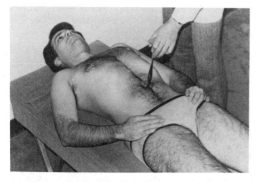

Figure 17.2. Testing abdominal reflexes.

evaluating muscle tone, age, sex, body structure, occupation, physical avocations, and nutritional status of the patient must be considered.

Paralysis. True paralysis is the complete inability to control a muscle or group of muscles. Spastic paralysis is commonly seen in lesions of upper motor neurons. Flaccid paralysis occurs in the peripheral type of nerve lesions affecting the lower motor neurons of the anterior horn cells. Peripheral nerve paralyses are especially apt to be accompanied by sensory symptoms, electrical changes, and wasting. Brain-originating paralyses have relatively few sensory symptoms (sometimes paresthesias) and relatively slight wasting; mental changes, coma, or convulsions often precede or follow. Cord paralyses may or may not show these associations but are often accompanied by disorders of the bladder and rectum.

The extent of the symptomatology frequently offers a clue to the location of the disorder. In most chronic pyramidal tract lesions, especially when the trauma has been sudden but not insidious, a partial recovery of control is expected. This occurs mostly in the large proximal muscles of the shoulder and hip. Disorders of the pyramidal tract commonly produce defects that are more conspicuous in the upper limb. This is possibly because highly skilled movements are more prevalent there in comparison to mass contractions.

Electrical Examinations. Electrical examination of muscles and nerves is often indispensible in affections of peripheral nerves. Such tests help to determine if disease of the upper or lower motor neuron is being dealt with, help to determine if the nerve is interrupted, and help to determine if the muscles are undergoing degeneration.

Lower Motor Neuron Lesion Characteristics

Lesions of the lower motor neurons result from fractures, trauma, infection, toxins, vascular disorders, tumors, congenital malformation, and degenerative processes. Lesions involving spinal nerves or peripheral nerves induce both motor and sensory losses. In this type of lesion, the neuronal impulse from the upper central level or from the anterior gray horn of the spinal cord cannot reach the appropriate muscle fibers; thus, the characteristic clinical picture is as follows:

- There is a loss of both superficial and deep reflexes. The stretch and tendon reflexes are abolished, thus producing a hypotonus state. No classic pathologic reflexes are present.
- Fibrillations and fasciculations are present only in the early stage during which muscles are undergoing atrophic changes.
- A flaccid type of paralysis is seen if there is no regeneration; the muscles involved eventually shrink and possibly are replaced by connective and adipose tissues. Muscle tone no longer exists because the peripheral nerve is unable to maintain it, and the muscles become limp.
- Severe atrophy of muscles is observed within a few weeks due to a lack of efferent impulses which results in a degeneration of muscle fibers.
- Reaction of degeneration is seen from 10–14 days after the injury. The nerve is unable to conduct the electrical current because of structural alterations.

Upper Motor Neuron Lesion Characteristics

Any lesion producing an interruption of connections between the motor cortex or subcortical levels and the motor axons found in the anterior horn of the spinal cord is considered to be an upper motor neuron lesion. Such a lesion may interrupt corticospinal fibers or extrapyramidal fibers, or both, since the pyramidal and extrapyramidal systems are so closely associated that lesions involving one will invariably encompass both. On the other hand, any lesion producing damage to motor neurons whose axons reach skeletal muscle fibers produces a lower motor neuron lesion, whether the destruction is in the anterior horns, ventral roots, or peripheral nerves.

Lesions of the upper motor neurons may occur anywhere along their course and may be the result of hemorrhage, thrombosis, trauma, inflammation, neoplasm, or a degenerative process. The classical clinical picture of an upper motor neuron lesion is portrayed as follows:

• A spastic type of paralysis or paresis is seen on the opposite side of the body and below the level of the lesion if the lesion is at or above the medullary pyramid. Weakness is especially pronounced in the muscles of the limbs, and there is great difficulty with movements of the hands. Increased muscle tone expresses as firmness and stiffness, especially in the arm flexors and the leg extensors.

• There is minimal or no atrophy of the muscles involved. However, there will be a later disuse atrophy. After a few days to a few weeks, stretch reflexes return in the involved muscles and usually become more active than usual. Muscle resistance to passive movements is exaggerated; often strong at the beginning of movement, then collapsing in a peculiar "clasp-knife" method as more force is applied.

• The superficial reflexes are abolished. There is an increase of deep reflexes since the normal operation of gravity against the weight of the body may initiate stretch reflexes. Reflex contractions are exaggerated due to a loss of the inhibitory mechanism from the higher central level. The combination of this effect with contractions resulting from continuous discharge of brain stem excitatory mechanisms leads to a hypertonic state.

• The flexor reflex or nociceptive reflex and the Babinski sign can be observed. The nociceptive reflex evokes withdrawal of a body part by action of flexor muscles at one or several joints, depending on severity of stimulus, in response to injurious stimuli such as pricking, pinching, or burning. In a patient with a pyramidal tract lesion, the Babinski reflex is positive. Hoffmann's sign is usually present but not a reliable sign since it is seen occasionally in normal individuals.

• No reaction of degeneration will be present in an upper motor neuron lesion; ie, no ability of the muscle or nerve to respond to galvanic or faradic current. If the peripheral nerve responds to electrical stimulation, it can be assumed that the lesion is in an upper motor neuron.

Evaluating the Cerebellar System

Once the cerebral cortex receives an afferent impulse and decides what task must be performed in response, the cerebellum coordinates the reaction so that the act will be carried out smoothly.

Malcoordination Tests. Test cerebellar function by the evaluation of gait, carriage, station, limb pronation/supination, hand patting, finger-to-nose tests, heel-to-knee, heel-to-toe, Romberg, and foot-to-buttock tests.

Signs of Cerebellar Lesions. The major motor signs seen in cerebellar lesions include tremor, nystagmus, ataxia, decomposition of movement, dysmetria, dysdiadochokinesia or adiadochokinesia, scanning speech, hypotonia, and asthenia. Other signs include vertigo, cerebellar fits presenting a rigid convulsion, and vocal dysarthria characterized by explosive, slurred speech peculiar to cerebellar lesions. Note any sign of skew deviation of the eyes where one eyeball is deviated up and outward and the other is deviated down and inward (brachium pontis lesion). In time, cerebellar defects are compensated for to a considerable degree by other brain mechanisms; thus, symptoms are less severe in slowly progressing diseases than in acute cerebellar disorders.

Keep in mind that the left side of the body is under the influence of the left cerebellar hemisphere, and vice versa. Any symptoms that occur unilaterally will then be on the same side as the cerebellar lesion. The opposite is true with cerebral lesions, where the lesion invariably produces contralateral symptoms and signs.

COMMON SYMPTOMS OF NEURAL DISORDER

Weakness, paralysis, nervousness, pain, tenderness, sensory loss, paresthesia, and abnormalities of muscle mass or tone are the most common signs and symptoms noted in neural disorders.

Weakness

Weakness (fatigue) and nervousness are frequently presented together, and can usually be attributed to psychologic or physical disorders or appear as a complication in organic disease. Weakness in the absence of further symptoms or signs is indicative of an emotional problem (eg, depression).

However, weakness may be the only symptom of an early systemic disease (eg, Guillain-Barre syndrome).

Weakness is characterized by feelings of lassitude, tiredness, weariness, depletion, exhaustion, malaise, loss of energy and motivation. It may be general or local. If local, the weakness may be described in lower or upper extremities, either distal or proximal. It may be localized in the trunk, in the head, or in respiration. It is important to analyze weakness in terms of body segments because weakness always follows a neuroanatomic distribution in organic disease.

Neuromuscular defects are usually marked by weakness, and fatigue may be an early symptom in the myopathies. A rule of thumb is that proximal weakness is the result of a myopathy, while a distal weakness is caused by a neuropathy. Weakness upon exertion that is progressive with muscular effort is called fatigability.

Pain

All pain is mediated by the nervous system, yet only some pain originates from neuropathology. When an inflammatory process involves the sensory fibers, neuralgia is often presented along the total nerve course. For example, in medial nerve entrapment (carpal tunnel syndrome), pain is rarely localized in the wrist; it often extends into the upper arm and shoulder. Hypersensitive points can often be located where touching a certain point only slightly initiates severe radiating pain.

Fortunately, nerve course is fairly predictable and varies little because of body type. The exception to this is that nerves which normally pass over or under a muscle, may pass through it, thus subjecting it to abnormal stress. The sciatic nerve, for example, may pass over, under, or through the piriformis, or it may be divided. Abnormal bone formation may also be a consideration such as a cervical rib encroaching upon a branch of the brachial plexus.

Dermatomes

Inflammation or compression of dorsal nerve roots irritate pain fibers and commonly produces pain felt along the anatomic distribution of the roots affected (dermatome). Myotomes are groups of muscles

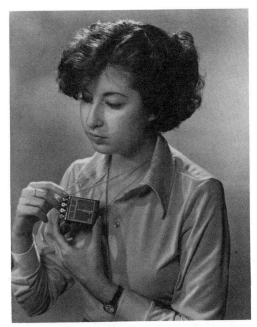

Figure 17.5. Microceptor II, battery-operated transcutaneous electrical nerve stimulator for pain control (with the permission of Ohio Chiropractic Equipment and Supplies).

innervated by a single spinal segment. Evaluation of the integrity of the neurologic levels rests upon the examiner's knowledge of dermatomes, sclerotomes, myotomes, and reflexes. Pain may be limited in distribution to one or more dermatomes (radicular pain).

Sensory changes other than pain may be associated with dorsal root irritation, eg, localized areas of paresthesia or hyperesthesia. If the pathologic process is a progressive one which gradually destroys fibers, dorsal roots finally lose their ability to conduct sensory impulses, resulting in hypesthesia which eventually leads to anesthesia.

Typical Causes of Pain and Paresthesia

Local paresthesia, as expressed by prickling, tingling, crawling, or burning sensations, is not uncommon in lesions of the cerebral cortex. Typical causative factors include:

• Obvious direct trauma or injury
• Reflex pain from visceral reflexes or reflex pain from musculoskeletal lesions,

which deep pressure often exaggerates, such as trigger points.

• Peripheral nerve injury (eg, causalgia) which results in an intense burning superficial pain. A history of injury usually helps to evaluate this disorder.

• Presence of nerve inflammations and degenerations of the peripheral or central nervous system. They frequently cause other changes indicative of such lesions.

• Vascular disease, which is usually associated with other changes such as swelling, redness, blanching, or other vascular disorder signs, depending upon whether it is an arterial or venous problem. Certain neurovascular syndromes may be associated with pain and paresthesia. Vasomotor disturbances may also be caused or aggravated by vertebral subluxations such as the deep congestive leg aches associated with upper-lumbar subluxations or the cranial vasomotor headaches and other symptoms of cervical subluxation.

• Sensory root pressure characterized by pain, paresthesia, and often by abnormal sensitivity to touch along the course of the involved nerve root's segmental skin supply. Thus, this becomes an important consideration and needs to be traced and demarcated with a skin pencil to see if the area corresponds to a specific dermatome.

Pain and other sensory disturbances caused by subluxations may be due to direct nerve root involvement and therefore of the nature mentioned above. They may also be due to reflex irritation of the paravertebral ligaments, tendons, or muscles and, like other myofascial trigger areas, refer pain into somatic areas that do not correlate to direct dermatomes or specific nerve roots

Extremity Pain

The origin of nerve root lesions may be traced during the history of trauma, herniated discs, compression, hypertrophic changes in the vertebrae, neoplasms, and inflammation of the nerve root. Peripheral nerve diseasse frequently indicates a history of trauma of the entrapment neuropathies. Rare nutritional disorders may result in a polyneuropathy because of unfavorable metabolic activities within the nerve cells. Peripheral neuritis, less common than peripheral neuropathy, can be classified into one of three types: infectious, allergic, or idiopathic.

Limb pain may be the result of any structural disorder of the extremities or a disturbance elsewhere wherein the sensory phenomena are referred to the limbs. Pain situated in various parts of the extremities will reveal the point of origin by its peculiar location and quality. The pain may be of mechanical, chemical, thermal, toxic, nutritional, metabolic, or circulatory origin, or a combination of some of these factors, depending upon the nature of the pathologic process involved. The most important clues toward determining cause—type of pain, its distribution, and its associated symptoms—are the result of a carefully taken case history.

Referred Pain and Reflexes

Pain in one region of the body may indicate disease elsewhere because nerve supply often overlaps; eg, pain associated with the ureter can result in reflex spasm of the lumbar muscles. Such pain radiates to distant parts of the body depending upon the intensity of the stimulus, amplitude of the afferent impulse, and the excitatory state of the spinal cord at the level into which the noxious impulses enter.

Visceral disease or dysfunction frequently

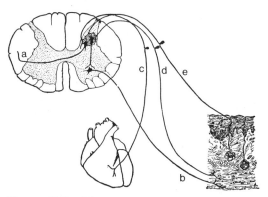

Figure 17.6.   Diagram to show a possible neural path for referred pain of cardiac origin. Nerve impulses (c) from disturbed heart bring about an "irritable" area in gray matter of cord. Nerve fibers from skin and muscle (d and e) enter this same region. Nerve fibers from this region carry impulses over path (a) to the spinothalamic tract and the cerebral cortex, and over path (b) to the chest muscles which contract in an exaggerated manner.

refers pain to the spinal segments supplying the involved viscera and also alters the function of other viscera sharing the same nerve supply. In addition, the probability should be considered of somatic dysfunction occurring in segmentally involved areas causing visceral dysfunction or of other somatic structures sharing the same nerve supply. The nervous system is not a one-way street: somatosomatic, somatovisceral, viscerovisceral, and viscersomatic reflexes must be considered.

Headaches. Headaches, the most frequent symptom in America today, are usually attributed to tension, migraine, abnormal sinus, tumor, vascular disorders, or hysteria. Often neglected causes are overall postural strain and trauma to the cervical spine. Headaches caused by viscerosomatic reflexes from the gallbladder, stomach, and duodenum are much more common than suspected. Nausea or vomiting with headaches is usually considered to have a neurologic basis of a vascular nature; however, a vagal disturbance due to upper cervical function may be the offender. .

Cervical Reflexes. Cervical reflexes can be easily overlooked. Vertigo makes basilar insufficiency or Meniere's syndrome suspect, but vertebral artery ischemia due to upper cervical dysfunction or an atlanto-occipital subluxation secondary to scoliosis may be the reason. In blackout spells of an unexplained nature, epilepsy and arterial occlusive disease are suspect, but cervical somatic dysfunction involving the cervical ganglia may be the cause. Numbness or tingling in the hands is seen in a number of neuropathies. However, the cause may be musculoskeletal in origin such as degenerative disease or somatic dysfunction of the cervical spine, brachial plexus entrapment due to clavicular and upper rib abnormality, or carpal tunnel syndrome. In a lower cervical motor-unit dysfunction resulting in brachial distribution symptoms, there are somatosomatic reflexes which have afferents from and efferents to the soma.

Shoulder Symptoms. Gallbladder disease associated with referred pain near the right scapular tip is an example of viscerosomatic reflexes having afferents from a viscus and efferents to a somatic area. Frequently overlooked is the gallbladder reflex causing cardiac arrhythmia. However, several diseases may refer pain to the shoulder or arm other than the gallbladder such as coronary artery disease, empyema, pneumothorax, pericarditis, mediastinal lesions, peptic ulcer, diaphragmatic hernia, perisplenitis, and subphrenic abscess. In coronary occlusion associated wtih nausea and vomiting, there are viscerovisceral reflexes which have afferents from a viscus and efferents to a viscus. Pain radiating to the arm may also be a reflex from brachial neuropathy caused by dysfunction or degenerative disease of the cervical spine or a trigger point.

Chest Symptoms. Several common chest symptoms may indicate visceral disease or as often referred musculoskeletal problems. Ventilatory impairment is usually suspected in dyspnea, but it may be the result of rib-cage dysfunction, spondylitis, or paravertebral muscle spasm and pain. Air hunger at rest is a cardinal sign of anxiety and often seen in chronic obstructive pulmonary disease; it is, however, also a reflex sign of rib-cage dysfunction of a musculoskeletal nature. Chest pains point to coronary insufficiency or a dissecting aneurysm, or they may be of esophageal or pleural origin; but chest pain may also be the result of somatic rib-cage dysfunction costochondral or costovertebral strain, or referred pain from the gallbladder, stomach, duodenum, or pancreas.

In chest pains associated with a cough, pulmonary infections, pneumonia, lung abscess, and bronchitis are usually suspected, along with pleuritis and lung or pleural tumors. Reflex considerations would include costovertebral dysfunction, costochondral dysfunction or separation, or costal fracture. In cough with chest pain, one normally thinks of acute or chronic infection, chronic bronchitis, bronchial tumor, pulmonary embolism, broncholith, bronchiectasis, postnasal discharge, or the inhalation of irritants. However, reflexes from clavicular strain affecting recurrent laryngeal nerves, cervical subluxation, or cerumen impaction should not be overlooked.

Hysterical Anesthesia or Palsy

Hysterical anesthesia or palsy following injury to an arm or leg is not rare. The involvement of the extremity in both sensory loss or motor control, ideational rather than neuroanatomic, is a characteristic feature of this neurosis. For example, a hysterically anesthetic arm will be insensitive as far as the shoulder line, whereafter normal sensation abruptly returns. This contrasts with sensory zones demarcated by injury to a peripheral nerve or spinal cord segment. Motor loss is similarly referred to the arm as a whole rather than to identically innervated muscle groups. These nonanatomic findings, as well as normal or hyperactive reflexes, prompt electric responses, and good muscle tone serve as signs differentiating functional from organic nerve, nerve root, and cord-segment lesions.

PERIPHERAL NERVE INJURIES

Damage to an individual peripheral nerve (eg, trauma) is characterized by (1) flaccid, atrophic paralysis of the muscles supplied by the involved nerve, and (2) loss of all sensation, including proprioception, in the skin areas distal to the lesion. When partial destruction to various peripheral nerves occurs, the effects are usually more prominent in the distal extremities. The condition is characterized by muscular weakness and atrophy and poorly demarked areas of sensory changes.

Trophic lesions of the joints, muscles (atrophy), skin, and nails are common. They blend and are somewhat explained as the results of vasomotor changes.

Classification of Nerve Trauma

Nerve trauma occurs from contusion, stretching, or laceration:

1. Contusion (neurapraxia). Recovery is usually within 6 weeks. Contusion may be the result of either a single blow or through persistent compression. Fractures and blunt trauma are often associated with nerve contusion and crush. Peripheral nerve contusions exhibit early symptoms when produced by falls or blows. Late symptoms arise from pressure by callus, scars, or supports. Mild cases produce pain, tingling, and numbness, with some degree of paresthesia. Moderate cases manifest these same symptoms with some degree of motor-sensory paralysis and atrophy.

2. Crush (axonotmesis). Recovery rate is about 1 inch/month between the site of trauma and the next innervated muscle. If innervation is delayed from this schedule or if the distance is more than 6 inches, surgical exploration should be considered.

3. Laceration (neurotmesis). Laceration follows sharp or penetrating wounds and is less frequently seen associated with tears from a fractured bone's fragments. Surgery is usually required. A traction injury typically features several sites of laceration along the nerve. Stretching injury is usually limited to the brachial plexus.

Nerve Pinch or Stretch Syndromes

Nerve "pinch" or "stretch" syndromes are especially common in sports. They are often seen in football "spearing" with the neck in flexion, but these syndromes appear throughout the cranium, spine, pelvis, and extremities in many sports. Hardly any peripheral nerve is exempt. Terms used synonymously include nerve compression, nerve contusion, nerve lesion, nerve pinch syndrome, nerve root syndrome, nerve stretch syndrome, radiculopathy, spinal dysarthria, subluxation, or traumatic neuritis.

A *nerve stretch syndrome* is commonly associated with sprains, lateral cervical flexion with shoulder depression (eg, football, blocking, tackling), or dislocations. Nerve fibers may be stretched, partially torn, or ruptured most anywhere in the nervous system from the cord to peripheral nerve terminals.

A *nerve pinch syndrome* may be due to direct trauma (contusion and swelling), subluxation, a protruded disc which results in nerve compression, or fracture (callus formation and associated posttraumatic adhesions). Any telescoping, hyperflexion, hyperextension, or hyperrotational blow or force to the spine may result in a nerve "pinch" syndrome where pain may be local or extending distally. In sports, nerve pinch syndromes are less common than nerve stretch syndromes, but more serious.

Examination

Painstaking examination is required as multiple nerve injury, related tendon or other soft-tissue damage, and fractured bones complicate the picture. The immediate site of injury should be first investigated, followed by the part's general appearance, voluntary motion, reflexes, and vasomotor changes. In addition to sensory and motor loss, the response to electrical stimulation should be evaluated.

Typical Examples of Findings. Sensation is lost on the ulnar side of the hand, including the little finger and medial half of the ring finger, in ulnar nerve damage. In median nerve damage, sensation of the remainder of the anterior surface of the hand is lost. As time goes on, the affected part assumes a posture and atrophy peculiar to the particular nerve involved; for example, "wrist drop" with the radial nerve, "claw hand" with the ulnar nerve, "flat hand" with the median nerve, "ape hand" with the ulnar and median nerves, and "foot drop" with the peroneal nerve.

Management

The effect of treatment depends largely upon early recognition of the nerve injury with removal of the initiating cause. Management consists of support of the affected part and normal regimens for severe contusions. As with most injuries, associated or concomitant subluxations or fixations must be adjusted to aid recovery, and sites of abnormal reflexes and stasis must be normalized. Cold is applicable in the acute stage to reduce adjacent swelling and bleeding. Heat, massage, passive and active exercises, electrical stimulation, and nutritional control are helpful.

A reaction of degeneration added to typical sensory and motor loss is indicative of complete anatomic or physiologic nerve damage, usually requiring surgical intervention. If surgery is required, careful attention must be given to postoperative care directed to maintaining as much as possible normal joint flexibility, fascia and ligamentous resiliency, muscle elasticity, and adequate nutrition to all tissues involved. Approximately one month before it can be detected clinically, an electromyogram will exhibit reinnervation.

When a peripheral nerve fiber is permanently destroyed by either trauma or disease, the portion distal to the nerve cell body completely degenerates, and the fiber loses its myelin sheath in the process. In time, the isolated fiber stump tries to sprout in random directions in an attempt to make a bridge with the severed portion of the nerve. Some of these sprouts may, apparently by chance, cross the gap and enter neurilemmal tubes leading to a peripheral motor or sensory terminal. Function may be restored if the connection is a suitable match. Fibers in the spinal cord and brain do not regenerate effectively; however, recent evidence discloses that some regeneration can occur.

MAJOR TYPES OF NEURITIDES

Local Neuritis

Acute Neuritis. Pain and hyperalgesia are witnessed in the area of nerve distribution along with tenderness on palpation of the nerve trunk and muscles supplied by the nerve. Trigger spots may be present. Reflexes are either unaffected or possibly increased.

Chronic Neuritis. Paresthesias are witnessed over the area of nerve distribution along with tenderness on palpation of the nerve trunk and muscles supplied by the nerve. Hypesthesia and hypalgesia are usually present. Diminished reflexes and motor weakness of the muscles supplied by the affected nerve are typical.

Radiculitis. The paresthesia and sensory changes are expressed similar to those present in typical neuritis, but the area affected corresponds to dermatome, myotome, and sclerotome of affected roots. Coughing, straining, jugular compression, and other causes of increased cerebral spinal fluid pressure will increase symptoms. In chronic cases, there may be paresis of muscles that are partly supplied by the affected root, but not complete paralysis.

Peripheral Neuritis

Rarely seen in the sportsperson, general peripheral neuritis is seen in such conditions as diabetes, anemia, and vitamin deficiency. Decreased sensation perception will be noted, with proprioception affected most. Stocking-like distribution with a poorly defined border is commonly witnessed. Glove-like distribution may appear later along with paresthesias in the most distal areas of sensory distribution. The clinical picture does not conform to either dermatome or nerve patterns of distribution.

Common Reflex Irritations

In addition to nerve root involvements and/or peripheral irritations, many sensory disturbances can be caused by reflex irritation to somatic musculoskeletal tissues. These symptoms lack the typical features of nerve root involvement such as observed in cervical compression tests and usually do not create compression tests and usually do not create significant motor changes. They may arise from inflammatory tissues or fibrotic muscles, tendons, or ligaments which characteristically act as trigger areas. That is, their stimulation such as with deep pressure initiates the reflex pain.

Peripheral Nerve Entrapment Syndromes

A peripheral entrapment syndrome represents a distinct type of neuropathy in which a single nerve is compressed at a specific site (eg, within fibrous tissue, a fibrous-osseous tunnel, or a muscle), either by external forces or by surrounding tissues. Local impairment of blood supply may further damage the entrapped nerve if associated vessels become stretched, kinked, or compressed.

So that a patient may avoid unnecessary pain and disability, it is important to identify a peripheral entrapment syndrome rapidly through careful examination and appropriate diagnostic studies such as electromyog-

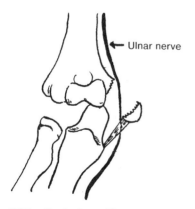

Figure 17.7. Illustration of how the ulnar nerve may be overstretched by an abduction force which dislodges the internal epicondyle of the elbow.

raphy, nerve conduction evaluations, and roentgenography. Severe impairment of nerve function is usually only reversible in its early stages.

The major features of upper-extremity and lower-extremity nerve entrapment syndromes are shown in Table 17.1. Specific entrapment syndromes will also be discussed in various chapters of Part Four.

AUTONOMIC IMBALANCE

In health, the autonomic divisions are tonically stimulated to maintain a physiologic balance. However, for various reasons, this balanced harmony may be shifted in favor of one or the other division and create visceral malfunction. An understanding of visceral neurology is indispensible to appreciate and explain the pathophysiologic processes involved. The vegetative nerves correlate and integrate action in the body and are often subjected to an amount of stimulation necessary to overbalance their normal function. When the autonomic system is involved, causalgic pain must be differentiated from somatic pain.

Physiologic Control of Body Activity

Vegetative imbalance implies visceral instability wherein the normal physiologic control of visceral activity throughout the body, or in some organ or system, is so unstable that a comparatively mild stimulus, when applied to the system of unstable cells, is sufficient to produce a marked effect to overcome all antagonistic forces and create a pathologic state. Patients having such an imbalance show reactions beyond what is natural for the stimulus applied. For instance, such factors as subluxations, emotions, fatigue, weather changes, and toxemia produce changes in such individuals which are far greater than would normally be expected.

Visceral nerve action varies according to (1) the state of activity of the organ when it receives the stimulus, and (2) the transmitter substances which are liberated into the circulation at the site of action. For the most part, parasympathetic effects in the visceral tissues are cholinergic and the sympathetic effects are adrenergic. But this is not exclusively true as there are some cholinergic

Table 17.1.
Common Nerve Entrapment Syndromes*

UPPER-EXTREMITY SYNDROMES			
Syndrome	Site	Nerve	Major Findings
Anterior interosseous	Proximal forearm	Anterior interosseous	Abnormal pinch sign; normal sensations; flexor pollicis longus, pronator quadratus, and flexor digitorum profundus weakness; poorly defined ache in forearm.
Carpal tunnel	Wrist	Median	Pain, paresthesiae, numbness, and poor two-point discrimination in thumb and radial 2½ fingers; hypoesthesia especially on palmar aspect of second digit; thenar weakness and wasting; positive Tinel's and Phalen's signs.
Cubital tunnel	Elbow	Ulnar	Sensory loss in ulnar 1½ fingers and ulnar aspect of the hand; weakness and wasting of ulnar intrinsic and flexor digitorum profundus; ache in medial elbow and forearm; little finger numbness; positive Tinel's sign.
Guyon's canal	Wrist	Ulnar	Sensory loss in ulnar 1½ fingers; weakness and wasting of ulnar intrinsic muscles.
Postcondylar groove	Elbow	Ulnar	Sensory loss in ulnar 1½ fingers and ulnar aspect of the hand; weakness and wasting of ulnar intrinsic and flexor carpi ulnaris muscles; elbow joint deformity.
Posterior interosseous	Proximal forearm	Posterior interosseous	Normal sensation; wrist drop; dull ache in dorsal forearm; difficult finger extension.
Pronator	Proximal forearm	Median	Proximal forearm pain and tenderness; flexor pollicis longus and abductor pollicis brevis weakness; paresthesiae in thumb and radial 3½ fingers; forearm and hand pain; positive Tinel's sign.
Radial	Midarm, spiral groove	Radial	Sensory loss in radial side of dorsal hand; wrist drop; weak wrist and finger extensors; possible sensory impairment in web of thumb.
Crutch or sleep palsy	Axilla, humeral groove	Radial	Sensory loss of radial forearm; loss of elbow extension; wrist drop.
LOWER-EXTREMITY SYNDROMES			
Syndrome	Site	Nerve	Major Findings
Femoral	Inguinal area or pelvis	Femoral	Sensory loss of anteromedial thigh; weakness and wasting of quadriceps femoris; local tenderness in groin; impaired knee jerk.
Meralgia paresthetica	Inguinal area	Lateral cutaneous of thigh	Sensory loss, paresthesiae burning pain, and numbness in anterolateral thigh; no motor weakness.
Obturator	Pelvis	Obturator	Sensory loss of superomedial thigh; thigh adductor weakness.
Peroneal	Neck of fibula	Common peroneal	Sensory loss of dorsal foot and lateral leg; foot drop; steppage gait; local tenderness; anterior and lateral compartment atrophy.
Tarsal tunnel	Ankle	Posterior tibial	Burning pain and paresthesiae of sole and toes; weakness of intrinsic foot muscles.

* Adapted from Reddy.

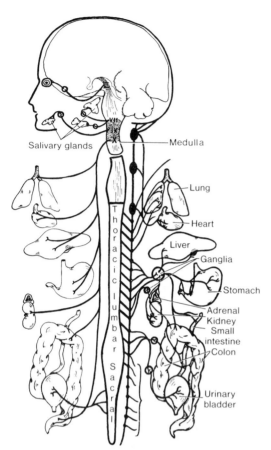

Figure 17.8. Schematic of the autonomic nervous system. The parasympathetic system is shown on the left and the sympathetic system on the right. Distribution of nerves is indicated by duplication of the organs.

sympathetic fibers and adrenergic parasympathetic fibers.

Factors Involved In Vegetative Imbalance

Through their innervation of blood vessels, sympathetic fibers reach almost every tissue of the body. They control blood vessel constriction, subdermal structures, heart muscle, sphincter system of the gut and urinary apparatus, parts of the bladder and genitalia and reproductive organs; inhibit many structures in the head and chest; and reach the enteral system's muscles and glands.

The parasympathetics activate the intrinsic eye muscles, glands of the peripheral head, bronchi muscles and glands, the entire enteral system, and body of the bladder; inhibit the heart; and provide vasodilation in many structures (especially the head and penis).

Vegetative functional activity and control are complex affairs conducted by the cells, the electrolytes, chemicals of the various hormones, and the sympathetic and parasympathetic nerves. The action of these systems is interdependent and can be understood only when considered together because imbalance in one may mean imbalance in all. Imbalance may have as its chief cause a disturbance in any one or more of these factors. The cells may be at fault, the electrolytes that have an important part to play in cellular activity may be abnormal in their proportions, or the chemical or nervous regulators may create too little or too much stimulation. Usually, the cells will do their job if the environment is right. This puts the onus on nerve supply, nutrition, electrolytes, and lymph circulation. Regardless, deviations from the norm result in abnormal function.

Sympathicotonia and Vagotonia

The two common deviations from normal are sympathicotonia and vagotonia (parasympathicotonia). These disorders may be general or limited to certain systems or organs. Although they are expressed in terms of sympathetic and parasympathetic action, this does not mean that the nervous system is primarily at fault. The fault may lie with the cells, electrolytes, hormones, or vitamins. Regardless of cause, there are large numbers of people who have a marked tendency to respond to stimuli which act on one or the other part of the vegetative system to such a degree that it amounts to malfunction or disease.

The disorders most commonly associated with a sympathetic predominance are hyperthyroidism effects, dryness and paleness of the mucous membranes of the head, deficient salivary secretion, tachycardia, dilatation of the stomach, hypochlorhydria, poor digestion, and atonic constipation. Pottenger states that sympathicotonics react more markedly than normal to cold, toxins, and emotions in an adrenalin-like manner. They readily produce reflexes wherein the sympathetics are involved. Contrary to this, parasympathicotonics are particularly susceptible to allergic excitants and respond in an atropine-like manner.

Stimuli to the sympathetic-accelerator side of the autonomic nervous system, are initiated frequently by anger, exercise, and emotions. Within a reasonable time, the symptoms created by the stimuli should return to normal. However, if these stimuli are too prolonged or too pronounced, then the balancing parasympathetic should be investigated to see why it is not exerting its proper opposition force.

Common disorders associated with a parasympathetic predominance are lacrimation, hay fever, urticaria, angioneurotic edema, intestinal allergies, sinusitis, rhinitis, pharyngitis, excessive salivary secretion, bradycardia, asthma, hyperchlorhydria, peptic ulcer, diarrhea, spastic constipation, mucous colitis, and anaphylaxis. Addison's disease is a classic parasympathetic disease.

Stimuli to the parasympathetic-brake side of the autonomic system are initiated frequently by bad news, fright, or shock. Again, within a reasonable time, the patient should recover from the effects of these stimuli and emotions return to normal. If these stimuli are too prolonged or too pronounced, then the balancing sympathetics should be investigated to see why they are not exerting their proper opposition force.

Syndromes may be produced by stimuli that act either centrally or peripherally. Toxins, for example, act centrally and result in widespread sympathetic effects. Inflammation in an organ, on the other hand, may act upon the nerve endings therein and create reflex sympathetic or parasympathetic effects only in the specific organs of tissues whose nerves receive the reflex stimulation.

A patient need not be sympathicotonic or vagotonic throughout the vegetative structures. He/she may have a sympathicotonic heart while the rest of the structures are normal or may express symptoms of vagotonia elsewhere such as hyperchlorhydria or spastic colon. The important thing during diagnosis is to assign these phenomena when they arise to the components of the vegetative nervous system to which they belong and determine the cause.

SPECIAL THERAPEUTIC CONSIDERATIONS

Irritability, a fundamental property of living tissue, governs an organism's ability to respond to a stimulus if applied with sufficient intensity to create a response. This property lies chiefly with the integrity of the nervous system. In injury or disease, nerve irritation results from an abnormal duration, quantity, or quality of stimulation resulting in an excessive physiologic response. Any interference with impulse generation or transmission must result in a degree of dysfunction.

In addition to osseous spinal adjustment and extremity manipulation, various forms of neurotherapy are worthy of mention. Once structural correction has been made, adjunctive therapy is often helpful in enhancing physiologic balance to speed recovery. That is, once structural interferences with normal nerve transmission have been corrected, peripheral neurotherapy or spondylotherapy may be utilized to inhibit pain or spasm or enhance healing by stimulation.

Neurotherapy and Spondylotherapy

Neurotherapy refers to the inhibition of overly active nerve function or the activation of sluggish function. Spondylotherapy is the treatment by physical methods applied to the spinal region. A nerve fiber may be stimulated artificially (ie, mechanically, thermally, chemically, electrically) anywhere along its course.

Certain nerve fibers function specifically for certain sensory and motor acts and may be stimulated at either their central or peripheral ends: efferent nerves are stimulated centrally and afferent nerves peripherally. The ability of sensory nerve stimulation to produce a motor or glandular response is readily demonstrated in eliciting any tendon reflex where superficial percussion produces the characteristic jerk, the muscle-spasm reflex resulting from skin exposure to a cool wind or proprioceptive excitement from strain or sprain, or the salivary response from seeing a person eat a lemon.

Neuroinhibition. Abnormal reflexes appear to be inhibited more by pressure and cold than by any other methods. For example, a painful splinting erector-muscle spasm can be relaxed by placing the muscle in a position of functional rest and then applying mild continuous stretching or pressure. Cold is an excellent neuroinhibitor, especially with nerves which are located not too deep. Functional inhibition can be gained by stimulating a nerve whose chief function is inhibitory. Pressure may be applied digitally or with a pressor instrument at or near the paravertebral spaces. Steady pressure on the surface of the body, usually applied digitally, over the course of a nerve tends to be a restraining influence. There also appears to be a reflex influence upon vessels and glandular secretions. Certain skin areas (eg, suboccipital, paraspinal, parasacral, perianal, peripheral meridian) are highly responsive to mild pressure from which reflexes of vasodilation and muscle relaxation can be initiated.

Neurostimulation. Deep and rapid short-duration percussion, applied either by hand or by a percussion-type vibrator, upon spinous processes at a rate 1-2/second for about 20 seconds with 30-second rest intervals can be used to stimulate a spinal center. Prolonged stimulation such as 3 minutes or longer fatigues excitability and produces an inhibitory effect. When a medium-strength electric current passes through a portion of nerve, an impulse is created at the instant the current is initiated and broken, as evidenced by muscle contraction. Experience has shown that sinusoidal current is the best method to contract involuntary muscle without irritation, but pulsating ultrasound is also effective in stimulating spinal centers. Therapeutic heat in most any form increases nerve conductivity.

Tissue Goading and Pressure

Deep tissue goading has been applied within the profession for many decades as a means to arouse driving impulses, break up areas of stasis, and stretch contractures and adhesions. A site of localized stasis or muscle contraction, approximately the size and shape of a small pea, is often the site of noxious reflexes and referred pain. Quite frequently, they are found in the deep tissues of the iliac crest and associated with sciatic-like pain that persists in spite of vertebral and disc correction, but they may be found almost anywhere in the musculoskeletal system.

A thumb, ball of a finger (never a finger-tip), or small-blunt instrument is used to deeply massage (up to patient tolerance) a localized tender site within subcutaneous tissues. During goading, with strokes about 1 inch in length, the skin should not be moved. The therapy is quite uncomfortable but often brings dramatic relief in a few hours when more conservative measures have failed.

Hanes feels that many disorders are the result of a posttraumatic neuritis, produced intrinsically or extrinsically, and has isolated several specific points of major irritation. The sites are palpated as excessively tender local spasms. He recommends a firm, constant pressure with no thumb motion which is easily bearable for the patient. The typical pressure duration is 10–30 seconds.

Neurovascular and Neurolymphatic Receptors

Lactic acid is a normal by-product of muscle contraction; ie, when a muscle contrasts, lactic acid is produced. Bennett and Goodheart base their work in this area on the hypothesis that any blockage (eg, inhibitory reflex) of the neurovascular receptors will prohibit the normal lactic acid response from occurring, leading to an accumulation of lactic acid in the muscles. This in turn causes further blood vessel dilation. As vascular dilation occurs through a vasomotor response, any blockage of the neurovascular receptor prohibits normal lactic acid response.

Neurolymphatic receptors are located singularly or in multiples on the anterior and posterior aspects of the body, varying in size from that of a pea to a bean. Most of the larger muscles have about four drainage points; ie, two anterior and two posterior. The neurolymphatic receptors do not correspond to the sites of lymph glands; however, they are related to the lymphatic system according to a hypothesis developed by Chapman and later expanded by Goodheart, who has correlated these receptors with the musculature system. It is believed that the neurolymphatic reflex points inhibit normal lymphatic flow when the system becomes "overloaded" and that neurolymphatic receptor "blockage" has the same effect as that of neurovascular blockage; ie, a prohibition of normal dilation and an abnormal lactic acid response.

CHAPTER 18

Basic Spinal Subluxation Considerations

The concept that an "off centered" vertebral or pelvic segment parallels a unique effect upon the neuromuscular bed which may be the cause of, aggravation of, or "triggering" of certain syndromes is a major contribution to the field of functional pathology and clinical biology by the chiropractic profession. This section discusses the basic biomechanics and effects of vertebral subluxations as related to the management of sports-related and recreational injuries.

SPINAL BIOMECHANICS

While the erect spinal column is a concern in static postural equilibrium, it is never actually in a static state in life. It is alternately changing from a state of "quiet dynamics" in the static postural attitude to a state of "active dynamics" in movement.

The Vertebral Motion Unit

An intervertebral motion unit consists of two vertebrae and their contiguous structures forming a set of articulations at one intervertebral level. Thus, what is called a vertebral "subluxation" in chiropractic is the alteration of the normal dynamics, anatomic or physiologic relationships of contiguous articular structures. The components of the spinal column (the vertebral motion units) confer a quality and quantity of motoricity to the relationship of two vertebrae. They are firmly interconnected by the intervertebral disc and restraining ligaments, which are activated by muscles which respond to both sensory and motor stimulation.

The biomechanical efficiency of any one of the 25 vertebral motor units, from atlas to sacrum, can be described as that condition (individually and collectively) in which each gravitationally dependent segment above is free to seek its normal resting position in relation to its supporting structure below, is free to move efficiently through

its normal ranges of motion, and is free to return to its normal resting position after movement. The motion unit has an anterior and a posterior portion, and each has peculiar characteristics; the articulations are actually the mobile or motor portion of the unit:

1. The anterior portion of the motion unit includes the vertebral bodies, the intervertebral disc, the anterior and posterior longitudinal ligaments, and the other associated soft tissues. This anterior portion is weight bearing and supportive. It has very little sensory innervation. Changes or pathology affecting these structures, though they may be quite spectacular in appearance on a x-ray film and alter biomechanics and spinal mobility significantly, are seldom accompanied by much pain or other subjective discomfort in the local area.

2. The posterior motion unit consists of the pedicles, neural foramina, articular processes and apophyseal articulations, the ligamenta flava and those which encapsulate the articulation, the interspinous and supraspinous ligaments, and all the muscles and other attached soft-tissue structures. The posterior portions of the motion units are rich with sensory and proprioceptive nerves. Thus, problems that affect these structures are usually painful.

Normal and Abnormal Vertebral Movements

Normal movements of a vertebral segment relative to its supporting structure below may be described by its ability to laterally flex on the coronal plane, rotate on the transverse plane, and anteroflex and retroextend on the sagittal plane. To some extent, all vertebrae are able to function in all three dimensions; however, the magnitude of such movements varies in degree in the lumbar, thoracic, and cervical spinal regions, as well as in the transitional areas.

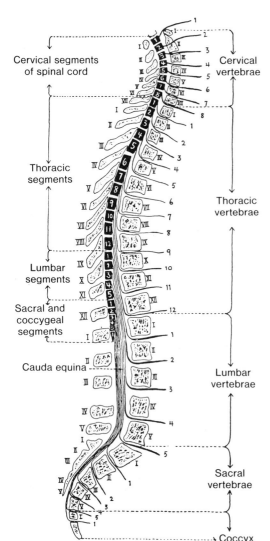

Figure 18.1. Illustration of spinal segments depicting the bodies and spinous process of vertebrae, the place of origin of the nerve roots from the spinal cord, and the roots exiting from the corresponding intervertebral foramina.

Abnormal spinal biomechanics primarily relate to the intervertebral subluxation and other spinal fixations that result in structural and functional inadequacies of the spinal column. This state is the condition of a vertebral motion unit which has lost its normal structural and/or functional integrity and is, therefore, unable to move from its normal resting position, unable to move properly through its normal range of motion, or unable to return to its normal resting position after movement.

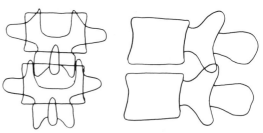

Figure 18.2. *Left*, schematic posterior view of the intervertebral motion unit in normal position. *Right*, lateral view of the intervertebral motion unit in normal position.

The degree of derangement of a bony segment within its articular bed may vary from a microtrauma to one that is macroscopic and quite readily discernible. It is always attended to some degree by articular dysfunction, neurologic insult, stressed muscles, tendons, and ligaments. Once produced, the lesion becomes a focus of sustained pathologic irritation: a barrage of impulses stream into the spinal cord where internuncial neurons receive and relay them to motor pathways. The contraction that provoked the subluxation initially is thereby reinforced, thus perpetuating both the subluxation and the pathologic process engendered.

MOTOR-UNIT CLASSIFICATION OF SUBLUXATIONS

There are numerous methods to classify vertebral subluxations. Each has its own rationale and each has had certain validity that has been a contribution to our understanding of this complex phenomenon. The biomechanical element of the vertebral motion unit subluxation is classified by Hildebrand and Howe in accord with its static or kinetic aspects and in accordance with the number of vertebral motion units involved. Following are the generally accepted characteristics and significance of the classified vertebral motion unit subluxation-fixations:

Static Intersegmental Subluxations

Flexion Subluxation. This is characterized by approximation of the vertebral bodies at the anterior and by separation of the vertebral bodies, facets, and spinous processes at the posterior (Fig. 18.3). When

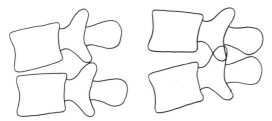

Figure 18.3. *Left*, flexion malposition. *Right*, extension malposition.

found, it is indicative of irritative microtrauma to the anterior intervertebral foramen (IVF); forced excursion of the nucleous pulposis and bulging of annular fibers; stretching of the posterior longitudinal, interspinal, and supraspinal ligaments; traction shearing stress of the synovia of the facet articulations; and biomechanical impropriety of the motion unit.

Extension Subluxation. This type of subluxation is featured by separation of the vertebral bodies at the anterior and approximation of the vertebral bodies, facets, and spinous processes at the posterior (see Fig. 18.3). Such a subluxation points toward irritative microtrauma at the posterior IVF, forced exclusion of the nucleous pulposis and bulging of the annular fibers, stretching of the anterior longitudinal ligament, imbrication of the facet articulations with compressive shearing stress to the synovia of the facet articulations, and biomechanical insult of the vertebral motion unit.

Lateral Flexion Subluxation. This is characterized by approximation of the vertebral bodies and facets on the side of flexion and separation of the vertebral bodies and facets on the side of extension (Fig. 18.4). This type of subluxation is suspicious of irritative microtrauma to the intervertebral disc (IVD) on the side of flexion, imbrication of the facets and compressive shearing stress to the synovia on the side of flexion, forced excursion of the nucleous pulposis with bulging of the annular fibers, stretching of the anterior longitudinal ligament at its lateral aspect, and biomechanical impropriety of the vertebral motion unit.

Rotational Subluxation. Such a subluxation is featured by rotatory displacement of the vertebral bodies laterally and posteriorly on the side of rotation with torsion of the facet articulations in the direction op-

posite to vertebral body rotation (see Fig. 18.4). This situation is significant of torsion binding of the annular fibers of the IVD, decreased resiliency of the IVD due to torque compression of the annular fibers, torsion stretching of the anterior and posterior longitudinal ligaments, rotatory imbrication of the facets with reverse shearing stress to the synovia, and biomechanical insult of the vertebral motion unit.

Anterolisthesis Subluxation Without Spondylolysis. This is characterized by an anterior-inferior excursion of the vertebral body at the anterior and by anterior-superior excursion of the vertebral body and facets at the posterior. It points toward irritative microtrauma at the anterior IVD, forward shearing stress to the annular fibers of the IVD, stretching of the anterior and posterior longitudinal ligaments, imbrication of facets with forward shearing stress to the synovia, and biomechanical impropriety of the vertebral motion unit.

Anterolisthesis Subluxation With Spondylolysis. This is featured by anterior excursion of the verebral body independent of the posterior division of the motion unit (Fig. 18.5). The posterior division of the unit remains in position with the structure below because of separation of the pars. It is characterized by irritative microtrauma to the posterior aspect of the IVD, forced excursion of the nucleous pulposis with bulging of the annular fibers, forward shearing stress to the annular fibers, stretching of the anterior longitudinal ligament, and biomechanical insult of the vertebral motion unit

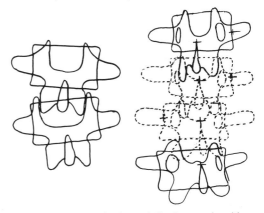

Figure 18.4. *Left*, lateral flexion malposition. *Right*, rotational malposition.

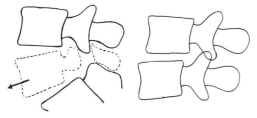

Figure 18.5. *Left*, anterolisthesis, or spondylolisthesis. *Right*, retrolisthesis.

Retrolisthesis Subluxation. Such a subluxation is featured by posterior-inferior excursion of the vertebral body and by posterior-inferior excursion of the facets (see Fig. 18.5). This subluxation signifies irritative microtrauma to the posterior IVD, posterior shearing stress of the annular fibers, stretching of the anterior and posterior longitudinal ligaments, imbrication of the facets with posterior shearing stress to the synovia, and biomechanical impropriety of the vertebral motion unit.

Laterolisthesis Subluxation. This is characterized by lateral, superior, and posterior excursion of the vertebral body on the side of deviation and by separation of the facets on the side of deviation with reverse torsion and approximation on the side opposite deviation (Fig. 18.6). This suggests irritative microtrauma to the IVD on the side opposite deviation, lateral and posterior shearing stress to the annular fibers on the side of deviation, imbrication of facets and anterior shearing of the synovia on the side opposite deviation, and biomechanical insult to the vertebral motion unit.

Decreased Interosseous Space Subluxation. This type is featured by narrowing of the IVF space and inferior excursion of the facets (see Fig. 18.6). It is characterized by degeneration of the IVD with approximation of the vertebral bodies, traumatic compression of the IVD with possible herniation of the nucleous pulposis through the end plate, imbrication of the facets with compressive shearing stress to the synovia, compression of the contents of the IVF, and biomechanical impropriety of the vertebral motion unit.

Increased Interosseous Space Subluxation. This is characterized by superior excursion of the vertebral body and the facets (Fig. 18.7). It results in inflammatory swell-

ing or pathologic enlargement of the IVD, traction shearing stress to the annular fibers of the IVD and the synovia of the facet articulations, stretching of the anterior and posterior longitudinal ligaments, and biomechanical insult to the vertebral motion unit.

Bony Foraminal Encroachment Subluxation. This type is featured by potential concomitant findings of other types of subluxations with a possible relationship to osteophytic interforaminal spurs in conjunction with other types of subluxations. It features associated microtraumas and macrotraumas to the vertebral motion unit; compression, irritation, and swelling of the foraminal contents; osseous and soft-tissue primary degenerative processes of the vertebral motion-unit structures; and interforaminal neurovascular insult effecting possible disseminated secondary pathophysiologic processes.

Kinetic Intersegmental Subluxations

Hypomobility and/or Fixation Subluxation. This common subluxation is characterized by fixation of the vertebral motion unit in relation to the supporting structure below and compensatory hypermobility of

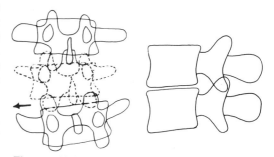

Figure 18.6. *Left*, laterolisthesis. *Right*, decreased interosseous spacing.

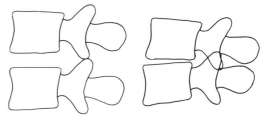

Figure 18.7. *Left*, increased interosseous spacing. *Right*, foraminal occlusion.

the vertebral motion unit above the level of fixation (Fig. 18.8). It is associated with irritative excessive function of the hypermobile vertebral motion unit resulting in microtrauma or macrotrauma to the IVD, anterior and posterior longitudinal ligaments, periosteum, etc; muscular irritation, spasticity, muscle trauma, fatigue, etc; neurologic insult within the confines of the neural canal and IVF; vascular insult to the paraspinal and interforaminal blood vessels; and biomechanical impropriety of all vertebral motion units involved.

Hypermobility Subluxation. This is featured by an excessively mobile vertebral

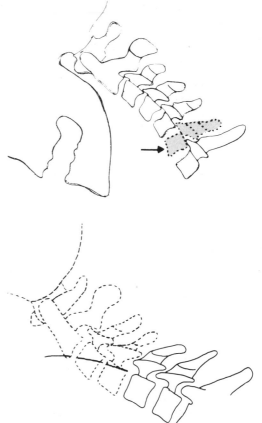

Figure 18.9. Stress film tracings. *Top*, aberrant mobility of a vertebra. *Bottom*, abnormal motion of a cervical section.

motion unit in relation to a normally functioning of hypomobile motion unit below (see Fig. 18.8). It has the same features as that of a hypomobile and/or fixation subluxation except for a possible traumatically loosened vertebral motion unit as opposed to compensatory hypermobility of a vertebral motion unit within its normal range of motion.

Aberrant Movement Subluxation. This type, frequently traumatic in origin, is characterized by movement of a vertebra "out of phase" with the segment above and below where two motion units are involved (Fig. 18.9). It points toward microtrauma to both of the vertebral motion units involved, occlusion of the IVFs above and below the aberrant segment, shearing stress to the IVDs and synovia of both vertebral motion units, restriction of the neural canal, and

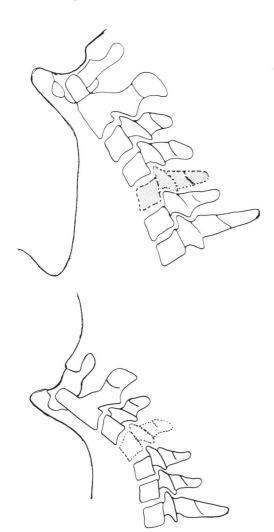

Figure 18.8. *Top*, vertebral hypomobility. *Bottom*, vertebral hypermobility shown on stress-flexion film tracing.

biomechanical impropriety of both vertebral motion units.

MECHANICS INVOLVED IN THE SPINAL EXAMINATION

During spinal analysis, the major motions evaluated are flexion, extension, right and left lateral flexion, and right and left rotation. Motion of a superior segment is described in terms of the segment beneath it. Motion evaluations, however, are just one part of the examination procedures. A larger scope of chiropractic procedures is roughly charted in Figure 18.10.

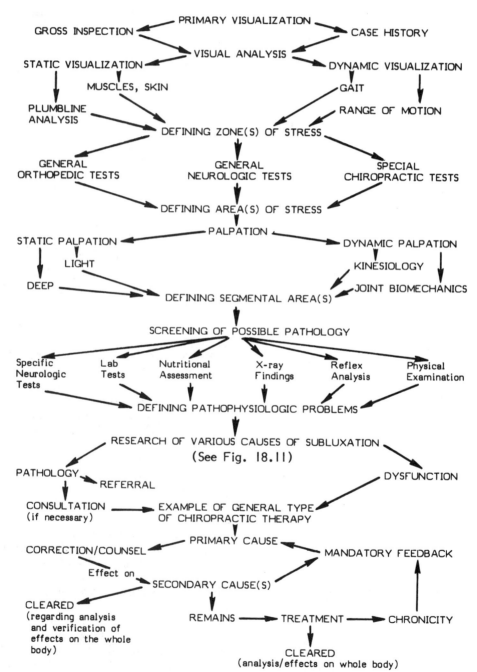

Figure 18.10. Determination of subluxations by chiropractic procedures. Based on charts prepared by B. Faucret, et al (reprinted with permission of the Los Angeles College of Chiropractic).

Spinal Motions

When the spine is in a neutral standing or sitting position, the anterior surface of a vertebral body will rotate to the side opposite the lateroflexion with the vertebral bodies tending to crawl out from under the load. This pattern of function usually takes place within multiple spinal segments, but dysfunction will occur when ligaments and muscles attached to and affecting the vertebral articulations are shortened or lengthened to effect restricted or excessive motion of one or more segments. The articular facets open during flexion, close during extension, and individual segments rotate and side bend to the same side. When the neutral position is resumed, the spinal joints should return to their "normal" position.

The direction of vertebral rotation is determined by inspection and dynamic palpation of the transverse processes, with the processes being more posterior on the side toward which the vertebrae have rotated. If one or more segments are rotated to one side in the neutral position, lateroflexion will usually be noted to the side opposite the rotation. In spinal flexion, the segment rotated will be side bent to the same side with a loss in its ability to bend forward. Likewise, during spinal extension, the segment is rotated to the same side and is unable to bend backward.

Motion Barriers

To keep measurements standardized, an understanding of the barrier concept is necessary. When a joint is passively tested for range of motion, the examiner will note increasing resistance to motion referred to as a "bind" or the physiologic motion barrier. When the joint is carried past this point, the added motion becomes uncomfortable to the patient. This point is referred to as the anatomic motion barrier. In evaluating the degrees of passive motion, the joints should be moved up to but not through the anatomic motion barrier. Thus, joint motion is accomplished by passively carrying the joint(s) through a range of motion until the motion barrier is encountered and recording the degrees of movement allowed. This is also true for extremity joints.

Spinal Joint Locking or Blocking

Good describes spinal joint blocking within a subluxation syndrome as an actively maintained, reversible, biomechanical phenomenon in which paravertebral spasm (especially unilateral multifidus and rotatore contraction) physiologically locks one or more motion segments, causing a shift of the axis of motion towards an apophyseal joint to the degree that the unsynchronized segment is unable to articulate about the new axis. Thus, any method that assists relocation (normalization) of the axis of movement which releases the nociceptor feedback or relaxes the unisegmental spasm will be effective in reducing acute joint hypomobility whose initial origin was that of strain.

The Apophyseal Joints

The posterior articular facets of the spine possess the histologic capability to account for many of the various phenomena found in the subluxation syndrome. Their close proximity to the IVF is of special interest since both structural and functional changes in these facets have been shown to affect the nerve root.

In writing of experimental studies on the apophyseal joints, especially that of normal joint structures and their reaction to injury, Reiter describes an anatomical study of 75 postmortem spines that revealed significant changes, many of which would not be visible on x-ray. The capsular changes included edema, granular ossification, calcification, and adhesion between the capsule and the meningeal covering of the nerve root adjacent to it. The intra-articular changes included hypertrophy of the menisci up to four times their normal size, occasional chondrification and ossification of the menisci, detached bodies, ulcerated areas of denuded hyaline cartilage, cartilage thinning, fibrillation, and osteophytic marginal proliferation.

Evaluating Joint Motion and Strength

The range of gross motion for any particular spinal area is usually recorded in degrees by a goniometer with comparable measurement of the opposite side noted. When asymmetry of motion range is observed, the examiner must determine whether the side with the greatest movement is weak or the side with less motion is restricted. A test of the strength of a muscle or group of muscles is made by carrying the joint or joints to the extreme of allowed movement permitted by the antagonist muscles, after which the examiner resists an active maximum effort by the patient to contract the muscles being tested. Strength is recorded bilaterally from Grade 5 to Grade 0.

PRECIPITATING FACTORS OF SPINAL SUBLUXATIONS

The spinal dysarthric subluxation may be either a cause or an effect, and the immediate causes may be divided into two major categories: the unequal or asymmetrical muscular efforts upon the joint structures and the inequality in the supporting tissues of a particular joint such as the cartilage, intervertebral disc, ligaments, etc. Some form of internal or external stress is necessary to produce a subluxation to a degree sufficient to cause a state of neurodysfunction.

The general cause-and-effect relationships involved in subluxation complexes are shown in Figure 18.11.

Inequality of Muscle Balance

Inequality in muscular balance may be initiated by trauma, postural distortion phenomena, biochemical reactions, psychomotor responses, paralytic affects, and somatic and visceral responses.

Trauma. Prank trauma may cause in-

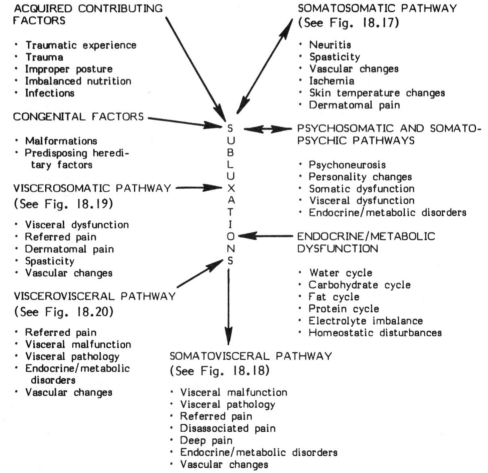

Figure 18.11. General overview of cause-and-effect relationships involved in subluxation complexes. Based on charts prepared by B. Faucret, et al (reprinted with permission of the Los Angeles College of Chiropractic).

flammation, degeneration, etc, and particularly the muscular splinting reaction that muscles make when their surrounding tissues are injured. This alters the position and motion of the structural tissues that are related. Sustained microtrauma, though of a less acute nature, may cause a slow continual irritation and eventually create degenerative pathologic changes which similarly alter muscular reaction. The obvious trauma of a fall or blow which surprises a joint with the intrinsic muscles unprepared will cause a joint sprain with ligament injury. A sudden slip during a lift is equally damaging to the unprepared or weak joint. Watkins reminds us that the slower trauma of occupational strain is not as easy to visualize. He reminds us of the game of youth in trying to hold an axe at arms length to the side for 1 minute. Within 2 minutes, the shoulder aches but the big "catch" is at the lumbosacral level in following hours and days.

Postural Distortion Phenomena. Postural compensations for either mechanical activity or structural changes in the skeleton itself are referred to as postural distortion phenomena. These changes, as well as other causes of subluxation, often result in a series or combination of minor mechanical errors which together may be termed scoliosis, kyphosis, lordosis, distortion, or similar terms. Such a distortion phenomenon is dependent upon the ability of the spine to adjust to any interference in the body's vestibular, visual, or proprioceptive adaptation which is incompatible with the normal balance of the musculoskeletal system to gravity. Whether this structural imbalance creates disturbances or appears asymptomatic is dependent upon the neurologic irritation developing within the tissues affected. They may not elicit apparent disturbance at a given time, but rather at a later date when they overcome the adaptation and resistance of the individual.

Biochemical Reactions. The acute or chronic hypo- or hypertonicity of musculature may be due to various biochemical changes within the above-mentioned tissues. This may be brought about by foreign bodies, by either local or general pathologies which may cause anoxia, ischemia, toxicity, etc, or by systemic fatigue-producing activities, nutritional deficiencies of excesses,

caustic chemical exposure, ingestion of harmful chemicals, inhalation of noxious gases, microorganism toxins, abnormal glandular activity, excessive heat or cold, or electric shock affecting the chemical environment of cells histologically.

Psychomotor Responses. These responses refer to the reaction of musculature to emotional effects on the nervous system as the body depicts its psychologic stresses. They may be environmentally, socially, or intrinsically initiated.

Paralytic Effects. Primary disease of the neuromuscular system itself (eg, paralytic diseases) affects musculoskeletal tone and strength, thus affecting position and quality of motion.

Somatic and Visceral Responses. These responses refer to the secondary reactions of the muscular system to somatic or visceral sensory irritation which may develop elsewhere in a given neurologic segment. Our embryologic nature is such that the various components of a given vertebral segment and its ramifications of neuromere may be influenced by sensory stimuli that arise from any tissue supplied by these components. The somatic or visceral sensory neurons that enter into a given neurologic segment and cause somatic or visceral motor response may cause a similar response throughout the various ramifications of that segment. This, of course, depends upon certain states of sensitivity or facilitation, certain convergencies or divergencies within the nervous system, and particularly upon the intensity and duration of the initiating stimulation. Therefore, it could well be a visceral sensory irritation in the intestinal tract or other viscus that is causing motor changes not only in the internal organs, but also in the vascularity and the musculature of the body. These changes may result in motor alterations in the tone of muscles, consequently resulting in a spasm or splinting action. If long standing, degenerative changes, atonicities brought about by atrophy, contractures, or other pathologic changes within the musculature may develop which can influence the mechanics of the vertebral segment(s) involved.

Abnormal Structural Support

Mechanical errors in position or motion

may also be brought about by structural alterations in the supporting tissues of the joint itself. These in turn may be brought about by: (1) Genetic and developmental abnormalities causing asymmetry of the vertebrae, cartilage, muscular structure, etc. (2) Various acquired disease processes within the joint such as arthritic degeneration, avascular necrosis, or a neuropathic process that causes the cartilage, bone, ligaments, or musculature to be structurally altered. (3) The resolution of macro- or microtraumas, strains, sprains, or other primary pathology may cause fibrosis, degeneration, or other retrograde changes of a structural nature within the joints themselves.

These same processes not only develop within the vertebral column and its paravertebral tissues but also in the musculoskeletal tissues of the appendicular skeleton. Thus, similar lesions may exist remote from the spine which perpetuate neuropathic responses by their presence. When the cause is within the structures of the vertebral column, the effects are more evident because of the close anatomical proximities and the functional importance of normal motion-unit function or the integrity to the various components of the nervous system.

Stress Factors Resulting in Subluxation

Depending on the degree of stress produced, any internal or external stress factor involves the nervous system directly or indirectly, resulting in decreased mobility of the vertebra of the involved neuromere. This decreased mobility may be the result of (1) muscle splinting, especially on the side of greatest stimulation according to Fluger's Law or (2) from abnormal weight distribution to the superior facets and other structures of the vertebrae involved. Fluger's law states that if a stimulus received by a sensory nerve extends to a motor nerve of the opposite side, contraction occurs only from corresponding muscles; and, if contraction is unequal bilaterally, the stronger contraction always takes place on the side which is stimulated. When affecting one or more vertebrae, this state of decreased mobility of the motion unit encourages nerve dysfunction leading to pathologic processes in the areas supplied by the affected nerve

root or neuromere, depending upon the degree and chronicity of involvement.

EFFECTS OF SPINAL SUBLUXATIONS

As a primary concept of chiropractic clinical science, spinal subluxations may result in the development of disease states locally within the vertebral motion unit itself or throughout the body (see Fig. 18.12). These primary and secondary effects of subluxations may be divided into three major categories:

1. The mechanical effect, motion, and balance of the local segment, or the effect upon the skeleton elsewhere, due to compensatory distortions and alterations as the proprioceptive mechanism would correct its mechanics to the presence of structural imbalance.

2. The effect of any localized condition occurring within the articulations due to interarticular stress and trauma (often microtrauma) such as irritation, inflammation, swelling, necrosis, and degenerative changes.

3. The neurologic effects of vertebral subluxation may be grossly differentiated as nerve pressure, nerve stretch, nerve torsion, circulatory changes, meningeal irritations,

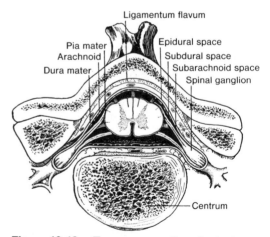

Figure 18.12. Transverse section of spinal cord and vertebra to show their relative positions. Note dorsal root ganglia lying in the IVF and the dorsal and ventral roots in the spinal canal. The spinal nerve is shown outside the vertebra, with branches to the dorsal body wall, ventral body wall, and viscera.

cerebrospinal fluid flow alterations, alterations of proprioceptive responses and reflexes, traumatic insult to the rami communicantes or sympathetic ganglia, etc. Neurologic effects are undoubtedly the more important of the three categories.

The projected neurophysiologic pathways that may be involved in a subluxation complex are shown in Figure 18.13.

Many spinal subluxations have more than one immediate cause and effect. Therefore, a complicated far-reaching series of interacting and interdependent changes occur which may be designated as a subluxation syndrome. As a cause-effect interrelationship, it is hypothesized that, once initiated, this biomechanical impropriety becomes an etiologic "vicious cycle" from cause to effect

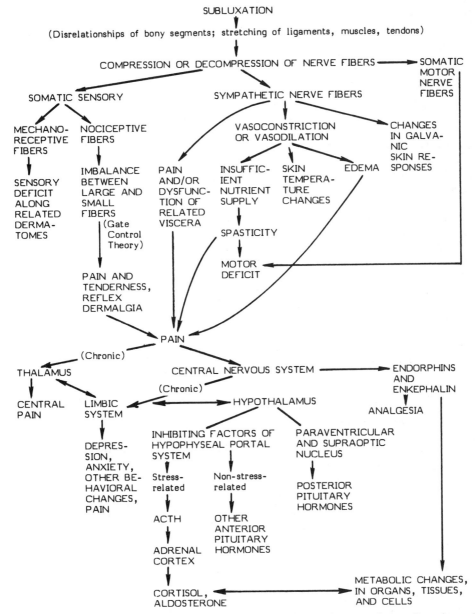

Figure 18.13. Projected neurophysiologic pathways of subluxation complexes. Based on charts prepared by B. Faucret, et al (reprinted with permission of the Los Angeles College of Chiropractic).

and from effect back to cause which, if not interrupted by corrective effort, will carry on to an ultimate and perhaps fatal conclusion.

Structural Alterations

The primary physical and mechanical factors that often negatively influence the body are gravity, pressure, weight load, inertia, compression, elasticity, leverage, movement, stretch, expansion, and contraction. With these forces in mind, a subluxation may be grossly determined by its structural alterations and manifestations.

Postural   Analysis.   Postural   faults, which may be either the cause or result of vertebral subluxations, are often readily visualized in postural analysis. Pressure or stretching stress of viscera leads to disturbed visceral function and abnormal reflexes. Abnormal body mechanics affecting the thoracic and abdominal cavities interfere with normal function by: (1) Abnormal efferent visceral stimuli reaching organs from the facilitated segment. (2) Abnormal tensions and stretching of visceral supports, nerves, blood and lymph vessels. (3) Venous pooling as the result of inactivity, diaphragm dysfunction, organ displacement, and sustained postural stress. (4) Abnormal vasomotor impulses to blood vessels. Blocking stress or irritation of blood vessels leads to ischemia or congestion. There are many general effects to the body as a whole besides these local effects because each abnormal stress results in abnormal discharges or afferent impulses to the central nervous system with consequent hormonal reactions systemic in character. Also considered must be the associated emotional stress as the result of the local stress which contributes to the clinical picture.

Physical Examination. Palpable alterations in the normal anatomic relationships of one joint to another are frequently found. These mechanical changes may occur in the static recumbent, sitting, or standing positions or in various ranges of motion as the segments and their supporting tissues are put through either active or passive positions of motion. Subluxations are also evident by the presence of certain objective or subjective signs and symptoms when the joint and tissues are put through certain

kinetic or orthopedic tests. Stress, strain, and sprain at the area of the zygapophyses and the attending inflammatory reaction may give rise to a radiculitis of moderate disposition.

Mechanical spinal disturbances can adversely affect the body in a number of ways such as (1) load stress on muscles leading to hypertrophy or atrophy and alterations of local muscle strength, (2) leverage stress at joints leading to weakness or sprain of ligaments, articular and intra-articular cartilage damage, and synovitis, and (3) compression stress or irritation of nerves leading to increase or decrease of conduction with consequent trophic changes.

Roentgenography. Subluxations visualized on x-ray films exist as disrelationships in the normal structural relationship of one joint to another. This may not be evident in a given view, but in the view best depicting the mechanical fault. Sometimes they may only be evident on views when an area is put through various positions of motion. Compression stress on bone leads to a sclerosis or alteration of its normal shape and internal architecture, and pressure stress on connective tissues leads to thickening or thinning. Combinations of factors influence cartilage degeneration such as severe isolated or repeated minor trauma, chronic mechanical stress or tension, local circulatory excesses or deficiencies, idiopathic biochemical factors, developmental anomalies or malformations, nutritional factors, and the inherited cellular quality of the cartilage.

Events at the Intervertebral Foramen

There are 115 diarthroses within the spine and pelvis vulnerable to the "off centering fixation" of subluxation. Each of these articulations is an organ of proprioceptive sensitivity which under articular strain is insulted and provoked to express pain. As mentioned, a working hypothesis regarding spinal dysarthrias is that the vertebral displacement-fixation causes adjacent areas of the spine to become hypermobile, resulting in stress of adjacent motor units. Neurologic feedback may cause the elicitation of ACTH and a resulting increase in the production of corticosteroids as an adaptive mechanism, according to the Hans Selye stress syndrome, and this may also be reflected by possible blood sugar changes.

Contents of the Intervertebral Foramen. Each foramen is dynamic: widening and expanding with spinal motion, serving as a channel for nerve and vascular egress and ingress, and allowing compression and expansion of the lipoareolar bed (see Fig. 18.14). The following structures are usually found in the IVF: anterior and motor nerve root, posterior or sensory nerve root, part of the dorsal nerve root ganglion, recurrent meningeal nerve, spinal ramus artery, intervertebral vein, lymphatic vessels, nervi nervorum, nervi vasorum, vaso vasorum, and vaso nervorum.

Factors Which Change the Diameter of the IVF. In review, the factors modifying the diameters of the IVFs are (1) the disrelation of subluxation, (2) changes in the normal curves of the spine, (3) the presence of induced abnormal curves of the spine, (4) degenerative thinning, bulging, or extrusion of the related IVD, (5) swelling and sclerosing of the capsular ligaments and the interbody articulation, and (6) marginal proliferations of the vertebral bodies and articulations.

Consequences of IVF Diameter Alteration. These factors mitigate the viable contents of the IVF and subject its contents to physiologic compromise which results in

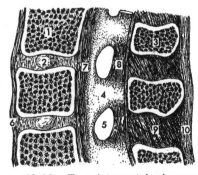

Figure 18.14. Two intervertebral symphyses seen in a longitudinal section through three segments of the vertebral column. *1*, body of the vertebra; *2*, intervertebral cartilagninous disc; *3*, spinous process; *4*, spinal canal; *5*; intervertebral foramen; *6*, anterior longitudinal ligament; *7*, posterior longitudinal ligament; *8*, ligamentum flavum; *9*, interspinous ligament; *10*, supraspinous ligament.

nerve root pressure, traction or torque, constriction of the spinal blood vessels, intraforaminal and paraforaminal edema, induration and sclerosing of the periarticular ligaments with incarcerating insult upon the contained receptors, forcing of the foraminal contents into protracted constriction and altered position, and such other consequences.

Effects of Microtrauma. Initially, subluxation is attended by the following aspects of microtrauma: (1) minute hemorrhage, transudation, and arterial-venous stagnation from the sluggish circulatory flow as the result of the motion unit's decreased mobility and arterial backup; (2) para-articular and paraforaminal traumatic edema; (3) eccentric compression stress upon the IVD and the zygapophyseal cartilages; (4) possible separation of minute fasciculi of the retaining fibers of the annulus, joint capsule, dural root sleeve, and nerve root sheath, (5) stress insult of the proprioceptive bed; (6) minute crushing of the periosteal margins with resultant proliferative irritation; and (7) minute tearing of the attachments of the dural root sleeves as they attach to the lining periosteum of the IVF.

In consequence, the following pathologic changes occur: (1) Extravasation and edema, along with the precipitation of fibrinogen into fibrin, result in interfascicular, foraminal, and articular adhesions that restrict fascicular glide, ingress and egress of the foraminal contents, and the competent motoricity of the vertebral segment within its articular bed. (2) Whenever there is extravasation, mineral salts are precipitated and infiltration and sclerosing result. (3) Binding adhesions may develop between the dural root sleeves and the nerve roots within the inter-radicular foramen and between the spinal nerve root sheath and the inner margins of the IVF. (4) When subjected to microtrauma, mesenchymal connective tissue undergoes a relative rapid and extensive degenerative change with loss of functional integrity and substance.

Altered Nerve Root Level. Induced disrelation between level and direction of nerve root origin (spinal cord) and nerve root exit (IVF) is an important factor. Whenever there is subluxation, change in normal curves, or presence of abnormal curves, the relative levels of points of nerve root origin and exit are altered. Hence, the position, direction, and course of the nerve roots and trunk within the IVF become abnormal. Compression or irritation is thus more likely. In addition, a vertebral column affected with partial fixation of several segments when subjected to flexion, extension, and circumduction efforts will be attended by marked tension upon the dural root sleeves and the related spinal nerve radicles, especially the cauda equina.

Proprioceptive Responses and Reflexes. Perhaps the most significant effect is that of proprioceptive irritation. The musculoskeletal tissues and particularly the ligaments and paravertebral or intervertebral musculature of the spine are richly endowed with proprioceptive neurons. First, when overly stimulated by stretching, these neurons interpret the stimuli as somatic sensory stimulation which may be perceived as pain. Second, they may also send reflexes to their motor components and cause muscular changes within the paravertebral muscles or elsewhere in the soma supplied by the segment. Third, they may be interpreted as visceral sensory stimuli, whose visceral motor response alters circulatory changes, smooth muscle activity, glandular secretions, or trophic activity in the musculoskeletal tissues or viscera supplied by a given neurologic segment or within the cord itself. It is this vast ability of the proprioceptive sensory beds to influence motor changes, both of a somatic-motor or visceral-motor nature, that is perhaps the most universal effect of vertebral subluxation.

Related Pain. The pain effected by a subluxation complex may be the result of mechanical, metabolic, or neurologic insults. The projected pain pathways involved in a subluxation complex are shown in Figure 18.15.

Intraneural Effects. It is probable that any interference with or abnormality of (1) the interstitial fluids in which the nerves lie and/or (2) the intracellular fluid of the nerve itself in the nerve axoplasm will cause a breakdown of the sodium pump mechanism that will prevent the normal flow of impulses along the nerve fibers concerned. These abnormal impulses refer to an overaction or underaction in the rate of impulse frequency along a nerve. Once a threshold stimulus has been reached, a nerve will fire in accordance with the all-or-none law.

Circulatory Changes. Decreased mobility (vertebral fixation) of a motion unit within its normal physiologic range of movement causes a sluggish circulatory lymphatic or vascular supply that may be influenced by mechanical pressure. This can cause chemical or physical changes within tissues such as anoxia, toxicity, swelling, edema, etc, and the consequent derangement of normal function brought about by these metabolic disorders. Local irritation at the site of misalignment and hypomotoricity causes an inflammatory reaction with edema leading to a disturbance in the normal exchange of nutrients and waste products between capillary and extracellular fluid. Added to this stasis is the probable factor of lactic acid buildup in the area as a result of acid leaking from the surrounding hypertonic musculature.

Local Toxicity Effects. The venous stagnation from arterial backup produces a local toxicity. While toxic metabolic end-products (eg, urea, uric acid, creatinine, lactic acid) accumulate in the stagnant tissue and congested capillary beds, there is also a corresponding decrease in nutrient and oxygen concentration in these fluids. Thus, the nerves emitting from the involved area will be deficient in necessary nutrients and quite possibly hypoxic as well. The buildup of metabolic waste products in the area of the IVF may also alter the normal pH of local fluids causing a breakdown of Krebb's cycle, due to decreased oxygen and toxicity, which causes a partial breakdown of the sodium pump mechanism, resulting in an ionic imbalance. As the sodium pump can no longer maintain a normal ionic balance, ionic imbalance results in some degree of erratic nerve conduction and edema in the tissues of the immediate area. This erratic nerve conduction may be exhibited in all nerves passing through the involved IVF and immediate area. When toxicity occurs in the central and peripheral nervous systems, the formation of acetylcholine at the level of involvement will be interfered with and result in further disturbances due to increased nerve conduction. This situation, along with

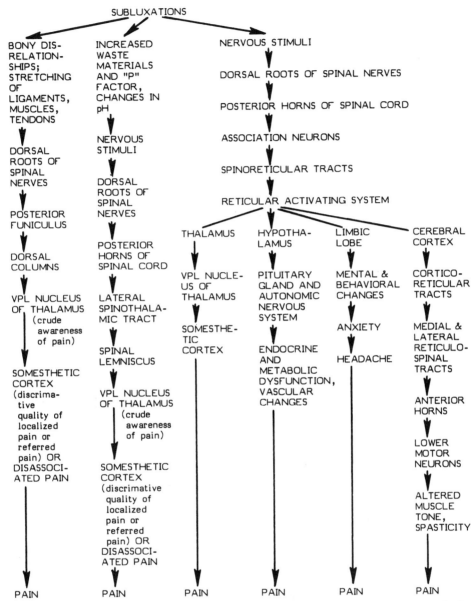

Figure 18.15. Projected pain pathways of subluxations. Based on charts prepared by B. Faucret, et al (reprinted with permission of the Los Angeles College of Chiropractic).

the toxicity effects upon the nerve, may well result in a disorder in membrane permeability leading to dysfunction.

Ganglion Irritation/Compression. Irritation/compression of the dorsal root ganglion may be a factor. The general sensory dorsal root ganglion of each spinal nerve lies within the upper medial aspect of the IVF. Whenever its position is altered or the diameters of positions of the IVF are modi-

fied, the ganglion may be subject to compression and irritation. For example, an acute whiplash-like mishap to the cervical spine, especially of the hyperextension type, may force the vagus and the superior cervical sympathetic ganglion against the transverse processes of the atlas and axis, provoking the bizarre autonomic reactions that not uncommonly attend this condition.

Meningeal Irritations. Mechanical errors in motion and position may cause tractional effects upon the meningeal coverings of the cord or dural-root sleeves which may produce mechanical pressure upon the neurons emitting from the cord itself. These may, therefore, cause the elicitation of abnormal motor effects or sensory interpretations.

Cerebrospinal Fluid Flow Alterations. These refer to the mechanical effect upon the flow of cerebral spinal fluid within the central nervous system and perhaps within the peripheral nerves themselves. Cerebrospinal fluid stagnation possibly occurs in association because of the intimate relationship between spinal fluid and venoid blood, contributing to toxicity in the nerve root area. According to some researchers, minute pressure on meninges alter the mechanics or flow of cerebrospinal fluid and interfere with its ability to remove wastes and provide nutritional substances to the cord and nervous system. This may be either the effect of direct mechanical pressure or impairment of motion necessary for proper inflow and outflow of this nutrient material.

Paraforaminal Adhesions. Paraforaminal adhesions in consequence to stress and traumatic edema often result in a painful restriction of the normal back-and-forth glide (¼–⅓ inch) of the nerve root within the IVF. Symptoms simulate a low-grade radiculitis: increased pain on movement, straining, and stretching; pain on changing positions and when placing the involved part in extension.

Distal Neurologic Manifestations

Because of the effects of the subluxation's microtrauma and the consequent pathologic changes involved, the neurologic insult may result in the following changes: (1) modification of the basic chronaxie, (2) alteration of normal impulse amplitude, wave length, force intensity, and/or (3) extension of the refractory period.

The neurologic manifestations of a subluxation are indicated by the response the nervous system makes to irritation not external to it (ie, discernible in its immediate area), but rather from within the body. Thus, it is an intrinsic source of neurologic irritation. This altered state of the nerve-fiber threshold and the impulse proper leads to dysfunction in the sensory, motor, vasomotor, and spinovisceral responses.

Somatic Responses. Dysfunctions in the somatic-sensory field include varying degrees of discomfort and pain, tension, superficial and deep tenderness, hyperesthesia and hypesthesia, haptic sensations, acroparesthesia, formications, flushing, numbness, coldness, and postural fatigue. Dysfunctions in the somatic-motor field include painful and especially proximal muscle spasms; abnormal muscular tone such as from hypotonicity to spasm and weakness, atrophy, or degeneration in long-standing cases; sluggish and incoordinated movements; paralyses; fasciculations, tics, and tremors.

Visceral Motor Responses. Visceral motor responses of the nervous system may be evidenced as follows:

1. Dysfunction in the vasomotor field includes local swellings, angioneurotic edema, flushing, blanching, mucous membrane congestion, urticaria and dermatographia. Minor changes in the circulation of the skin can be measured by various heat sensitive devices, thermography, galvanometers, or infrared photography. Such changes often parallel circulatory changes in the deeper tissues as they too are affected by similar vasomotor responses.

2. Changes in the ability of the skin to secrete oils or perspiration which can be measured by various electrical means. These secretory errors may also be indicative of similar changes in deeper visceral tissues. Hyperhidrosis or dryness, as well as hyperesthesia or hypesthesia, in a local area near the spine implies altered vasomotor activity in the subsequent spinal segment. Hyperesthesia and hyperhidrosis are usually associated with an increased "red response" to scratching and a decrease in electrical skin resistance.

3. Dysfunction in the spinovisceral field including visceral musculature abnormalities, glandular and mucous membrane secretory malfunctions, and sphincter spasms of the detrusor muscles and myocardium.

4. Changes in the quality of tissue from torphic disturbances such as atrophies, degenerations, thinning or discoloration of the skin, or other changes that reflect viscerotrophic abnormalities.

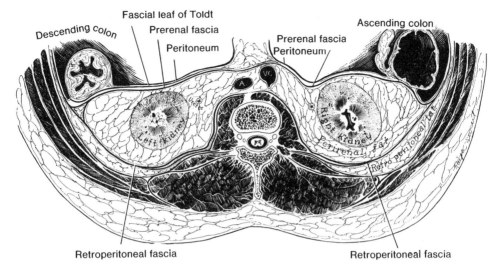

Figure 18.16. Transverse section of body at L2 level demonstrating the perirenal fascia. Support of anterior surface of left kidney is reinforced by fascial leaf of Toldt. On the other side, prerenal fascia is not reinforced, which weakens support of right kidney.

The Perplexing Reflexes

The human body exhibits an astonishingly complex array of neural circuitry. While the study of reflex communication between tissues under "voluntary" control and tissues under "autonomic" control (and their excitatory and inhibitory effect on one another) is still in its infancy, the answers to why so many visceral disorders mimic musculoskeletal disorders and why so many musculoskeletal disorders mimic visceral disorders appear to be on the horizon. Hypotheses are also being presented that help to explain the progressive reaction spread of some disorders that fail to respond to conventional therapies.

These reflexes can be classified into four broad categories; ie, those communicating from (1) a site on the body wall, cranium, or limb to another site on the body wall, cranium, or a limb (somatosomatic reflex); (2) a site on the body wall, cranium, or a limb (cutaneous, subcutaneous, musculoskeletal) to an internal organ or gland (somatovisceral reflex); (3) an internal organ or gland to a site on the body wall, cranium, or a limb (viscerosomatic reflex); and (4) an internal organ or gland to another internal organ or gland (viscerovisceral reflex). It must also be considered that these reflexes usually have segmental, propriospinal, and/ or suprasegmental implications.

Inasmuch as many reflexes are modulated within the spinal cord, their potential interrelationship with a subluxation complex, and vice versa, cannot be ignored when we consider that a vertebral lesion can be a focus for neuronal hyperexcitability or hypoexcitability. Thus all structures receiving efferent fibers via the IVF and all afferent fibers entering the IVF are potentially exposed to excessive stimulation or inhibition by some factor producing irritation, pressure, or tension at this vulnerable gateway.

Somatosomatic Reflexes. A somatosomatic reflex develops when a sensory receptor in the skin, subcutaneous tissue, fascia, striated muscle, a tendon, ligament, or a joint is stimulated to trigger a volley of reflex impulses to another anatomical location of this type via efferent sensory, motor, or autonomic fibers. Therapeutically, these reflexes are commonly evoked by manipulation, superficial heat or cold, electrotherapy, meridian therapy, hydrotherapy, traction, compression, vibration/percussion, applied kinesiology, and massage. The projected effects of spinal subluxations on the somatosomatic pathway are shown in Figure 18.17.

Somatovisceral Reflexes. A somatovisceral reflex develops when a sensory receptor in the skin, subcutaneous tissue, fascia, striated muscle, a tendon, a ligament, or a joint is stimulated to trigger a volley of reflex impulses to an internal organ, a gland, or a vessel via efferents of the autonomic nervous system. Therapeutically, these reflexes are commonly evoked by manipulation, superficial heat or cold, electrotherapy, meridian therapy (possibly), hydrotherapy, traction, compression, vibration/percussion, and massage. The projected effects of spinal subluxations on the somatovisceral pathway are shown in Figure 18.18.

Viscerosomatic Reflexes. A viscerosomatic reflex develops when a sensory receptor in an internal organ, a gland, or a vessel is stimulated to trigger a volley of reflex impulses to the skin, subcutaneous tissue,

fascia, striated muscle, a tendon, a ligament, or a joint. It essentially operates through motor or sensory efferents (eg, the abdominal spasm overlying peritonitis, angina pectoris). Therapeutically, these reflexes are commonly evoked by biofeedback therapy, spinal manipulation, spondylotherapy, and spinal traction or compression. The projected effects of spinal subluxations on the viscerosomatic pathway are shown in Figure 18.19.

Viscerovisceral Reflexes. A viscerovisceral reflex develops when a sensory receptor in an internal organ, gland, or vessel is stimulated to trigger a volley of reflex im-

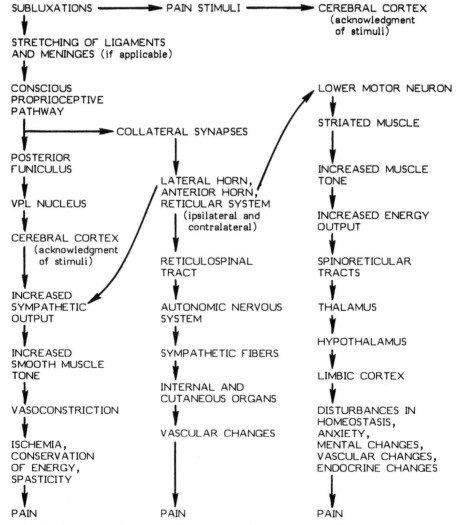

Figure 18.17. Projected effects of subluxations on the somatosomatic pathway. Based on charts prepared by B. Faucret, et al (reprinted with permission of the Los Angeles College of Chiropractic).

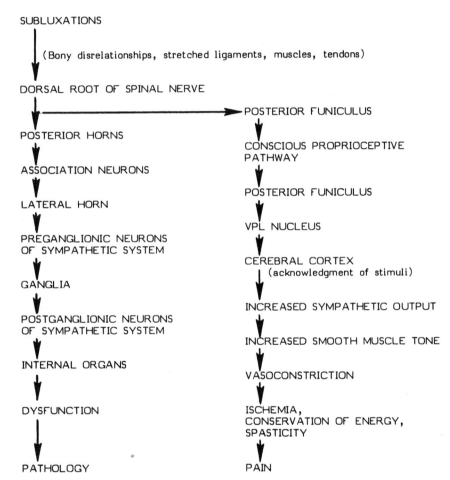

SUBLUXATIONS

(Bony disrelationships, stretched ligaments, muscles, tendons)

DORSAL ROOT OF SPINAL NERVE

POSTERIOR HORNS

ASSOCIATION NEURONS

LATERAL HORN

PREGANGLIONIC NEURONS
OF SYMPATHETIC SYSTEM

GANGLIA

POSTGANGLIONIC NEURONS
OF SYMPATHETIC SYSTEM

INTERNAL ORGANS

DYSFUNCTION

PATHOLOGY

POSTERIOR FUNICULUS

CONSCIOUS PROPRIOCEPTIVE
PATHWAY

POSTERIOR FUNICULUS

VPL NUCLEUS

CEREBRAL CORTEX
(acknowledgment of stimuli)

INCREASED SYMPATHETIC OUTPUT

INCREASED SMOOTH MUSCLE TONE

VASOCONSTRICTION

ISCHEMIA,
CONSERVATION OF ENERGY,
SPASTICITY

PAIN

Figure 18.18. Projected effects of subluxations on the somatovisceral pathway. Based on charts prepared by B. Faucret, et al (repprinted with permission of the Los Angeles College of Chiropractic).

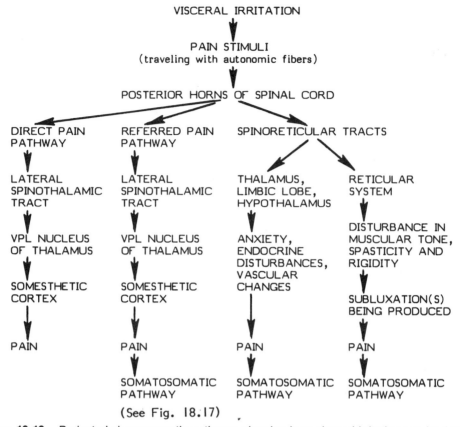

Figure 18.19. Projected viscerosomatic pathway, showing how visceral irritation can lead to pain and the development of subluxations. Based on charts prepared by B. Faucret, et al (reprinted with permission of the Los Angeles College of Chiropractic).

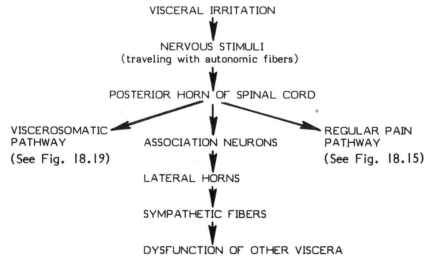

Figure 18.20. Projected viscerovisceral pathway, showing how visceral irritation can lead to viscerosomatic syndromes and regular pain. Based on charts prepared by B. Faucret, et al (reprinted with permission of the Los Angeles College of Chiropractic).

pulses to another anatomical location of this type via efferents of the autonomic nervous system. Rarely, however, does this reflex exist alone; ie, it usually has a segmental somatic component. Therapeutically, these reflexes are commonly evoked by spinal manipulation, deep heat, and hypnosis or other forms of psychotherapy. The projected effects of spinal subluxations on the viscerovisceral pathway are shown in Figure 18.20.

Suggested Readings: Part 3

CHAPTERS 12-18

ACA Council on Physiotherapy: Physiotherapy Guidelines for the Chiropractic Profession, *ACA Journal of Chiropractic*, June 1975.

Albright, JA and Brand, RA: *The Scientific Basis of Orthopaedics*, New York, Appleton-Century-Crofts, 1979.

Andreoli, G: Neurological Implications of Sports Injuries, *New England Journal of Chiropractic*, Winter 1979.

Andrews, FW: Discussion of Ice Therapy, *ACA Journal of Chiropractic*, April 1968.

Ariel, GB et al: Biomechanical Considerations in Resistive Exercise Equipment Design, Biomechanics and Kinesiology in Sports, Colorado Springs, an Olympic Sports Medicine Conference sponsored by the U.S. Olympic Committee, January 1984.

Betge, G: *Physical Therapy in Chiropractic Practice*, published by the author, Via Tesserete 51, Switzerland, 1975.

Butler, R, Jr: Cardiopulmonary Resuscitation (CPR), *Newsletter of the Florida Chiropractic Association*, February 1978.

Cailliet, R: *Soft Tissue Pain and Disability*, Philadelphia, F.A. Davis Company, 1977.

Chun, JJ: Determination of the Anatomical Movers of Human Movement, Biomechanics and Kinesiology in Sports, Colorado Springs, an Olympic Sports Medicine Conference sponsored by the U.S. Olympic Committee, January 1984.

Copass, MK and Eisenberg, MS: *The Paramedic Manual*, Philadelphia, W.B. Saunders Company, 1980.

Costrini, NV and Thomson, WM (eds): *Manual of Medical Therapeutics*, ed 22, Boston, Little, Brown, and Company, 1977.

Craig, TT (ed): Athletic Injuries and First Aid, in *Comments in Sports Medicine*, Chicago, American Medical Association, 1973.

Daube, JR and Sandok, BA: *Medical Neurosciences*, Boston, Little, Brown, and Company, 1978.

Dolan, JP and Holladay, LJ: *First-Aid Management*, ed 4, Danville, IL, Interstate Printers & Publishers, Inc, 1974, chapters 10 and 12.

Faucret, B et al: Determination of Bony Subluxations by Clinical, Neurological and Chiropractic Procedures, *Journal of Manipulative and Physiological Therapeutics*, 1:3, September 1980, pp 165–176.

Fitz-Ritson, D: Therapeutic Traction: A Review of Neurological Principles and Clinical Application, *Journal of Manipulative and Physiological Therapeutics*, 7:1, March 1984, pp 39–48.

Frishberg, BA: Practical Anatomy Laboratory Experiences, Biomechanics and Kinesiology in Sports, Colorado Springs, an Olympic Sports Medicine Conference sponsored by the U.S. Olympic Committee, January 1984.

Gitelman, R et al: The Archives: *An Anthology of Literature Relative to the Science of Chiropractic*, Vol 1, Abstracts; Vol 2, Index; Toronto, Canadian Memorial Chiropractic College, date unknown.

Goldstein, M (ed): *The Research Status of Spinal-Manipulative Therapy*, Monograph No. 15, U.S. Department of Health, Education, and Welfare, Public Health Service, Bethesda, MD, National Institutes of Health, DHEW Publication No. (NIH) 76-998, 1975.

Good, AB: Spinal Joint Blocking, *Journal of Manipulative and Physiological Therapeutics*, 6:1, March 1985, pp 1–7.

Goodheart, GJ: Reactive Muscle Patterns in Athletes, Biomechanics and Kinesiology in Sports, Colorado Springs, an Olympic Sports Medicine Conference sponsored by the U.S. Olympic Committee, January 1984.

Guyton, AC: *Medical Physiology*, 4th ed, Philadelphia, W.B. Saunders, 1971, p 557.

Hains, G: *Post-Traumatic Neuritis*, published by the author, Trois-Rivieres, Quebec, Canada, 1978.

Haldeman, S: Referred Pain: Extra Spinal Symptoms of Spinal Origin, *The Texas Chiropractor*, July 1974.

Hill, LL: *Parameters of Physiotherapy Modalities*, class notes, Lombard, IL, National Chiropractic College, date not shown.

Hirata, I, Jr: *The Doctor and the Athlete*, ed 2, Philadelphia, J.B. Lippincott Company, 1974, chapters 7, 21.

Hirschberg, G., et al: Rehabilitation, Philadelphia, J.B. Lippincott Company, 1964.

Hirschy, LD: Utilization of TENS in Conjunction with Chiropractic Methodology in the Treatment of Acute and Chronic Pain, *Ortho-Briefs*, ACA Council on Orthopedics, April 1984, pp 23–29.

Irving, RE: Pain and the Protective Reflex Generators: Relevance to the Chiropractic Concept of Spinal Subluxation, *Journal of Manipulative and Physiological Therapeutics*, 4:2, June 1981, pp 69–71.

Iversen, LD and Clawson, DK: *Manual of Acute Orthopaedic Therapeutics*, Boston, Little, Brown, and Company, 1977, chapters 1–4, 6.

Jahn, WT: Stress Fractures, Orthopedic Brief, ACA Council on Chiropractic Orthopedics, January 1985.

Janse, J: The Intergrative Purpose and Function of the Nervous System: A Review of Classical Literature, *Journal of Manipulative and Physiological Therapeutics*, Vol 1, No 3, September 1978.

Jaquet, P: *An Introduction to Clinical Chiropractic*, ed 2, published by the author, Grounauer, Geneva, Switzerland, 1976.

Jaskoviack, PA and Schafer, RC: *Applied Physiotherapy*, prepublication manuscript, Arlington, VA, American Chiropractic Association, scheduled to be released in 1986.

Johnson, AC: *Chiropractic Physiological therapeutics*, published by the author, Palm Springs, CA, 1977.

Judge, RD and Zuidema, GD (eds): *Methods of Clinical Examination: A Physiological Approach*, ed 3, Boston, Little, Brown and Company, 1968.

Kaesberg, NT: *One Doctor on High Voltage Modalities*, Belleville, IL, Erwin Printing Company, 1979.

Kennedy, WJ: Medical Aspects of Sports for the School-Age Athlete, in Haycock, CE (ed): *Sports Medicine for the Athletic Female*, Oradell, NJ, Medical Economics, 1980.

Korr, LM: The Spinal Cord as Organizer of Disease Processes: Some Preliminary Perspectives, *Journal of the American Osteopathic Association*, September 1976.

Kraus, H: Evaluation and Treatment of Muscle Function in Athletic Injury, *American Journal of Surgery*, vol 98, September 1959.

Krusen, FH et al: *Handbook of Physical Medicine and Rehabilitation*, ed 2, Philadelphia, W.B. Saunders Company, 1971.

Leon, AS: Cardiovascular Considerations, in Haycock, CE (ed): *Sports Medicine for the Athletic Female*, Oradell, NJ, Medical Economics, 1980.

Levy, AM: Medical Illness, in Haycock, CE (ed): *Sports Medicine for the Athletic Female*, Oradell, NJ, Medical Economics, 1980.

Lowe, JC: Calcium, Magnesium, and Muscle Spasms, *The Chiropractic Family Physician*, ACA Council on Diagnosis and Internal Disorders, 3:6, September 1981, pp 18, 20–21.

Lucy, JM, et al: New Developments in Cardiopulmonary Resuscitation, *ACA Journal of Chiropractic*, February 1981.

MacBryde, CM and Blacklow, RS: *Signs and Symptoms*, ed 5, Philadelphia, J.B. Lippincott Company, 1970.

Markovich, SE: Painful Neuro-Muscular Dysfunction Syndromes in the Head: A Neurologist's View, presented at the American Academy of Cranio-Mandibular Orthopedics Meeting, New Orleans, September 1976.

Mayer, DJ and Price, DD: Central Nervous System Mechanisms of Analgesia, *Pain*, 2:279–404, 1976.

Melzack, R and Wall, P: Pain Mechanisms: A New Theory, *Science*, 150:971, 1975.

Mennell, JMcM: Spray-and-Stretch Treatment for Myofascial Pain, *Hospital Physician*, December 1973.

Miller, GF: Clinical Evaluation and Treatment of Common Musculoskeletal Disorders, *ACA Journal of Chiropractic*, April 1963.

Morehead, JJ and Ludlum, WD, Jr: Traumatic Surgery, in *The Cyclopedia of Medicine, Surgery and Specialities*, Philadelphia, F.A. Davis Company, 1948.

Naval Educational and Training Support Command, *Standard First Aid Training Course*, NAVEDTRA 10081-C, SN 0502-LP-050-4060, Washington, DC US Printing Office, 1978.

Nielsen, AJ: Spray and Stretch for Myofascial Pain, *Physical Therapy*, Vol 58, No 5, May 1978, pp 567–569.

Pottenger, FM: *Symptoms of Visceral Disease*, St. Louis, C.V. Mosby Company, 1953.

Reddy, MP: Peripheral Nerve Entrapment Syndromes, *American Family Physician*, 28:5, November 1983, pp 133–143.

Reiter, L: Apophyseal Joint Functional Anatomy and Experimental Findings: A Literature Review, *PCC Research Form*, 1:2, Winter 1985, pp 49–52.

Ryan, AJ and Allmann, FL (eds): *Sports Medicine*, New York, Academic Press, 1974.

Sandman, KB: Myofascial Pain Syndromes: Their Mechanism, Diagnosis and Treatment, *Journal of Manipulative and Physiological Therapeutics*, 4:3, September 1981, pp 135–139.

Schafer, RC (ed): Basic *Chiropractic Paraprofessional Manual*, Des Moines, 1A, American Chiropractic Association, 1978.

Schafer, RC (ed): *Basic Chiropractic Procedural Manual*, ed 3, Des Moines, IA, American Chiropractic Association, 1980, chapter X.

Schafer, RC (ed): *Chiropractic Physical and Spinal Diagnosis*, Oklahoma City, OK, American Chiropractic Academic Press, 1980, chapters II, IV, V.

Schafer, RC: *Symptomatology and Differential Diagnosis*, Arlington, VA, American Chiropractic Association, 1985.

Siegele, D: The Gate Control Theory, *American Journal of Nursing*, March 1974.

Simons, DG: Myofascial Triggerpoints: A Need for Understanding, *Archives of Physical Medicine and Rehabilitation*, Vol 62, March 1981.

Sola, AE: Myofascial Trigger Point Therapy, *Medical Times*, January 1982, pp 70–77.

Snyder, D: Chiropractic on the Field, *Journal of Clinical Chiropractic*, Special Edition: Athletic Injuries, Vol 1, No 6, 1974.

Speransky, AD: *A Basis for the Theory of Medicine*, translated by CP Dutt, New York, International Publishers, 1943.

Travell, J: Basis for the Multiple Uses of Local Block of Somatic Trigger Areas, *Mississippi Valley Medical Journal*, 71, January 1949, pp 13–21.

Travell, J: Referred Pain from Skeletal Muscle, *New York State Journal of Medicine*, February 1, 1955.

Travell, J: Myofascial Trigger Points: Clinical View, in Bonica JJ and Albe-Fessard, D (eds): *Advances in Pain Research and Therapy*, Vol 1, New York, Raven Press, 1976.

Turek, SL: *Orthopaedics: Principles and Their Application*, ed 3, Philadelphia, J.B. Lippincott Company, 1977.

US Department of the Air Force: *Physical Therapy Technician*, AF Manual 160-21, Washington, DC, US Government Printing Office, 1977.

US Department of the Army: *Army Medical Department Handbook of Nursing*, Washington, DC, US Government Printing Office, No. 008-020-00336, 1970.

Vazuka, FA: *Essentials of the Neurological Examination*, Philadelphia, Smith, Kline, & French Laboratories, 1962.

Voss, DE et al: Traction and Approximation, *Proprioceptive Neuromuscular Facilitation: Patterns and Techniques*, 3rd edition, Harper & Row, Philadelphia, 1985, pp 294–314.

Wallis, C: Unlocking Pain's Secrets, *Time*, June 11, 1984, pp 58–66.

Watkins, RJ: Monitoring Subluxation Inter-relationship, *The Journal of Clinical Chiropractic*, date unknown.

Wilkins, RW and Levinsky, NG: Medicine: *Essentials of Clinical Practice*, Boston, Little, Brown and Company, 1978.

Williams, JGP and Sperryn, PN (eds): *Sports Medicine*, ed 2, Baltimore, Williams & Wilkins, 1976, chapters, 7, 14, 15, 26.

Zimmermann, M.: Physiological Mechanisms in Chronic Pain, in *Pain and Society*, report of Dahlem Workshop, Berlin, November 1979, Verlong, Chemic Weinbeim and Deerfield Park, Florida, Basle, 1980, pp 283–298.

Part 4

INJURY CASE MANAGEMENT

CHAPTER 19

Head and Facial Injuries

Potentially fatal injuries in athletics are almost exclusively confined to the head, neck, and vital organs, and they demand great diagnostic skill and clinical judgment. Other musculoskeletal injuries are easy to diagnose in comparison. Any physician, regardless of specialty, may be faced with the problem of initially caring for such cases; thus it is vital to have knowledge of at least the general principles involved in cranial trauma.

TRAUMA TO THE HEAD AND SCALP

All head injuries are potentially dangerous, not only because of the immediate tissue damage and increased susceptibility to infection, but also because of the probability that some vital area or special sense is or will become involved. Orderly analysis of the skull is imperative after any severe injury to the head presenting suspicious clinical symptoms. Except for minor injuries, orthopedic or neurologic consultation should be sought.

Head and neck injuries comprise the third highest incidence in sports-related trauma. Probably the most dangerous accidents in sports are those of head injuries—the primary killer in competitive sports. They have insidious beginnings and disastrous potential.

Assessment of Head Injuries

Begin by noting the shape of the patient's head, facial bones, teeth, etc. Check the scalp for lacerations, lumps, and depressions. Look for "battle signs" such as blood or cerebrospinal fluid flowing from the ear, blood behind the ear drum, ecchymosis over the mastoid process, and possible basal skull fracture. Seek signs in the face of swelling, edema, cyanosis, bleeding, and lesions. In adults, auscultate the flow of blood over the carotid, temporal, suboccipital, and parietal areas, and the eyeballs. Auscultate the pa-

tient's skull as he says "99" (green-joint sign). Percuss the head for areas of tenderness and "cracked pot" sound. Evaluate signs of anxiety, lid malfunction or puffiness, mouth breathing, unilateral facial palsy, tongue protrusion deviation, skin color, and abnormal movements of the head and face. Check lips and mouth for color, lesions, edema, and bleeding. Unless signs warn against it, have the patient carefully flex, extend, and rotate the head, and note special limitations of neck motion. Then examine each of the 12 cranial nerves according to the standard tests.

Particular concern should be given to the state of consciousness, pupil size, muscles, vital and localizing signs.

State of Consciousness

The patient may appear dazed, stunned, drowsy, irritable, irrational, or delirious. For this purpose, certain descriptive adjectives should be used, as appropriate, to define the state of consciousness observed:

1. The *conscious* patient is alert and oriented in time and space.

2. The *confused* patient is alert but disoriented and excited, presenting some coherent conversation. The disorientation and excitement, which are not in keeping with the total situation, may be temporary and have a psychologic basis in addition to or instead of brain injury. The confused patient is often irritable, impatient, angry. He may refuse to talk or cooperate.

3. A *somnolent* patient is excessively drowsy, but responds to stimulation.

4. A *semiconscious* patient responds to painful stimuli but makes no spontaneous movements. For the purpose of taking fluid, the semiconscious patient should be considered unconscious.

5. *Irrationality*, which usually precedes delirium, is characterized by loquaciousness and belligerence. Blunt forehead trauma may be sufficient to injure the frontal lobes

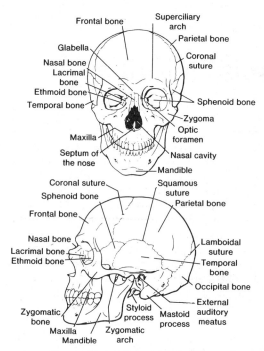

Figure 19.1. Bones of the skull.

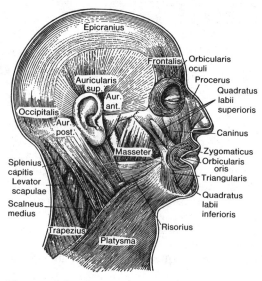

Figure 19.2. Superficial muscles of the head and neck.

of the brain and cause marked behavioral changes, irritability, and seizures (rare).

6. *Delirium* is a state of extreme irrational unrest which often follows unconsciousness. The delirious patient is irritable, aggressive, and noisy.

7. *Stupor* is a borderline state from which a patient may sink into coma or enter when recovering from coma. In stupor, there are few sensible answers obtained; but the patient will often respond to simple forceful commands.

8. In *coma*, the patient does not respond to a stimulus; he is unconscious in the usual sense.

Pupil Size and Visual Disturbances

Unequal pupils indicate possible brain injury. Dilation of pupils in the presence of strong light indicates central nervous sytem impairment. When neither eye is obviously injured and the pupils are of unequal size, brain impairment should be assumed until proven otherwise. Posttraumatic strabismus and diplopia are also indicative of brain damage, as are signs of possible visual field defects.

Muscles

The musculature on one or both sides of the face may droop due to lack of stimulation through the cranial nerves serving the facial muscles. There may be loss or impairment of speech. Paralysis and lack of firmness in the muscle mass of any part or region where there is no damage in the part nor suspicion of spinal cord damage are presumptive evidence of impairment of the brain area offering motor control.

Vital Signs

Temperature, blood pressure, and respiration are especially important in head injuries because changed indices frequently indicate the onset of complications. When signs of shock appear, they suggest that inapparent injuries may be present such as hidden abdominal or thoracic bleeding. Pyrexia of 38°C or over, developing a few hours after injury, indicates primary damage to the thermoregulating mechanism; usually other signs of a midbrain lesion (decerebrate rigidity) are present. Hyperpyrexia developing at a later date is probably due to hematoma or infection. Rapid respiration associated with restlessness accompanies intracranial hemorrhage. Stertorous breathing with the cheeks puffing in and out usually indicates an advanced stage of cerebral compression.

Localizing Signs and Symptoms

These may include speech difficulties which suggest a lesion of the parietal lobe and/or adjacent areas of the frontal, occipital, and temporal lobes. Nasal speech is indicative of palatal paralysis; slurred speech, upper or lower motor lesions; irregular explosive speech, cerebellar involvement. Personality changes suggest involvement of the prefrontal region of the frontal lobe. Loss of memory for recent events and disturbances in recognition of sounds and their significance suggest a temporal lobe lesion. Visual disturbances of recognition relate to the occipital lobe. Difficulty of movement with spastic paralysis and/or hypertonicity and rigidity of the contralateral side imply a lesion of the precentral gyrus and adjacent frontal gyri. Disturbances of recognition of ordinary sensations suggest postcentral gyrus lesions. Vasomotor and autonomic disturbances appear with lesions of the hypothalamus. Severe, intractable, poorly localized pain appears with thalamic lesions.

Mechanisms of Injury

Injury to the craniocerebral mass results from compression (compaction), tension (stretching or tearing), or shear (sliding). In acceleration injuries, the brain is damaged by sudden contact with bony prominences; and a pressure wave transverses the skull with the highest pressure at the point of impact and a negative pressure (cavitation) occurs directly opposite the point of impact. Deceleration injuries result when a moving head strikes a fixed object. Rotation injuries occur from hyperflexion, hyperextension, lateral flexion, and rotational movements that produce shearing forces in the brain with tissue tearing.

Velocity Vs Momentum Forces

In blunt blows and falls involving the head, it is less the velocity than the momentum of forces impacted to the skull and brain which determines the severity and type of brain injury. Velocity determines the type of fracture involved. The position of the head and the changes of the brain relative to the skull are determined by momentum. Most blows and falls involving the head produce complex movements (linear and rotational) in brain position as it is jerked around and twisted within its fluid bath within its bony encasement. Severe traction is produced at any point of fixation. The most damaging effects are produced by the rotational (shearing) stresses. An associated neck injury is presumed until it is ruled out.

Major Vs Minor Head Injury

Major trauma within the skull essentially includes brain contusions and lacerations, nerve damage, compound skull fractures, and hemorrhage or edema within the closed space. Bleeding is rarely a problem in open head wounds; most will be from superficial vessels. If brain tissue is exposed, it should be covered with a sterile pad, and no attempt should be made to push it back into the skull. Fixed dilated pupils and respiratory impairment suggest a dire prognosis.

Treatment is the specialty of the neurosurgeon. Once major head injury is an evidence, immediate transport by stretcher and ambulance to the nearest hospital is indicated for detailed diagnosis, management of shock, and surgical care. Stretcher transportation, in cases of head injury, should be made with the patient's head and upper body slightly raised.

Fortunately, instances of major head injury are rare as compared to the effects of accumulated minor trauma to the head. Minor impacts resulting in variable degrees of stuns, black-out, and headache are often the responsibility of the team or family doctor who must recognize the potential dangers and noxious signs and symptoms. While loss of consciousness or posttraumatic headache are common in contact sports and do not represent diagnostic significance in themselves, they do offer a starting point for observation and thorough investigation.

Degrees of Injury

Mild head injuries do not usually give rise to unconsciousness, cranial nerve palsies, or focal contusion. If the injury is a little more severe, the patient feels momentarily dazed and may have a headache for some hours thereafter but, as a rule, suffers no other ill effects. Relatively trivial injuries can also produce disproportionately severe symptoms in patients who have had previous trauma to the head. With more severe injuries, consciousness is lost instantly. Respirations may cease, and all reflexes are lost. Within a few seconds, breath returns but unconsciousness continues. This stage may last minutes or days and may be followed by deepening coma and a rise in blood pressure or by a phase of cerebral irritability from blood in the cerebrospinal fluid. Seizures may occur. In the absence of massive intracranial bleeding, deepening coma usually means increasing intracranial swelling impairing cerebral circulation. A return of consciousness features irritability, confusion, disorientation, and a degree of amnesia.

Closed Skull Wounds

Except for a possible bruise or contusion, there is no obvious external damage in closed wounds. Injury may be to the brain itself or to the pia or arachnoid meninges. Rupture of blood vessels in the pia is particularly important in closed injury. Blood spilled onto brain cells is a foreign substance that disturbs the functioning of these tissues, and blood collecting within the cranium exerts pressure against the brain. If there is no skull fracture or if skull fracture is such that the integrity of the dura is not disturbed, the cranium is unyielding. If the skull is depressed or displaced inwardly, it may exert direct pressure on brain tissues even without formation of a hematoma. Frequently, a fall upon the back of the head will cause much more internal damage than a blow to the anterior head.

Symptoms of Closed Head Injuries

Headache, nausea, dizziness, and loss of consciousness (which may be brief, intermittent, or extended) often accompany a closed head injury, depending upon the particular injury and its severity. If injury is from impact with a blunt surface (common in sports), an elevated contusion forms when blood and other fluids collect in a pocket in the subcutaneous tissue between the skin and the skull. There may be a fracture in which part of the skull is displaced inwardly.

In the more severe injuries, vomiting and paralysis of some muscle groups may occur. The patient may bleed from the nose, mouth, or ears in the absence of obvious injury to these parts. Cerebrospinal fluid coming from the nose or ears indicates a grave injury. Normally clear cerebrospinal fluid becomes cloudy when mixed with small quantities of blood. Signs of increasing intracranial pressure include elevated blood pressure, slow pulse, restlessness, dilation of one or both pupils, decreased respiration, cyanosis, delirium or irritability, and paralysis. Unless a surgeon is available soon to relieve pressure by opening the skull, increasing respiratory failure, heart failure, and death may be expected.

Contusions and Lacerations

Scalp Injury

Scalp contusions are apt to be circumscribed or localized (producing a hematoma of the scalp) and sometimes accompanied by brain concussion. A depressed skull fracture may be falsely suspected because most of these blood pools are depressible in the center and offer the sensation of indentation of the skull. In scalp lacerations associated with compound fractures, the prevention of sepsis leading to meningitis is the principle aim in emergency care.

Cerebral Injury

Cerebral contusion is a bruising of the brain that is difficult to distinguish from concussion unless it is to the degree that there is an increase in intracranial pressure. Contralateral localizing signs are usually seen opposite the bruise or hematoma. If the bruise is situated on the same side of paralysis, there is the possibility of contrecoup injury.

In definite injury to the surface of the brain, edema and ecchymosis with loss of function of the area involved result. Shock is commonly associated, unconsciousness and amnesia are more prolonged, and headache is more severe in the acute stage. Disorientation and mild confusion are usually exhibited and may exist for many hours or days following injury. General or focal convulsions may be present, and paresis or paralysis of the cranial nerves or extremities are seen, depending upon the area of the brain involved. Giddiness and transient postural unsteadiness may be seen. Intracranial pressure is usually increased, and the spinal fluid is blood-tinged. Blood in spinal fluid interferes with the circulation and absorption, encouraging mechanical hydrocephalus, confusion, and increased headache. In severe cases, a permanent intellectual defect may persist, varying from minor memory failure to profound dementia.

Cerebral laceration often follows severe trauma, particularly contracoup injuries. Shock is almost always present, confusion and disorientation are severe, wild restlessness is pronounced, and deep stupor may prevail. General muscle flaccidity and loss of sphincter control are common. Marked neurologic changes are characterized by abnormal reflexes, pupillary changes, paralysis, aphasia, and cranial nerve disorders. Other features include respiratory irregularity, increased pulse pressure, slow pulse, fever, meningismus, possible convulsions, bloody spinal fluid, increased intracranial pressure, slow return to consciousness, prolonged headache, and amnesia.

Emergency Treatment of Head Wounds

Assure an open airway, and keep the patient's vital signs carefully monitored. Prevent or treat shock, but do not put the patient in the head-low position. Control bleeding and protect the wound with a sterile dressing. Do not remove or disturb any foreign material which may be in the wound.

Cranial Hemorrhage and Hematoma

The dura mater of an adult does not adhere to the entire skull. Thus it is possible for fluid to be forced between the cranium and the dura, and the increased pressure tends to dislodge attached dura from its points of skull connection. As branches of the middle meningeal artery nourish both the dura and the surrounding bone of the skull, if torn, bleeding forms between the skull and the dura and forms an extradural hematoma. It is controversial whether this condition is commonly associated with trauma: opinions vary from frequently to rarely. Intracerebral hemorrhage can be associated with either extradural or subdural

hematoma, or it may be the sole lesion. Lateralizing signs are usually absent.

Extradural Hemorrhage   *Epidural*

Extradural hematoma results when a fracture tears the middle meningeal artery. It features early but brief unconsciousness, followed by drowsiness, headache, vomiting, and hemiparesis. Immediate surgical intervention is required. Extradural hematoma is suspected by hematoma of the temporalis muscle, gradual onset of hemiplegia, deepening coma, Hutchinson's pupils, and a lucid interval.

The common picture is a patient who has received a head injury, suffered a momentary loss of consciousness followed by complete or partial recovery. This *lucid interval* of recovery may last from a few hours to 2 days. Then, rather abruptly, a focal convulsion or rapidly progressing stupor, slow pulse and respirations, unilateral pupillary dilation, and weakness of face and extremities offer evidence of a localized and expanding lesion. This important lucid interval is sometimes obliterated if the initial injury causes prolonged unconsciousness.

A characteristic feature of an extradural hematoma is the appearance of paralysis of the arm, leg, and face on the contralateral side of the lesion. The semiconscious patient will not respond to supraorbital pressure on the affected side. When hemiplegia is suspected, corroborating signs must be sought such as increased deep reflexes, absent abdominal reflexes, and positive Babinski. In early cases, the arm is more affected than the leg. In cases of intracranial hemorrhage, Babinski's sign is most significant and the one most frequently present. It usually denotes a hematoma on the opposite side of the brain. Aphasia may be the first lateralizing sign in a left side lesion in a right-handed person. Broca's area usually is on the left side.

Subdural Hemorrhage

Subdural hemorrhages are caused by a rupture of the bridging veins crossing the space between the dura and the arachnoid and are characterized by headaches, drowsiness, poor concentration, mild confusion, progressively decreasing level of consciousness, and motor deficits (eg, hemiparesis). These symptoms may be immediate or delayed for weeks or months after injury. Although larger in size than an extradural hemorrhage, a subdural hemorrhage is confined unilaterally because the dura is firmly fixed to the falx between the hemispheres.

Acute subdural hematoma is the most frequent cause of death in sports injuries. Unconsciousness is the major physical sign. This is much more common than extradural hematoma and shows no lucid interval. Lateralizing signs are similar. Inequality of pupils (anisocoria) is of considerable localizing value. Hutchinson's pupil from compression of the 3rd cranial nerve against the free edge of the tentorium is often seen. Frequent examinations of the pupil are mandatory. Widely dilated and fixed pupils bilaterally indicate that death is near.

Severe acute subdural hemorrhage is usually associated with cerebral laceration. Symptoms include pronounced and progressive headache, drowsiness, stupor, epileptic attacks, temperature increase, reduced pulse and respiratory rates, increased pulse pressure, progressive contralateral paralysis, sphincter relaxation, severe shock, and coma. Bleeding from the brain itself seeps into the subdural space, adding to probable dura, pia, and arachnoid bleeding.

In the late stage, signs of herniation and oculomotor paralysis appear. The incidence is high in the elderly because cortical atrophy increases the space in which the veins must traverse. The incidence is also high in boxers, other contact-sport athletes, and alcoholics because of increased head trauma.

Differentiation

Differentiation between hematoma and a depressed fracture is made by evaluating the edges of the lesion. The edges are usually smooth in hematoma and the circumference is rather regular. In depressed fractures, the edges are usually rough, irregular, and sloping. Careful pressure over a hematoma will ordinarily push aside any central indentation; but in fracture, no such shifting of the depression occurs. Roentgenography, however, offers the only reliable evidence.

In cerebral contusion or laceration, weakness or paralysis of the face or extremities appears immediately after injury and increases very little if at all. Thus, this time of findings and lack of progression are an important differentiation from an intra- or extradural hemorrhage.

Extradural and subdural hematomas may be associated with either opened or closed head wounds and possible fractures. For example, a hematoma discovered in the temporal area suggests possible temporal fracture with meningeal artery laceration and associated epidural hematoma.

Cranial Concussion

Cerebral concussion is a syndrome in which there is an immediate impairment or neural function following a blow to the head which may result in disturbances of consciousness, memory faults, visual disorders, or equilibrium problems. It is the most common injury to the brain following a cranial blow.

Concussion is defined as an essentially transient state due to head injury which has an instant onset, manifests widespread purely paralytic (flaccid) symptoms without neurologic evidence of gross brain injury, and is always followed by a degree of transient unconsciousness and amnesia for the

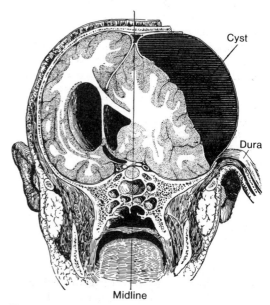

Figure 19.3. Diagrammatic cross–section of brain showing relative size and position of subdural hematoma resulting from head injury; also mechanical effects produced upon ventricular system.

actual moment of the accident. The degree of posttraumatic amnesia appears to be a guide to the severity of the concussion. The spinal fluid is always clear, and intracranial pressure is rarely elevated. Headache is often the sole posttraumatic complaint, but shallow breathing, pallor, feeble pulse, reduced reflexes, and other signs of surgical shock may result. The period of short-duration unconsciousness after concussion is attributed to the momentary compression of brain capillaries resulting in cerebral ischemia/anemia. Any prolonged period of unconsciousness or inequality in pupil size indicates the need for neurologic consultation.

Pure concussion is rare. Most head injuries are accompanied by some degree of brain injury with a reaction similar to injury found in other tissues. Edema and congestion occur that are coupled with a moderate rise in cerebral venous pressure, although the cerebrospinal fluid may be clear. Unconsciousness may be prolonged, memory loss more pronounced, and reflex changes and even convulsions may manifest (especially in children).

Grades of Cerebral Concussion

Cerebral concussion produces a temporary disturbance in brain function that is not the result of overt structural damage. Schneider classifies the severity of a cerebral concussion syndrome into three major groups:

1. First-degree concussion. This mild form of cerebral concussion features slight mental confusion and possible trauma-related memory loss, tinnitus, and dizziness. There is no unsteadiness, lack of coordination, gait deficit, or loss of consciousness. Recovery appears to occur within minutes, but such postconcussion symptoms as headaches, inability to concentrate, and photophobia may persist for 1–2 weeks.

2. Second-degree concussion. This moderate type of cerebral concussion is characterized by a loss of consciousness up to 4 minutes that is followed by (1) a loss of memory for the immediate events that led up to the injury; (2) transient mental confusion and disorientation; and, most likely, (3) degrees of dizziness, tinnitus, and unsteadiness. Recovery appears to occur within 24 hours, but residual symptoms may persist for several weeks.

3. Third-degree concussion. This severe form of cerebral concussion exhibits a loss of consciousness over 5 minutes that is followed by prolonged retrograde amnesia, marked unsteadiness, and severe confusion, disorientation, dizziness, and tinnitus. Recovery is much slower than that seen with first- and second-degree syndromes, and residual symptoms may persist as long as a few months.

Cranial Impact in Sports

In most cranial impacts, the injury forces result from acceleration, deceleration, or compression of the head or a combination of these factors. The nonyielding plastic suspension football helmet has done much to reduce cranial injuries in football, but at the same time it has created an effective battering ram. A. C. Larcher, DC, who has developed and patented several excellent types of athletic equipment designed to reduce injury, describes the effect of cranial collision in football essentially as follows:

• The sudden setting of the head (acceleration) or stopping of the head (deceleration) may result in the generation of intracranial pressures and intracranial lesions such as hemorrhages, contusions, and concussions.

• The lines of force, or energy, of impact are transmitted through the vault and base of the cranial cavity, and should a fracture develop as the result of impact, serious subdural or extradural hematomas may occur. At the moment of great traumatic impact, the skull is pressed against the brain and this may cause contusions of the meninges and brain, especially if the head is held firmly and cannot roll. Should the head be free a fraction of a second after the impact, the momentum of the blow throws the brain forcibly against the skull opposite the point of impact. If an artery is not torn, it may be stretched and weakened to an extent to cause aneurysm and probable stroke.

• A blow on the posterior region of the skull causes contrecoup contusions on the tips of the frontal and temporal lobes when the brain is forced against the irregular bone of the anterior and middle cranial fossae. If the sharp sphenoid ridge is struck by the brain in contrecoup injury, injury to the meningeal artery that passes through the sphenoid is likely, resulting in an extradural hematoma.

• Response to any severe injury causes edema and hemorrhage or both. This means an increase in the size of the brain within a bony cavity of limited size and hence an increase in intracranial pressure.

Hirata of the University of South Carolina feels that by the time he arrives on the field at the side of an injured player (20–30 seconds), if the player is awake, able to think and answer questions, recognize others, and follow instructions, the player has not had a true concussion. A slight tap on the side of the face of a dazed player often results in arousal. If cranial nerve tests shown normality, careful questioning receives rational answers, and responsibilities in play are alertly discussed, a return to action (under careful observation) can be made after a short rest. On the other hand, if the player is disoriented 20–30 seconds after impact, he can be considered to have had a degree of concussion. This requires restriction from play for 1–10 days wherein neurologic tests, vital signs, and subjective complaints are carefully monitored. Return to play can be made only after clinical signs are normal, the player is completely free of headache, and verbal-congnitive responses are normal. Skull films and cerebrospinal taps are never routinely ordered.

The typical athlete will shortly recover consciousness after a "knock out." There will be no retrograde headache, vomiting, or abnormal neurologic signs. Still, such a player should be accompanied home, be strongly advised to go to bed immediately, and seek follow-up examination the next day. Any player that must be carried from the field or ring deserves hospitalized observation and neurologic evaluation for at least a day or two.

The Punch-Drunk Syndrome

Cumulative head trauma results in many boxers who fight professionally or as sparring partners for 5 years or more. It is expressed as the punch-drunk syndrome and sometimes referred to as dementia puglistica or progressive posttraumatic encephalopathy. Bowermann describes the early symptoms as mental confusion and slight unsteadiness of gait. Progressively, the individual may develop leg dragging, jerky responses, hesitant and slurred speech, hand tremors, head nodding, expressionless facial features of Parkinsonism, vertigo, deafness, euphoria or aggressiveness, and finally, marked mental deterioration. More than half of all boxers with 5 years experience or more develop some degree of mental and emotional changes obvious to close associates. The syndrome may be either cerebellar or extrapyramidal oriented.

On autopsy of such an individual, the hippocampus may show senile plaques, changes within its vessels, neuron degeneration (Alzheimer's), decreased cortical neurons, subarachonoidal adhesions, increased gliosis, an encysted hematoma, frontal lobe atrophy, many aged extradural and extra-arachnoid clots, fibrous thickening and localized scarring, defects in the deep layers of the septum pellucidum, and possible thrombosis of the superior longitudinal sinus and its parietal afferents. Headache and vomiting are early signs of chronic inflammation and thickening of any of the three brain coverings (pachymeningitis).

While the point of impact in boxing may be the chin, the greatest damage is probably produced by concussive forces transmitted to the area of the brain stem at the base of the skull. This is also true with blows to the side of the head which result in a sharp lateral or rotational shearing near the atlanto-occipital joint. With a knock-out blow to the head, brain damage may result from the blow itself or just as easily and more seriously from the fall to the floor or canvas. Subdural hemorrhage, areas of diffuse small hemorrhages within the brain, cerebral edema, and/or thrombosis of superficial and deep vessels may result.

The above findings are the opinion of most authorities. However, Kaplan, who for many years conducted pre- and postfight electroencephalographic studies of boxers for the New York State Athletic Commission, feels that the "punch-drunk" syndrome is a myth. He states that more than 6,000 EEG records on boxers (many repeat recordings over several years) show no changes of altered brain electrical activity to suggest any degree of diffuse petechial brain hemorrhage. Other EEG studies of boxers have shown that interval alpha-rhythm increases do not persist after 4 minutes following a fight. However, if persistent focal changes do occur on EEG graphs (eg, incipient epilepsy signs), boxing should be permanently banned for the athlete.

Posttraumatic Cranial Signs and Symptoms

A team physician should be especially cognizant of those clinical signs that indicate progressively deteriorating brain malfunction, a state requiring immediate emergency action. These signs include:

- Increasingly severe headache
- Disorientation
- Nausea and vomiting
- Unequal pupil size
- Speech impairment
- Gradually falling pulse rate
- Gradually rising blood pressure
- Deepening state of unconsciousness

Such signs mandate immediate hospitalization because hourly observation is necessary for at least 24 hours. This means that (1) the patient must be talked with for a few minutes every hour (day and night) to ascertain any signs of progressive thought, speech, or memory deficit and (2) the vital signs must be closely monitored. Such precautions, which on the surface may appear extreme in some cases, may mean the difference between life and death.

Skull Fractures

Carefully palpate the skull and look for small lacerations hidden within the hair. Skull fractures may be divided into two major groups:

1. Linear fractures, whether single or multiple fissures. A subgaleal hematoma may form at the site of injury where the firm clot at the edges of the hematoma and the soft clot at its center may easily simulate a depressed fracture. No treatment except rest and careful observation is usually necessary for a simple linear or multiple fissured fracture of vault or base.

2. Depressed fractures. Be prepared that sometimes the inner table may be depressed and broken inward separately from the other table without leaving a palpable

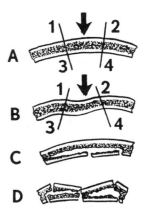

Figure 19.4. Mechanical principles of bending skull fractures. In *A* and *B*, *arrow* shows the direction of force and site of impact. Points *3* and *4* become separated until tensile strength of inner table is overcome. Possible effect on inner table shown in *C*; on both tables, *D*.

defect on the skull. A depressed fracture should always be surgically elevated if it involves the bone over the motor cortex to prevent epilepsy. Slight depressions in young children, prior to ossification of the sutures, will usually spontaneously elevate with the gentle expansion of the cranial contents with each heart beat.

Signs and Symptoms

Although x-ray proof of fracture is important, many fractures are difficult to demonstrate and clinical evidence may be more important. There may be bleeding or leakage of spinal fluid from nose, mouth, or ears; difference in size of pupils; blackening of tissues under the eyes; changes in pulse and respiration that are not necessarily compatible with the blood picture; and paralysis or twitching of muscles. Head and/or neck injury should be suspected in any unconscious person.

A fracture of the temporal area is often associated with deafness and facial nerve injury. Bleeding from the ear with a subcutaneous hemorrhage over and below the mastoid area (*battle sign*) appearing 24–48 hours after injury is highly suspicious of a temporo-occipital fracture at the base of the skull. Periorbital ecchymoses (*raccoon sign*) may indicate a basilar skull fracture. A tight ecchymosis of the eyelids indicates a fracture through the corresponding orbital plate. Rhinorrhea is proof of a fracture through the cribriform plate or into one of the paranasal sinuses in the anterior of middle fossa. Cerebrospinal fluid escaping from the ear signifies a fracture through the temporal bone at the base of the middle fossa.

Roentgenographic Considerations

In film analysis, abnormally lucent (overlapping bony margins) or dense lines (two thicknesses of bone in a focal area) should be sought as both occur with skull fracture. Bright view-box illumination of the scalp margins helps to locate a site of injury and to detect soft-tissue swellings.

The skull is subject to linear fractures which appear on the film as thin black lines with ragged edges that may run in any direction. They must be differentiated from suture lines, diploic veins, and other blood-vessel grooves—all of which have fairly definite courses and smooth margins but are lighter in color. Vascular markings are normally shaped as gentle arcs, while fracture lines appear as straight lines or sharply angled lines that are more lucent than vascular grooves. Fractures split the entire thickness of bone, while vascular grooves occupy only a part of the bone's thickness. Fracture lines may open sutures or follow blood vessel markings, but they can usually be traced beyond the course of these normal lines. A fracture extending through the distribution of the middle meningeal artery can produce epidural hemorrhage within a few hours.

Both dislocation or separation may also occur through suture lines. In adolescents and young adults, suture lines are still present and measure less than 3 mm. Potential arterial or venous bleeding or thrombosis of the dural sinuses may be found at the lamboidal and sagittal sutures. In rare cases, a meningeal cyst may protrude through a dural tear and herniate into a fracture, gradually eroding bony margins and inhibiting healing.

Comminuted and stellate fractures are generally obvious. A depressed fracture offers an appearance of a white line because of the overlapping margins of the break. Fractures of either the outer or inner table appear as thin black lines or areas of slightly irregular density and structure of the bone. A tomogram may be necessary for detection. A basilar skull fracture is the most difficult skull fracture to detect, and most always requires a basal view. It is frequently overlooked.

A slight collection of air (pneumocephalus) progressing along the meningeal margins is a sign of skull fracture seen in roentgenography. The air pocket appears on the film as an area of markedly diminished density (usually frontal).

The pineal gland, located in the central portion of the brain, is calcified in 60% of adults, and it may calcify as early as 6 years. Displacement of this gland, noted on either A-P or lateral views of the skull, may be the only indicator of a hematoma producing structural shifts within the cranium.

Cranial Nerve Injury

The cranial nerves represent a variety of functions and often become involved in combined lesions because of their close proximity to each other. Cranial nerve injuries usually result from and are treated with brain and skull injuries; eg, penetrating wounds often damage the 5th, 7th, 11th, and 12th cranial nerves. Cranial nerve disorders often give clinical evidence of a cranial fracture. The prognosis for functional return is often good, with gradual recovery, because the involved nerve is usually contused rather than severed. If a nerve is severed, repair is difficult if not impossible and prognosis is poor.

Olfactory and Optic Nerve Injury. While accidental injury to the olfactory nerve (1st cranial) is rare, the loss of function which follows first trauma may be prolonged or permanent (rare). Injury to the optic nerve (2nd cranial) is not uncommon. Loss of vision accompanies a fracture through the sphenoid involving the orbital foramen.

Injury to the Oculomotor, Trochlear, and Abducens Nerves. Injury to the 3rd, 4th, or 6th cranial nerves are frequent but seldom persistent. Trochlear paralysis usually indicates a fracture of the petrous ridge.

Facial Palsy. The 7th cranial nerve is occasionally injured in deep neck, jaw, and mastoid wounds. Facial palsy may follow injury. If neurologic examination reveals that the paralysis is peripheral as evidenced by inclusion of forehead muscle palsy, review the history to determine the pathogenesis of symptoms. A facial nerve injury frequently indicates a basilar fracture through the facial canal. A blow striking the front of the ear may cause swelling in the parotid gland with consequent 7th nerve involvement. In such cases, improvement is usually slow but complete. Patients with central facial paralysis, as shown by absence of forehead-muscle palsy, have suffered injury to the corticobulbar pathways. Here, outlook is less favorable. Paralysis of half the face rarely interferes with performance in itself, but weakness of the obicularis oculi often proves disabling because of the lacrimation, photophobia, and danger of corneal ulceration. The physician should always examine the general motor system to determine the nature and site of the lesion. The not uncommon combination of a Bell's palsy (peripheral) unilaterally with a Babinski sign on the opposite indicates a lesion, usually hemorrhage or edema, in the brain stem near the exit of the 7th cranial nerve.

Injury to the Vestibulocochlear Nerve. Disability of the 8th cranial nerve is computed on the basis of loss of hearing function. Some authorities feel that this nerve is involved in head injuries more frequently than any other (see Table 19.1).

Glossopharyngeal, Vagus, and Accessory Nerve Injury. An occipital injury may tear through the posterior foramen and paralyze the 9th, 10th, and 11th cranial nerves. Injury of the 10th nerve is extremely rare. When seen, it is usually from damage to the recurrent laryngeal branch following neck trauma.

Hypoglossal Nerve. Injury to the 12th cranial nerve is not infrequently seen from fracture. Major signs are deviation of the tongue and difficult speech. Differentiation must be made from involvement of the carotid artery above its bifurcation or an injury to the recurrent nerve of the high vagus.

Prognosis

There are four general signs helpful in determining outcome of brain injury: (1) the degree of initial subnormal temperature and shock, (2) the amount of blood in the cerebrospinal fluid, (3) the degree and length of stupor, and (4) the neurologic signs indicating the amount and location of cranial damage.

The initial examination of an unconscious patient is always unsatisfactory. Pupil size and reaction, however, should be noted. Fixed and dilated pupils present a poor prognosis. A unilaterally dilated pupil usually indicates a unilateral brain lesion and sometimes is more serious than bilaterally dilated pupils. Tendon reflexes and clonus can be noted. Raising the extremities and letting them fall by gravity offers a fair opinion as to comparative limb power and tone. Complete muscular relaxation in all four extremities suggests a widespread injury, as does a bilateral Babinski sign and ankle clonus. The eye grounds exhibit few clues in acute cases.

IMPLICATIONS, COMPLICATIONS, AND SEQUELAE OF HEAD INJURY

Some authorities feel that trivial head injury may have serious sequelae while others insist on objective evidence of organic damage before acknowledging the likelihood of grave results. Some deny the possibility of permanent damage from a head injury with normal neurologic responses, normal spinal fluid, and normal ocular fundi or believe that a really serious injury is rare except in the presence of a fractured skull.

Even the pathogenesis of the sequelae is controversial. Some authorities have found actual cerebral hemorrhage, often gross, as the substratum of the unconsciousness accompanying concussion. Others report hemorrhage in the areas supplied by the terminal vessels, and still others attach major importance to cerebral hydraulics, pointing out that the gnostic areas suffer more than the vital zones because the former are more recent in development, less important, and highly vascularized.

Prognosis is also controversial. Some authorities predict a gloomy outcome from minor injuries, stressing degenerative changes. Others reflect a more hopeful verdict, feeling that only in a small minority of instances do patients have lasting effects from head trauma. A claimant's attorney stresses the serious sequelae as it is impossible to make any infallible estimate of the nature and duration of the sequelae. Convulsions, photophobia, vertigo, weakness, and persistent headaches are sequelae common enough to merit consideration in any

Table 19.1.
Correlated Index to Neurologic and Orthopedic Maneuvers, Reflexes, Signs, or Tests Relative to Sport and Nonsport Cerebellar, Cerebral, and Cranial Nerve Syndromes

CEREBELLAR SYNDROME SIGNS AND PROCEDURES

Andre-Thomas sign	Heel-to-knee test	Pronation-supination test
Finger-to-finger test	Heel-to-toe test	Rebound test
Finger-to-nose test	Homes' sign	Toe-to-finger test
Finger tapping test	Patting test	

CEREBRAL SYNDROME SIGNS AND PROCEDURES

Adie's sign	Glabella reflex	Quinquad's sign
Baillarger's sign	Grasp reflex	Saeneer's sign
Barany's pointing test	Jaw jerk	Setting sun sign
Berger's sign	Kleist's sign	
Fundi signs	MacEwen's sign	

CRANIAL NERVE SYNDROME SIGNS AND PROCEDURES

1. *Olfactory*	6. *Abducens*	9. *Glossopharyngeal*
Odor differentiation	Ballet's sign	Carotid sinus reflex
2. *Optic*	Cantelli's sign	Gag reflex
Consensural reflex	Disconjugate gaze	Laryngoscopic signs
Dazzle reflex	Red glass test	Palatal reflex
Field of vision	7. *Facial*	Swallowing test
Ophthalmoscopic	Chvostek's sign	Taste test (posterior
signs	Consensural reflex	third)
Gunn's sign	Corneal reflex	10. *Vagus*
Pupillary reflex	Facial motion tests	Carotid sinus
Visual acuity	Glabella reflex	flex
3. *Oculomotor*	Jaw jerk	Erben's reflex
Accommodation reflex	Jaw reflex	Gag reflex
Argyll-Robertson's	Taste test (anterior	Nasal speech sign
sign	two-thirds)	Oculocardiac reflex
Arroyo's sign	8. *Auditory Nerve*	Saliva pH test
Ballet's sign	Cochlear Division:	Salivation response
Cantelli's sign	Auditory reflex	Somagyi's reflex
Consensural reflex	Bing's test	11. *Spinal accessory*
Disconjugate gaze	Gelle's test	Active cervical rota- ✓
Gower's sign	Gruber's test	tion test
Pupillary reflex	Otoscopic signs	Cervical range of
Red glass test	Rinne's test	motion test
4. *Trochlear*	Schwabach's test	Shoulder elevation ✓
Ballet's sign	Weber's laterali-	test
Cantelli's sign	zation test	Shoulder posture
Red glass test	Vestibular Division:	evaluation
5. *Trigeminal*	Babinski-Weil's	12. *Hypoglossal*
Bite test	test	Protruding tongue
Consensural reflex	Barany's test	Speech test
Corneal reflex	Caloric test	Tongue tremor sign
Oculocardiac reflex	Cantelli' sign	
Orbicularis reflex	Cochleopapillary	
Sneeze reflex	reflex	
Snout reflex	Mittlemeyer's test	
Zygomatic reflex	Past-pointing tests	

case. Insanity is a rare result (less than 0.01%), and the incidence of transient convulsions from severe head injury is about 4–5%.

The distinguishing features of organic brain damage include (1) *hyperglycemia*, which occurs in the early stages of cerebral injury, thus offering a tentative diagnostic

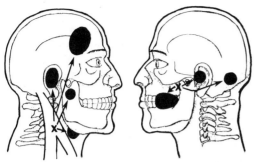

Figure 19.5. *Left*, sternocleidomastoideus trigger point; *X*, common site. *Blackened areas* indicate typical areas of referred pain. *Right*, masseter trigger point.

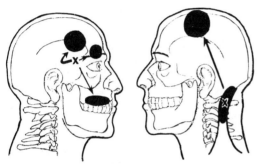

Figure 19.6. *Left*, temporalis trigger point; *X*, common site. *Blackened areas* indicate typical sites of referred pain. *Right*, splenius cervicis trigger point.

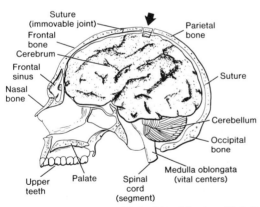

Figure 19.7. View of left side of brain with left side of skull and mandible removed. *Arrow* indicates fracture site.

sign; (2) *pupil inequality*, an important sign; (3) *headache*, when due to cerebral contusion, and characteristically worse on stooping or during excitement; and (4) the

promptness with which the organic signs appear. The absolute criteria of brain injury include bloody spinal fluid, local palsies, and positive x-ray findings.

Headaches

While cranial nerve involvement, weakness, or paralysis frequently follow severe head injury, the most frequent and annoying posttraumatic symptoms are headache and vertigo. These purely subjective complaints are most difficult to judge.

Mechanisms. Six major mechanisms are involved in headaches: traction, distention, inflammation, pressure, spasm, and referred pain or vasomotor dysfunction. There can be traction on veins and displacement of the venous sinuses producing headaches, or traction on or distention of the meningeal arteries and large arteries at the brain base. An inflammatory process or a pressure mass involving any of the pain-sensitive brain structures will result in headache. Spasm of the cranial or cervical muscles will result in headaches quite frequently and often be of a reflex nature.

Chronic or Recurrent Headaches. Chronic or recurrent headaches require a detailed case history. The site of pain is important, as a general rule of thumb holds that pain originating above the tentorium moves across the 5th cranial nerve and is perceived in the forehead, temples, and parietal areas of the skull. Pain that has its origin in the posterior fossa is carried across the 9th cranial and upper cervical nerves and is perceived in the occipital area.

Acute Headaches. Recently acquired headaches may elicit associated symptoms of subdural hematoma, subarachnoic hemorrhage, systemic infection, seizures, and focal nerve deficits lending suspicion to meningismus, meningitis, brain abscess or tumor. Inflammations such as meningitis produce headache by direct involvement of the brain's pain-sensitive structures. The first concern is to see if the headaches are in any way associated with a life-threatening situation. Most life-threatening conditions have a short headache history of acute, severe pain with associated systemic symptoms. Virulent bacterial meningitis is characterized by acute illness, rapid advancing signs of meningeal irritation, and systemic infection. Symptoms are similar in viral meningitis, but the severity of symptoms is less. In granulomatous meningitis, signs of chronic organic disease stand out.

Tension Headaches. Tension headaches, which frequently have an emotional base, are rarely present upon arising but increase in severity as the day progresses and stress accumulates. Two types are seen: the occipital type and the "hat-band" type. The occipital type exhibits severe contraction in the muscles of the neck and scalp which can be palpated and demonstrated in electromyography. Trigger points can often be found in the suboccipital area. During suboccipital spasm, the nerves in the area are vulnerable to irritation from C1 to C2 subluxations. Upper neck pain, stiffness, tension, and tingling in the occipitoparietal region are typically associated. Passive upper cervical stretching reproduces the pain and possibly the paresthesia, and palpation of the area elicits tenderness. Anxiety symptoms and hyperactive deep reflexes are commonly associated. The atlanto-occipital joint is inevitably hypomobile indicating a fixation. Prior to adjustment of the subluxation, Schoenholtz suggests a cold pack under the neck during intermittent traction (30° angle) to help open the posterior facets. In the "hat-band" type with a history of a constriction feeling around the circumference of the scalp, the cause can usually be found in a history of emotional stress. Symptoms of chronic anxiety and/or depression are often found.

Migraine Headaches. In migraine headaches, there is an initial vasoconstriction from amine release that produces prodromal neurological symptoms in 10% of the cases from the ischemia which initiates a period of vasodilation that causes the headache. In regular migraine, the headache is unilateral in onset, occurs early in life, and is frequently associated with a family tendency.

Cluster Headaches. In cluster migraine (Horton's histamine cephalgia), the pain is unilateral, has a nocturnal onset, and is very intense. It begins initially in the temporal-supraorbital area and progresses to the occipital area, or the opposite may appear; occiput to temple. The pain may be so intense that suicide is contemplated. Pain usually lasts 30–90 minutes, reappearing in clusters in from a day or two to several months, then is remiss for several months or years. Cluster headaches are frequently found associated with "silent" peptic ulcers in which the duration of severe pain may be extended to several hours. Such conditions are frequently aggravated by huge consumption of aspirin for relief of pain but which increases the gastritis that is producing the noxious reflex mechanism. Nothing appears to help until the pain runs its course. Medication of any type, even morphine, has little effect; yet treatment to the hidden gastrointestinal fault will often show relief in a short time.

Syncope

Syncope is caused by three main reversible disturbances in cerebral function: (1) transient ischemia, (2) changes in composition of blood in the brain, and (3) changes in central nervous system activity by stimuli entering the central nervous system. When syncope results from arteriolar dilatation, it can be classified into three general types: (1) vasopressor syncope (common faint), (2) carotid sinus depressor reflex, or (3) postural hypotension from some disorder of the sympathetic nervous system.

Although fainting is often a fault of the cardiovascular system, neurogenic syncope is differentiated in that a warning symptom (prodrome) usually precedes the faintness. Coughing or something to elicit orthostatic hypotension may be a precipitating factor. Hysterical syncope is differentiated by the fact that there is no history of injury, and the hysteric will always try to protect himself while falling if at all possible

Vertigo

Vertigo implies a hallucination of turning or rotating either of the self or the surroundings. The fault is often anywhere from the middle ear (semicircular canals, labyrinthitis) to the brain stem through the 8th cranial nerve. Pallor, sweating, and nausea are commonly associated. A related hearing loss or sensitivity to noises points to involvement of both divisions of the vestibulocochlear nerve. Dizziness in sports is often caused simply by anxious overbreathing, which causes reduced blood carbon dioxide that inhibits nutrition of the balancing center.

Dizziness is caused by some vestibular system dysfunction. One or both parts of the system may be involved. The history and examination will help determine the anatomic site of the lesions and the disease process involved. The significance of vertigo cannot be judged until the cause has been determined. It may represent a benign self-limiting condition, or it might represent a life-threatening condition. *Central vertigo* can be traced to one of six major types: (1) vascular (infarcts, postural hypotension plus vascular disease), (2) tumors in cerebellopontine angle, (3) seizures from temporal lobe lesion, (4) multiple sclerosis, (5) trauma (cranial, whiplash), and (6) inflammatory (eg, meningitis). *Peripheral vertigo* is one of five major types: (1) vestibular apparatus lesion (Meniere's disease, benign positional vertigo), (2) peripheral nerve lesion (acoustic neuroma, vestibular neuronitis, diabetic neuropathy), (3) skull fracture and trauma, especially of the temporal bone, (4) vascular (acoustic artery occlusion), and (5) various eye disorders.

The causes of vertigo are head injury, viral labyrinthitis (aural vertigo), lesions of the 8th cranial nerve, lesions of the brain stem, temporal lobe, or cerebellum, disorders of the forebrain (eg, migraine, epilepsy), cerebrovascular disease, psychogenic dizziness (eg, anxiety and hyperventilation syndromes), ocular vertigo, and motion sickness. Many drugs (eg, alcohol, barbiturates) give rise to disequilibrium sensations. Infrequently, a metabolic process such as hypothyroidism may be involved.

Diver's Vertigo. Two uncommon types of vertigo are commonly associated with divers. One is called "whiteout" when a diver cannot see the bottom and becomes disoriented. Closing the eyes during an attack or following air bubbles up helps in reorientation. The second type is that of alternobaric vertigo occurring during a diving ascent, where eustachian tube blockage causes middle-ear pressure buildup.

Meniere's Disease. The vertigo associated with Meniere's disease is almost always associated with a hearing loss, tinnitus, and a peripheral vascular disorder. Neuropathy (eg, diabetic), multiple sclerosis, tumors in the cerebellopontine angle, and temporal masses may be involved. In the elderly patient, vertigo is often associated with vascular insufficiency of the peripheral acoustic artery or secondary to vertebrobasilar disease.

Lewit writes of the relationship of the cervical spine to Meniere's disease (review in *Czechoslovak Medicine*, VII:2, 1961) after 120 cases of Meniere's disease and similar forms of vertigo were sent by leading ear departments of Prague for manipulative treatment. The conclusions reached were "(1) The results of manipulative treatment in Meniere's disease whether there is any noticeable symptomatology from the cervical spine at the same time or not and in cases of vertigo (Barre-Lieou syndrome) are practically the same. (2) There are gradual transitions between all the groups of vertigo, sometimes even in one and the same patient. (3) The vertebral origin of Meniere's disease can frequently be directly proved by the aid of tests; ie, experimentally. Thus, cases of cervical origin can be diagnosed from the start. And (4) although Meniere's disease (labyrinthine vertigo) may be provoked by other ways than that of the cervical spine, by labyrinthitis for example, it appears that we have to cope with a syndrome that in the large majority of cases is connected with functional disturbances of the cervical spine; therefore, it should be indicated for manipulative treatment."

Seizures

Seizures can sometimes be linked to a history of head trauma when the trauma is recent. Convulsive seizures may be the first sign of something more serious than simple concussion. Determine where the seizure began if possible as it is helpful in the localization of the various cerebral centers. Small subdural hematomas can easily be overlooked which result in a meningocerebral cicatrix. Seizures rarely result when skull fracture does not injure the dura.

Focal seizures result from anatomic lesions, while generalized seizures from the start are caused by metabolic or unknown (but presumed functional) lesions such as grand mal and petit mal. Psychomotor seizures, often denoting temporal lobe pathology, are characterized by episodes of behavioral changes and perception alterations.

Delirium, Coma, and Convulsions

The causes of coma are nearly identical with the causes of convulsions. Almost every disorder that causes the one may cause the other; hence, all that is said of one applies equally as well to the diagnosis of the other. Either or both may result from cerebral concussion or compression (skull fractures), sun stroke, apoplexy, epilepsy, toxemia, diabetes, drugs, and Stokes-Adams's syndrome.

Coma is a medical emergency, and at no time should it be ignored. Life-sustaining measures always have precedence over diagnostic procedures. Quickly evaluate the status of the respiratory and cardiovascular systems. See if the patient has an adequate airway, that he is not hypotensive, in shock, or bleeding. Institute proper emergency procedures if any of these conditions exist.

Cerebrospinal Fluid Circulatory Disturbances

Impairment to normal cerebrospinal fluid circulation results in a backup in the ventricles leading to an increase in intracranial pressure. Severe facial or skull trauma, edema, meningitis, brain mass, or anything that will cause blockage along the passageways will produce fluid accumulation in the system, resulting in a degree of hydrocephalus. Signs of early increased intracranial pressure include yawning, hiccuping, and projectile vomiting. In a few days or weeks, high pressure inside the sleeve of the dura surrounding the optic nerve may cause the retinal veins to dilate and the pale pink optic nerve head to exhibit papilledema and a choked disc. A mass compressing part of the ventricular system is the most common cause of papilledema. It is commonly associated with headaches (dura mater stretching) and vomiting (parasympathetic center reflex).

Infection

Meningitis. Meningitis is the most dreaded complication of cranial trauma. It frequently follows a compound fracture with cerebrospinal leakage but sometimes follows poorly treated scalp lacerations which suppurate. The features are headache, stiff neck, positive Kernig's sign, rapid temperature rise, and cloudy spinal fluid from bacteria and white cells.

Brain Abscess. Brain abscess is a late and infrequent complication of head injury which usually results from a depressed fracture or penetration of a foreign body. Features include a period of mild chilliness and malaise which is followed by a normal or subnormal temperature as the abscess forms, dulled mentality, slowly progressing signs of intracranial pressure, slight or severe headache, possible vomiting and choked disc, and neurologic evidence of an expanding lesion.

Cerebral Fungus. In a compound fracture with considerable bone and dura loss, a cerebral fungus infection not infrequently follows. This serious complication, often unavoidable, is characterized by spreading infection, edema, herniation, and abscess formation.

Aerocele

The prerequisite for the formation of a typical aerocele is a compound fracture with a ruptured dura. This is especially common with a fracture that involves the base of the skull or the sinuses, particularly the frontal sinus. The aerocele is produced by the increased air pressure within the nasal cavity when the patient sneezes or blows the nose. During these events, bacteria may be forced through the fracture into the cranial vault. A combination of symptoms practically pathognomonic for this condition is a history of cranial trauma followed by sneezing which produces a sudden rhinorrhea. Coughing, sneezing, or nose blowing may force air within the cranium with the torn dura over the fracture line acting as a flap valve to prevent air from escaping. In roentgenography, air may be seen in the subdural space near the fracture, fill the subarachnoid spaces and reach ventricles, or be found within the substance of the brain itself. Symptoms suggest slowly increasing intracranial pressure.

Chronic Subdural Hemorrhage

Chronic subdural hemorrhage frequently offers symptoms of anorexia, vomiting, blurred vision, drowsiness, personality changes, and gait disturbances. These not infrequent sequels of head injury are often related to a mild initial cranial trauma, insufficient to cause loss of consciousness. The accident is often forgotten by the patient. Headache, mental changes, and drowsiness develop some months later. This is caused by the clot attracting nonprotein fluids which cause gradual enlargement of the mass; ie, the osmotic tendency of any fluid of lighter density to pass through a semipermeable membrane to join fluid of greater density. Symptoms are often marked on one occasion, disappear, and return later with greater severity. Albuminuria is a striking concomitant finding, and a xanthochromic spinal fluid is frequent. Motor involvements, emotional disturbances, and greatly altered deep reflexes are found. Less frequently, cranial nerve involvement, Jacksonian convulsions, aphasia, vomiting, slow pulse, and choked disc are exhibited.

INJURIES OF THE FACE, NOSE, AND SINUSES

On-field examination has an advantage over office or hospital evaluation because analysis can be made before swelling and bleeding obliterate many palpable signs of fracture-line tenderness, abnormal angulation, bony crepitus, and structural continuity or irregularity.

Facial Wounds

The incidence of facial wounds has been greatly reduced in athletics through the mandatory use of protective equipment in some sports, yet they commonly arise when protection is not provided.

Background. Bleeding from wounds of the face is usually profuse because of the many blood vessels in the region. Hemorrhage is difficult to control. The upper airway may become obstructed by blood, mucus, or foreign matter causing respiratory failure and death. Maintenance of an open airway and control of hemorrhage are the emergency procedures which take priority.

First Aid in Face Wounds. Clear the airway if necessary. Check for signs of closed head injury. More than any other area of the body, injuries to the face and jaws are likely to produce upper airway obstruction. In jaw fracture, the tongue may fall backward or blood may gather in the hypopharynx. Place the patient in the semiprone position to allow drainage of the airway. Prevent or treat for shock, which is always a danger, and prevent chilling or overheating. If the patient prefers, he may sit on the ground with knees drawn up and with his head resting on his arms folded across his knees. Except for minor wounds, surgical consultation should be sought immediately. Apply digital pressure to appropriate pressure points to control hemorrhage. In minor abrasions of the face or skull, bleeding can be stopped with cold and compression, and the wound can be washed with a warm saline solution. In stubborn cases, fibrin foam under the pressure pad may be necessary. Many recommend dusting the wound with an antibacterial powder. Apply a sterile pressure dressing and cold pack over skin wounds, but never place a dressing within the mouth.

Facial Bruises

Severe pain, swelling, heat, redness, and subcutaneous bleeding may result even when fracture is ruled out. Cryotherapy therapy is the treament of choice during the first 48 hours, and this may be followed by any physiotherapy procedure that tends to reduce the edema and promote healing.

Proteolytic Enzymes. Because posttraumatic inflammatory processes of the face and other areas of the body often proceed far greater than necessary (ie, overact), Cichoke feels that proteolytic enzymes (eg, trypsin and papain) and enzyme mixtures (eg, chymotrypsin) are effective agents in accelerating the rehabilitative process by decreasing the time loss from athletic injuries and increasing the rate of soft-tissue repair. Hasselberger, Wolf and Ransberger, and others have discussed several advantages of combined proteolytic enzymes in accelerating the rehabilitative process in sports and nonsport injuries. These investigators report that the healing time of a posttraumatic inflammatory process may be reduced up to half that normally seen when proteolytic enzymes are not utilized.

Facial Fractures

Severe facial injuries are usually the result of high-speed collisions in vehicles (eg, snow-mobiling, auto racing), thrown objects (eg, baseball, basketball), an elbow blow, or a kick. The most common facial fractures in sports occur to the nose, mandible, and supraorbital margins. Progressive swelling of the face (pumpkin face) or depressions in the upper cheek may indicate a midface fracture.

In any facial fracture, always check the mouth and tongue for bleeding. Severe bleeding from the nasopharynx or hypopharynx suggest a fracture that has lacerated vessels near the ethmoidal sinus. Direct pressure and suctioning may be required to maintain an open airway.

The incidence of facial injuries is high in an individual with a long history in boxing. The most common injuries seen are nosebleeds, eye contusions, lacerations, nose fractures, and concussion. Boxing contributes few facial fractures apart from nasal bone injuries; the skull and neck have a much higher injury incidence in most other contact sports (eg, football).

Roentgenographic Considerations. Due to the confusing picture of overlapping and oddly contoured structures, close examination must be made. Both Waters (chin up) and Caldwell (standard facial) views are frequently necessary. Close scrutiny of the orbital margins is necessary, with particular attention paid to the normal air space in the maxillary and ethmoid sinuses. After trauma, soft-tissue effusion often obliterates the inferior and medial orbital margins. Bone fragments may be noted near a fracture site, and old injuries may be evidenced by ossification consequences or hemorrhage.

Zygomatic and Trimalar Fractures. Fractures of the zygomatic arch are usually caused by a direct blow to the cheek that results in mechanical impingment upon the coronoid process of the mandible. There is severe swelling and trismus when attempting to open the mouth. The sunken cheek only becomes apparent after swelling subsides. Cheek trauma may cause trimalar fractures presenting fracture lines through the infraorbital and lateral orbital rim or the zygomatic arch. Displacement depends upon the direction of force. Again, early swelling obliterates displacement. Eye injury, diplopia, and infraorbital anesthesia are common complications.

Orbital Blow-Out Fractures. Blunt trauma to the eye may result in a hydrostatic blow-out fracture of the eggshell-thin margins of the orbital floor, altering the upper maxillary sinus margin and bulging soft tissues through the orbital floor. The dense orbital rim is usually intact. These fractures often result from a direct blow to the eye by an elbow, knee, fist, ball, or some other blunt object. In evaluating the lower orbital margin in roentgenography, the overlapping anterior rim of the orbit and the deeply seated posterior-inferior rim of the orbit must be located. In most cases of fracture, a third line may be seen, representing a bony fragment. A soft-tissue bulging of periorbital tissue may be the sole indication of a fragment hinging laterally or medially. In doubtful cases, tomography is most helpful. Trauma to the infraorbital nerve results in anesthesia of the cheek. Enophthalamos and diplopia result from displacement of extra-ocular muscle and fat or supplying nerve entrapment within fracture fragments.

Fracture of the Jaw

A fractured mandible (often multiple) is a common facial fracture, second only to nasal fracture. A mandible with an impacted fracture heals slowly as compared to long-bone fractures. Symptoms may include abnormal closure of teeth, inability to swallow or talk, point tenderness, abnormal palpable bony motion, abnormal deviation of the jaw upon opening, bleeding and drooling from the mouth, and ear pain (especially in condyle fracture). In case of fracture of both jaws, especially, the soft tissues may drop back

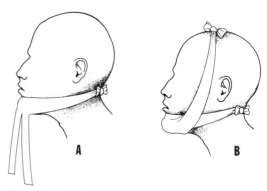

Figure 19.8. Four-tailed bandage for a fractured jaw.

into the throat and strangle the patient, requiring early tracheotomy. The most frequent and most overlooked fracture site is at the condyle.

Temporomandibular Joint (TMJ) Dysfunction

TMJ dysfunction usually presents a unilateral dull ache of gradual onset, pain aggravated by chewing, a joint click felt or heard, deviation of the jaw to one side, tenderness and muscle spasm, a nervous bruxism, and pain on opening and closing the mouth.

The adult range of motion is usually normal (1) if the examiner is able to insert three finger widths between the incisor teeth when the mouth is opened; and (2) if the patient is able to jut his jaw forward and place his lower teeth in front of his upper teeth. Yet, these signs may be present and there still be a degree of fixation resulting in chronic local or reflex symptoms. If there is any doubt as to the presence of crepitus, auscult the joint for clicks or grating sounds.

Berkman points out that the jaw has been proven to influence the holding power of the atlas and axis, and, in turn, subluxations of the atlas and axis effect the stability of the TMJ. The fascia colli binds the jaw and cervical spine into a unit where a fault of any one part affects the entire mechanism. Osteopathic research suggests that a subluxated temporal bone is often at fault. This is grossly indicated by flattening (temporal internal rotation) or protrusion (temporal external rotation) of an ear from the skull. A blow to the jaw is easily transmitted to the temporal bones.

Joint Strain and Sprain

In sports, this type of strain is sometimes seen in underwater swimmers who clench their teeth tightly on a mouthpiece. Poor occlusion and the habit of teeth grinding are often predisposing factors. The stressed temporalis and pterygoid muscles become chronically spastic and cause localized pain at muscular attachments or refer pain and/or paresthesias (eg, itching) to one or both ears, face, temples, or forehead. There is usually joint clicking and transient locking. If not properly treated, a subluxation-fixation may result.

Joint sprain may be the result of improper dentition or a spontaneously reduced luxation. Relative muscle strain, capsule and ligament sprain, muscle spasm, and soft-tissue swelling may be involved depending upon the extent of injury. Poor occlusion leads to a chronic sprain or strain as does bruxism. Overstretch causes pterygoid spasm and an asymmetrical lateral motion of the jaw. Restricted joint motion is the result of subluxation, muscle spasm, arthritis, ankylosis, scar tissue, or trismus of the elevating muscles of mastication from local inflammation, hysteria, tetanus, or underlying congenital defects.

Adjunctive Care

Trigger Points and Spasm. Several trigger points have been isolated which frequently refer pain and deep tenderness to the TMJ. The most common points are within the masseter (see Fig. 19.5, *right*), temporalis, internal and external pterygoid muscles. Prior to correcting isolated subluxations, it is quite helpful to spray the located trigger areas with a vapocoolant. The patient's mouth should be comfortably propped open with a roll of gauze. The patient's eyes and nose are draped, and the

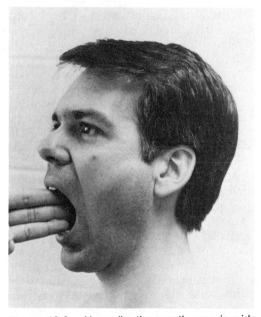

Figure 19.9. Normally, the mouth span is wide enough to accommodate the width of three fingers between the incisor teeth.

patient's neck is laterally flexed away from the involved side. A few slow, even, interrupted sweeps of the spray in one direction only from jaw angle to temple should reduce any spasm and referred pain present. Do not frost the skin. Two or three applications, a few days apart, are usually sufficient. High-voltage galvanic current over spastic masseter or temporal muscles for 15 minutes is an alternative approach.

Exercises. It is helpful to instruct the patient in opening his jaw against resistance for 3–5 minutes 4–5 times a day.

Dislocation Reduction Technique

The most common example of mandibular dislocation is the anterior displacement of the mandibular condyle from its temporal articulation into the infratemporal fossa. The patient presents the classic "mouth-agape," anxiety and helplessness, aching and spastic temporal and masseter muscles. The mouth cannot be closed. It is often caused in a lax joint by a jaw blow or simply by a yawn, laughing, or eating an apple.

During reduction of uncomplicated luxation confirmed by x-ray, take care to well pad the thumbs before placing them firmly on the molar and premolar surfaces. The patient should be supine. The thumbtips should be firm against the coronoid processes while the eight fingers are extended around the lower jaw. Apply an inferior-

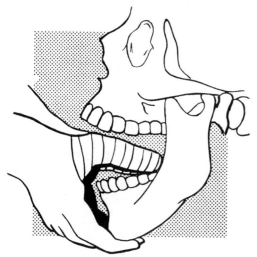

Figure 19.10. Position for reducing a dislocated jaw.

posterior thrust against the molars with the thumbs while the fingers tilt the mandible superior-anterior upward with a rotatory motion. Thumb padding is essential during leverage because reduction is usually immediately followed by an involuntary contraction of the masseter and temporal muscles in unison, causing the jaws to sharply snap shut. If only one side is involved, one contact thumb is used within the mouth, and the other hand is applied against the patient's forehead for counterpressure. After successful reduction, the chin should be mobilized for several seconds and then supported for 1–3 days.

Unilateral TMJ Anterior-Inferior Subluxation Adjustment

A fixation anterior-inferior misalignment of the TMJ may be found on one side with the other side normal. During correction, place the patient in the sitting position facing forward. Stand behind the patient, and cup the patient's chin within your clasped fingers. Ask the patient to stabilize his occiput against your chest. The adjustment is made from the anterior-inferior to the posterior-superior. The thrust should be short, rapid, well-controlled, and in accord with normalizing the anatomic misalignment.

In some cases, there will also be a degree of medial misalignment associated. If this be the case, the line of correction should be diagonal towards the patient's eyes on the side of misalignment rather than directly posterior-superior (ie, posterior-superior-lateral). This will require the doctor to slightly rotate his shoulder anteriorly on the side contralateral to the lesion.

Unilateral TMJ Lateral Subluxation Adjustment

A TMJ joint may be found to be subluxated-fixated in an abnormal lateral position. This misalignment is usually accompanied by some superior jamming. During correction, place the patient in the sitting position facing forward. Stand behind the patient, slightly to the side of the lesion. If the lesion is of the patient's right TMJ, place your right palm on the right side of the TMJ so as your thenar eminence is directly over the head of the affected condyle and the rami of the mandible above the angle. The left stabilizing hand is placed in a like position on the patient's left mandible. Lean slightly forward so your head is over the patient's head. In this position, your elbows will be bent and your wrists extended. The adjustment is from the superior-lateral to the inferior-medial against the stabilizing hand.

Unilateral TMJ Inferior Subluxation Adjustment

A TMJ may become subluxated (separated) and become fixed in a straight inferior position with the other side normal. During correction, place the patient in the sitting position facing forward. Stand behind the patient, slightly to the side of the lesion. If the lesion is of the patient's left TMJ, make contact on the medial aspect of the mandible under the angle with the fingertips of your left hand. Your right stabilizing hand should be cupped under the patient's right ramus. Ask the patient to stabilize his occiput against your chest. The adjustment is made by asking the patient to force his mouth open while you apply pressure from the inferior to the superior.

Nose Trauma

Nose injuries and fractures are invariably accompanied by profuse bleeding. In the typical broken nose, the bridge of the nose will be bruised and show a definite depression (if not obliterated by swelling). When viewed from the front, the nose will deviate from the midline.

Epistaxis. Facial contusions and nosebleeds are common in sports and exhibit an excellent need for ice, compression, and elevation (I-C-E). Apply ice or another source of cold, compress the nostrils together, and elevate the part by having the patient sit with his neck hyperextended. In severe cases, pack the nose with several feet of ribbon gauze, and refer to cauterization or to surgical attention. In cases other than direct trauma, cracking of dry nasal mucous membranes, coagulopathy, hypertension, Weber-Rendu-Osler syndrome, or barotrauma may be a factor. The latter situation is seen in scuba divers where poor pressure equalization within sinuses causes facial pain followed by nonfrothy sinus bleeding into the nose and/or mouth.

Fractures. These are rarely viewed in roentgenography during the early stages because severe damage is usually restricted to cartilaginous structures. Nasal fracture with displacement requires quick reduction. Later, positive x-ray findings are the result of healing by fibrous union between fragments. Examination must be made immediately before swelling takes place or after swelling subsides. Deformity is difficult if not impossible to correct without refracturing after 2 weeks from the time of injury. Associated hematoma and/or infection are always a threat. Rarely, an acute hematoma develops between the cartilage and perichondrium, requiring cold, pressure by a nose pack, and aspiration. Infection offers the danger of cavernous sinus thrombosis and its life-threating potential.

DENTAL INJURIES

Contact sports have a high incidence of injuries to the teeth when protection is not mandatory. Over 20% of fractured molars have been traced to sports injuries, and front teeth are even more vulnerable.

Background. Pain on biting indicates decayed dentine, pain on eating sweets is usually due to decay, and pain on temperature changes points to pulpitis (eg, abscess). Gum tenderness dorsal to the molars suggest pericoronitis from an impacted wisdom tooth. A painful dental disorder may be brought out and isolated by lightly tapping the suspected tooth with a mirror handle. A blue-gray tooth is likely dead from an old infection. In any case, dental referral should be made for evaluation and treatment.

Trigger points within the temporalis muscle frequently refer pain similar to facial neuralgia. Points within the anterior aspect tend to refer pain to the front teeth; the middle aspect, the incisor area; the posterior aspect, the molars and TMJ area.

Concussion results in little loosening or displacement of teeth, but sensitivity to biting pressure or temperature extremes may be present for a period. However, a comparatively mild force against the upper front teeth can lead to fracture and dislocation. Tooth injury may vary from (1) cracked enamel of one or more teeth resulting in slight loosening (subluxation) and sensitivity to cold, (2) crown fracture involving tooth pulp, or (3) injury of one or more tooth roots. Severe pain usually indicates that fracture has exposed the pulp. During severe trauma to the teeth, the force may extend to the periodontal tissues. A displacement of a tooth involves socket fracture.

First Aid. Temporary support can be given to a loose tooth with soft paraffin or candle wax heated to the form of masticated chewing gum. The player should be instructed not to apply finger pressure to test the looseness of a damaged tooth. If complete avulsion occurs, the tooth should only be wrapped in gauze and the patient and tooth immediately referred to a dentist for possible reimplantation. The dentist will wash and prepare it. Replacement in the socket must be done as soon as possible to be successful. The quicker implantation and splinting are made, the better the results; and the younger the patient, the better the results. A replanted tooth is not permanent, but it may last 10–15 years.

CHAPTER 20

Traumatic Eye and Ear Disorders

This chapter discusses sports-related injuries to the lids, conjunctiva, lens, cornea, orbit, and retina of the eye, and injuries of the outer, middle, and inner ear.

INJURIES OF THE EYE AND VISION

Badminton and racketball, especially, have a high incidence of eye injuries, usually occurring in inexperienced or nearsighted players nor wearing safety glasses. Eye injuries also have a high incidence in basketball, especially where jumps under the backboard place the eye in jeopardy of an opponent's fingers or elbow, or even of the ball.

Concussion to an eye frequently results in anterior and/or posterior chamber hemorrhages. These may be noticed on gross inspection, but any complaint of blurred vision requires careful ophthalmoscopy. Slow bleeding may require several hours to obscure vision. Except for the most minor eye or visual injuries, ophthalmologic consultation should be sought.

Basic Assessment of Eye Injuries

The equipment generally considered minimum to assess the integrity of the eye and vision is a penlight, an ophthalmoscope, an eye chart, and sterile eye pads, fluorescein strips, and Q-tips. The basic procedural recommendations of Pashby and Gorman for examining an injured eye are shown in Table 20.1. Such procedures must be conducted quickly and in good light before swelling precludes proper examination.

During evaluation, it is just as important to know what not to do as what to do. Normally, if the patient refuses to open an injured eye for inspection, it should not be forced. The patient should be rused to an opthalmologist for examination and treatment. One exception to this rule is in the case of a chemical burn such as seen from the lime used on various playing fields and courts. If this is suspected, the lid must be forced open and the eye flushed with water for at least 5 minutes before rapid referral to the nearest emergency facility to assess the severity of the damage.

The Lids and Conjunctiva

Inspect lids for cuts, edema, and skin changes. Note position of the lid relative to the anterior orbit and record degree of ptosis. Evaluate degree of exophthalmos or enophthalmos and the distance between orbits. Inspect for conjunctival edema, pallor, foreign bodies, petechiae, and vascular injection both of the anterior eyeball and posterior lid surfaces. Note any conjunctival congestion, bogginess, and episcleritis.

Abrasions and Lacerations. Conjunctival abrasions usually result from dirt or an opponent's fingers. A severe concussion to the orbital area usually results in injury and edema to the affected lid. Swelling may be so severe that the lid cannot be opened by either the patient or doctor. If this be the case, the patient must be referred to an opthalmologist without further evaluation. Hematomas of the lid always require the exclusion of an associated orbital fracture. Proptosis after injury may be associated with retrobulbar hemorrhage.

Traumatic splits in the lid may expose deep tissues. These require immediate cleaning, covering with a sterile pad, and referral for suturing. Linear splits in the lid or a torn tear duct usually require the attention of a plastic surgeon because they take special surgical experience to avoid touble for many years. If a vertical split through the circular lid muscles and the palpebral cartilage is not repaired expertly, a troublesome V-notch lid scar may result.

Subconjunctival Hemorrhage. When the eye is struck with a fist, elbow, knee, ball, puck, or any blunt object larger than the eyeball itself, the result is usually swelling, eyelid ecchymoses, and bright-red subconjunctival hemorrhage. Other causes include severe rubbing with a finger or nicking

Table 20.1.
Basic Assessment of Sports Eye Injuries

1. Inspect the brows, lids, and temples for cuts, bruises, swelling, bleeding, and hematoma. Eversion of a lid will often show a cut, rupture, or foreign object (eg, grit, displaced contact lens) that would not otherwise be visible.

2. Note the eye generally for enophthalmus (a sunken eye), which makes the palpebral fissure appear narrow (eg, in fracture of the orbital floor), or proptosis (protrusion), which makes the fissure appear wide because the eye is pushed anteriorly (eg, retrobulbar hemorrhage).

3. Examine the conjunctival sacs for cuts, rips, hemorrhage, and foreign bodies.

4. Inspect the involved cornea for signs of abrasion, laceration, or a foreign body. An abrasion may not be noticed unless the lid is pulled down and a sterile fluorescein strip is dipped into the tear pool of the lower fornix and then allowed to cover the cornea by blinking.

5. Evaluate the depth and clarity of the anterior chamber and compare with the uninjured eye.

6. Assess pupil size, roundness, and reaction to light and compare with the uninjured eye.

7. Note the color of iris of the injured eye and compare with the uninjured eye.

8. Bilaterally, test visual acuity of with an eye chart or card.

9. Evaluate ocular motion and peripheral vision bilaterally (a) by having the patient look upward, to the right, downward, and then to the left with both eyes; and (b) with the opposite eye covered, by having the patient identify the number of fingers extended in all quadrants peripherally. Diplopia should not be present with both eyes moving together in all quadrants. The minimal visual fields are generally 65° downward, 60° nasally, 45° upward, and 85° temporally.

10. With an opthalmoscope, seek signs of damage to the lens, vitreous, and retina.

the conjunctival with a sharp object. There is usually no visual disturbance or eye pain. Although frightening in appearance, the patient should be reassured that subconjunctival hemorrhage is not serious and will disappear in about 10–14 days. As with any subcutaneous bleeding, cold packs should be applied initially, followed by warm compresses in the later stage. Specific medications are not required according to Grant and Cinotti and Williams and Sperryn.

Contusion Injuries of the Eyeball

It is not unusual to have rupture of the eyeball just outside the corneoscleral margin where the sclera is thinnest. A rupture here is often associated with subconjunctival dislocation of the lens. Hemorrhage is a frequent complication of rupture. Mild injuries may produce traumatic keratitis, and severe injuries may produce rupture of the cornea. Rupture of the sphincter of the iris is also common and diagnosed by first finding that the iris is dilated and then by detecting a slight notch in the pupillary margin. Temporary dilation of the pupil may result from

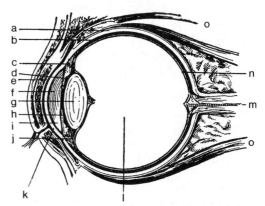

Figure 20.1. Vertical section through the eyeball: *a*, sclera; *b*, choroid; *c*, ciliary muscle; *d*, iris; *e*, cul-de-sac of conjunctiva; *f*, anterior chamber and aqueous humor; *g*, crystalline lens; *h*, posterior chamber; *i*, angle of anterior chamber; *j*, suspensory ligament of lens; *k*, cornea; *l*, vitreous body; *m*, optic nerve with central artery of retina; *n*, retina; *o*, ocular muscles.

sphincter stretching. Sometimes the iris is torn from its attachment to the ciliary body, producing iridodialysis. Detachment of the ciliary body may occur, thus deepening the anterior chamber at the point of separation. Paresis of accommodation, sometimes observed after injuries, may show improvement when acute symptoms subside. The lens is frequently partly dislocated due to partial rupture of the suspensory ligament.

Several other complications may arise. Prolapse of the vitreous may occur into the anterior chamber, usually producing a shallow anterior chamber in this area. The lens may be dislocated into the anterior chamber, with resulting secondary glaucoma requiring extraction. A traumatic cataract may also result, which requires surgical intervention. Rupture of the choroid is not uncommon and usually appears as a crescentric lesion between the optic nerve and the macula. Glaucoma frequently follows eyeball contusion and is one of the most serious complications. It may occur at the time of injury or later. Traumatic enophthalmos appears as a lifeless eyeball in its sunken orbit. The motility of the eye is sometimes seriously reduced. Sympathetic ophthalmia is a rare complication of eyeball contusion.

The retina may be ruptured or detached with or without tear. Commotio retinae may follow injury, resulting in edema of the retina which appears gray and cloudy while the macular region assumes a dark red color in comparison to the surrounding retina. In traumatic retrobulbar neuritis, the optic nerve suffers a low-grade traumatic retrobulbar inflammation which may be so slight as to be noted only by careful study of the blind spot (which may be enlarged). Evulsion of the optic nerve may also occur. A well-defined hole may be seen occupying the position of the nerve, corresponding in size to that of the disc.

The Lens

Traumatic Cataract and Complications

Traumatic cataract usually reacts from a rupture or disturbance of the capsule or lens from any injury which allows the aqueous or vitreous fluid to come into contact with the lens fibers. The result is a partial or complete loss of transparency of the crystalline lens or of its capsule.

Traumatic cataracts are usually caused by penetrating foreign bodies, but a blunt blow on the orbit or even to the side of the head may cause cataract. Soon after capsular laceration, the lens fibers near the tear begin to swell and cloud. Later, after injury, the lens substance oozes into the anterior chamber and appears as gray fluffy-appearing masses which are dissolved and eventually absorbed on coming in contact with the aqueous. In time, the major portion of the lens substance may be absorbed and the pupil again becomes almost black. In most cases, however, the capsule scars and closes, stopping the process of absorption before liquefaction is fully accomplished.

Septic matter may also be introduced into the eye either at the time of injury or later, which gives rise to an iridocyclitis, a panophthalmitis, and even an orbital inflammation. If not prevented, a secondary glaucoma may supervene.

Contact Lenses in the Unconscious Athlete

Contact lenses offer a special hazard with the unconscious or injured athlete. Here, a warning bracelet or identification card helps to alert first-aid attendants of the presence of the lenses. When possible, ask the injured player to remove the contacts, as an awkward search by another party may do more harm than good.

With the unconscious player who is unable to remove the lenses himself, first examine the eye with a small flashlight. By focusing the beam of light from the side, the edge of the lens will often become visible. Most disengaged contact lenses will be found under the upper eyelid. Place the tip of a finger on the athlete's lower eyelid, pull down and laterally, then push the upper lid against the top of the lens. The lens should eject; if not, a small suction cup can be on hand for assistance.

The Cornea

Corneal Abrasions. In the typical athlete, protective reflexes tend to prevent extensive corneal abrasions, but even minor lesions are quite painful, result in blurred vision, photophobia, excessive lacrimation, and usually require some hospitalization. They are commonly the result of scratches from a fingernail, ball, or piece of equipment in close contact sports, and they always present a threat of possible visual impairment. A topical dye is required for positive diagnosis, but uncomplicated cases often heal in about 4 days with only first-aid treatment. The clinical picture is one of an extremely red eye, pain, photophobia, and excessive lacrimation. First aid consists of an eye ointment, a firm pad over the closed lid, and mild cold.

Corneal Lacerations. Lacerations of the eyeball from sharp or pointed objects result in eye pain and visual impairment. On examination, the cornea will appear cut, present an irregular corneal reflex, or possibly exhibit a tear-shaped pupil with a small ebony tip at the apex of the tear; or the iris may exhibit a hole from perforation. A cold pack should be applied immediately, followed by a protective shield, a loose patch, and referral to an ophthalmologist.

Traumatic and Striate Keratitis. Injuries to the cornea may set up a general inflammation of the membrane, but more frequently they cause loss of substance of the cornea and thus cause corneal ulcers. These ulcers heal quickly if small and not affected. They present little pain and leave only a temporary opacity proportionate to their extent. If they are extensive, even if superficial like a severe abrasion, they may be extremely painful if the corneal epithelium is removed. Once becoming infected, they exhibit characteristics of a suppurating ulcer. An injury causing bending of the cornea may exhibit a number of fine gray streaks (striate keratitis), more or less perpendicular to the corneal injury, noticed from a few hours to a week or more after the trauma.

Hyphema and Hematic Corneal Infiltration. After eye trauma, the patient may complain of eye pain and fuzzy vision and present red or black blood over all or just the inferior aspect of the iris or pupil. Referral should be made to an ophthalmologist, who usually suggests hospitalization, sedation, and careful observation for several days until the hemorrhage clears. Prior to referral, an eye pad should be applied over the closed lid.

Cases of hematic discoid infiltration of the cornea are nearly always of traumatic origin. Contusions of the anterior segment of the eye or penetrating wounds may be followed by a disturbing picture of "blood

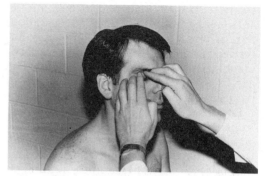

Figure 20.2. One method of testing facial nerve strength. The examiner tries to forcefully open the eyelid against patient's resistance.

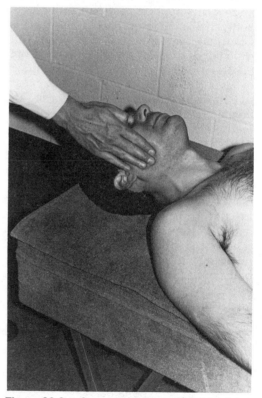

Figure 20.3. Screening for potentially high intraocular pressure with light thumb palpation.

stain." After 10 or more days, it may simulate an anterior dislocation of the lens. The cornea slowly recovers its transparency in 3–24 months.

Concussion injuries (eg, a ball) may result in hyphema with hemorrhage between the cornea and iris from damage to the small vessels of the iris. It should always be considered serious. The clinical picture is one of blurred vision, aching eye pain, severe eye redness with intense dilatation of the pericorneal vessels, and photophobia. In a short time, the blood settles below from gravity to form a "fluid level." There is danger of secondary hemorrhage into the anterior chamber, which may be more dangerous than the initial hyphema. If secondary hemorrhage does not occur, absorption usually takes place in a week.

Sun or Snow Blindness. Ultraviolet injury is often seen in skiing and yachting when glasses with filtering lenses do not prevent sustained reflection of the sun's rays from snow or water. Considerable ultraviolet exposure results in small multiple corneal epithelial erosions.

Foreign Bodies

In sports, foreign bodies within the eye are especially common under windy and/or dusty conditions.

Background. Foreign bodies are frequently imbedded in the cornea because it occupies nearly two-thirds of the space between the opened eyelids and a much larger proportion of that space when the eyes are partly closed as during squinting in bright sunlight or when the entrance of a foreign body is anticipated. The tissue of the cornea tends to retain particles which may penetrate it, but the conjunctiva and subconjunctival tissues are so loose that imbedded particles easily work out spontaneously.

Once a foreign body becomes imbedded in the cornea, it causes irritation and usually a suppurative inflammation by which it becomes loosened and easily drops out or is wiped away by the lids. If, however, it lies at the bottom of a considerable loss of substance, it may lie there for some time, although quite detached from corneal tissue. Under these circumstances, it becomes a source of painful irritation causing chronic eye muscle weakness, blurred vision, photophobia, excessive lacrimation, conjunctival redness, and the development of vessels in the adjoining pericorneal space which press against the seat of the foreign body and give an appearance of a chronic phlyctenular ulcer or superficial vascular keratitis.

Management. Most superficial unimbedded debris can be washed out with clean

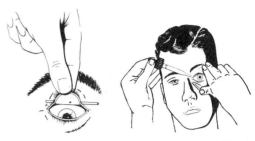

Figure 20.4. *Left*, turning the upper eyelid back over a wooden applicator for inspection. *Right*, syringing loose debris from within the eye lids.

water, a weak saline solution, or a commercial eye wash (eg, Cramer's). For this purpose, a bulb lavage is a helpful tool in the emergency kit. If gentle irrigation is not adequate, a light patch should be applied and immediate referral to an ophthalmologist should be made.

Orbital Lacerations

One of the most common facial injuries in sports is that of laceration in the bony-prominent orbital area. The typical face mask protects the other areas quite sufficiently. Injuries in the orbital areas are often deeper than first thought, frequently exposing the bony ridge. While cleaning the wound, never shave an eyebrow for, in about 25% of cases, it does not grow back or grows back most scantily. Proper suturing often requires a plastic surgeon, as the scar increases vulnerability and each additional scar encourages the accumulation of dense scar tissue (eg, boxer's brow).

Eye Injuries Produced by Indirect Trauma

Papilledema. Papilledema following skull fracture, especially a depressed fracture, is sometimes seen, but swelling of the disc and hemorrhage are rare. Vision is usually not affected, and visual fields are typically normal. The papilledema usually disappears in 1–3 weeks after the intracranial pressure is reduced.

Occipital Injuries. Complete blindness may be a temporary result in occipital injuries because of physical shock affecting the neurons correlated with the damaged cortical neurons. There is usually complete restoration of function of all but the definitely destroyed neurons. Vision may be permanently lost if hemorrhage involves the visual centers.

The Retina

Concussion injuries of the eye may result in retinal hemorrhages, retinal tears and disinsertions, choroid ruptures, and optic nerve avulsion (rare).

Retinal Hemorrhage and Choroidal Ruptures. Retinal edema and bleeding usually occur in the macula or temporal area, and resolution usually occurs in a few weeks without radical treatment. A choroidal rupture appears as a whitish circumscribed area near the disc in ophthalmoscopy because the herniation allows underlying sclera to be viewed. Strenuous physical activity must be restricted for 2–3 weeks.

Retinal Dialysis and Detachment. While disinsertion of the retina probably occurs at the time of concussion, retinal detachment may not occur for weeks or even months after the time of injury. Initially, the area of retinal dialysis will appear red, well defined, and near the periphery of the retina, usually on the lateral aspect.

Early diagnosis of retinal dialysis may save the patient's vision if cryotherapy or photocoagulation can be effectively applied. In the later stage, the detached retina will present a gray appearance with dark vessels and require surgical intervention. Once retinal detachment has been corrected, further contact sports are ill-advised as recurrence is quite frequent.

A review of various neurologic reflexes, signs, or tests pertaining to disorders involving the eye and/or vision are shown in Table 20.2.

INJURIES OF THE EAR AND RELATED DISORDERS

The Outer Ear

All sports have their share of injuries to the external ear. Even in mandatory-helmet sports, lacerations and abrasions are seen. These may be due to an opponent's fingernail or a player bending the ear during the placement of a helmet. This latter injury may not be uncomfortable at first, but after hours of practice, the folded ear may swell and bleed at the crease, producing intense pain and many months of sensitivity.

Table 20.2.
Review of Neurologic Reflexes, Signs, or Tests Relative to Eye and Visual Syndromes (Sport and Nonsport)

Syndrome Manifestation	Procedures/Signs	
Optic nerve (Cranial 2)	Consensual reflex Dazzle reflex Field of vision Ophthalmoscopic signs	Gunn's sign Pupillary reflex Visual acuity
Oculomotor nerve (Cranial 3)	Accommodation reflex Argyll-Robertson's sign Arroyo's sign Ballet's sign Cantelli's sign	Consensual reflex Disconjugate gaze Gower's sign Pupillary reflex Red glass test
Trochlear nerve (Cranial 4)	Ballet's sign Cantelli's sign	Red glass test
Trigeminal nerve (Cranial 5)	Bite test Consensual reflex Corneal reflex Oculocardiac reflex Orbicularis reflex	Rooting reflex Sneeze reflex Snout reflex Zygomatic reflex
Abducens nerve (Cranial 6)	Ballet's sign Cantelli's sign	Disconjugate gaze Red glass test

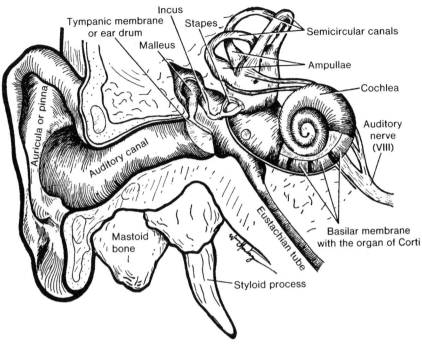

Figure 20.5. Diagram of the general anatomy of the ear.

Caulifower Ear

While cauliflower ear has in past years been commonly associated with boxing, its incidence is much higher in wrestling. The condition itself is the result of untreated or poorly treated hematoma. The clinical picture progresses through (1) trauma to the ear causing persistent, throbbing pain which lasts long after the athletic event; (2) possible fibrocartilage fracture, (3) swelling, local heat, tenderness, followed by the development of a hematoma after several hours, initially between cartilage and overlying skin, visible to the naked eye; (4) tissue hardening and the development of early fibrous tissue in about 14 days; and (5) the resulting keloid mass, development of new cartilage, and permanent deformity of the external ear characterized by skin wrinkling, thickening, and contraction at the site of injury.

First aid consists of ice packs and pressure bandages during the healing stage. Hirata condemns straightforward incision, although a common practice, as it opens the area to secondary infection, chondritis, and perichondritis due to the relative avascularity of the cartilage. Referral for aspiration, several if need be, is preferred. Following aspiration, some authorities recommend irrigating the aspirated area with a solution of hyaluronidase to reduce swelling and edema of injured tissues.

Prevention lies essentially in the use of proper headgear, but care must be taken that the earcap is properly fitted or this in itself creates a hazard.

Miscellaneous Disorders

Lacerations. In any case of laceration of the pinna, secondary infection is always a danger due to the poor resistance of the relatively avascular cartilage exposed. Appropriate care must be made to avoid permanent and ugly scarring.

Otitis Externa. External otitis (swimmer's ear) is commonly seen in competitive surface swimmers. The cause is a breakdown of the normal cerumen barrier due to constant exposure to warm water. Itching and discharge are the first symptoms. Infection in the skin of the external auditory canal quickly leads to inflammation, erythema, edema (which hides the drum), acute tenderness, and a mild cellulitis that matures rapidly to a firm furuncle that is extremely painful and tender, usually requiring antibiotics and sedation. Each attack destroys some cerumen glands, which encourages further attacks. A chronic mild itching encourages "ear picking" that tends to spread the infection. Diffuse otitis externa is typically a bacteria, fungi, or allergic disorder. Pool work must be restricted until healing is complete. Many otolaryngologists recommend careful monitoring of the pool chorine content and the instilling in each ear of half-strength Burrow's solution after each pool session to prevent infection. Others suggest a commercial antifungal preparation or a solution of 90% isopropyl alcohol and 10% vinegar or 5% glacial acetic acid for irrigation.

Canal Collapse. Due to relaxation of soft-tissue support, the medial end of the condral cartilage may drop forward to narrow the lateral end of the external canal. The resulting slit can easily be opened with a speculum, but normal cerumen passage is inhibited, leading to infection and possible otitis externa.

External Barotrauma. During a diving descent below 30 feet when the ear is protected by ear plugs or a hood, a negative pressure develops which causes the drum to bulge outward, usually without discomfort or rupture. Capillaries within the external canal may break to form small blisters in the skin of the exterior canal which present a roughened surface. People so afflicted should be advised to avoid scuba diving. If diving is continued, some help can be obtained by avoiding ear plugs or cutting a hole in the hood to allow water to enter the exterior ear.

Exostoses. Exostoses are another afflic-tion often seen in swimmers, especially cold water swimmers, which often predispose to otitis externa. The superior aspect of the canal just lateral to the pars flaccida of the drum is a favorite site of these benign bony tumors of the exterior canal. They are neither the cause or the effect of the otitis directly. They are usually asymptomatic and rarely cause complete canal blockage, but they do encourage otitis externa because they interfere with cerumen passage and inhibit water within the ear to drain out. Ear plugs may help in prevention and avoid continued growth, but surgical removal may be necessary.

Insects in the Ear. An uncommon but frightening experience is an insect buzzing within an ear. Treatment can be provided by placing the patient in the side position with the affected ear up and syringing or pouring warm vegetable oil or warm water into the external auditory meatus. This will usually float out the insect.

The Middle Ear

Hearing depends upon the integrity of the external canal, the drum, the air chamber of the middle ear, the windows, the mobile chain of ossicles, the auditory nerve, and the perceptive higher centers in the brain. Any abnormality of one or more of these factors can impair hearing. Treatment of most all middle-ear disorders consists of keeping the ear dry (difficult with swimmers and divers), using preventive irrigations, using an appropriate therapy to decongest the tissues, managing any infection present by appropriate means, and seeking otological consultation when necessary (see Table 20.3).

Table 20.3.
Review of Neurologic Reflexes, Signs, or Tests Relative to Ear, Hearing, and Equilibrium Syndromes (Sport and Nonsport)

Syndrome Manifestation	Procedures/Signs	
Auditory nerve (Cranial 8)	Cochlear division: Auditory reflex Bing's test Gelle's test Gruber's test Otoscopic signs Rinne's test Schwabach's test Weber's lateralization test	Vestibular division: Babinski-Weil's test Barany's test Caloric test Contelli's sign Cochleopapillary reflex Mittlemeyer's test Past-pointing tests

Otitis Media. Otitis media is the result of the normally air-filled middle ear chamber with an intact drum becoming filled with fluid because of impaired eustachian tube function. This is usually the result of an inflammation spreading from a sore throat via the eustachian tube. A feeling of fullness in the ear progresses to pain and a degree of deafness. As pressure builds within the chamber, the drum appears thick and red (blood) or yellow (pus) prior to possible rupture. The common cause in swimmers is poor technique; ie, not expelling air when the nose is under water. The water irritates the nasal mucosa, resulting in nasal congestion and infection. For the same reason, scuba divers should never let water enter the mask. An ear where fluid leakage is seen should never be plugged, just lightly covered with a sterile pad.

Middle-Ear Barotrauma. In rapid pressure changes such as in diving or airplane descent, the drum herniates inwardly if the eustachian tube does not afford pressure equalization. The negative pressure within the middle ear causes slight hemorrhages and extracts fluids from adjacent tissues. A weakened drum may rupture in a deep descent, resulting in severe vertigo as water enters the middle chamber. Prevention is made by avoiding clogged ears or nasal congestion prior to descent. When on the surface, a diver may help unblock an eustachian tube by laterally flexing the neck away from the affected side and pulling the skin of the neck up and down on the affected side or by manipulating the pinna.

Alternobaric Vertigo. Alternobaric vertigo sometimes occurs during a rapid diving ascent where eustachian tube blockage causes middle-ear pressure buildup. In severe cases, the drum may rupture. The associated rotary vertigo, vertical nystagmus, and severe disorientation may produce panic. An experienced diver will usually recognize the early signs of dizziness and slow his ascent accordingly.

Drum Perforation. In addition to the barotraumatic forces mentioned, a concussive blow to the ear may result in a traumatic perforation of the drum and possible ossicle damage. Special audiometric tests are usually required to determine the exact degree of resulting deafness. Slightly perforated drums usually heal spontaneously if kept dry. There is slight scar development. During healing, care must be taken while blowing the nose. Flying and deep diving should be avoided.

Ruptured Round-Window Membrane. An aqueduct connects the cochlea and the subarachnoid space. In some people, this aqueduct is large enough to allow a free flow of cerebrospinal fluid within the scala tympani. As the aqueduct's opening is near the round-window membrane which separates the inner and middle ear, a forceful Valsalva maneuver or an attempt at autoinflation (causing transient increase in blood and cerebrospinal pressure) can transmit cerebrospinal fluid pressure to such an extent as to rupture the round-window membrane. Once this occurs, fluid escape causes the hair cells to become malfunctional, the ear feels full or "dead," a loud tinnitus is heard, deafness (unnoticed when under water) occurs especially with high tones, and vertigo and nausea usually manifest and are associated with spontaneous nystagmus and a staggering gait. During diagnosis, differentiation must be made from Meniere's disease or a viral infection of the middle ear.

The Inner Ear

Inner-ear disorders are characterized by vertigo, tinnitus, and hearing loss.

Inflammation. Acute viral labyrinthitis is usually secondary from a cold or gastrointestinal infection. Hearing loss is rarely associated, but vertigo is usually severe. It is usually self-limiting in 1–2 weeks.

Referred Earache. A common cause of earache is often not within the ear itself but from the adjaent temporomandibular joint, especially in gum-chewers and brace-wearers who have a subclinical arthralgia of the joint. Chronic tonsil, pharynx, or larynx inflammations are also common causes of referred pain to the ear. Other causes include cervical subluxation, sternomastoid and masseter trigger points, dental problems, and an abnormally long styloid process.

Inner-Ear Barotrauma. Injury to the inner ear is usually of an intrinsic nature as it is well protected by surrounding bone. Impairment is usually the result of abnormal pressure changes or fistulae.

Meniere's Syndrome. The syndrome features endolymphatic hydrops from pressure changes in inner-ear fluids. Symptoms include paroxysmal dizziness, tinnitus, and a degree of deafness. The latter two may originate unilaterally and progress to both ears. It is often secondary to a number of metabolic disorders, but a common cause (primary or secondary) often overlooked is a cervical or upper thoracic subluxation. Differentation must be made from central nervous system vertigo and benign paroxysmal postural vertigo.

Motion Sickness

Motion sickness from swinging or travel (air, land, sea) is particularly common in migrainous patients and usually absent in deaf mutes. While the exact cause is unknown in susceptible individuals, it appears to be related to an adverse reaction from repetitive stimulation of the vestibular apparatus. Symptoms include headache, faintness, nausea, vertigo, and sometimes vomiting. The attacks may vary in duration from a few minutes to several days. Travell feels that pyridoxine deficiency with trigger points in the clavicular division of the sternocleidomastoideus are often involved. However, cervical subluxations, inner-ear disorders, genetic susceptibility, and subacute brain and brain stem pathology also must be excluded.

Mayes reports that ginger, which is available at most health-food shops, has been found to be at least as effective in controlling idiopathic motion sickness as are the powerful antimotion drugs, and it does not induce drowsiness. The typical recommended dosage is 2–3 gelatin capsules containing 500 mg of powdered gingerroot taken about 30 minutes before the expected motion.

CHAPTER 21

Neck and Cervical Spine Injuries

The anterior and lateral aspects of the neck contain a wide variety of vital structures, yet have no bony protection. Partial protection is provided by the cervical muscles, the mandible, and the shoulder girdle. Williams and Sperryn report that back and neck injuries form 10–20% of sports injuries. The peak incidence occurs in the third decade, with 90% of the accidents occurring in males. Body build does not appear to be a major factor. High-speed sports such as seen with vehicle accidents, football backs and ends, gymnastics, diving, skiing, surfing, and horseback riding have the highest injury rate.

EMERGENCY CARE

In general, trauma anteriorly to the neck implies soft-tissue damage and possible airway obstruction; trauma posteriorly suggests cervical spine and cord damage; and lateral trauma indicates possible vascular and musculature damage. Due to relative head weight to neck strength and other anatomic differences, neck injury is more critical in the very young.

Initial Assessment

Stabilize the neck before assessment of severity. The patient should never be asked to sit or stand until major disability has been ruled out. The first point in analysis is knowing the mechanism of injury. Without moving the patient, check vital signs and palpate for swelling, deep tenderness, deformity, and throat cartilage stability. When logical, another person should apply gentle bilateral traction on the cervical area via the skull during palpation.

Are there bleeding, spasm, pain, motion restrictions, sensory changes, signs of shock? Limb weakness or dysesthesia indicates nerve root compression. Injuries of the upper airway or alimentary canal feature ventilation abnormalities, stridor, bubbling wound, subcutaneous emphysema, hoarse-ness and dysphagia, bloody sputum, nosebleed, bloody vomitus, or unexplained wound tenderness. Injuries to the cervical nerves are suggested by deviation of the tongue, drooping mouth corner, sensory deficits, and Horner's syndrome. Cervical fractures are commonly associated with severe pain, spasm, and joint stiffness.

Vascular injuries feature vigorous bleeding, absent superficial artery pulsations, an enlarging or pulsatile hematoma, and stroke signs. If there is any suggestion of injury to the carotid artery, palpation should be avoided. Such an injury should be suspected if there is a diagonal erythematous contusion on the side of the neck. Palpation may encourage complete carotid occlusion.

If there are no severe complaints or recognizable signs of major disability, ask the patient to conduct mild active movements if able to do so without discomfort. If slight straight axial compression on top of the head produces unilateral or bilateral radiating root pain, deep injury must be suspected and precautions taken immediately. After the neck has been evaluated, check possible injury to other parts of the body.

For a review of neurologic, orthopedic, and peripheral vascular tests, see Table 21.1.

Emergency Management

Establishment of an adequate airway takes priority over all other concerns with the exception of spurting hemorrhage. After injury to the anterior neck, tenderness and crepitus in the thyroid area associated with hoarseness or signs of respiratory distress signal the need for probable emergency intubation. The airway in the neck region may be obstructed by blood, mucus, edema, and broken parts of the trachea and larynx. Clearing, the mouth (not the pharynx) with the fingers, together with postural drainage in the semiprone position, may be successful, but care must be taken not to force debris further down the airway with probing fingers. If not successful, an emergency surgical airway must be made promptly by the most experienced person available.

Whenever spinal injury is suspected, a backboard should be used before transporting the patient. Gentle constant hand traction should be applied to the chin and occiput while transfer is being made to a board. The head should be laterally fixed with sandbags or rolled cloth and the rest

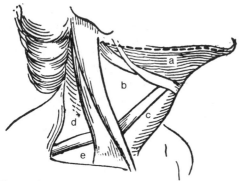

Figure 21.1. Triangles of the neck: *a*, submaxillary triangle; *b*, superior carotid triangle; *c*, inferior carotid triangle; *d*, occipital triangle; *e*, supraclavicular triangle.

of the body with straps. A cervical collar should not be used as it interferes with examination and tracheostomy. See that the neck is never flexed.

Hemorrhage from a neck wound, unless treated at onset, is rapidly fatal. Dressings applied to the neck must be tied over the head or downward under the opposite armpit, but never around the neck. Avoid pressure on the trachea, carotids, and deep veins.

After severe neck injury, return to play should not be allowed until after roentgenography indicates proper healing, the neck is stable and painless during passive and active motion, and the neck has been strengthened by progressive therapeutic exercises.

SOFT-TISSUE INJURIES OF THE ANTERIOR NECK

After attending to all life-threatening possibilities, a more thorough examination may proceed, but required transportation should never be delayed for this purpose. Seek gross abnormalities, then check for details.

Table 21.1.
Review of Neurologic, Orthopedic, and Peripheral Vascular Maneuvers, Reflexes, Signs, or Tests Relative to the Neck and Cervical Spine (Sport and Nonsport Disorders)

Disorder	Procedures/Signs	Disorder	Procedures/Signs
Cervical syndromes	Active rotary compression test		Pectoral reflex
	Bakody's test		Percussion test
	Barre-Leiou's test		Radial reflex
	Biceps reflex		Range of motion tests
	Bikele's test		Ruggeri's reflex
	Brachioradialis reflex		Rust's sign
	Bradburne's sign		Scapulohumeral reflex
	Brudzinski's test		Shoulder depression test
	Cervical distraction test		Soto-Hall's test
	Ciliospinal reflex		Spurling's tests
	Deltoid reflex		Swallowing test
	George's tests		Triceps reflex
	Head retraction reflex		Ulnar reflex
	Infraspinatus reflex		Valsalva's maneuver
	Inverted radial reflex		Vertebrobasilar maneuvers
	Kernig's test		Wrist reflex
	Lhermitte's test	Thoracic outlet and related syndromes	Adson's test
	Light touch/pain tests		Allen's test
	Muscle strength grading		Costoclavicular maneuver
	O'Donoghue's maneuver		Eden's test
	Passive cervical compression tests		Traction test
			Wright's test

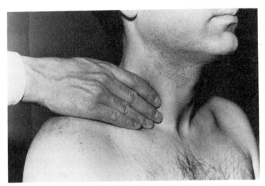

Figure 21.2. Palpating the supraclavicular area.

When the patient swallows, note the action of the cricoid cartilage area. Check the trachea for midline alignment. Evaluate abnormal contours, curvatures, and restricted movements. Venous thrombosis, masses, and exudates may produce visible and palpable edema in the neck. Palpate the neck with the patient supine so that the muscles are relaxed and the head may be passively controlled.

Direct Vascular Injuries

With the exception of spinal cord damage, injuries of the major blood vessels comprise the highest mortality and morbidity of all neck trauma. The most serious consequences are those of airway obstruction from blood, air embolism, spurting hemorrhage, cerebral infarct, and neurologic deficits consequent to cerebral hypoxia. Seek signs of bleeding, discoloration, swelling, lack of superficial pulses, or auscultated bruits. Pressure will control almost any hemorrhage.

Laryngeal, Cricothyroid, and Tracheal Injuries

Obstruction within the upper airway is the second most common cause of death resulting from head and neck trauma. Thus, the priority concern in any anterior neck injury is impairment of the airway. In this regard, the cricoid and thyroid cartilages are quite vulnerable to direct trauma of the neck. Any injured person tends to hyperventilate. Thus, ventilation is not difficult to assess. A minor airway obstruction may soon become suddenly life threatening or be delayed for several hours after injury.

Laryngeal Injuries. The larynx may be crushed between a blunt object and the anterior cervical spine, leading to cartilaginous fracture, subluxation, and/or dislocation. The most common fracture of the thyroid cartilage is that of a vertical anterior split between the thyroid notch and the cricothyroid membrane producing avulsion of the anterior vocal cord attachments and hematoma. Laryngeal injury usually produces a louder stridor than tracheal injury, but stridor may be absent if the obstruction is severe enough to completely obstruct the airway. Besides stridor, other signs and symptoms of laryngeal fracture are loss of cartilaginous landmarks from edema, dyspnea, dysphonia from paresis or hematoma, pain increased by neck motion, dysplagia, subcutaneous emphysema (sometimes from scalp to clavicle), and local tenderness. Otolaryngeal consultation should be quickly sought. Less severe bruises are the result of a fist, elbow, baseball, racket, or stick. Hoarseness and point tenderness are exhibited, but edema and airway obstruction are absent. An overnight ice collar is usually sufficient.

Cricothyroid and Hyoid Injuries. Displaced fractures of the cricoid, especially, must be quickly openly reduced as the cricoid encircles the airway. Subglottic stenosis is a common result of associated lacerations and mucosal tears not being carefully reapproximated. Hyoid injuries are rare, extremely painful, and seldom affect the integrity of the airway.

Tracheal and Thyroid Injuries. Tracheal injuries are fortunately rare, usually resulting from a clothesline-type injury or a "chop" to the base of the neck just below the "Adam's apple." Possible airway obstruction requires quick and careful evaluation. Tracheal rupture causes air to leak into neck tissues (balloon neck) and connective tissues of the shoulder girdle. Fracture is also characterized by emphysema and breathing difficulties. A similar blow above the sternum may cause a thyroid hematoma, characterized by severe hoarseness. After any neck or thorax injury, the trachea should be checked for its midline position. Indirect whiplash injury to the cervical spine is also a possibility with any blow to the anterior neck.

Emergency Care. The first-aid priority is to assure an adequate airway. The problem becomes complex when endotracheal intubation is necessary (requiring extension of the neck) and possible cervical spine and/ or cord damage may be present, making extension of the neck contraindicated. This requires "blind" endotracheal intubation, cricothyreotomy, or tracheotomy by an experienced person. Also, if the larynx has separated from the trachea or separated between two tracheal rings, attempts at endotracheal intubation may be fatal. This situation requires inserting the tube below the separation if possible.

Thyroid Cartilage Mobilization. Chronic pain or ache may occasionally arise from a fixated thyroid cartilage. This is usually from previous trauma resulting in immobilization and stasis. For correction, place the patient on a table in the supine position without a pillow. Stand to the side of the patient, and grasp the upper and lower margins of the thyroid cartilage with the fingers of your caudad hand while your cephalad hand supports the patient's chin. Gently manipulate in a clockwise and counterclockwise motion with the fingers using the thumb as a pivet. The action should come from your elbow rather than your wrist or fingers. Several movements should show increased cartilaginous mobility after 1–3 sessions.

Hypopharyngeal and Esophageal Injuries

The esophagus is normally collapsed and shielded by surrounding structures. However, because it has extremely delicate walls, it can be easily injured by internal (eg, foreign body ingestion, exploration) or external penetrating wounds. Simple tears of the oropharynx or nasopharynx respond well to saline irrigation, solid food restriction, and precautions against infection. More severe injuries require surgical repair and antibiotics.

THE CERVICAL SPINE

Cervical spine injuries can be classified as being (1) *mild* (eg, contusions, strains), (2) *moderate* (eg, subluxations, sprain, occult fractures, nerve contusions, neuropraxias), (3) *severe* (eg, axonotmesis, dislocation, fracture without neurologic deficit), and (4) *dan-

gerous* (eg, fracture and/or dislocation, spinal cord injury).

Roentgenologic Considerations of the Neck

If routine cervical views are normal, then oblique, open-mouth odontoid, flexion, and extension views with most extreme care should be taken to verify symptoms. Flexion and extension views will indicate the extent of ligament rupture and bony displacement, but the danger of causing further damage is great. A complete radiographic study of the cervical spine can usually be accomplished with the views of the Davis or the modified-Davis series. Such a series is recommended when there is a history of trauma to the cervical spine and adjacent tissues or a history of chronic complaint and symptoms of possible pathology. Subtle fractures are often elicited only on laminagrams or tomograms.

Soft Tissues

In an injured player who is conscious, any neck spasm should be considered the expression of a cervical fracture or dislocation until proved otherwise. Dislocation or severe subluxation of C1 at the occipital junction may be seen, especially on the lateral view, and be associated with widening of the prespinal soft-tissue space following hemorrhage. The soft-tissue shadows anterior to the upper cervical vertebrae are normally narrowest in the upper cervical area and seldom wider than a C6 vertebral body's A-P dimensions in the lower cervical area. The retropharyngeal space should not exceed 7 mm, and the retrotracheal space should not exceed 22 mm. Signs of free air, edema, or hemorrhage may be seen in the prespinal and anterior area of the neck. After trauma, an increase in soft-tissue width is presumptive evidence of hemorrhage or edema from fracture.

With close inspection, one may sometimes note a lucent line tracking along the anterior margin of the cervical vertebrae, representing fatty tissue between the esophagus and anterior longitudinal ligament. This strip may be displaced anteriorly in spinal trauma and present the only evidence of injury.

The space available for the spinal cord

(diameter of spinal canal) is the narrowest distance between the posterior edge of a vertebral body and the anterior edge of the posterior vertebral arch. This measurement should not exceed 14 mm from C1 to C7 in adults or children. The width of the odontoid is approximately equal to the width of the spinal cord at the C1 level, and thus is a guide to the space available for the cord. If the space is less than the width of the odontoid, the cord is likely compromised.

Up to 3 mm of displacement of the atlas on the axis infers that the transverse ligament is intact, while ligament rupture is implied if displacement is from 3–5 mm. When displacement exceeds 5 mm, it may be assumed that the ligament has ruptured and the accessory ligaments has ruptured and the accessory ligaments are stretched and partially deficient. Atlantoxial instability is commonly caused by odontoid fracture, rheumatoid arthritis, and odontoid anomalies.

An acute rupture is often indicated by collapse of the disc space. Keep in mind that severe neurologic damage may be present without roentgenographic evidence (eg, brachial plexus injury), thus indicating a possible need for myelography after acute injury to elicit evidence of an avulsed nerve-root sleeve, intramedullary hemorrhage, bone fragments, or edema.

Osseous Tissues

Bony spurs are common in the cervical spines of male wrestlers, although adjacent intervertebral disc spaces are usually normal. Check for possible vertebral compression fractures by evaluating the anterior aspects of the vertebral bodies for collapse and comparing their margins. Posterior vertebral margins are compared for signs of subluxation or dislocation; ie, a continuous line passing through each posterior vertebral margin should be smooth and unbroken.

Carefully evaluate the relationships of the apophyseal joints and spinous processes for possible injury. The joints may show possible slippage. On an oblique view, the facets will be shingle-like and the end-on images of the lamina will appear as a chain of ovals. Whether or not a subluxation appears, a fracture may be located in the neural arch

or facet joint. Fractures of a spinous process frequently occur without displacement.

Intervertebral joint dislocation, unilateral or bilateral, may result from severe flexion trauma. Lamina fracture may or may not be associated. Facet locking is particularly common in unilateral dislocations, and it is usually associated with severe root and/or cord involvement.

Clinical Compression Tests

There are several syndromes to consider under the classification of neurovascular compression syndromes (also termed thoracic outlet or inlet syndromes), each of which may produce the symptom complex

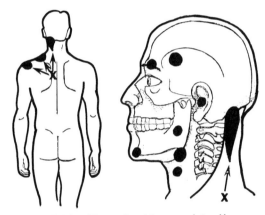

Figure 21.3. Trapezius trigger points; *X*, common sites. *Blackened areas* indicate sites of referred pain.

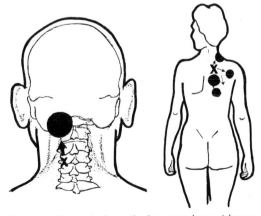

Figure 21.4. *Left*, splenius cervicus trigger point; *X*, common site. *Blackened areas* indicate typical sites of referred pain. *Right*, levator scapulae trigger point.

or radiating pain over the shoulders and down the arms, atrophic disturbance, paresthesias, and vasomotor disturbances. These syndromes do not necessarily give the cause of the problem. In some cases, poor posture, anomalies, muscle contractures, or other factors may be responsible. In addition, subluxation syndromes may initiate these and other disturbances of the shoulder girdle and must be further evaluated. Always x-ray before performing a cervical compression or traction test, especially when the patient has been involved in trauma, to rule out possible arteriosclerosis, disc compression, fracture, avulsion, gross subluxation, dislocation, or bone disease.

Active Cervical Rotary Compression Test. With the patient sitting, observe while the patient voluntarily laterally flexes his head toward the side being examined. With the neck flexed, the patient is then instructed to rotate his chin towards the same side, which narrows the intervertebral foramina diameters. Pain or reduplication of other symptoms probably indicates a physiologic narrowing of one or more intervertebral foramina.

Passive Cervical Compression Tests. With the patient sitting, stand behind the patient. The patient's head is laterally flexed and rotated slightly towards the side being examined. Place interlocked fingers on the patient's scalp and gently press caudally. If an intervertebral foramen is physiologically narrowed, this maneuver will further insult the foramen by compressing the disc and narrowing the foramen, thus causing pain and reduplication of other symptoms. In the second test, the patient's neck is extended by the examiner who then places interlocked hands on the patient's scalp and gently presses caudally. If an intervertebral foramen is physiologically narrowed, this maneuver mechanically compromises the foraminal diameters bilaterally and causes pain and reduplication of other symptoms.

Spurling's Tests. With the patient in the seated position and the examiner standing behind, the patient's head is rotated and laterally flexed to one side. With the patient actively holding the head and neck in this position, the examiner places a palm on the patient's scalp and vertically strikes it with the other fist. The patient's head is then rotated and laterally flexed to the opposite

side, and the test is repeated. If these tests can be tolerated by the patient without undue discomfort, the procedure is repeated with hyperextension added. In radiculitis, sensitive spondylosis, IVD syndromes, and other inflammatory or space-occupying conditions in or near the IVF or posterior facets, pain will be increased by the induced compression.

Shoulder Depression Test. With the patient sitting, stand behind the subject. The patient's head is laterally flexed away from the side being examined. This is done by the doctor stabilizing the patient's shoulder with one hand and applying pressure alongside the patient's head with the palm of the other hand, thus stretching the dural root sleeves and nerve roots or aggravating radicular pain if the nerve roots are adhered to the foramina. Extravasations, edema, encroachments, and conversion of fibrinogen into fibrin may result in interfascicular, foraminal, and articular adhesions and inflammations that will restrict fascicular glide and the ingress and egress of the foraminal contents. Thus, pain and reduplication of other symptoms during the test probably indicate adhesions between the nerve roots and the capsular structures within the intervertebral foramen.

Cervical Distraction Test. With the patient sitting, stand to the side of the patient, place one hand under the patient's chin and the other hand under the base of the occiput. Slowly and gradually lift the patient's head to remove its weight from the cervical spine. Such a maneuver widens the intervertebral foramen, decreases the pressure on the joint capsules around the facet joints, and stretches the paravertebral musculature. If the maneuver decreases pain and relieves other symptoms, it is a probable indication of narrowing of one or more intervertebral foramen, cervical facet syndrome, or spastic paravertebral muscles.

Adson's Test. With the patient sitting, palpate the radial pulse and advise the patient to bend the head obliquely backward to the opposite side being examined, take a deep breath, and tighten the neck and chest muscles on the side tested. The maneuver decreases the interscalene space (anterior and middle scalene muscles) and increases any existing compression of the subclavian artery and lower components (C8 and T1)

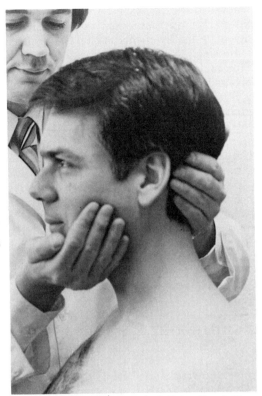

Figure 21.5. The cervical distraction test.

of the brachial plexus against the 1st rib. Marked weakening or loss of the pulse or increased paresthesias indicate a positive sign of pressure on the neurovascular bundle, particularly on the subclavian artery as it passes between or through the scaleni musculature, thus indicating a probable cervical rib or scalenus anticus syndrome.

Eden's Test. With the patient sitting, palpate radical pulse and instruct the patient to pull shoulders backward and throw the chest out in a "military posture" and to hold deep inspiration as the pulse is examined. The test is positive if weakening or loss of pulse occurs, indicating pressure on the neurovascular bundle as it passes between the clavicle and the 1st rib, thus a costoclavicular syndrome.

Wright's Test. With the patient sitting, the radial pulse is palpated from the posterior in the downward position and as the arm is passively moved through an 180°C arc. If the pulse diminishes or disappears in this arc or if neurologic symptoms develop, it is suspect of pressure on the axillary artery and vein under the pectoralis minor tendon

and coracoid process or compression in the retroclavicular spaces between the clavicle and 1st rib, thus a hyperabduction syndrome.

Vertebrobasilar Artery Maneuvers. 1) With the patient seated and the head placed in the neutral position, the carotid and subclavian arteries are palpated for abnormal pulsations and auscultated for bruits. If pulse abnormalities or obstruction (stenosis or compression), and the second maneuver should not be conducted. (2) If palpatory and auscultory signs are negative in the neutral position, the patient is asked to slowly rotate and hyperextend the neck first in one direction and then the other to place a motion-induced compression on the vertebral arteries. Positive signs include dizziness, faintness, nausea, nystagmus, vertigo, and/or visual blurring.

Other Pertinent Tests

Mankopf's Procedure. This is the only objective test for pain, and it is not restricted to musculoskeletal complaints of the cervical spine. The patient is placed in a relaxed position and the pulse is taken. The examiner then precipitates the pain (eg, by probing, applying heat or electrostimulation, etc). The pulse rate is then re-evaluated. In situations of true pain, the pulse rate will increase a minimum of 10%.

George's Tests. With the patient seated, blood pressure and the radial pulse rate are taken bilaterally and recorded. Stenosis or occlusion of the subclavian artery is suggested when a difference of 10 mm Hg between the two systolic blood pressures occurs and a feeble or absent pulse is found on the involved side. Even if these signs are absent, a subclavian deficit may be exhibited by finding auscultated bruits in the supraclavicular fossa.

Traction Test. With the patient seated and the arm held in the anatomical position, the radial pulse is determined while traction is firmly applied to the patient's wrist. If a decreased pulse is found on one side but not the other, a cervical rib should be suspected on the side of the decreased pulse.

Swallowing Test. The seated patient is asked to drink some water. If a pharyngeal lesion is ruled out (eg, tonsillitis), painfully difficult swallowing may suggest a space-occupying lesion at the anterior aspect of the cervical spine (eg, abscess, tumor, osteophytes, etc).

Brudzinski's Test. With the patient in the relaxed supine position, the examiner's slowly flexes the patient's neck toward the chest. If a spinal cord inflammatory process (eg, meningitis) is present, the neck will become painfully rigid and the patient will automatically flex the knees to lessen the traction forces being placed on the cord. Meningeal irritation is rarely seen in sports; however, this does not eliminate the possibility of a professional or amateur athlete becoming involved with such a disorder. Also see Kernig's and Soto-Hall's tests.

Valsalva's Maneuver. The seated patient is asked to bear down firmly (abdominal push), as if straining at the stool. This act increases intrathecal pressure, which tends to elicit localized pain in the presence of a space-occupying lesion (eg, IVD protrusion, cord tumor, bony encroachment, etc) or of an acute inflammatory disorder of the cord (eg, arachnoiditis). Coughing will produce the same effect under like circumstances.

Bikele's Test. The seated patient is asked to raise the arm laterally to a horizontal and slightly backward position, flex the elbow, and laterally flex the neck to the opposite side. If active extension of the elbow, which stretches the brachial plexus, produces resistance and increased cervicothoracic radicular pain, the test is said to be positive for a nerve root or spinal cord inflammatory process (eg, brachial neuritis, meningitis).

Bakody's Test. The seated patient is asked to raise the arm laterally to a horizontal position, flex the elbow, and then place the open palm upon the top of the head. This maneuver should relieve traction on the ipsilateral lower cervical roots and offer reliev of nerve root irritation in cases of an IVF syndrome.

SOFT-TISSUE INJURIES OF THE POSTERIOR NECK

Cervical Contusions, Strains, and Sprains

Contusions in the neck are similar to those of other areas. They often occur to the cervical muscles or spinous processes. Painful bruising and tender swelling will be found without difficulty, especially if the neck is flexed. Phillips points out the necessity of normally lax ligaments at the atlanto-axial joints to allow for normal articular gliding, thus making tonic muscle action the only means by which head stability is obtained.

Strains (1–3 Grades) or indirect muscle injuries are common, frequently involving the erectors. Flexion and extension cervical sprains are also common in sports (1–3 Grades) and usually involve the anterior or posterior longitudinal ligaments, but the capsular ligaments may be involved. In the neck especially, strain and sprain may coexist. Severity varies considerably from mild to dangerous. Anterior injuries are more common to the head and chest as they project further anteriorly, but a blunt blow from the front to the head or chest may result in an indirect extension or flexion injury of the cervical spine. Many cervical strains heal spontaneously but may leave a degree of fibrous thickening or trigger points within the injured muscle tissue (refer back to Figs. 21.3 and 21.4). Residual joint restriction following acute care is more common in traditional medical care than under mobilizing chiropractic supervision.

Cervical sprain and disc rupture are associated with severe pain and muscle spasm and are more common in adults because of the reduced elasticity of supporting tissues. Pain is often referred when the brachial plexus is involved. Cervical stiffness, muscle spasm, spinous process tenderness, and restricted motion are common. When pain is present, it is often poorly localized and referred to the occiput, shoulder, between the scapulae, arm, or forearm (lower cervical lesion), and it may be accompanied by paresthesias. Radicular symptoms are rarely present unless a herniation is present.

Diagnosis and treatment are similar to that of any muscle strain-sprain, but concern must be given to induced subluxations during the initial overstress. Palpation will reveal tenderness and spasm of specific muscles. In acute scalene strain, tenderness and swelling will usually be found. When the longissimus capitis or the trapezius are strained, they stand out like stiff bands.

O'Donoghue's Maneuvers. The cervical spine of a seated patient is passively flexed, extended, laterally flexed to both sides, and rotated in both directions against patient resistance. Pain precipitated by such iso-metric contraction indicates cervical strain. The test is then repeated without patient resistance. Pain precipitated by passive un-restricted motion signifies cervical sprain.

Rust's Sign. A seated patient is asked to lie back to a recumbent (supine) position. A positive sign is seen when the patient au-tomatically places the palm of one hand behind his neck to support the cervical spine. This sign is thought to be indicative of a lesion leading to weakness in the cer-vical flexors.

Extension Injuries. When the head is violently thrown backwards (eg, whiplash), the damage may vary from minor to severe tearing of the anterior and posterior liga-ments. Severe cord damage can occur which is usually attributed to momentary pressure from the ligamentum flavum and lamina posteriorly, even without roentgenographic evidence. A facial injury usually suggests an accompanying extension injury of the cer-vical spine as the head is forced backward. Management of minor injuries requires re-duction of subluxations, traction, physio-therapeutic remedial aid, a supporting collar for 10–12 weeks, and graduated therapeutic exercises.

Flexion Injuries. Slight anterior sublux-ation is usually not serious, but neurologic symptoms may appear locally or down the arm. Disc degeneration may follow, leading to spondylosis. An occipital injury usually suggests an accompanying flexion injury of the cervical spine as the skull is forced for-ward. Management is similar to that of ex-tension injuries except required support is often shorter (6–8 weeks).

Torticollis, Spasms, and Similar Disor-ders. Bolton describes torticollis (wryneck) is a state (acute or chronic) of one or more contracted cervical muscles that produces an unnatural, unsightly, twisted, disabling position of the head. It may or may not be painful. The acute forms are usually precip-itated by trauma, infection, unaccustomed postures, trigger point arousal, transient cer-vical vascular disturbances, aberrant tonic reflexes (local or referred), an acute apophy-seal or IVD syndrome, exposure to a unilat-eral cold draft, or hysteria. The chronic forms are usually spastic, dependent upon nerve irritation, and usually find their cause in congenital and habitual malposition (eg,

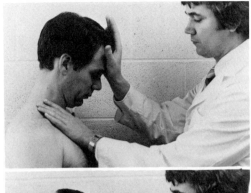

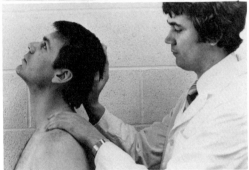

Figure 21.6. *Top*, testing cervical flexion strength. *Bottom*, the testing of extension strength.

ocular defect) and biomechanical, neoplas-tic, and psychogenic etiologies. In addition, torticollis may be a complication of basilar impression, vestibular dysfunction, cerebel-lar disease, hyperthyroidism, parkinsonism, drug toxicosis, pulmonary disease, visceral disease, and other disorders that may reflect upon cervical segments and/or musculature. Wryneck spasm (tonic, rarely clonic) of the sternocleidomastoideus and trapezius may be due to irritation of the spinal accessory nerve by swollen glands, abscess, acute up-per respiratory infections, scar, or tumor, but it more often occurs from traumatic cervical subluxations or idiopathically in "rheumatic" or "nervous" individuals. The muscles are rigid and tender, the head tilts toward the spastic sternocleidomastoideus, and the chin is rotated to the contralateral side. Common trigger points involved in "stiff neck" are in the trapezius (usually a few inches lateral to C7) or the levator scap-ulae and splenius cervicus lateral to C4–C6 cervical processes (see Figs. 21.3 and 21.4). These points are often not found unless the muscle is relaxed during palpation.

Wryneck may also be the result of subdiaphragmatic irritation being mediated reflexly into the trapezius and cervical muscles. Subclinical visceral irritation is sometimes the factor involved.

Dislocations of upper cervical vertebrae cause a distortion of the neck much like that of torticollis. A fracture-dislocation of a cervical vertebra will produce neck rigidity and a fast pulse, but fever is absent. Local and remote trigger points are frequently involved. In suspicious cases, the neck should always be x-rayed before it is examined. Neck rigidity may also be the result of a sterile meningitis from blood in the cerebrospinal fluid. Thus, if a patient has slight fever, rapid pulse, and rigid neck muscles, subarachnoid hemorrhage is suspected. Lateralizing signs are often indefinite.

Management. The correction of any spinal subluxation-fixation complex should never be attempted by the unskilled. In the context, Carrick wisely warns that "manipulation of the cervical spine is not to be considered conservative therapy, but rather a most aggressive noninvasive procedure by which the normal mechanical attitudes of the motion segments can be restored if aberrant. In all cases of cervical radiculopathy where there is demonstrable pathomechanics, it is recommended that manipulation be the primary treatment of choice, and that this therapy be prescribed and administered by qualified clinicians who have had extensive training in this science.

To relieve muscle spasm, heat is helpful, but cold and vapocoolant sprays have shown to be more effective in acute cases. Mild passive stretch is an excellent method of reducing spasm in the long muscles. Heavy passive stretch, however, destroys the beneficial reflexes. For example, place the patient prone on an adjusting table in which the head piece has been slightly lowered. Turn the patient's head toward the side of the spastic muscle. With head weight alone serving as the stretching force, the spasm should relax within 2–3 minutes. Thumb pressure, placed on a trigger area, is then directed towards the muscle's attachment and held for a few moments until relaxation is complete.

Isotonic exercises are useful in improving circulation and inducing the stretch reflex, especially in the cervical extensors. These exercises should be done supine to reduce exteroceptive influences on the central nervous system.

Peripheral inhibitory afferent impulses can be generated to partially close the presynaptic gate by acupressure, acu-aids, acupuncture, or transcutaneous nerve stimulation. Most authorities feel deep sustained manual pressure on trigger points is the best method, but a few others prefer brutal short-duration pressure (1–2 seconds). Deep pressure is contraindicated in any patient receiving anti-inflammatory drugs (eg, cortisone), as subcutaneous hemorrhage may result. The effects of cervical traction are often dramatic but sometimes short lived if a herniated disc is involved. In chronic cases, relaxation training with biofeedback is helpful.

During rehabilitation, a cervical pillow is recommended to provide proper postural support while sleeping. Grade 2 injuries should invariably be provided with an immobilization collar to provide support assistance and protection during the early stages of healing. This support should remain until pain-free motion is obtained. Any activity that induces discomfort should be avoided.

Nerve Stress

"Hot Shots" and Brachial Plexus Traction

After lateroflexion injuries of the neck, a sharp burning pain may radiate along the course of one or more cervical nerves, the result of nerve contusion due to stretching. Scalenus anticus syndrome may be exhibited. This is often referred to as a "hot shot" or "pinched nerve" by players and sports writers. Recurring injury is common, especially in football from "spearing." The syndrome is also seen in wrestling, squash (sidewall collision), and collisions in basketball.

Immediate pain may radiate to the back of the head, behind the ear, around the neck, or down towards the clavicle, shoulder, arm or hand. There are frequent arm paresthsias, severe arm weakness if not lack of active motion, often decreased biceps and triceps reflexes, forearm numbness, and cervical movement restriction. These signs and symptoms may disappear and reappear with greater severity. Roentgenography may show spur formation on cervical vertebrae.

If the symptoms appear on the opposite side of the forceful bending, undoubtedly a nerve has been "pinched" within the powerful muscles dorsal to the sternocleidomastoid. If this be the case, symptoms usually subside in a few minutes with only slight residual tenderness and paresthesia which disappear within a few hours. On the other hand, if symptoms appear on the same side as the direction of the forceful bending, deep skeletal injury such as fraction, dislocation, severe rotary subluxation, or nerve compression may be involved.

Prevention of aggravation requires correction of associated subluxations, strengthening cervical muscles, wearing a plastic roll within a stockinet as a cervical collar or applying a Thomas-type collar, and avoiding dangerous techniques of play.

A similar but more severe nerve injury common in sports is injury to the brachial plexus or its roots which is usually caused by a fall on the shoulder, a blow to the side of the neck, forceful arm traction, or a combination of these mechanisms. The injury is essentially caused by acute shoulder depression which stretches the brachial plexus, especially in the supraclavicular area. The effect may be root tear near the vertebral foramen, spinal cord damage, dural-cuff leaks of cerebrospinal fluid, and/or vertebral fracture or dislocation. But such severe manifestations are rarely seen in well-conditioned athletes where the picture is usually limited to pain radiating into the arm and/or hand.

The Stinger Syndrome

Albright describes the "stinger" syndrome as an apparently mild athletic brachial plexus injury that reflects a transient radiculopathy at the time of impact. Football "spearing" and head butting are common causes. The injury usually occurs when the neck is forcibly hyperextended and laterally flexed, and symptoms can usually be precipitated in this position during examination.

The condition is initially felt as a painfully severe electrical shock-like dysesthesia that extends from the shoulder to the fingertips. This feeling passes within a few moments and is replaced by sensations of numbness and upper extremity weakness that may last from a few seconds to several minutes.

The most common site of injury is at the C5 or C6 root level; and because of this, the most persistent sign will be weakness of the proximal shoulder muscles. An initial attack rarely leaves residual neurologic symptoms. Repetitive injuries of this nature, however, tend to have an accumulative effect that may lead to axonotmesis and chronic muscle weakness, which may take up to 6 months for full recovery.

The most common lesion associated with the stinger syndrome is cervical sprain with traumatic compression neuritis. Infrequently, an acute cervical disc rupture or a spontaneously reduced hyperextension dislocation may be associated. These later disorders are far more serious and usually require hospitalization until the severity of the injury can be properly assessed.

Trigger Points

The cervical and supracapsular areas of the trapezius frequently refer pain and deep tenderness to the lateral neck (especially the submastoid area), temple area, and angle of the jaw. The sternal division of the sternocleidomastoideus refers pain chiefly to the eyebrow, cheek, tongue, chin, pharynx, throat, and sternum. The clavicular division refers pain mainly to the forehead (bilaterally), back of and/or deep within the ear, and rarely to the teeth (see Fig. 19.5). Vapocoolant sprays to isolated sites often produce rapid spasm reduction of affected areas.

Vertebral Artery Deflection

The vertebral artery is a captive vessel from C6 upward. Extremes of rotation and flexion occur at the upper cervical region, but the four normal curves in the vertebral artery help to compensate for neck movements. Deflection may be caused by any stretching or elongation of the artery during neck injury. In later years, it is commonly associated with bony spurs from covertebral joints or grossly hyperplastic posterior vertebral articulations from arthrosis.

In discussing this situation, Smith explains that extension of the cervical spine allows the tip of the superior articular process of the posterior joint to glide forward and upward. If sufficiently hyperplastic, the motion may cause encroachment on the vertebral artery and/or the intervertebral foramen. Deflection of the artery and any resulting symptoms are exaggerated by rotation and/or extension of the neck. As a result of pressure against the artery, there may be temporary lessening in the volume of blood flow. Atheromatous changes may occur later within the vascular wall. The Barre-Lieou syndrome may be exaggerated by cervical extension. Sometimes symptoms are aggravated by dorsal extension and relieved by forward flexion with cervical traction.

The Barre-Lieou Syndrome. This syndrome frequently occurs from trauma to the cervical spine, and an underlying cervical arthritis and/or IVD lesion (eg, spondylosis) are often present. Although the symptomatology is nonspecific, Kimmel describes the common features to be earache, eye pain, facial vasomotor disturbances headache, temporary blurred vision, tinnitus, and vertigo. Dysphagia, phonation defects, and laryngeal and pharyngeal paresthesiae are often associated. If chronic cervical arthritis is a cause of sympathetic irritation, especially in the midcervical area, corneal hyperesthesia and small persistent ulcers usually appear that are confined to the exposed conjunctiva.

The vertebral nerve has its origin in the middle cervical sympathetic ganglion, and it offers vasomotor control over the vertebral artery. The Barre-Lieou syndrome is thought to be the result of vertebral nerve irritation that causes a circulatory impairment in the area of the cranial nuclei, especially those of the trigeminal and auditory nerves.

Barre-Leiou's Test. The seated patient is asked to slowly but firmly rotate the head first to one side and then to the other. Crawford reports that transient mechanical occlusion of the vertebral artery may be precipitated by simply turning the head, and this phenomenon is attributed to the compressive action of the longus colli and scalene muscles on the vertebral artery, just prior to its course through the IVF of C6. A positive sign in Barre-Leiou's test is exhibited if dizziness, faintness, nausea, nystag-

mus, vertigo, and/or visual blurring result, indicating of buckling of the vertebral artery.

Roentgenologic Considerations. When the vertebral bodies of the midcervical region are involved, the process of vertebral artery deflection may be visualized either by oblique or A-P projections. Smith feels stereoscopic studies are especially valuable. The midcervical region shows a predilection for this process. An aneurysm-like condition occurs not uncommonly within the cancellous lateral mass of C2. The tortuosity is visualized in both A–P and lateral views. Since the erosion develops slowly, there is a radiolucency surrounded by a white curvilinear line in the osseous structures adjacent to the vertebral artery. The significance of the erosions is the implication of vessel wall changes, but these erosions may be mistaken for the results of tumor pressure or other destructive processes involving bone.

Disc Disorders

Cervical Disc Herniation. Specific signs of acute disc herniation are:
- *C4–5 disc rupture*: shoulder and arm pain and paresthesia, hypesthesia of 5C root distribution, deltoid or biceps weakness.
- *C5–6 disc rupture*: hypesthesia of lateral forearm and thumb, biceps and supinator weakness.
- *C6–7 disc rupture*: hypesthesia of the index and middle fingers, triceps, and grip weakness.
- *C7–T1 disc rupture* (uncommon): ulnar hypesthesia and intrinsic muscle weakness in the hand.

Lhermitte's Test. With the patient sitting, flexing of the patient's neck and hips simultaneously with the knees in full extension may produce sharp pain radiation down the spine and into the upper or lower extremities. When pain is elicited, it is a sign suggesting irritation of the spinal dura matter either by a protruded cervical disc, tumor, fracture, or multiple sclerosis.

Degenerative Disc Disease. The cervical spine is readily subject to degenerative disc disease because of its great mobility and regional biomechanical stress and because it serves as a common site for various bony congenital defects. Bone changes are more common posteriorly in the upper cervicals and anteriorly in the lower cervicals. Cervical degenerative changes can be demonstrated in about half the people at 40 years of age and 70% of those at 65 years, many of which may be asymptomatic.

Management. Adjustive treatment consists of specific manipulation performed, with manual traction at the involved motion units to free impinged synovial fringes and reduce intra-articular subluxations and disc displacement, but this should never be performed with the neck in extension. Therapy includes immobilization of the neck with a cervical collar, sleeping with the head between sand bags or in traction, heat (diathermy, infrared, moist hot packs), massage, ultrasound to cervical paraspinal muscles, and periodic bed rest with cervical traction (10–20 lb). Supplementation with 140 mg of manganese glycerophosphate six times daily has proven helpful. Refer for radical treatment if one of the following occurs: (1) conservative treatment fails to produce remission of symptoms; (2) attacks reappear after a short period; (3) severe nerve-root compression with paralysis is indicated by muscle wasting and/or a sensory deficit has developed.

Spinal Cord Injury

While only about 6% of spinal cord injuries occurring within sports result in permanent paralysis, even this number is unacceptable inasmuch as many are preventable. Most injuries are caused by extreme flexion where subluxation, fracture and dislocation may be associated. Hemorrhage may occur at the site with the same reaction as brain injury (liquefaction, softening, disintegration). Congenital fusions and stenosis may predispose a child to spinal cord trauma during a sporting activity.

There are direct and indirect classes of injuries:

• *Direct injury* to the cord, the nerve roots, or both may be caused by impact forces or shattered bone fragments. The cord may be crushed, pierced, or cut. This type of injury is generally an open wound.

• *Indirect injury* to the cord may be caused by the disturbance of tissues near the spine by violent forces such as falls, crushes, or blows. This type of injury, which

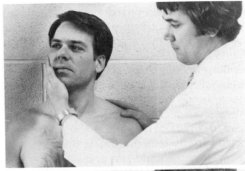

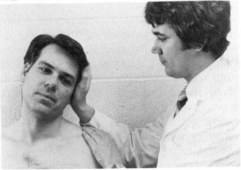

Figure 21.7. *Top*, testing cervical rotation strength. *Bottom*, testing lateral flexion strength.

is normally closed with respect to the spinal column and cord, is of a lesser degree than direct injury. It takes the form of concussion, hemorrhage, or edema of the cord. The cord may cease to function below the site at which the force was applied even if the cord itself received no direct injury. Such dysfunction may be temporary or long standing. Injuries to the spinal column in which the cerebrospinal fluid is rapidly depleted may be fatal.

If the cervical cord is injured, there is loss of sensation and flaccid paralysis. The lower limbs exhibit a spastic paralysis. If the space in which the spinal fluid flows between the spinal cord and the surrounding vertebral column is either compressed or enlarged, severe headache occurs. Posttrauma penile erection strongly suggests either cervical or thoracic cord injury.

Emergency Care. Immediate and obvious symptoms of spinal cord injury parallel those of a fracture of the spinal column. In the emergency-care situation, the patient with spinal cord injury must be treated as if the spinal column were fractured, even when there is no external evidence. Shock must be prevented or reduced. If the player is conscious, ask the location of pain. Ask if the player can move arms and legs. Pinch the skin and check for pain perception. Clothing should be loosened and everything removed from the pockets. Shoes and moist socks should be removed. Knee and ankle reflexes can be tested, but do not move the head and neck. The patient should be protected from temperature extremes, but heavy covers should not press against paralyzed parts.

On-Field Evaluation. Schneider warns that the initial examination of a player on the field with cord damage can be quite deceiving. Rarely is a deformity palpable in a muscular athlete. If cord damage has occurred, the player may complain of little or no pain even if paralysis or sensory loss are present (see Table 21.2).

Bradburne's Sign (Thorburn's position). During the acute stage of cervical cord contusion, compression, or shock (with or without vertebral fracture), a sign of spinal cord damage in the area of C5 and C6 is exhibited by bilateral abduction of the arms and flexion and external rotation of the forearms.

BONE AND JOINT INJURIES AND RELATED DISORDERS

Cervical Spondylosis

Cervical spondylosis is a chronic condition in which there is progressive degeneration of the intervertebral disc(s) leading to secondary changes in the surrounding vertebral structures, including the posterior apophyseal joints. It is the result of direct trauma (ie, disc injury), occupational stress, or aging degeneration, or found in association with and adjacent to congenitally nonsegmented vertebrae. Incidence is high in the second half of life with increasing severity in advancing years; 60% at 45 years, 85% at 65 years. It is most often seen at the C5–C6 disc level, and next in frequency at the C6–C7 level.

Background

Spondylosis may produce compression of either the nerve root or spinal cord. Deep tendon reflexes in the area are decreased or absent. Pre-existing spinal stenosis, thickened ligamentum flavum, protruding disc, and spur formation not uncommonly complicate the picture of cervical spondylosis. There is almost no correlation between the degree of perceived pain in the neck and the degree of arthritic changes noted in x-ray films.

The onset is usually rapid and insidious but may be subjectively and objectively asymptomatic. Whiting lists the symptoms which develop to include neck stiffness; cervical movement limitations; neck crepitus, subjective or objective; local neck pain and tenderness; headaches; neck pain radiating to the scapulae, trapezius, upper extremities, occiput, or anterior thorax; extremity muscle weakness; paresthesia of the upper and/or lower extremities; dizziness and fainting; impaired vibration sense at the

Table 21.2.
Quickly Determined On-the-Field Cord Signs

Injury Level	Paralysis	Loss of Pain to Pin Prick
C3–C4	Trunk, extremities, diaphragm	Below clavicle, upper extremities
C4–C5	Arms, lower extremities, trunk, only abdominal breathing	Numbness to the level of the outer border of the upper extremity between the shoulder and elbow
C5–C6	Fingers, impaired arm extension	Thumb and Index finger
C6–C7	Impaired grasp, weak elbow flexion and extension, loss of finger spread	Middle finger, radial half of ring finger

ankle; hyperactive patellar and Achilles reflexes; and positive Babinski responses.

Roentgenographic Considerations

Due to the constant weight of the head, postural strains, occupational insults, degrees of congenital anomalies, and post-traumatic or postinfection effects with or without an associated disc involvement, the development of chronic degenerative spondylosis offers some distinct progressive characteristics: (1) flattening of the cervical spine from muscular spasm and adhesion development, (2) anterior-posterior fixation and restricted mobility, (3) thinning of the atlanto-occipital and atlantoaxial articular plates resulting in motion restriction, (4) middle and lower cervical disc wearing and thinning which narrows the intervertebral foramina, (5) disc thinning and weakness encouraging disc herniation contributing to nerve encroachment, (6) osseous lipping and spurs with extensions into the intervertebral foramina, and (7) infiltration and ossification of perivertebral ligaments adding to inflexibility and pain upon movement. The Davis series may suffice, but special views, tomography, myelography, or discography may be necessary for firm diagnosis.

It is important to avoid the pitfall of assuming that all the patient's symptoms involving the neck and upper extremities are caused by a cervical spondylosis when it is found radiographically. Cervical spondylosis is common, and symptoms may thus be associated with unrelated neurologic disease which may coexist with the spondylosis, making the diagnosis more difficult.

Case Management and Prognosis

Whiting brings out that it is fortunate that most people with cervical spondylosis are asymptomatic because there is no correction per se. Treatment is aimed at reducing symptoms of neurologic vasoneurologic involvement or treating the soft-tissue injury superimposed on the pre-existing spondylosis. A trial of conservative treatment is preferred in cases demonstrating signs of either cervical radiculopathy and/or myelopathy.

There is a natural tendency for a patient suffering with symptoms of radiculopathy related to cervical spondylosis to improve regardless of the treatment regimen. Unfortunately, the degenerative changes of the intervertebral disc, vertebral bodies, and associated diarthroidial joints are permanent and, in most cases, progressive. Treatment is therefore aimed at reducing symptoms and future attacks by proper case management and prophylaxis. Exacerbation of symptoms are quite common, but months or years may elapse between attacks. With age and the gradual increase in degenerative changes, atttacks are more closely spaced, and recovery from each attack is prolonged. Any superimposed trauma on silent cervical spondylosis can result in permanent partial disability of the cervical spine with symptoms out of proportion of the severity of the injury.

In cervical myelopathy, there is a gradual increase in the neurologic signs and symptoms until a leveling off occurs and symptoms remain stationary, unless superimposed trauma ensues. Although conservative care does produce remission of subjective symptoms, especially in early diagnosed cases, objective signs are very rarely changed and sensory symptoms return and progress to a plateau. Thus, suggests Whiting, surgical intervention is probably the treatment of choice in severe myelopathy once the symptoms return following a trial of conservative care or if there is evidence of paralysis.

Reversal of the Normal Cervical Curve

A pathologic loss of the normal anterior curve of the cervical spine, characterized by a straightening of the spine, results in mechanical alteration of normal physiologic and structural integrity. The condition occurs more frequently after the age of 40, and the sexes appear equally affected. The cause is usually the result of trauma-producing whiplash injury, herniated disc, subluxation, dislocation, fracture, or ligamentous injury. Torticolis, arthritis, malignancy, tuberculosis, osteomyelitis, and other pathologies may be involved.

Symptoms and signs include headaches (occipital, occipital-frontal, supraorbital), vertigo, rigidity due to cervical muscle spasm, limited extension and flexion, tenderness elicited on lateral C4–C6 nerve

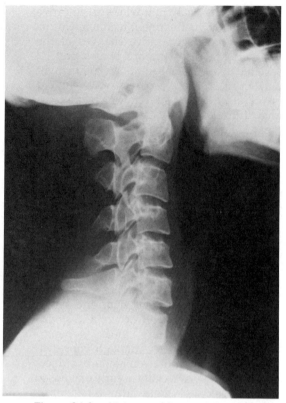

Figure 21.8. Male, age 30, complained of acute pain in the cervical area following a touch football game to which he was unaccustomed. Later cervical view showed a reverse (kyphotic) cervical curve with possible dyskinesia at C3 and C4 which had not been previously present (with the permission of Shu Yan Ng, D.C.)

Case Management and Prognosis. Specific correction of offending vertebral subluxation(s) should be accomplished. Adjunctive care includes massage, intermittent traction, and methods to reduce muscle spasm such as ultrasound, diathermy, hydrocolator packs, reflex spinal techniques, and a rolled towel placed under the neck in the supine position to increase the cervical curve. The individual should be instructed to sleep without a pillow. Cervical muscle re-education is quite helpful. Rehberger feels that the prognosis is excellent if the condition is treated early and the case is not complicated by fracture or dislocation, but guarded if the trauma is severe. In cases of minimal cervical discopathy, symptomatic relief can be expected. Prognosis is poor in advanced degenerative osteoarthritis.

Cervical Rib

Anomalous development of extraribs in the region of the cervical vertebrae may be a single unilateral rib, be bilateral, or be multiple bilaterally. The condition is usually seen at C7, and the cause is a variation in the position of the limb buds. It may vary from a small nubbin to a fully developed rib. A small rudimentary rib may give rise to more symptoms than a well-developed rib because of a fibrous band attached between the cervical rib and sternum or 1st thoracic rib. Incidence is more frequent in females in the ratio of 3 to 1.

A cervical rib arising from C7 and ending free or attached to the T1 rib appears in the neck as an angular fullness which may pulsate owing to the presence of the subclavian artery above it. It rarely produces symptoms, often encountered when percussing the apex of the lung. The bone can be felt behind the artery by careful palpation in the supraclavicular fossa and demonstrated by roentgenography. Pain or wasting in the arm and occasionally thrombosis may occur.

Differentiation. Symptoms usually occur at age 12 or later, after the ribs have ossified. Two groups of symptoms are seen, those of scalenus anticus syndrome and those due to cervical-rib pressure. The symptoms of cervical rib and scalenus syndrome are similar, and the scalenus anticus muscle is the primary factor in the production of neurocirculatory compression whether a cervical rib is present or not.

roots, neuritis involving branches of the brachial plexus due to nerve-root pressure, hyperesthesia of one or more fingers, and loss or lessening of the biceps reflex on the same or contralateral side. In rare cases, the triceps reflex may be involved. One or more symptoms are frequently aggravated with an abnormal position of the head such as during reading, sleeping, or driving.

Roentgenographic Considerations. Rehberger reports the typical radiographic findings to include loss of cervical curve with straightening of the cervical spine (78% cases), anterior and posterior subluxation on flexion and extension views, narrowing of intervertebral disc spaces at C4–C6 (46% cases), discopathy at the affected vertebral level as the injury progresses, and osteoarthritic changes which are often accompanied by foraminal spurring.

When symptoms are presented, they are usually from compression of the lower cord of the brachial plexus and subclavian vessels such as numbness and pain in the ulnar nerve distribution. Pain is worse at night because of pressure from the recumbent position. Pain of varying intensity, tiredness and weakness of the extremity, finger cramps, numbness, tingling, coldness of the hand, areas of hyperesthesia, muscle degeneration in the hand, a lump at the base of the neck, tremor, and discoloration of the fingers are characteristic. Work and exercise accentuate symptoms, while rest and elevation of the extremity relieve symptoms.

Adson's and other like signs will be positive. The 4th and 5th decades mark the highest incidence, probably because of regressive muscular changes. Trauma is a common factor in sports. Aneurysms of the subclavian artery are rare. Differential diagnosis must exclude infectious neuritis, arthritis of the shoulder joint, cervical arthritis, subachromial bursitis, deformities, and cardiac disease. Compression of nerve tissue results in numbness, pain, paralysis, and loss of function. Compression of vascular structures results in moderate pain, edema, swelling, and obstruction of circulation resulting in clotting within the vessels with possible consequent infarction in the tissues supplied. These unilateral phenomena are limited to the cervicobrachial distribution.

The etiologic theories of the cervicobrachial syndrome are compression of the nerve trunks, trauma to nerve trunks, injuries to the sympathetic and vasomotor nerves, trauma to the scalenus anterior muscle, embryologic defects, postural or functional defects, narrowing of the upper thoracic cap as a result of adjacent infections or anatomic defects, acute infection producing myositis, intermittent trauma to the subclavian artery, or a cervical rib.

Case Management. It has been Claypool's experience that some palliative relief can be obtained in some cases by correction of posture, gentle manipulation of the upper dorsal and lower cervical spine, cervical traction, and other relaxing physiotherapy. Those cases which don't respond to conservative treatment require surgery, and those cases treated conservatively usually show a recurrence of symptoms periodically.

CERVICAL FRACTURES

Fractures of the cervical spine are usually the result of blows, falls, or vehicular accidents. Most cervical fractures are characterized by neck pain that tends to radiate into the trapezius and upper extremities. The neck is rigid because of a protective spasm. Localized tenderness, upper extremity motor and sensory disturbances, and easy fatigue of involved musculature is common. Referred pain may radiate to the scalp, and upper extremity pain and paresthesiae may be present. In many cases, however, the patient will be asymptomatic except for mild symptoms.

Fractures and Dislocations of the Atlas

Atlanto-occipital dislocations, often bilateral, are usually quickly incompatible with life. Any severe subluxation in the upper cervical area can lead to quadriplegia or death, often with little warning and few symptoms to differentiate it initially from a mild strain. Thus, it is always better to be extra cautious (and be accused of being overly concerned in mild injuries) to insure against a possible disaster. Signs and symptoms vary from subtle to severe pain and gross motor involvement. Tenderness may be acute over the posterior atlas, aggravated by mild rotation and extension.

Classes. There are three major types of severe injury, all of which are serious: (1) The atlas may displace on the axis and fracture the odontoid process. The patient usually survives if extreme care is taken in transportation to the hospital. (2) A vertical blow may split the atlas and force the lateral masses outward, disrupting the ring. Severity depends upon fragment displacement relative to the cord and vital tissues. (3) If the odontoid is displaced posteriorly, the situation is usually fatal because of injury to the cord. The spontaneous fusion of C1 to the occiput is always a potential complication.

Roentgenographic Considerations. In C1–C2 dislocations, C1 often displaces anteriorly relative to C2. This will alter a line connecting the cortices of the anterior parts of the spinous processes from C1 to C7, unless the process of C2 is fused with the occiput or congenitally short. If this is suspected, flexion-extension views or a C1–C2 tomogram should be considered.

The atlas may be fractured on the posterior arch, ring, or anterior arch. Of all atlantoid fractures, most literature states that those of the posterior arch are the most common yet easily overlooked as the displacement is usually mild. The common site is at the narrowest portion just posterior to each lateral mass. The typical mechanism is hyperextension with compression of the posterior atlantal arches between the occiput and axis pedicles. Retropharygeal swelling is usually absent, and oblique views are often necessary for demonstration. Ring fractures are frequently produced by blows on top of the head where forces are dispersed laterally, fracturing the arches of the atlas and spreading them sidewards. Overhang of the atlantal lateral masses and widening of the paraodontoid space will be associated. Most authorities state that fractures of the anterior arch are rare, minimally displaced, usually comminuted, and frequently require tomography to be detected. However, Iversen and Clawson feel that fractures to the anterior arch are quite common and found either in the midline or just lateral to the midline.

Fractures and Dislocations of the Axis

Odontoid fractures are often produced by severe forces directed to the head, and the direction of force usually determines the direction of displacement. Suboccipital tenderness may be present. A severe extension force may fracture the odontoid at its base, with possible odontoid posterior displacement. The danger of cord pressure is great. Open-mouth views, flexion-extension x-ray views, or tomography may be necessary for accurate determination.

Roentgenographic Considerations. The atlantal-dens interval should be 3 mm or less in adults even during cervical flexion. The interval is slightly more (eg, as much as 4 mm during flexion) in children under the age of 8 years.

Many years ago, Anderson and D'Alonzo classified fractures of the axis into three types that are still applicable:

• *Type I:* Avulsion of the upper part of the odontoid (rare).

• *Type II:* Fracture through the base of the odontoid at or below the level of the superior articular facets of the axis. This is the most common type of axial fracture, and the cruciate ligaments on the posterior aspect of the odontoid may remain intact. Occasionally the odontoid will not be displaced but slightly angulated as a result of a toggle effect on flexion-extension films. This type of fracture is quite unstable and leads to nonunion.

• *Type III:* Fracture of the body of the axis. Displacement may not occur. A small bone chip separated from the anterior-inferior rim of the axis at the point of rupture of the anterior longitudinal ligament may be a clue. About 36% of these fractures occur through the cancellous bone of the body of the axis, are stable, and heal without difficulty.

Care must be taken not to confuse odontoid nonunion with os odontoideum. In os odontoideum, the process is about 50% smaller than normal, round, and separated from the hypoplastic odontoid by a wide gap. The remnant hypoplastic odontoid appears as a hill, forming upward from the slope of the superior articular facets. The fracture line in nonunion is narrow and at or below the level of the superior articular facets, and the process is normal in size and shape.

Severe C3–C7 Injuries

Cervical fractures and dislocations are not common in sports. They are usually the result of a football, trampoline, gymnastic, vehicular, or diving injury. Bruises on the face, occiput, and shoulders may offer clues as to the mechanism of injury. Seek signs of vertebral tenderness, limitation in movement, muscle spasm, and neurologic deficits. As in upper-cervical damage, careful emergency management is necessary to avoid paralysis and death. Severe fracture and/or dislocation of any cervical vertebra require orthopedic referral for reduction, bone traction, and casting. Keep in mind that overdiagnosing instability of C2–3 is a common pitfall.

Compression or flexion damage is sometimes seen, but extension injuries (eg, whiplash) are more common. Spinous process fractures usually occur at the C6 or C7 level after acute flexion or a blow to the flexed neck producing ligamentous avulsion. There is immediate "hot" pain in the area of the

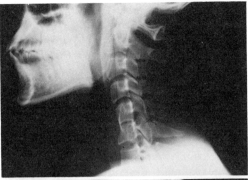

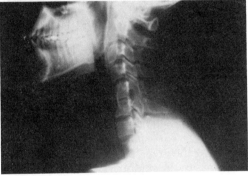

Figure 21.9. *Top*, male, age 22, complained of paresthesia in both hands immediately after diving into shallow water. X-ray films taken 2 months following the injury showed fusion of bodies of C5 and C6, with C5 slightly flexed upon C6. The fusion was probably not congenital as disc space was clearly seen. *Bottom*, radiograph taken 3 years later showed no significant changes (with the permission of Shu Yan Ng, D.C.)

profile. Fractures are frequently quite apparent when preesnt.

Flexion Injuries. During forceful cervical flexion, a unilateral facet dislocation and/or fracture may occur with the contra-lateral side remaining intact, or bilateral dislocation or fracture-dislocation may occur. Unilateral dislocation is more common in the lower cervical area.

Hyperextension "Whiplash" Syndrome. Forceful extension produces tearing of the anterior longitudinal ligament which may coexist with an avulsion fracture at the anterior vertebral bodies. Pedicle fracture or severe posterior subluxation may also occur. Tenderness will usually be shown along the lateral musculature. Upper extremity pain or numbness and restricted cervical motion at one interspace during flexion-extension may be exhibited. Symptoms may be prolonged without demonstrable evidence.

Cervical Spinal Percussion Test. The head of a seated patient is moderately flexed while the examiner percusses each of the cervical spinous processes and adjacent superficial soft tissues with a rubber-tipped reflex hammer. Evidence of point tenderness suggests a fractured or acutely subluxated vertebra or localized sprain or strain, while symptoms of radicular pain suggest radiculitis or an IVD lesion.

CERVICAL SUBLUXATION SYNDROMES

Vertebral subluxations are difficult to classify under normal categories of injury because they can involve bone, joint, muscle, ligament, disc, nerve, cord, spinal fluid, and vascular tissues.

Functional Anatomy Relative to Cervical Subluxations

Loss of mobility of any one or more segments of the spine corresponding influences its circulation. The resulting partial anoxia has a harmful influence upon nerve function. The artery and vein supplying a spinal nerve are situated in the foramen between the nerve and the fibrous tissue in the anterior portion of the foramen. It is unlikely that circulation to the nerve would be disrupted without first irritating or compressing the nerve because the arteries and veins

spinous process which is increased by flexion. Any injury to C6–C7 is difficult to view on film because of overlapping structures.

Compression Fractures. Vertebral body crush fractures are rare, and less common in the cervical spine than elsewhere. Compression fractures of articular processes occur in extension (eg, rear-end whiplash) injuries to the neck. They are not common in sports, with the exception of those occurring in divers, and are not demonstrable on A–P or lateral films until deformity is severe. Oblique views will often demonstrate them, but they are best seen on "pillar views." The pillar view is taken with the trunk A–P and the head turned 45° to the side, exposure factors are the same as those for the AP exposure. These views, taken bilaterally, will show the articular pillar in are much smaller, blood pressure within the lumen makes them not easily compressed, and nerve tissue is much more responsive to encroachment irritation.

Once a vertebra loses its ideal relationship with contiguous structures (subluxation) and becomes relatively fixed at some point (fixation) within its normal scope of movement, it is no longer competent to fully participate in ideal coordinated spinal movement. The affected area becomes the target for unusual stresses, weight bearing and traumatic. In addition to the attending circulatory, neuromechanical, and static changes in the involved area, there is disturbed reflex activity which may be exhibited as changes in superficial and deep reflexes, hyperkinesia, pupillary changes, excessive lacrimation, tremors and spasms. Frequent anomalies in the cervical area predispose subluxations from minor stress. The weight of the head along with activity stress may contribute to chronic degenerative spondylosis often superimposed upon asymptomatic anomalies. Clinically, a vicious cycle is seen where subluxation contributes to degenerative processes and these processes contribute to subluxation.

The Cervical Plexus

The dura mater of the spinal cord is firmly fixed to the margin of the foramen magnum and to the 2nd and 3rd cervical vertebrae. In other spinal areas, it is separated from the vertebral canal by the epidural space. Since both the C1 nerve and the vertebral artery pass through this membrane and both are beneath the superior articulation of the atlas and beneath the overhanging occiput, atlanto-occipital distortion may cause traction of the dura mater, producing irritation of the artery and nerve unilaterally and compressional occlusion contralaterally. This helps us understand those cases of suboccipital neuralgia where a patient upon turning his head to one side increases headache and vertigo that are relieved when the head is turned to the opposite side. In addition, there is a synapse between the upper cervical nerves and the trigeminal which also supplies the dura mater. This explains why irritation of C1 results in a neuralgia not only confined to a small area at the base of the skull but is also referred to the fore-

head or eye via the supraorbital branch of the trigeminal. The greater occipital (C2) does not tend to do this, but emitting as it does between the posterior arch of the atlas and above the lamina of the axis, it refers pain to the vertex of the head.

The superficial sensory cutaneous set of the cervical plexus (C1–4) is frequently involved in subluxations of the upper four segments, particularly when there are predisposing spondylotic degenerative changes. Janse describes four resultant neuralgias: (1) *Lesser occipital nerve neuralgia*: involving the area of the occipitalis muscle, mastoid process, and upper posterior aspect of the auricle. (2) *Greater auricular nerve neuralgia*: extending in front and behind the auricle, skin over the parotid gland, paralleling the distribution of the auriculo-temporal branch of the trigeminus and easily misdiagnosed as chronic trifacial neuralgia. (3) *Cervical cutaneous nerve neuralgia*: involving the area of the middle third of the platysma to the midline, possibly extending from the chain to the sternum. (4) *Supraclavicular nerve neuralgia*: depending upon which rami are affected, the neuralgia may involve the suprasternal area, pectoral area, or deltoid area. Thus, sternoclavicular and acromioclavicular neuralgias may originate in the spinal levels of the supraclavicular nerve.

De Rusha points out that dysphagia and dysarthria may at times be due to upper cervical involvement rather than a central nervous system situation. The C1 joins the hypoglossal cranial nerve which supplies the intrinsic muscles of the tongue. It then descends to join the descending cervical which is derived from C2 and C3. A loop of nerves, the ansi hypoglossi which supplies muscles necessary for deglutition and speaking, is derived from C1–C3.

Irritative lesions involving the cervical region and its articulations may in turn irritate the sympathetic nerve plexuses ascending into the head via the vertebral and carotid arteries. Some cases of visual and aural symptoms are related to upper cervical distortion where the arch of the atlas snugly hugs the occiput, thus possibly irritating the sympathetic plexus of nerves on the vertebral arteries as well as partial compression of the vessels. To appreciate this, note that

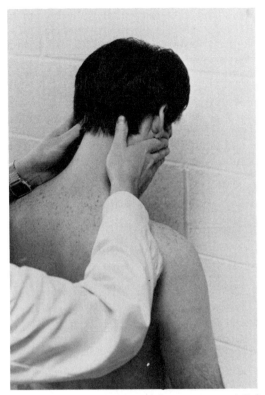

Figure 21.10. Palpation of the greater occipital nerve.

the visual cortical area of the occipital lobe requires an ideal blood supply dependent on the sympathetics ascending the great vessels of the neck, and this holds true for the inner ear as well. To test this syndrome, De Rusha suggests having the supine patient read some printed matter while the examiner places gentle traction on the skull, separating occipital and atlantal articulations. A positive sign is when the patient, often to his surprise, experiences momentarily enhanced visual acuity or a reduced tinnitus.

Disturbances of nerve function associated with subluxation syndromes manifest as abnormalities in sensory interpretations and/or motor activities. These disturbances may be through one of two primary mechanisms: direct nerve or nerve root disorders, or of a reflex nature.

Nerve Root Insults

When direct nerve root involvement occurs on the posterior root of a specific neu-

romere, it manifests as an increase or decrease in awareness over the dermatome. A typical example includes foraminal occlusion or irritating factors exhibited clinically as hyperesthesia, particularly on the (1) dorsal and lateral aspects of the thumb and radial side of the hand, when involvement occurs between C5–C6; and (2) dorsum of the hand, the index and middle fingers, and the ventroradial side of the forearm, thumb, index and middle fingers, when involvement occurs between C6–C7. In other instances, this nerve root involvement may cause hypertonicity and the sensation of deep pain in the musculature supplied by the neuromere—for example, (1) C6 involvement, with deep pain in the biceps; and (2) C7 involvement, with deep pain in the triceps and supinators of the forearm. In addition, direct pressure over the nerve root or distribution may be particularly painful.

Nerve root insults from subluxations may also be evident as disturbances in motor reflexes and/or muscular strength. Examples of these reflexes include the deep tendon reflexes such as seen in the (1) reduced biceps reflex when involvement occurs between C5–C6; and (2) reduced triceps reflex when involvement occurs between C6–C7. These reflexes must also be compared bilaterally to judge whether hyporeflexia is unilateral. Unilateral hyperreflexia is pathognomonic of an upper motor neuron lesion. Prolonged and/or severe nerve root irritation, not seen in the active athlete, may also cause evidence of trophic changes in the tissues supplied.

Subluxation-Induced Reflex Syndromes

Certain spinosomatic and spinovisceral syndromes may result from cervical subluxation. For example, the involvement may be in the area of C1–C4. This area includes the cervical portion of the sympathetic gangliated chain and the 9th–12th cranial nerves as they exit from the base of the skull and pass into their compartments within the deep cervical fascia. The syndrome may include (1) suboccipital or postocular migraine; (2) greater occipital nerve extension neuralgia; (3) mandibular, cervical, auricular, pectoral, or precordial neuralgia; (4) paroxysmal torticollis; (5) congestion of the upper respiratory mucosa, paranasal sinuses, or eustachian tube with hearing loss; (6) cardiorespiratory attacks; (7) ocular muscle malfunction; (8) pathologic hiccups; (9) scalenus anticus syndrome; and (10) painful spasms in the suboccipital area.

Phillips states that if a subluxation produces a stretching of the paravertebral musculature, there will be a continuous barrage of afferent impulses in the Ia fibers. "These afferent impulses monosynaptically bombard the alpha motor neurons causing the paravertebral musculature to go into tetany (spasm). There is a cessation of this afferent barrage when the stretch is released. The muscle stretching also initiates afferent impulses in the Group II afferents from flower spray endings which may reinforce the spastic muscle condition." He goes on to say that trauma to facet joints, disturbed articular relationships, spasms of closely related muscles, and overlying trigger points—all the results of a subluxation—set up a barrage of flexor-reflex afferent impulses via the Group II–IV fibers that converge upon the internuncial pool in lamina seven of the spinal cord. "This abundant supply or flexor-reflex afferent impulses excites the alpha motor neurons through multisynaptic connections causing an excess of excitation of paravertebral muscles resulting in spasm."

Occipital and Cervical Subluxations

Disturbances in this area usually arise from muscular spasm of one or more of the six muscle bundles which have attachments on the occiput, atlas, or axis. Unequal tension and ultimate fibrotic changes within the paravertebral structures can readily influence the delicate nerve fibers and vascular flow. The vertebral artery is frequently involved by compression of the overlying muscles in the suboccipital triangle. In fact, West points out that the vertebral artery has been completely occluded by turning the head backward and to the opposite side during postmortem studies.

Background

Neurologic disturbances may result from muscular and fibrotic changes along the cranial nerve pathways which emit from the skull and pass intimately between and un-

der suboccipital fasciculi. Five of the cranial nerves are thus vulnerable: the facial, glossopharyngeal, vagus, spinal accessory, and hypoglossal. In addition, circulatory impairment of major and minor nerves of the neck may alter the function of those cranial nerves that do not exit from the skull proper such as the olfactory, optic, oculomotor, trochlear, trigeminal, abducens, and auditory, but which are contained within the cranium and remote from vertebral subluxation encroachment effects. We should not overlook the fact that it is essentially muscle which produces and maintains the subluxation. Concern must be given to why the subluxation is produced.

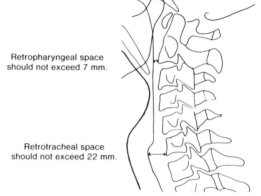

Retropharyngeal space should not exceed 7 mm.

Retrotracheal space should not exceed 22 mm.

Figure 21.11. Case history, focal neoplasm: a 47-year-old male consulted a medical physician with a complaint of localized upper-neck pain. A cursory physical examination was performed, and a radiographic report was issued as "essentially normal." Based on this report, the MD administered spinal manipulation to the patient's upper cervical spine which exacerbated the symptoms. Bed rest was advised, and analgesics were given. This offered no relief, and chiropractic care was sought by the patient. DC radiographs, taken 4 days after the MD's manipulation, showed a pathologic fracture through the body of the axis along with an increase in normal retropharyngeal space. Loss of bone density of the axis was evident on both neutral-lateral and close-up views. The chiropractic physician referred the patient for further evaluation. Biopsy revealed the lesion to be a solitary focus of multiple myeloma (plasmacytoma). This case demonstrates the consequence of failing to detect early subtle alterations in bone density and to carefully measure retropharyngeal and retrotracheal spaces (with the permission of the ACA Council on Roentgenology).

Inasmuch as all freely movable articulations are subject to subluxation, the atlanto-occipital diarthrosis is no exception. The stress at this point is unusual when one considers that the total weight of the cranium is supported by the ring of the atlas about 1/20th the circumference of the skull and a variety of spinal muscles, subject to spasm, have their attachments on the occiput.

If subluxation of a vertebra occurs in a superior direction, the contents of the intervertebral foramen become compressed. Anatomic disrelationship by elongating the short diameter of the intervertebral foramen will cause indirect pressure upon the nerve trunk from compression between the fibrous tissue in the anterior portion of the foramen. If there is movement in an inferior direction, enlargement of the foramen occurs. Because the nerve sheath is firmly anchored by tissues connecting it to the borders of the foramen, a stretching effect is exerted on the nerve sheath, altering its shape. It can thus be appreciated that enlarging the intervertebral foramen can cause as much trouble as a reduction in the size of the intervertebral foramen. In addition, it is impossible to subluxate a vertebra between C2 and L5 inclusive without changing the shape of the intervertebral disc in compensation.

Common Occipital Subluxations

Right or Left Condyle Inferior or Superior. A unilateral suboccipital muscle spasm causes the affected condyle to be pulled onto the articulating concavity of the atlantal lateral mass on one side (sunken condyle). This may not be attended by a degree of rotation. Inspection from the back shows a low medially inclined mastoid process on the side of involvement. Palpation discloses the mastoid riding close to the transverse process of the atlas, tension and tenderness in the groove between the mastoid and the lower jaw, and fullness in the groove between the occiput and the posterior ring of the atlas on the side of involvement. A right or left condyle superior may be considered the converse aspect of a right or left condyle inferior. That is, as one condyle is pulled inferior and anterior, the other

condyle presents a superior and posterior picture, or vice versa. There are certain situations, however, which indicate a unilateral abnormality without converse adaptation.

Right or Left Inferior Condyle with Associated Anterior Rotation. All occipital-atlantal movements tend to be associated with a degree of rotation because the occipital condyles and the articulating surfaces of the lateral masses of the atlas approximate each other more at the anterior than the posterior. Thus, most sunken condyles will be associated with a relative amount of rotation. On the side of involvement, inspection from the back reveals a medial head tilt. Palpation reveals approximation of the mastoid and transverse process of the atlas and approximation of the inferior nuchal ridge and the posterior arch of the atlas on the involved side. These points are widened on the opposite side. A right or left superior condyle with associated posterior rotation is often considered the contralateral aspect of a right or left inferior condyle attended by an anterior rotation. Illi feels it is always attended by a degree of arthritis and determines the primary subluxation roentgenologically by the side showing the greatest degree of degenerative articular alteration.

Right or Left Inferior Condyle with Associated Posterior Rotation. This type of subluxation or its contralateral representation is less common than that associated with posterior rotation. It usually results from vigorous twisting trauma such as in athletic activities. On the side of involvement: (1) inspection from the back shows the head held in a stiff inferior position with some posterior deviation, and (2) palpation discloses a mastoid that is inferior and posterior in relation to the transverse process of the atlas and the inferior nuchal ridge approximating the posterior arch of the atlas.

Suboccipital Jamming. This common subluxation of a trigeminal (ophthalmic division) reflex nature is often seen in people under severe visual or mental stress. Irritative impulses cause contraction of suboccipital muscles which pulls the occiput upon the posterior arch of the atlas creating a painful bilateral condylar jamming. A vertex blow is a rate cause. Palpation reveals suboccipital spasm, tenderness, nodular swellings, and a closing of the inferior nuchal ridge on the posterior arch of the atlas.

Common Atlas Subluxations

Right or Left Lateral Atlas. This atlantal sideslip between the atlas and axis articulations is usually attended by a degree of superiority and anteriority on the side of laterality because of the inclination of the articulating surfaces. Only in cases of severe twisting trauma or force will this not be the case. Ipsilaterally, palpation will reveal the transverse process of the atlas to be more lateral and slightly superior and anterior than its counterpart.

Bilateral Superior or Inferior Atlas. In this type of subluxation, the atlas tips up or down bilaterally in its transverse plane without an attending sideslip. Deep palpation may reveal the posterior arch of the atlas either approximating the occiput with a gap between the posterior tubercle of the atlas and the spinous of the axis or approximating the spinous process of the axis with a gap between the posterior tubercule and the occiput.

Right or Left Anterior Rotations of the Atlas. These subluxations are often associated with vagal syndromes because the anteriorly rotated transverse of the atlas may easily cause pressure on the vagus nerve. In such a rotatory state, the counterpart of an atlas listed right anterior would be left posterior. On the side of involvement, inspection from the back reveals suboccipital fullness. Bilateral palpation of the posterior ring of the atlas reveals a prominence of the side of posteriority, with the transverse process of the atlas being closer to the mastoid and its counterpart closer to the lower jaw. A clinical test, suggested by Goodheart, is to have the patient lying supine, then passively rotate the head right and left. If the anterior atlas exists on the left, the atlas has already turned to the right so that the patient's head will turn much further to the right. But when it is turned from right to left, the atlas has to first come out of its relatively anterior position on the left; thus motion is relatively restricted.

Common Axis Subluxations

With the possible exception of L5, no other vertebra is probably subluxated more frequently than C2. The most common symptom is a unilateral suboccipital neuralgia on the side of posteriority. On the side of posteriority, palpation discloses a tender prominence over the articulating process and a deviation of the spinous process away from the midline. Posterior axial subluxations are sometimes misdiagnosed as anterior atlantal subluxations.

Rotary subluxations of the axis are common biomechanical causes of cervical migraine. This cervical neuralgia is invariably unilateral, beginning in the upper neck and extending over the skull into the temporal and possibly orbital areas by myalgia extension. The greater occipital nerve (C2) is affected.

Rotary subluxations of one or more of the upper three vertebrae (particularly the axis) may cause pressure upon the superior cervical ganglion. The syndrome produced may incorporate excess facial and forehead perspiration, dry mouth and nasal mucous membranes, dryness and tightness of the throat, dilated pupils tending towards exophthalmos, pseudomigraine attacks due to unilateral angioneurotic edema, fascial vasomotor disturbances with possible angioneurotic swelling, and moderate tachycardia with functional arrythmias.

Lower Cervical Subluxations

A subluxation of one or more of the lower cervical vertebrae often involves the brachial plexus (C4–T1). Inasmuch as the distribution of the brachial plexus is so extensive, a multitude of abnormal reflections may be seen in areas of distribution which must be appreciated by knowledge of the pathophysiology involved. A few of the more common disturbances caused by lower cervical subluxations would include shoulder neuralgias such as "frozen shoulder," neuralgias along the medial arm and forearm or elbow, unclassified wrist drop and hand dystrophies, acroparesthesia, weak grip strength, and vague "rheumatic" wrist or hand complaints. A subluxation of one or more of the C3, C4, or C5 segments may involve the phrenic nerve and produce symptoms of severe chronic hiccup and other diaphragmatic disorders.

In any vertebral, occipital, or pelvic subluxation, neither physiotherapy, traction,

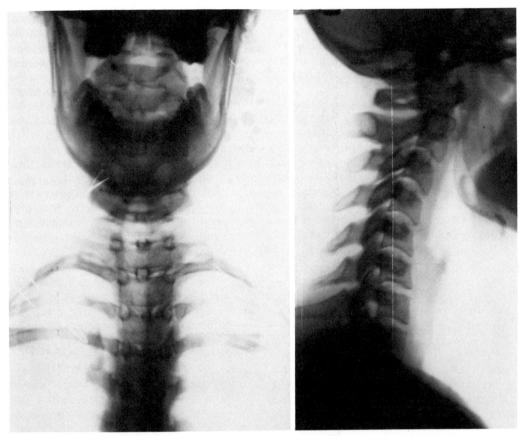

Figure 21.12. An enthusiastic female tennis player, age 21, became overheated during play on an extremely hot day. After taking a forceful swing with her tennis racket, she swung completely around and felt a pain in her neck and upper back. This was followed by recurrent headaches and pain in the neck and shoulder that radiated into the right shoulder and arm. Pain in the right elbow was severe. A medical physician treated her for carpal tunnel syndrome. After 1 year of recurrent symptoms, she sought chiropractic care with a major complaint of pain and stiffness of the neck and upper back, recurrent headaches, and pain radiating along the right arm. X-ray films (positive prints shown) revealed rotary subluxations in the lower cervical and upper thoracic region. On the lateral cervical view, a loss of the normal cervical curve with a tendency toward reversal was evident. The upper cervical vertebrae were in a position of forward flexion and anterior to the rest of the cervical spine. Chiropractic management consisted of spinal adjustments, cervical traction to reduce pressure on the IVDs and cervical nerves, and electronic muscle stimulation to enhance muscle tone. Ultrasound was employed for pain relief and the elimination of fibrositis which existed in the cervical paraspinal musculature (with the permission of the New York Chiropractic College).

muscle relaxants, gross manipulations, muscle stretching, injections, or other like methods will offer much relief by themselves unless the fixated articulation is correctly adjusted.

CERVICAL INSTABILITY SYNDROMES

Traumatic cervical instability exists when the ligamentous straps are so severely disrupted that an attempt by the neck to actively support the head results in malalignment of one or more cervical motion units to the degree that nerve roots or the spinal cord become injured. In contact sports, such a Grade 3 sprain is typically caused by an axial compression force when the neck is in hyperflexion or hyperextension.

Moderate Positional Instability. This state is characterized by weakened support of the head, segmental hypermobility, a flattened cervical curve, sharp posterior pain on movement, mild neurologic deficits, potential subluxation or dislocation (if not immobilized), and possible, associated fracture (eg, clay shoveler's, tear drop).

Severe Positional Instability. This variety features complete loss of support of the head in certain positions; overt structural damage (ligamentous and/or skeletal), either anteriorly or posteriorly; severe neck pain and moderate–severe neurologic deficits; possible cord signs; and, possibly, associated facet dislocation or burst fracture.

The Weakened Link Syndrome. This is a clinical picture of potential catastrophy, where previous injury or injuries have increased the vulnerability of the cervical spine to damage if further trauma is applied. Albright describes the situation as a neck that features mild compression fractures with angulation seen in flexion, in elastic posterior ligaments as the result of healed sprains, eroded and remolded facets that poorly restrict subluxation, and stiff IVDs that are thin and degenerated. A silent hemangioma of a vertebral body may be present. The patient may be completely asymptomatic and sometimes roentgenographically negative, even under stress tests, until moderate trauma produces a dramatic collapse and probable death.

CHAPTER 22

Shoulder Girdle Injuries

This chapter concerns injuries of and about the scapula, clavicle, and shoulder. In sports, the shoulder girdle is a common site of minor injury and a not infrequent site of serious disability. It is second only to the knee as a chronic site of prolonged disability. Upper limb injuries amount to about 20% of sport-related injuries. They can be highly debilitating, require considerable lost field time, and easily ruin a promising sports career.

INTRODUCTION

The regional anatomy offers little to resist violent shoulder depression, and the shoulder tip itself has little protection from trauma. The length of the arm presents a long lever with a large head within a relatively small joint. This allows a great range of motion with little stability. The stability of the shoulder is derived entirely from its surrounding soft tissues.

History and Initial Care

A careful history recording the mechanism of trauma and the position of the limb during injury, careful inspection and palpation of the entire region, muscle and range-of-motion tests, and other standard neurologic-orthopedic tests will often arrive at an accurate diagnosis without the necessity of x-ray exposure. Forceful manipulations should always be reserved for late in the examination to evaluate contraindications.

Contusions, strains, sprains, bursitis, and neurologic deficits must be alertly recognized and treated. Fractures and dislocations, obviously, take precedence over soft-tissue injuries with the exception of severe bleeding. Always check for bony crepitus, fracture line tenderness and swelling, angulation and deformity. Because the shoulder readily "freezes" after injury, treatment must strive to maintain motion as soon as possible without encouraging recurring problems. The key to avoiding prolonged disability is early recognition and early mobilization.

Posttraumatic Assessment

As in any musculoskeletal disorder, evaluation should include muscle strength grading, joint ranges of motion, sensory perception, appropriate tendon reflexes, and various other clinical tests (eg, laboratory, roentgenography), depending upon the situation at hand. A review of pertinent neurologic, orthopedic, and peripheral vascular maneuvers, reflexes, and tests relative to the shoulder girdle and arm is shown in Table 22.1.

Referred Pain

As the shoulder lies between the neck and the hand, pain from the neck or distal upper extremity may be referred to the shoulder, and a shoulder disorder may refer pain to the neck or hand. In shoulder disorders, differentiation must include cervical problems, superior pulmonary sulcus tumor, and referred pain from viscera. Pain can also be referred to the shoulder by brachial plexus involvement, pectoralis minor syndrome, anterior scalene syndrome, claviculocostal syndrome, suprascapular nerve entrapment, dorsal scapular nerve entrapment, cervical rib, spinal cord tumor, arteriosclerotic occlusion and other vascular disorders.

The origin of shoulder pain may be a viscerospinal reflex such as seen in some diaphragmatic, gallbladder, aortic, pleural, and coronary diseases. If you are able to reproduce pain during joint motion, the condition is most likely neuromuscular in origin. Pain that cannot be reproduced points towards a visceral origin.

In cases of a herniated cervical disc (common at C5–6), pain may radiate from the neck into the arm, forearm, and hand. The head and neck will be deviated to the affected side with marked restriction of movement. The shoulder will usually be elevated

Table 22.1.
Review of Neurologic, Orthopedic, and Peripheral Vascular Maneuvers, Reflexes, Signs, or Tests Relative to the Shoulder Girdle

Disorder	Procedures/Signs	
Thoracic outlet and related syndromes	Adson's test Allen's test Costoclavicular maneuver	Eden's test Traction test Wright's test
Shoulder and arm syndromes	Abbott-Saunders' test Apley's scratch test Arm drop test Biceps reflex Biceps stability test Bikele's sign Booth-Marvel's test Brachioradialis reflex Bryant's sign Calloway's sign Codman's sign Dawbarn's test Deltoid reflex Dugas' test Gilcrest's sign Hamilton's ruler sign Hueter's sign Impingement syndrome test Infraspinatus reflex Inverted radial reflex	Lax capsule test Light touch/pain tests Lippman's test Locking position test Muscle strength grading Pectoralis flexibility test Pectoral reflex Radial reflex Range of motion tests Scapulohumeral reflex Schultz's test Shoulder abduction stress test Shoulder apprehension test Subacromial button sign Supraspinatus press test Teres' sign Triceps reflex Ulnar reflex Wrist reflex Yergason's stability test

on the same side with the arm slightly flexed at the elbow (protective position). Biceps and triceps reflexes will be lost or diminished. Paresthesias and sensory loss in the dermatome distribution will be found corresponding to the disc involved.

Myofascial Shoulder Syndromes

In most cases of post-traumatic shoulder pain, its origin can generally be localized to a small area by palpation or reproduced at some point in active or passive motion. This is typical of many common disorders—capsulitis, bicipital tendinitis, dislocations, impingement syndromes, rotator cuff strains, subacromial bursitis, and supraspinatus injuries, for example.

Trigger point pain differs from that associated with most structural injuries in that the physical findings are few. Rather than being localized, the pain is described over a broad area that does not coincide with specific segmental patterns. Associated paresthesiae are described in extremely vague expressions. Range of motion tests and mus-

cle strength grading offer little help, even after referred pain from the cervical spine, lungs, or viscera is ruled out. While trauma may be involved, it may be only a precipitating rather than a causative factor.

The muscles of the shoulder girdle are highly susceptible to trigger point formation because they are anatomically susceptible to fatigue, easy victims of the stresses of poor posture and biomechanical faults, and the target for many psychosomatic reflexes. Michele and Eisenberg state that no less than one-third of their middle-aged patients with shoulder pain had the myofascial pain syndrome.

The focal point of pain in a myofascial syndrome will be found as one or more small areas of muscle fiber degeneration that feel fairly firm and ropey to the touch. Further probing will usually elicit the characteristic involuntary "jump sign" as the patient reacts and the physiologic "twitch sign." This latter sign is the result of a brief contraction of the surface fibers near the trigger point.

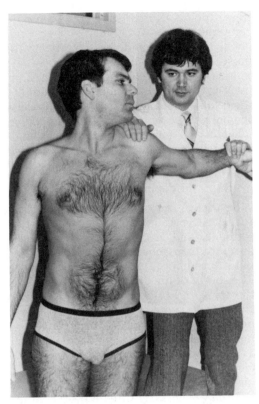

Figure 22.1. Performing Adson's test.

Although a trigger point may develop in any muscle, certain sites appear to be favorite locations. A point in the superior medial aspect of the scapula, near the insertion of the levator scapulae, is a common site, as are points in the supraspinatus and trapezius. Weed describes frequently occurring points over the heads of the 2nd, 3rd, or 4th ribs, just lateral to the spinous processes.

Management. As in other areas, goading, acupuncture, high-volt stimulation, spray-and-stretch, and deep percussion/vibration are generally the conservative therapies of choice in trigger point therapy.

INJURIES OF THE SCAPULAR AREA

For every 3° of arm abduction, 1° occurs at the scapulothoracic articulation for every 2° at the glenohumeral joint. If you wish to check solely glenohumeral joint passive abduction, the stabilizing hand should anchor the scapula while your active hand passively abducts the patient's arm with the forearm horizontal. The shoulder blade will normally not be felt to move until about 20° of abduction has occurred. Abduction should normally continue in this position to about 120° where the surgical neck of the humerus meets the tip of the acromion. In the "frozen shoulder" syndrome, scapulothoracic motion will be normal and glenohumeral motion will be absent. Then turn the patient's forearm so to externally rotate the humerus and turn the surgical neck away from the acromion, and continue abduction to its maximum. Abduction is quite painful against resistance in tendonitis.

Trapezius Strains and Contusions

Most trapezius injuries will be seen at the proximal portion, rarely distal to the scapular spine. That aspect between the occiput and the shoulder is the only significant muscle that can resist forceful shoulder depression. It is also this aspect that suffers contusion from a blow to the body from above that strikes lateral to the neck.

Management. The grade of trapezius strain determines its disability, from minor to crippling, depending upon the degree of related spasm and pain. Treatment consists of correction of concomitant subluxations, radiant heat, frequent hot showers, trigger-point therapy, and massage to reduce spasm and encourage healing.

Fibrositis

Strains and associated fibrositis are often seen in the musculature attachments to the vertebral border of the scapula from throw-

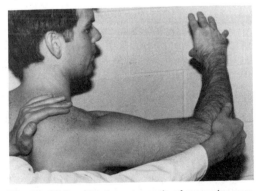

Figure 22.2. Testing strength of scapular protraction.

ing heavy objects (eg, shot put). The initial trauma may not be remembered.

Signs and Symptoms. Fibrositis is a generalized term which refers to a syndrome featuring spasm, stiffness through the range of motion without limitation, a dull gnawing ache at rest which is aggravated by exercise, localized tenderness, possible soft-tissue crepitus, and one or more palpable trigger points. The disorder is most often seen in the rhomboids and trapezius. However, the levator scapulae, scalene group, or erector spinae are often involved. Fibrofatty nodules herniate through the superficial fascia of the involved muscles. Palpation and movements may cause pain to radiate up the posterior neck and/or over the shoulder and sometimes down the arm. Cervical motions cause a vague soreness in the affected tissues. This is usually worse in the morning after arising and during cold, damp weather.

Management. Trigger-point therapy may be applied and a search made for the primary pathology such as a postural defect, chronic subluxation, or disc lesion. Once primary trigger nodules are normalized, several secondary sites may appear which require therapy. Bony and soft-tissue adjustive techniques, heat, massage, progressive passive manipulation, and active exercise will usually show excellent results. Initially, some soreness always follows musculature adjustments, which will be quickly relieved by a hot bath. The affected tissues enjoy warmth and use. Chilling of the part should be avoided by use of sweaters, etc. Instructions should be given for isometric exercises and to help develop proper postural and sleeping habits.

Postural Disorders

Shoulder girdle pain and discomfort are often seen in people who work overhead and use repetitive arm motions for long durations with little postural change. Trigger points will inevitably be found along the vertebral borders of one or both scapulae. Most feel the cause can usually be traced to muscular overuse leading to lower cervical or upper thoracic subluxations. Subluxations may be found in the shoulder girdle itself, especially when the scapulae are chronically affected. Acute or chronic fibrositis of the trapezius and rhomboids with trigger points is often superimposed or inconsequential.

On the other hand, Nelson doubts the muscular "overuse" concept. "The more a muscle is used, the stronger it gets. Certainly there may be a subluxation, but it would be the result of the muscle spasticity. The cause then must be a nervous or circulatory defect wherein the muscle cannot do sustained work without spasticity. A normal muscle merely tires."

Scapular Fixations

Restricted movements are sometimes found in the scapular area. They affect performance and posture. Their usual causes are (1) the consequence of injury, (2) trigger-point spasm, or (3) viscerosomatic reflexes. The source of the difficulty may be local, at the spine, or at the shoulder. The common sites to search are a costovertebral or upper dorsal subluxation or contractions of any muscle that has a scapular attachment such as the rhomboids, trapezius, levator scapulae, supraspinatus, infraspinatus, teres major and minor.

Management. Treat with deep heat followed by muscle therapy and passive manipulation to a degree just below pain expression to stretch and relax the shortened connective tissues involved. Follow this with chronic sprain therapy.

Scapular joint play should be found in all directions: superiorly, laterally, inferiorly, medially, and slightly clockwise and counterclockwise. If not, corrective manipulation is usually necessary. The adjustive procedure is conducted with the patient prone. Pressure is made with the base of the contact hand, the stabilizing hand is positioned on the wrist of the contact hand as in a toggle recoil, and the direction of thrust is into the fixation (restriction) on almost a horizontal plane so that the underlying thoracic cage is not greatly disturbed. To inhibit recurrence, therapeutic exercises should be prescribed that will stretch the shoulder in flexion, extension, adduction, and horizontal abduction.

Scapular Fractures

Scapular fractures are not frequently seen, but in severe trauma, fractures of the body and spine of the scapula can occur.

The strong muscular attachments usually prevent significant displacement. All that is usually required is rest in a sling until acute pain subsides, then early mobilization. In rare cases, the brachial plexus or axillary nerve may be injured. Fractures of the scapular neck (uncommon) are usually impacted and present little displacement. Acromion fractures are the result of a downward blow on the shoulder, often leading to avulsion of the brachial plexus. Fractures of the coracoid process, easily confused with an ununited epiphysis, are uncommon; and when they occur, they are usually associated with acromioclavicular separations.

INJURIES OF THE CLAVICLE

At the acromioclavicular and sternococlavicular joints, a wide range of injury and displacement may occur.

Contusions, Strains, and Sprains

Distal Trapezius Contusion

The tip of the shoulder, near the lateral aspect of the clavicle, is a common site of extremely painful and tender contusions to the trapezius.

Signs and Symptoms. Localized swelling is easily seen and palpable. The patient will depress the entire shoulder girdle in an attempt for relief. Care must be taken not to confuse this contusion with acromioclavicular separation.

Management. Treatment consists of cold packs and an arm sling for 24 hours, followed by moist heat, passive manipulation, and progressive active exercises. Attending cervical, upper dorsal, or shoulder girdle subluxations and muscle spasms should be corrected. Normal activity can usually be achieved in a few days.

Acromioclavicular Sprain

The acromioclavicular joint is relatively weak and inflexible, yet must bear constant stress in contact sports. Those who expose the joint to excessive and repeated trauma risk contusion, sprain, and separation. Posttraumatic arthritis is a typical consequence. Any force which tends to spring the clavicle from its attachments to the scapula is bound to cause severe sprain to the acromioclavicular, coronoid, and trapezoid ligaments un-

less the clavicle fractures beforehand. Keep in mind that the acromioclavicular ligament can be considered a part of the acromioclavicular joint capsule, thus sprain must involve a degree of capsule tear.

Signs and Symptoms. Signs in minor sprain are minimal local swelling and tenderness, moderate pain on motion, and no signs of diminished joint mobility. This is a simple reactive synovitis which responds well to cold packs, shoulder-cap strapping, and arm sling for 24 hours, followed by passive manipulation and progressive exercises (1–2 weeks).

Major sprain consists of a degree of severe stretching and tearing of the tough coracoclavicular ligaments. Carefully palpate for evidence of coronoid or trapezoid sprain. Acute tenderness and possible swelling will be found in the area of the coracoclavicular ligament below the clavicle. There is distinct abnormal mobility of the clavicle relative to the acromion process. After a week or more, a subcutaneous discoloration may appear. An aftermath of an old injury may be exhibited by laxity of the acromioclavicular joint without localized tenderness.

Management. As injury varies from slight laxity to complete disruption of all ligaments where the distal clavicle projects upward at a wide angle, treatment must be varied accordingly. Major sprain requires careful strapping (eq, a modified Velpeau bandage) with a downward pull on the clavicle and an upward pull on the elbow to assure immobilization for 3–6 weeks, followed by a period of intensive rehabilitation. Supplementation with 140 mg of manganese glycerophosphate six times daily is most helpful in most any ligamentous injury. Exercises of the shoulder should give particular attention to the pectoralis major and deltoid. Surgical fixation may be required in gross displacements.

Acromioclavicular Separation

The acromioclavicular joint serves as a roof for the head of the humerus. It is one of the weakest joints of the body but assisted by the strong coracoclavicular ligament. The ends of the joint are bound loosely so the scapula can raise the glenoid fossa.

Background. During shoulder injury,

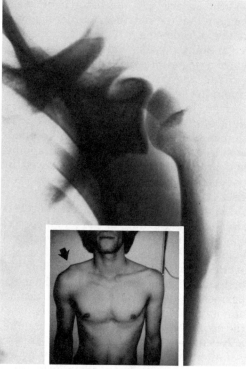

Figure 22.3. Case history, acromioclavicular separation-dislocation. The patient was a soccer goalkeeper who in the course of a game had to dive to make a save. Both arms were extended over his head to catch the ball. As he fell to the ground and tucked in the ball, he landed on his right shoulder. There was instant separation of the clavicle with immediate pain and swelling at its distal aspect. Rupture of the acromioclavicular and coracoclavicular ligaments with sprain of the sternoclavicular ligament were evident. Without weights, radiographs (positive P-A print shown) showed dramatic upper displacement of lateral clavicle with a wide space between the coracoid and clavicle. The clavicle rode high above the acromion. Treatment consisted of reduction by downward pressure of the distal clavicle with superior alignment along the shaft of the humerus. However, since there was significant muscle spasm in the area, trigger points were treated with high-voltage galvanic stimulation prior to reduction. The shoulder was immobilized by strapping after reduction, with the arm held in a flexed internally rotated position in a sling to prevent movement and further separation of the articulation. Follow-up treatment consisted of muscle stimulation with ultrasound for its palliative effects along with cervical and upper-dorsal adjustments. A weight-bearing sling was then used to hold the clavicle in place while healing continued. Once localized pain subsided and rel-

the scapula often rotates around the coracoid which acts as a fulcrum. The intrinsically weak superior and inferior acromioclavicular ligaments give way and the joint dislocates. In other instances, a downward force of great intensity lowers the clavicle onto the 1st rib which acts as a fulcrum, tearing the acromioclavicular and coracoacromial ligaments, resulting in complete acromioclavicular separation. Continued force can fracture the clavicle. Incomplete luxation can tear the intraarticular meniscus and lead to degenerative arthritis of the joint.

Initial Evaluation. In any acute separation, the most significant sign is that of demonstrable and significant false motion of the acromioclavicular joint from joint laxity. If examination (with patient sitting) can be made before swelling develops, evaluation can be made by pivoting the joint after the scapula has been stabilized by the nonpalpating hand. The swollen joint may give a false impression of a tender but stable joint. Injury can be graded as follows:

• *Grade I Injury:* This sprain is with some tearing but no subluxation or step-off. The joint is intact, but quite tender. The patient will complain of discomfort upon raising the arm and rotating the shoulder. There is point tenderness over the acromioclavicular area but not over the coracoclavicular area. Swelling is mild. Physical findings are often more reliable than x-ray films in Grade I separations to demonstrate laxity, even if weights are held. The joint should be immobilized and activity restricted until symptoms subside and abduction can be made without pain.

• *Grade II Injury:* The coracoclavicular ligaments are at least partially intact. There are signs of subluxation and a slight step-off. Symptoms and disability are more severe than Grade I. The shoulder may droop. The elevated lateral clavicle will exhibit a visible and palable knob. The weight of the

ative painless motion occurred, the shoulder was passively exercised for range of motion. Weight was added after range of motion normalized. Since there will be a predisposition to future dislocation, intensive exercise was recommended (copyright 1981, with the permission of Phillip and Joseph Santiago, DCs, postgraduate faculty, New York Chiropractic College).

dangling arm may intensify pain. Immobilization is required for 3 weeks and strenuous activity restricted for another 3 weeks. Subluxation and joint widening may be confirmed by stress roentgenography.

• *Grade III Injury*: Complete dislocation and coracoclavicular ligament rupture. The joint capsule is disrupted. The above mentioned symptoms and signs are greatly exaggerated. The skin appears tent-like at the lateral clavicle. Step-off is significant. Open or closed surgical care is inevitably required.

Schultz's Test. Standing behind the sitting patient, face the affected side. Place one hand under the flexed elbow and push up while the other hand placed over the acromioclavicular joint applies firm pressure. The more "give" that is felt in the joint, the greater the separation.

Chronic Cases. Signs of posttraumatic arthritis may appear, such as pain over the shoulder region with little or no radiation to the arm, tenderness over the acromioclavicular joint, and pain-free movement until the scapula begins to move. Shrugging the shoulders usually elicits pain.

Basic Management of Grade I and II Separations. A recent displacement can be reduced simply by applying downward pressure to the clavicle while the elbow is carefully lifted. Prior to strapping, a 3-inch × 4-inch piece of foam rubber should be placed over the articulation, secured by cross strips. Overlapping 1½-inch tape is applied horizontally with front to back tension, starting below the neck and working to well below the shoulder cap. A simple sling should be used for added support for several days. A more secure method is a modified Velpeau bandage. Immobilization is required for 10–20 days, depending upon the severity of injury. Treat as any severe sprain.

Sternoclavicular Sprains

Sternoclavicular sprains vary from minor to complete dislocation, either posteriorly (retrosternal) or anterior-inferior to overlap the 1st rib. Injury can be graded as follows:

• *Grade I Injury*: Sprain and slight tearing of the costoclavicular and sternoclavicular ligament fibers. There is usually no separation. Tenderness is found over and around the articulation.

• *Grade II Injury*: Severe subluxation of the clavicle exhibiting partial tear of the costoclavicular ligament and rupture of the sternoclavicular ligament.

• *Grade III Injury*: Dislocation exhibiting complete rupture of the costoclavicular and sternoclavicular ligaments. Above signs and symptoms are exaggerated. Displacement is demonstrated in roentgenography on oblique views and tomography.

Schultz's Strapping Procedure. A splint can be improvised by cementing a strip of foam rubber to a tongue depressor. Place over the joint horizontally, foam side against the skin, so it is centered over the affected articulation. Secure it with a few strips of tape so it will not move during strapping. Next, place a piece of cotton padding or felt large enough to cover the sternoclavicular joints and most of the sternum. The superior aspect of the pad should be cut in a V-notch or curve to avoid pressure on the throat. Prepare 10 strips of 1½-inch tape, long enough to extend from just above the nipple anteriorly to a few inches below the opposite scapula posteriorly. Start on the back of the injured side; bring the first strip up diagonally over the shoulder close to the neck and then slightly above the affected joint and towards a point midway between the axilla and the nipple. The tension on the tape is from back to front. The second strip is placed on the opposite side in the same manner. Place the remaining eight strips in a crisscross overlapping manner, moving downward. During strapping, the injured clavicle should be depressed firmly with the free hand as the tape covers it. For greater restriction and to anchor the criss-crossed tape ends, place several horizontal strips across the anterior thorax from the clavicles to the nipples. The arm of the affected side is then placed in a simple sling. Follow with standard treatment for a sprain. Rehabilitative exercises of the shoulder should give particular attention to the pectoralis major and deltoid.

The Costoclavicular Syndrome

This syndrome is due to the neurovascular bundle being compressed between the 1st rib and the clavicle at the point where the brachial plexus joins the subclavian artery and courses over the 1st rib. Symptoms are similar to those of the scalenus anticus syndrome and reproduced by the costoclavicular maneuver.

Costoclavicular Maneuver. With the patient sitting, monitor the patient's radial pulse from the posterior on the side being examined. Extend the patient's shoulder and arm posterior, and then depress the shoulder on the side being examined. This maneuver narrows the costoclavicular space by approximating the clavicle to the 1st rib, tending to compress the neurovascular structures. When the shoulder is retracted, the clavicle moves backward on the sternoclavicular joint and rotates in a counterclockwise direction. An alteration of the radial pulse or a reduplication of other symptoms is a probable sign of compression of the neurovascular bundle (costoclavicular syndrome).

Sternoclavicular Disc Injury

In some injuries to this joint which are just below the severity of a dislocation, the intraarticular disc may be pulled from its sternal attachment in a manner similar to a semilunar tear of the knee. The patient will complain of localized pain on movement. A "catch" may be felt by the patient, especially during ipsilateral shoulder flexion and circumduction. As in the knee if the cartilage is fragmented, surgery may be required if conservative measures fail.

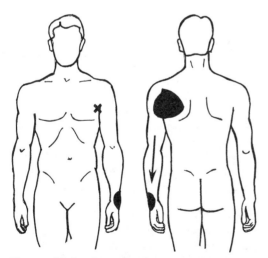

Figure 22.4. Subscapularis trigger point; *X*, common site is in the axilla. *Blackened areas* indicate typical sites of referred pain.

Subluxations

During correction of a subluxation, even mild dynamic thrusts should be reserved for nonacute, fixated situations. When subluxation accompanies an acute sprain, correction should be more in line with gentle traction pressures after the musculature has been relaxed. Obviously, the probability of fracture fragments or osteoporosis must be eliminated prior to any form of manipulation.

Anterior Medial Clavicular Subluxation

The mechanism of force is one of posterior-lateral impact which drives the shoulder anterior and medial. If sternoclavicular subluxation does not occur in the young, a green-stick midshaft fracture often results.

Signs and Symptoms. Acute disability results, and sometimes false joint motion can be palpated. Pain is acute and aggravated by joint motion. There is severe tenderness at the sternoclavicular joint. Secondary capsule injury may be expressed by intracapsular swelling, edema, and generalized tenderness. Exhibited crepitus suggests attending fracture fragments or articular comminution, thus making adjusting procedures contraindicated. Evaluate the integrity of the pectoralis major and subclavius. In older cases, a degree of fixation will inevitably be present. This is easily determined by placing two finger pads upon the sternoclavicular joint and widely circumducting the patient's abducted arm.

Adjustment. Place the patient supine on a low table. Stand at the side opposite the subluxation, about perpendicular to the patient. Place your cephalad pisiform securely against the medial clavicle the grasp the patient's arm of the affected side with your caudal hand. Give a slight thrust that is directed posteriorly and laterally while simultaneously applying traction on the patient's arm medially toward yourself (see Fig. 22.5).

Alternative Adjustment Procedure. The patient is seated on a low stool. If the patient's left shoulder is involved, abduct his arm and flex his elbow. Stand behind the patient toward the involved side. Hook your left arm under the patient's axilla and take contact with two or three finger pads on the medial eminence of the clavicle. The

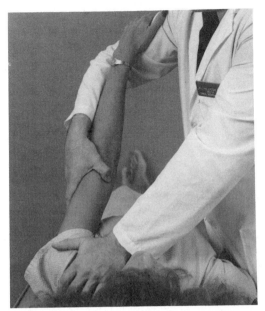

Figure 22.5. Adjustment procedure of subluxated anterior medial clavicle.

patient's proximal arm will rest upon your forearm. Next, reach your right arm around the right side of the patient's neck and place two or three stabilizing fingers upon your contact fingers. If possible, apply stabilization to the back of the patient's dorsal spine by firm contact against your chest. The adjustment is made by applying posterior-superior leverage traction on the patient's shoulder joint by lifting your left elbow back and up, while simultaneously applying posterior and lateral pressure with your contact and stabilizing fingers (see Fig. 22.6).

Management. Treat as a severe sprain with initial cold packs for 24 hours, aided by a pressure pad and stable strapping. Follow with physiotherapeutic measures such as diathermy and hydrotherapy. Mild progressive exercises of the shoulder girdle may begin in 5–7 days, but earlier for the trunk and lower limbs. Full activity can be expected in 10–14 days, but support should continue for about a month. During the last 2 weeks, the pressure pad is not necessary during nonactive periods. Hurried recuperation will likely invite recurrence and extend convalescence. Supplementation with 140 mg of manganese glycerophosphate six times daily speeds healing.

Posterior Medial Clavicular Subluxation

This is a most difficult subluxation to correct once it has become fixated. Fortunately, it is rare. Place the patient supine with a small firm pillow between his scapulae. The object is to try to "spring" the clavicle forward by applying bilateral posterior pressure against lateral structures. The doctor stands on the side of involvement facing the patient. His lateral hand firmly cups the patient's shoulder cap and the other hand takes contact on the patient's upper sternum as far away from the involved joint as possible without contacting the contralateral sternoclavicular joint. Using the pillow as a fulcrum, several gentle posteriorly directed thrusts are made simultaneously with both hands while your elbows are locked.

Anterosuperior Lateral Clavicular Subluxation

Acromioclavicular subluxations are common in contact sports, usually accompanying new or old joint separations.

Signs and Symptoms. The patient will complain of an ache within the joint, tenderness at the lateral end of the clavicle, and loss of some arm function. A partial ligamentous tear will be demonstrated by looseness of the joint during Schultz's test. The subluxation can be detected by bilateral palpation of the lateral end of the clavicle

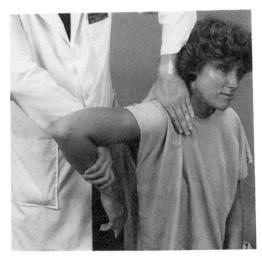

Figure 22.6. Alternative adjustment of subluxated anterior medial clavicle.

for the characteristic "step down." Bilateral comparison is necessary because some people normally have enlarged clavicle ends laterally which can be mistaken for subluxated clavicles. When subluxated, the clavicle tends to move superior and anterior. Evaluate the integrity of the clavicular division of the pectoralis major, anterior and middle deltoid, subclavius, and upper trapezius. In older cases, a degree of fixation will inevitably be present which can be determined by placing two finger pads upon the acromioclavicular joint and circumducting the patient's abducted arm.

Adjustment. The patient is placed on a low stool with the palm of his hand on the involved side on the back of his neck. Stand behind the patient and place the web of your medial contact hand on the patient's lateral clavicle. Stabilize the patient's abducted elbow with your lateral hand, and apply as much traction as possible. Apply pressure inferiorly with your contact hand. Then, make a short thrust inferior and posterior while simultaneously elevating the patient's elbow superior and medial with your stabilizing hand. Conclude by maintaining contact pressure and gently circumducting the abducted humerus (see Fig. 22.7).

Alternative Adjustment Procedure. The doctor-patient position is the same as

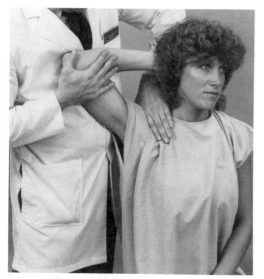

Figure 22.7. Adjustment of subluxated anterosuperior lateral clavicle.

above, and the doctor's contact is the same. The patient's arm is abducted, his elbow is flexed, and his hand points somewhat inferior and medial towards the floor. Rather than stabilizing the patient's elbow, place your stabilizing forearm under the patient's abducted elbow and grasp the dorsal surface of his wrist. Apply pressure inferiorly on your contact hand. Then, make a short thrust inferiorly and posteriorly while simultaneously elevating the patient's elbow superiorly and medially with your stabilizing forearm.

Management. The treatment formula is similar to that for sternoclavicular subluxation. Following adjustment, tape should be applied to force the humerous up tightly within the socket to relieve the gravitational pull on the tendons and ligaments. The strapping procedure is identical to that described for separation. If taping offers good support, a simple arm sling is necessary for only 3–4 days. The strapping should remain for 10–14 days. Frequent mild mobilization between tapings is necessary to avoid adhesions during healing.

Dislocations

Clavicular dislocations are most often seen in football, soccer, horse racing, bicycling, gymnastics, and wrestling. Analysis of complications should be made by roentgenography prior to considered reduction.

Acromioclavicular Dislocation

Signs and Symptoms. In injuries to the lateral clavicle, the clavicle is elevated, which increases the distance between the clavicle and the coracoid process. Thus, a distinct palpable and visible "step" will be noted in the supraspinatus region. If the prominent lateral clavicle is depressed, it will only spring back to its elevated position once pressure is released. The scapula falls away from the clavicle, and the acromion lies below and anterior to the clavicle. Fracture of the coracoid process is often associated.

Roentgenographic Considerations. Dalinka states that an increase of the coracoclavicular distance by 5 mm of greater than 50% of the contralateral side indicates a true acromioclavicular dislocation. Complete dislocation cannot occur unless the conoid and trapezoid ligaments are severely torn. The soft tissues within this area frequently ossify after injury. After chronic injury, signs of erosion or tapering may be observed, along with indications of soft-tissue calcification subsequent to old hematoma.

Management. Early treatment is necessary to avoid a persistent step deformity even in severe subluxations. Reduction is usually not difficult, but maintenance is. Recurrent displacement is common. Ice packs should be applied for 24 hours. Proper strapping assures that the shoulder is elevated while the acromion is depressed. The typical procedure is to use a webbing harness or a modified Velpeau bandage for 6–7 weeks. Another method is to pass non-stretch zinc oxide strapping over the clavicle, down the anterior upper arm and under the elbow, and then up behind to cross the clavicle again. A simple wrist sling is also necessary. Felt pads should be used under the strapping to protect bony prominences. To avoid a large joint knob, a plaster cast is preferred. In most cases of pure dislocation with ruptured ligaments (extremely painful), orthopedic reduction and surgical coracoclavicular fixation may be necessary.

Anterior Sternoclavicular Dislocation

Shoulder girdle movement at the sternoclavicular joint is slight but essential. At the medial end of the clavicle, displacement may occur either anterior, as is more common, or posterior in relation to the sternum. The latter is often associated with dyspnea and cervical edema from vasculature compression.

Background. The sternoclavicular joint is the least stable major joint of the body, although complete dislocations are rare. Coned-down x-ray views, tangential views, or tomograms are often necessary to clearly show displacement. When dislocations occur and are reduced, a deformity often persists. The displacement of the clavicle in anterior dislocation is typically anterior, superior, and medial.

Management. The best method of reduction is a two-man approach. One applies lateral traction to the patient's abducted arm while the other applies pressure to the medial clavicle. Once reduction has been made, a reverse figure 8 bandage is applied. As

pain and disability are severe, reduction usually requires the care of an orthopedist.

Posterior Sternoclavicular Dislocation

These luxations are often hidden by soft-tissue swelling. In chronic cases, a distinct depression is palpable. Acute posterior dislocations can be a medical emergency requiring the attention of a thoracic surgeon. Pure dislocations should be reduced by a specialist because of the vital tissues behind the sternum.

Emergency Care. For temporary aid, place the patient supine with a sandbag between the scapula to help pull the clavicle out of the retrosternal area and relieve the vital substernal structures. Mild, steady, posteriorly directed pressure over the lateral clavicles by one person while another attempts to grasp the medial end of the clavicle with a light towel and apply traction is helpful. In some cases, this may be all that is necessary. A figure 8 harness such as used for clavicular fracture is then applied to hold the shoulders back during healing.

Fractures

Fractured ends sometimes can be felt under the skin. The involved shoulder may be lower than the other, and the patient is unable to raise the involved arm above shoulder level. He usually supports the elbow of the involved side with the opposite hand.

Background. The most common site of clavicular fracture is near the midpoint, but both ends also deserve careful evaluation. In midshaft fracture, there is sometimes inferior, anterior, and medial displacement of the lateral section. Fractures of the inner third are uncommon and often represent an epiphyseal injury as the medial clavicular epiphysis doesn't close until about the age of 25 years. Most fractures (66%) of the outer third of the clavicle present intact ligaments with no significant displacement. About a third of outer-third fractures present detached ligaments medially and attached ligaments distally, with displacement inferior and medial on the trapezius muscle. Early active shoulder movements should be encouraged.

If the injury is due to a fall on an outstretched hand, the impact is transferred from the palm to the carpals, to the radius and ulnar, to the elbow and humerus, to the scapula and clavicle, and to the spine and thoracic cage. Thus, all structures involved in the line of impact deserve careful evaluation—not just the immediate area of obvious fracture (see Fig. 22.8).

Roentgenographic Considerations. Contralateral x-ray views are almost mandatory, and it frequently helps to have the subject hold a weight (10–15 lb) in each hand. Quite frequently, an angled view is necessary to show evidence of displacement because overlapping fragments may be hidden in the A-P view.

Management. Support should be provided by padded rings that hold the shoulder posteriorly or with figure 8 strapping. Immobilization is usually necessary for 20–30 days before abduction can be made without pain. In uncomplicated "greenstick" fractures, a simple arm sling with thorax stabilization may be all that is necessary. Mild shoulder motions are advised from the onset. Healing should be confirmed by roentgenography. To avoid a large callus formation for cosmetic purposes, a plaster cuirass is applied after orthopedic reduction, and 3 weeks of supine bed confinement against a high pillow between the shoulders is required. Most clavicular fractures heal quickly, and complications infrequently include supraclavicular nerve or subclavian

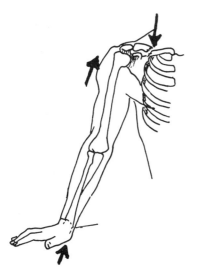

Figure 22.8. The typical mechanism of shoulder injury and lateral clavicle fracture.

vessel injuries that are rarely a problem. Nonunion is rare.

INJURIES OF THE SHOULDER JOINT

Most shoulder injuries are not single-entity injuries. They are composed of a variety of contusions, strains, sprains, and possible fracture. Dislocations, spontaneously reduced dislocations, and subluxations also complicate the picture. Thus, any painful shoulder syndrome requires careful differentiation.

Shoulder Injuries in Sports

The shoulder is at the forefront among high-incidence athletic injuries. Tears of the rotator cuff, usually without humeral displacement, are common in a large number of sports. Most are the result of throwing injuires, falls on the shoulder point, and vertical forces directed along the humerus. Careful evaluation of the soft tissues is necessary. Subclavian and axillary vessel injury may be the result of direct trauma or a sudden and violent shoulder movement. Rarely, just muscular hypertrophy may produce venous insufficiency or thrombosis. Brachial plexus and coracoid injuries are sometimes seen in recoil injuries such as in rifle sports. Epiphyseal injuries of the proximal humerus are rare, heal well, and are usually treated closed.

Throwing Injuries. Throwing includes an initial smooth sequence of elevation, abduction, and external rotation of the upper arm which quickly leads to a sudden, forceful, forward flexion, anterior abduction, and internal rotation of the shoulder associated with elbow, wrist, and finger extension. Crucial to the initial motion is the integrity of the rotator cuff. Unfortunately, the cuff muscles are well beneath overlying muscles, thus difficult to palpate and differentiate. Inasmuch as the path of the ulnar nerve is quite close to the medial epicondyle, strenuous pitching can readily result in traumatic ulnar neuropathy. Cases frequently present paresthesias associated with fragmentation and partial avulsion of the medical epicondyle.

The shoulder girdle is a multiaxial, intricately synchronized joint complex that has considerable power and an extreme range of motion. The anterior, superior, and posterior shoulder muscles provide the great power, and the collateral ligaments do not appreciably limit motion in any plane. Thus, stability must be provided by the musculature: essentially the rotator cuff and subscapularis muscles, which are aided somewhat by the glenohumeral ligaments. Muscle forces must act through four relatively unique joints (glenohumeral, scapulothoracic, acromioclavicular, sternoclavicular) to achieve the normally graceful coordination required of shoulder motion. Because of this, alterations of the throwing mechanism about the shoulder produce a clinical picture that is often difficult to diagnosis and effectively treat.

For the purposes of analysis, Tullos and King divide the throwing mechanism into three separate, independent stages, each of which is associated with specific shoulder injuries:

1. *The Cocking Phase.* During windup, the shoulder is brought into extreme external rotation, abduction, and extension. The biceps, triceps, and internal and external rotators are highly tensed. For this reason, a professional baseball pitcher will invariably exhibit abnormal external humeral rotation and subnormal internal rotation. Overstress makes the proximal arm vulnerable to biceps tendinitis, triceps tendinitis, and humeral subluxation (see Table 22.2).

2. *The Acceleration Phase.* The actual throwing phase is a two-stage process: (A) With the forearm and hand stationary, the shoulder is brought forward, the elbow is placed into extreme valgus strain as the muscular forces multiply on the shaft of the humerus, and the elbow is stabilized by the flexors of the forearm. (B) In the second stage, the forearm is rapidly whipped forward by internal shoulder rotation produced by severe contraction of the pectoralis major and latissimus dorsi. This stage ends when the hand is near ear level and the ball is released. Overstress makes the shoulder complex vulnerable to pectoralis and latissimus tendinitis, along with the effects of the mechanical forces upon the humerus.

3. *The Follow-Through Phase.* The last phase begins as the ball is released near head level and ends when the pitch is completed. Its major function is involved with deceleration of the arm and forearm and,

Table 22.2.
Typical Throwing Injuries

Throwing Phase	Especially Vulnerable Structures	Clinical Picture
Cocking	Biceps, long head	Tendinitis; localized pain in the anterior shoulder and bicipital groove, aggravated by resisted forearm supination.
	Triceps, long head	Tendinitis; pain in the posterior aspect of the shoulder, which radiates to axilla or deltoid area.
	Rotator cuff	Impingement syndrome during abduction and external rotation, involving entrapment against either the acromion or coracoacromial ligament.
	Humerus	Abduction subluxation during internal or external rotation.
	Axillary artery	Occlusion by the pectoralis minor when the arm is brought into hyperabduction, extension, and extreme external humeral rotation, leading to intimal damage and subsequent thrombosis.
	Subdeltoid bursa	Bursitis and the development of fibrous adhesions.
Acceleration	Pectoralis major	Strain, tendinitis, rupture.
	Latissimus dorsi	Strain, tendinitis, rupture.
	Humerus	Fatigue fractures, coracoid process avulsion, epiphysitis in the young.
Follow-through	Glenohumeral joint	Posterior capsulitis or tear; traction spurs.
	Quadrilateral area	Strain, myositis ossificans; occlusion of the posterior humeral circumflex vessel.

usually, some type of ball rotation. Great stress is applied to the glenohumeral joint and its adjacent tissues.

Roentgenographic Considerations. Keep in mind that everything within the film area must be evaluated. This includes rib, thoracic outlet, and pulmonary abnormalities in addition to osseous and soft-tissue structures related to a specific sports injury. Normally, the margins of the glenohumeral joint are parallel arcs. The cartilage space should be clear and uniform.

Anterior abnormalities may be found with the long head of the biceps tendon within the intertuberous groove or the supraspinatus. In rupture of the biceps brachii, a mass of soft tissue may appear at the anterior or anterolateral aspect of the mid or lower humerus. The long head of the triceps originating from the scapular at the infraglenoid tubercle may present an avulsion throwing injury detectable on roentgenography.

Less common throwing injuries include avascular necrosis of the head of the radius; thrombosis of the axillary artery; stress fracture of the olecranon process, the first rib (usually the contralateral midrib), and the front tips of the lower three ribs; and humeral fracture. Fracture of the humerus, a spiral fracture of the mid or lower third of the shaft (sometimes comminuted), appears to be associated with the sudden stopping of the throwing movement by the deltoid. While it is most common in the unconditioned baseball player, it is sometimes seen in softball, javelin, shot put, and handball.

Fracture of the proximal humeral epiphyseal cartilage is sometimes seen in adolescent baseball pitchers. Roentogenography may show irregular ossification of the capitellum, abnormalities of the medial epicondyle, accelerated closure of the epiphyseal cartilage, or fragmentation of the medial epicondylar epiphysis resulting from avulsion injury.

In heavy throwing sports such as shot put, hammer throw, and javelin, tears of the interscapular, scapulocostal, and rotator cuff muscles are often seen. In javelin activity, overstress may lead to elbow abnormalities such as bony-surface irregularities, soft-tissue calcification, para-articular ossification, capitellar erosion, rupture of the collateral ligaments, and intra-articular loose bodies at the lateral epicondyle and olecranon area. Bursal or tendon ossifications are best shown in coned-down views taken during external and internal rotation.

Swimming Injuries. Shoulder pain is a common complaint in swimmers, especially with the freestyle and butterfly strokes and during underwater pushoffs. The symptomatic picture is one of pain and discomfort after activity, tenderness over the supraspinatus or biceps tendon, and a painful arc (often restricted) of shoulder motion. Shoulder subluxation is sometimes seen in backstrokers.

Contusions, Strains, and Tears

The pain from strain implies (1) abnormal strain on a normal joint, (2) normal strain on an unprepared joint, or (3) normal strain on an abnormal joint.

Shoulder "Pointer"

This is a contusion, by a blow from above, in the prominent upper-deltoid area at the tip of the shoulder. It is easily mistaken for an acromioclavicular separation.

Signs and Symptoms. The trapezius medially and the deltoid laterally are simultaneously bruised between the impact force and bone. Acute disability, swelling, and extreme tenderness are exhibited in the trapezius and/or deltoid. The acromioclavicular joint is not lax, nor is tenderness found in the area of the trapezoid, coracoclavicular, or conoid ligaments.

Management. Initial treatment is by cold packs, shoulder-cap strapping, and a sling for support for 48 hours. For the next 3–4 days, moist heat, passive manipulation, and progressively active exercises should be offered. When the player returns to competition, a protection pad should be applied to the area to reduce impact forces for 1–3 weeks.

The Bicipital Syndrome

In shoulder injury, after possible dislocation and fracture have been eliminated, attention should be given to the bicipital muscle. The biceps is the most powerful flexor of the elbow and a strong supinator. Within the shoulder area, proximal strains and tears along the long head's course within the bicipital groove to the glenoid rim are frequently found.

Background. Acute rupture of the biceps tendon occurs as a result of forceful contraction of the biceps muscle or forceful movement of the arm with the biceps contracted. The injury may be avulsion of the tendon from the muscle belly anywhere along its course or be pulled free from its glenoid attachment. It is often a crippling problem in sports, often accompanied by tenosynovitis. The condition is called "golfer's shoulder" but occurs in almost any sport.

Signs and Symptoms. An acute tendon tear may be felt by the patient as a "snap," followed by swelling, tenderness, and ecchymosis over the bicipital groove and bulging of the biceps near the antecubital fossa at the lower half of the humerus. Pain is usually felt on the anterior shoulder about 2 inches below the humeral head at the site of the thecal tunnel. If the long head is torn, the contracted muscle belly moves distally and bulges even if the short head is intact. This is an important sign in differentiating a proximal biceps problem from other shoulder problems. A hollow in the upper humeral area can be both seen and felt. Flexion and supination, especially against resistance, increases the bulging at the lower half of the upper arm. Strength of forearm supination is decreased.

Yergason's Stability Test. The seated patient flexes the elbow, pronates his forearm, and attempts elbow flexion, forearm

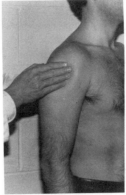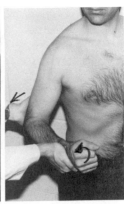

Figure 22.10. *Left*, palpating the bicipital groove. *Right*, Yergason's test to evaluate the stability of the long head of the biceps tendon within the bicipital groove.

supination, and humeral external rotation against the resistance of the examiner. The doctor stabilizes the patient's elbow with one hand while offering resistance to the patient's distal forearm with his other hand during the maneuver. Severe pain in the shoulder is a positive indication of a bicipital tendon lesion, a tear of the transverse humeral ligament, or bicipital tendinitis (see Fig. 22.10)

Loose-Tendon Syndrome. In some chronic bicipital disorders, the tendon may appear slack and actually glide from side to side on palpation during repeated adduction and external rotation. To further test this condition, place the patient's affected forearm on your knee. Palpate the bicipital groove with one hand while the other hand moves the patient's elbow laterally and anterior while the patient resists the movement. If the tendon is slack, it will be felt to "jump" during the motion. Injury to the transverse humeral ligament is often involved.

Gilcrest's Sign. The patient is instructed to lift a 5-lb weight (eg, dumbbell) overhead and then to externally rotate the arm and slowly lower it to the lateral horizontal position. Pain and/or reduplication of symptoms during this maneuver (with or without tendon displacement from the groove) is said to indicate instability of the long head of the biceps and probable tenosynovitis.

Hueter's Sign. If pain and/or reduplication of other symptoms appear when the

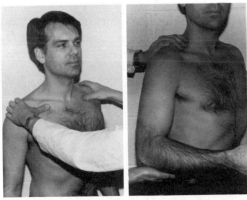

Figure 22.9. *Left*, testing the strength of scapular retraction against resistance; *right*, of shoulder adduction.

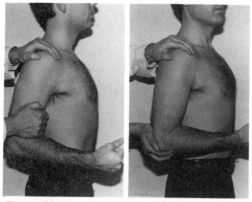

Figure 22.11. *Left*, testing strength of shoulder flexion against resistance; *right*, of shoulder extension.

patient's supinated forearm is flexed against resistance, partial rupture of the biceps is suggested.

Management. Bicipital injury with or without tenosynovitis requires careful strain therapy. Rest in an arm sling is necessary until all symptoms subside. Graduated exercises can be initiated once the tissues appear stable to clinical testing. Impatient pitchers must be advised against "testing" throws, as progress may be completely destroyed. Steroid injections are rarely helpful in the athlete, although frequently employed by habit by some medical physicians. Complete tear or rupture requires surgical approximation.

Rupture of the Transverse Humeral Ligament

An important function of this ligament is to hold the long head of the biceps within its humeral groove. The mechanism of injury is usually heavy lifting, "Indian" arm wrestling, or a slip while carrying a heavy object. Injury occurs, especially in young adults, when the contracted biceps meets an overload.

Signs and Symptoms. Extreme tenderness will be found at the superior aspect of the bicipital groove, with some tenderness along the groove distally. A slack tendon will be found on palpation of the upper groove as the humerus is abducted and internally rotated. A "jumping" sensation from the tendon is felt if the transverse ligament is partially torn. A gliding sensation is felt if the ligament is completely torn.

Management. Mild partial tears will respond to strapping and sling, and the usual physiotherapeutic measures for sprain. Supplementation with 140 mg of manganese glycerophosphate six times daily speeds healing. Severe ruptures require surgical attention.

Bicipital Tendon Dislocation

A stable tendon may be found to be dislocated or at least partially subluxated from its groove and express symptoms of a bicipital syndrome. This is due to rupture or loosening of the transverse ligament which holds it within the bicipital groove.

Background. The disorder is often a consequence of painful strains, sprains, capsule tears, and contractures. The subluxated tendon will be felt and/or heard to snap as the patient forward flexes and abducts his arm, then returns it to its natural position. The patient is unable to place the ipsilateral hand on the sacrum. As time passes, motion restrictions indicate cuff degeneration. Yergason's test is positive on resisted external rotation (see Fig. 22.10).

Abbott-Saunders Test. This is a modification of Yergason's test which forces the biceps tendon against the lesser tuberosity which will stress an unstable tendon. Bring the arm of the seated patient into full abduction, rotate it externally, and then lower the arm to the patient's side. A "click" felt or heard, frequently accompanied by pain and a reproduction of symptoms, is a positive sign of subluxation or dislocation of the biceps tendon.

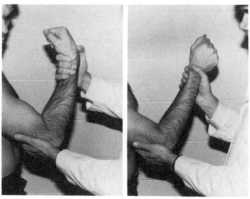

Figure 22.12. *Left*, testing the flexion strength of arm against resistance; *right*, testing extension strength.

Biceps Stability Test. The seated patient is asked to flex his elbow so that the forearm is held forward and horizontal. As the patient attempts to externally rotate the arm, the examiner applies resistance. Localized pain indicates an inflammatory instability of the long head of the biceps and/or displacement of the tendon from the bicipital groove.

Lippman's Test. In the relaxed seated position, the seated patient is asked to flex the elbow on the involved side and rest the forearm in the lap. The examiner palpates for the tendon of the long head of the biceps about 3 inches distal from the glenohumeral joint. An attempt is made to displace the tendon laterally or medially from its groove. Pain, reduplication of other symptoms, and a palpable displacement of the tendon from its groove signifies tenosynovitis with instability.

Booth-Marvel's Test. The examiner abducts the patient's arm laterally to the horizontal position, flexes the elbow to a right angle, and deeply palpates the bicipital groove as the humerus is passively rotated internally and externally. If the transverse humeral ligament has been stretched, a painful and palpable snap wil be felt as the tendon of the long head displaces from the bicipital groove.

Adjustment. To reset, stand behind the sitting patient towards the side of involvement. If the right shoulder is involved, place your left hand over the shoulder cap and grasp the patient's right wrist with your right hand. The patient's arm is allowed to hang loose, the elbow should be flexed about 45°, and the arm should be abducted about 45°. Press the thumb of your left hand against the back of the tendon, and wrap your fingers under the short head of the biceps and coracobrachialis to compress the tendon of the biceps. Advise the patient that the adjustment is not painful and not to resist. With firm contact on the shoulder muscles, quickly bring the patient's flexed arm anterior and medial to internally rotate the humerus. This usually brings immediate relief. If not, a steady lateral (rarely medial) pressure is applied to the slipped tendon while the elbow is drawn posterior and held close to the chest until the limit of motion is reached. Then with continued pressure on the tendon, abduct the elbow, bring it forward, and return it to its original position.

Management. Follow adjustment with traction strapping, sling, and the usual treatment of sprain depending upon the history. Efforts to elongate the tendon with weight exercises following the acute stage are most helpful. If the ligament is severely torn, it will not remain in place; surgery is required for permanent correction.

Rotator Cuff Injuries

Five deep muscles are around the glenohumeral joint. They comprise the rotator cuff. The infraspinatus and teres minor work as external rotators of the humerus. The subscapularis and teres major rotate the humerus medially. The supraspinaturs pulls the humerus into the glenoid fossa and abducts the humerus initially (10–15°) before the deltoid becomes effective. In further abduction, the supraspinatus stabilizes the humerus as the deltoid, during full abduction, tends to displace the humerus from the glenoid. The mechanism of injury may be a fall with outstretched hand, a blow on the shoulder, throwing, or heavy lifting.

Background. In pitching "round house" curves, the tendon is whipped against the outer edge of its groove, initiating an inflammation and degenerative process ("glass arm" syndrome). The injury is essentially a localized tendinitis from intrinsic overload particularly at the subscapularis insertion on the lesser tuberosity. This creates disability on elevation and external rotation of the arm in the early stages of throwing. The cause is found in overstretch of the subscapularis at the end of "draw back" which is instantly interrupted by a sudden force on the tendon as the throw takes place. Examination shows limited motion and pain on abduction and external rotation of the shoulder. Pain is increased when active internal rotation is resisted. Tenderness will be found over the lesser tuberosity.

Stages. Three stages are commonly recognized and related to age: (1) Edema and hemorrhage resulting from overuse (eg, swimming, tennis, baseball) are characteristically seen in young athletes before 25 years but may be seen at any age. (2) With repeated episodes, the subacromial bursa becomes fibrotic and thickened. The patient is usually 25–40 years old. (3) There is wearing of the bone and rupture of the tendon in individuals over 40 years, associated with anterior acromial erosion and spurs. However, these stages fail to recognize the effect of a reflex-produced ischemia so often seen in practice.

Supraspinatus tears (full or partial rupture) are characterized by a total loss of initial abduction. The tendon of the supraspinatus may be the site of peritendonitis or ectopic calcification.

Rotator cuff strain can be classified as follows:

• *Grade I Injury:* Minor pain and weakness; tenderness over upper end of humerus, weakness and loss of normal shoulder rhythm on flexion and abduction.

• *Grade II Injury:* Pain with moderate disability; exaggerated signs of Grade I; unpalpable tear site.

• *Grade III Injury:* Pain at tear site (partial or complete) with severe disability; weakness with inability to actively abduct shoulder. A tear is possibly palpable. Later signs of atrophy appear. A supraspinatus tear is characterized by a dull ache on rest which is aggravated by abduction. It is usually sited in the rotator cuff or common tendinous insertion, rather than within the tendon itself. Complete ruptures are rare in comparison to partial tears.

The degree of injury is determined by the degree of pain or weakness on passive motion or active motion against resistance. Differentiation must be made from bicipital tenosynovitis by a positive Yergason's sign and severe pain on palpation. Roentgenograms are usually negative; but, in chronic cases, the anterior edge of the acromion may show spur formation or a displaced fracture of the tuberosity.

Signs and Symptoms. On examination, the patient's arm is held to the side and cannot be abducted actively without pain; however, nearly a full range of passive movement can be obtained with care. The arc of pain is generally located between 45°–90° as the tuberosity of the humerus passes under the acromion process. Pain may also be noticed during adduction from 120°–170° with subacromial crepitus, varying amounts of weakness, and recurrent "bursitis" episodes. When the patient is asked to raise his arm, the shoulder hunches in support and a short motion may be made but the arm quickly collapses to the side in pain. While passive motions of the shoulder are unrestricted, pain may be felt when the humeral head presses under the acromial arch. When the shoulder is extended, the front and back of the humerus will be tender but not as acute as at the greater tubercle. Extreme tenderness is found where the cuff inserts into the tuberosities. A superior subluxation of the humerus is often associated.

Subacute Cases. An important sign in 1–2 weeks after injury is an area of thinning or depression at the fossae of the supraspinatous and infraspinatus (especially) musclers. If this is the site of rupture, a "catch" and clicking sound may be felt and heard at the site during passive movements if swelling is minimal.

Arm Drop Test. Hold the patient's arm at 90° abduction and then ask him to hold that position without assistance. If this cannot be done actively for a few moments without pain, it is a positive indication of a torn rotator cuff. In lesser tears, the patient may be able to hold the abduction (a slight tap on the forearm will make it drop) and slowly lower it to his side, but the motion will not be smooth.

Supraspinatus Press Test. With the patient in the relaxed seated position, the examiner applies strong thumb pressure directed toward the midline in the soft tissues located superior to the midpoint of the scapular spine. The production of pain signifies an inflammatory process in the supraspinatus muscle (eg, strain, rupture, tendinitis).

Apley's Scratch Test. This is a two-phase test: (1) The patient (seated or standing) is asked to raise the arm on the involved side overhead, flex the elbow overhead, and then place the fingers as far down on the opposite shoulder blade as possible. (2) The patient is then asked to relax his arm at the side, then place the hand behind the back and attempt to touch as far up on the opposite scapula as possible. If either of these manuevers increases shoulder pain, inflammation of one of the rotator cuff's tendons is indicated. The supraspinatus tendon is most commonly involved. Restricted motion without sharp pain points to osteoarthritis or shortened soft tissues.

Shoulder Abduction Stress Test. The seated patient is asked to abduct the arm laterally to the horizontal position with the elbow extended while the examiner applies resistance. If this causes pain in the area of the insertion of the supraspinatus tendon, acute or degenerative tendinitis should be suspected.

Codman's Sign. This is a variation of the shoulder abduction stress test and the arm drop test. If the patient's arm can be passively abducted laterally to about 100° without pain, the examiner then removes support s othat the position is held actively by the patient. This produces sudden deltoid contraction. If a rupture of the supraspinatus tendon or strain of the rotator cuff is present, the pain elicited will cause the patient to hunch the shoulder and lower the arm.

Teres's Major Spasm Sign. When the relaxed staining patient is viewed from behind, the arms normally rest so that the palms face the thighs. If the palm faces distinctly backward (toward the examiner) on the involved side, a spastic contraction of the teres major muscle is suggested.

Management. The chief therapy for small tears is rest. Any taping technique should be designed to assist the action of the rotator cuff tendons or the joint capsule. This requires strapping from just above the elbow to the neck. Horizontal strips should be laid "in line" at the base of the neck to cover the entire shoulder to stabilize the clavicle and scapula. Early rehabilitation exercises should emphasize flexion, extension, adduction, and adduction in the later stage. Moderate or large tears usually require surgery.

Impingement Syndrome of the Supraspinaturs and/or Bicipital Tendon

Locking Position Test. The patient's arm is extended and internally rotated. If a painful reduplication of the patient's symptoms occurs on this maneuver, an impingement syndrome of the supraspinatus and/or bicipital tendon is suggested.

Impingement Syndrome Test. The patient is placed supine with the arms resting loosely at the sides. The elbow on the involved side is then flexed to a right angle and the arm is rotated internally so that it rests comfortably on the patient's upper abdomen. The examiner places one hand on the patient's shoulder and the other hand on the patient's elbow. A compressive force is then applied, which pushes the humerus against the inferior aspect of the acromion process and the glenohumeral fossa. Pain and/or a reduplication of symptoms indicates an impingement syndrome of the supraspinatus and/or bicipital tendon.

Deltoid Contusion and Strains

This powerful abductor is a frequent site of acute and chronic disability. Injury may be intrinsic. Powerful contraction of the deltoid has been known to fracture its attachment from the clavicle or humerus.

Anterior deltoid strain is often seen in football following an attempted one-arm tackle. Symptoms arise slowly, often peaking 6–8 hours after injury. Pain and weakness increase on forward abduction. Evidence of swelling and tenderness appear in the anterior third of the muscle (see Fig. 22.13).

Middle deltoid strain follows forceful abduction against resistance in the lateral plane. Symptoms arise slowly. Pain and weakness increase on lateral abduction. Evidence of swelling and tenderness appear in the midthird of the muscle.

Dorsal deltoid strain is the result of a posteriorly directed strain such as seen in swimmers using the butterfly stroke. Symptoms arise slowly. Pain and weakness increase on posterior abduction. Evidence of

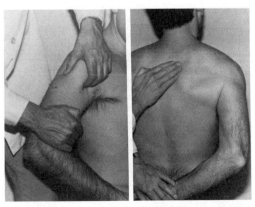

Figure 22.13. *Left*, palpating the deltoid and the lesser tuberosity areas. *Right*, palpating the rhomboids.

swelling and tenderness appears in the posterior third of the muscle.

Management. Cold packs, shoulder-cap strapping, and an armsling are necessary during the first 2 days, followed by moist heat and passive manipulation. Active exercises should be conducted during a warm shower. Full activity can usually be allowed (with support) in 3–5 days.

Brachialis Contusion and Strain

Brachialis strain is common in contact sports. It is continually subjected to bruises in football as it is exposed to contusion just below the epaulettes of the shoulder pad.

Signs and Symptoms. In sprain of the proximal radioulnar joint, there is often a related injury to the brachialis anticus muscle with contracture, or, especially in children, a strip of periosteum may be torn from the anterior aspect of the humerus, followed by callus formation and blocked joint motion. The athlete will present a highly developed muscle belly on the anterolateral aspect of the upper arm which is easily found between the deltoid and the lateral head of the triceps

Management. Treat for acute sprain with ice and pressure, and follow with typical physiotherapeutic procedures such as heat and progressive exercises.

Posttraumatic Trigger Points

The source of many shoulder pains sited in the front of the shoulder will be found at the insertion of the infraspinatus muscle at the scapula. In other cases, a localized trigger point may be found in the anterior deltoid with pain referred to the subdeltoid bursa. Other common trigger-point sites in shoulder pain include the lesser tuberosity at the insertion of the subscapularis, the greater tuberosity at the insertion of the supraspinatus tendon, at the glenohumeral joint space, within the bicipital groove, at the acromioclavicular joint, or at the sternoclavicular joint. The levator scapulae, scaleni, pectoralis major and minor, sternalis, and seratus anterior are less common sites. (see Figs. 22.14 and 22.15).

Muscle Technique

No physical therapy will strengthen a muscle or shorten a lax muscle. Only exer-

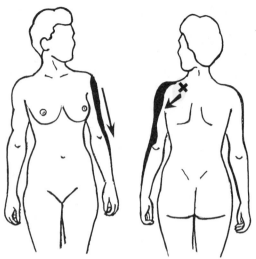

Figure 22.14. The supraspinatus trigger point; *X*, common site. *Blackened areas* indicate typical sites of referred pain.

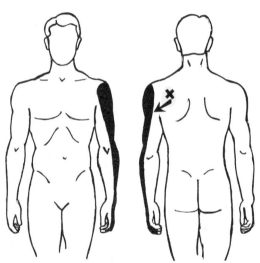

Figure 22.15. Infraspinatus trigger point; *X*, common site. *Blackened areas* indicate typical sites of referred pain.

cise will do that. Various techniques may be applied to relax a muscle, but only active or passive stretching exercises will lengthen a shortened muscle.

After a muscle has been strained, Goodheart's research found that heavy pressure over the origin or insertion of the affected muscle will elicit a normalization response in the comparatively weakened muscle. This state of weakness after strain appears to be the result of a microavulsion of the tendoperiostela connection. The following technique is essentially used on weak hypertonic muscles created by overstretch injuries:

1. Test the isolated muscle, and note comparative weakness, hypertonia, and/or shortening.

2. If strain to the tendoperiosteal site has occurred, the muscular origin and insertion will be tender. Select the site which appears to be the most tender, origin or insertion. Apply the pads of two or three fingers on the muscle's tendon or point of attachment. Direct pressure from the muscle towards the point of origin or insertion. If partial rupture has occurred, it may be necessary to strap the muscle somewhat prior to therapy. If relaxation of a reactive muscle is desired, apply pressure gently at first, and slowly increase it to just below the patient's tolerance (2–3 lb). Initial heavy pressure can be extremely painful and tends to increase spasm. The pressure utilizes the Golgi tendon receptor reflex to induce muscle relaxation. Maintain pressure for several (30–60) seconds until the muscle relaxes and allows lengthening, then for approximately 10 seconds after the muscle has relaxed.

3. Re-examine the muscle unless severity prohibits retesting. In some cases, small sensitive nodules noted on palpation near the affected muscle's origin and/or insertion usually disappear within 24 hours after successful treatment. When normalized, conclude by giving the patient instructions in proper stretching exercises.

Spasm Management

The benefits of vertebral and rib adjustments are well known within the chiropractic profession. To relieve muscle spasm, heat is helpful, but cold and vapocoolant sprays have shown to be as effective. The effects of cervical traction are often dramatic but sometimes short-lived if a herniated disc is involved.

Mild passive stretch is an excellent method of reducing spasm in the long muscles, but heavy passive stretch destroys the beneficial reflexes. For example in rhomboid spasm, have the prone patient place his hand on the involved side behind his back to "wing" the scapula. This slightly stretches the muscle fibers by pulling the scapula from the midline. It may be assisted by the doctor offering a slight tug upward on the scapular angle. The muscle should relax within 2–3 min. Thumb pressure, placed on a trigger area, is then directed towards the muscle's attachment and held for a few moments until relaxation is complete. When pain has subsided, good home progressive exercises are gravity-assisted pendulum exercises holding a weight or iron while prone and holding a broom stick in front with both hands and doing elevations.

Other methods may prove helpful. Peripheral inhibitory afferent impulses can be generated to partially close the presynaptic gate by acupressure, acupuncture, or transcutaneous nerve stimulation. Isotonic exercises are useful in improving circulation and inducing the stretch reflex when done supine to reduce exteroceptive influences on the central nervous system. An acid–base imbalance from muscle hypoxia and acidosis may be prevented by supplemental alkalinization. In chronic cases, relaxation training and biofeedback therapy are helpful.

General Sprains

Overtreating an upper humeral fracture or sprain is a common pitfall according to some orthopedic authorities.

Background. The symptoms of sprain of the shoulder are pain, tenderness on pressure, and, rarely, swelling. Passive motion is comparatively painless, but active motion induces severe pain. Differentiation must always be made from rupture of the supraspinatus tendon, subdeltoid bursitis, fracture, and inflammation of other bursae about the shoulder.

Management. During the acute hyperemic stage, structural alignment, cold, compression, strapping, positive galvanism, ultrasound, and rest are indicated. An application of hyaluronidase is helpful to reduce tissue swelling and edema, especially if it is "driven in" with ionotophoresis or phonophoresis. After 48 hours, passive congestion may be managed by contrast baths, light massage, gentle passive manipulation, sinusoidal stimulation, ultrasound, and a mild range of motion exercise initiated. Immobilization may be required if effusion and swelling persists. Vitamin C and 140 mg of manganese glycerophosphate six times daily may prove helpful throughout care. During the stage of consolidation, local moderate heat, moderate active exercise, moderate range of motion manipulation, and ultrasound are beneficial. In the stage of fibroblastic activity, deep heat, deep massage, vigorous active exercise, negative galvanism, ultrasound, and active joint manipulation speed recovery and inhibit postinjury effects.

Subluxations

Shoulder subluxations may be primary conditions after injury, or they may occur weeks or months after reduction of a primary dislocation. Thus, in cases of chronic shoulder pain, probe the history for possible shoulder dislocation and reduction. Most shoulder subluxations are not acute, exhibit little or no swelling, but they present chronic (often episodic) pain, movement stiffness or "blocks," and other signs of tissue fibrosis and joint "gluing." Mild to moderate local muscle weakness and possible atrophy are characteristic. Postural distortions of the lower cervical and upper dorsal spine and musculoskeletal abnormalities of some aspect of the shoulder girdle are invariably related.

During correction of a shoulder subluxation, dynamic thrusts should be reserved for nonacute, fixated situations. Whne subluxation accompanies an acute sprain, attempts at correction should be more in line with gentle traction pressures after musculature has been relaxed. Obviously, the probability of fracture fragments or osteoporosis must be eliminated prior to any form of manipulation.

Severe Subluxation of the Humeral Head

This acute condition is probably a dislocation which has partially reduced itself spontaneously.

Background. It occurs when the greater tuberosity has been displaced upward as a whole to lie between the humeral head and the glenoid. The capital part is rotated to a degree but has not completely escaped from its capsular envelope. The outer border of the shaft is impacted firmly into the cancellous tissue of the head of the humerus.

Management. The chief obstacle in obtaining reduction is in the difficulty of re-

moving the tuberosity from within the joint and overcoming the very firm impaction of the two main fragments. It is rarely possible to overcome these obstacles by manipulation, especially without anesthesia: thus immediate referral should be made for orthopedic attention.

Superior Humerus Subluxation

Because of its bony arch, the humerus cannot dislocate much superiorly unless there is severe fraction involved. However, several authorities believe that superior subluxation can often be demonstrated on bilateral rentgenography.

Background. Schultz feels this is the most common shoulder subluxation seen. This writer, however, believes the term to be a misnomer as the suprahumeral joint is not an articulation in the true sense of the word but is a structure that serves as a protective and supportive mechanism. Most likely what is referred to as a superior humeral subluxation is the result of contractures within the superior humeral area which prevent the greater tuberosity from gliding smoothly under the coracoacromial ligament during abduction. The result is chronic compression and irritation of the enclosed tissues. Keep in mind that the acromioclavicular meniscus progressively thins with age. It is quite thick in the young and may be completely gone by the sixth decade.

Adjustment. Determine if correction is necessary for any associated internal or ex-

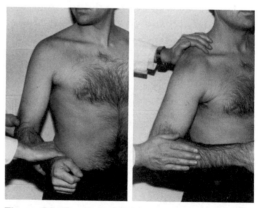

Figure 22.16. *Left,* testing strength of shoulder internal rotation against resistance; *right,* of shoulder abduction.

ternal rotation in addition to the superior displacement. The doctor sits on the affected side facing the head of a supine patient. A shoeless foot is placed in the patient's axilla for counterpressure and stabilization of the shoulder girdle. Straight axial traction is then applied with both hands on the patient's arm. The traction is towards the inferior and slightly lateral. After a few seconds and with steady traction, the patient's arm is rotated internally (usually) or externally as need be, and a short tug is applied inferiorly towards the doctor's body to correct any rotational deficiency present. Strapping is sometimes, but not always, necessary for a few days to rest the joint. Follow with therapy for chronic sprain, frequent mobilization, and progressive stretching exercises. Evaluate the integrity of the pectoralis major and the latissimus dorsi for associated dysfunction.

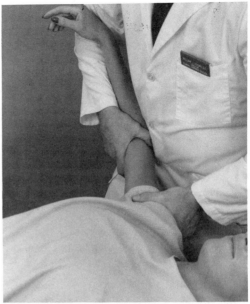

Figure 22.17. Alternative adjustment of subluxated superior humerus.

Alternative Adjustment Procedure. Determine if correction is necessary for any associated internal or external rotation in addition to the superior displacement. The patient is placed supine if there is any internal rotation, prone if there is any external rotation. The doctor sits relatively perpendicular to the patient's affected side. The patient's elbow is flexed 90°, and his shoulder abducted 90°. The doctor takes contact with the web of his cephalad hand on the lateral proximal humerus (cephalad aspect) and with the web of his caudad hand on the medial distal humerus (caudad aspect). Pressure is made against the proximal humerus in a caudal direction, and a thrust is made while the doctor's caudad hand stabilizes the distal humerus (see Fig. 22.17).

Anterior Humerus Subluxation

This is also a frequently seen shoulder subluxation. The mechanism of injury is that similar to anterior humeral dislocation.

Background. There is difficulty in raising the arm overhead. Fullness will be noted on the upper anterior arm that will be tender on palpation. The deltoid will feel taut and stringy. A sensitive coracoid process will be found higher than the head of the humerus. Signs of acute or chronic sprain will be found depending upon the history. Check infraspinatus, teres minor, and rhomboid major for possible strain.

Adjustment of Externally Rotated Anterior Humerus. Stand behind the patient sitting on a low stool. Instruct the patient to place his hand on his opposite shoulder near his neck to internally rotate his humerus. The elbow will be fully flexed and the arm will be almost horizontal to the floor. Reach around the patient with both arms and clasp your fingers over the patient's elbow. Brace your chest against the patient's dorsal spine for counterpressure. Ask the patient to relax, and as this is done, lift the elbow slightly and apply pressure followed by a short quick thrust (pull) posterior and slightly inferior towards yourself. Follow with sprain therapy and rehabilitation measures to assure against joint looseness or restrictions (see Fig. 22.18).

Adjustment of Internally Rotated Anterior Humerus. The procedure is essentially the same except that prior to the adjustment, the patient is instructed to grasp the back of his neck on the ipsilateral side with the palm of his hand on the affected side to externally rotate his humerus.

Inferior Humerus Subluxation

Background. A slight hollowness may be found at the joint space, indicating that the humeral head has dropped from its nor-

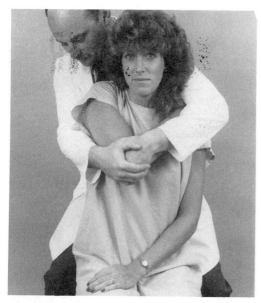

Figure 22.18.   Adjustment of subluxated anterior humerus: anterior humerus with external rotation.

mal position. The deltoid will often feel firm and stringy, indicating a chronic disorder. Evaluate the integrity of the supraspinatus, long head of the triceps, deltoid, coracobrachialis, and clavicular division of the pectoralis major. Signs are often vague and should be confirmed by bilateral roentgenography.

Adjustment.   Determine if correction is necessary for any associated internal or external rotation in addition to the superior displacement. The patient is placed supine if there is any internal rotation, prone if there is any external rotation. The doctor sits relatively perpendicular to the patient's affected side. The doctor takes contact on the patient's medial proximal humerus (caudad aspect) with the web of his caudad hand and on the patient's lateral distal humerus (cephalad aspect) with the web of his cephalad hand. Pressure is made cephally, and then a short thrust is made with the doctor's contact hand while his cephalad hand stabilizes the patient's humerus (see Fig. 22.19).

Alternative Adjustment Procedure. Correction is by abduction, moderate traction, and then superior pressure. The patient is placed supine and the doctor sits perpendicular to the affected side. The patient's

flexed elbow of the affected extremity is placed in the doctor's axilla for control. The doctor grasps the humerous high with both hands and pulls the head of humerus first laterally towards himself and then cephally in one smooth quick movement. Counterpressure is applied by the doctor's knee against a pillow placed in the patient's axilla. This is a "reseating" procedure which must be followed by temporary immobilization to encourage the lax tissues to tighten and then rehabilitation procedures to strengthen weakened musculature and lax supporting tissues.

Posterior Humerus Subluxation

Background.   Physical signs of this rare disorder are usually negative; bilateral roentgenography is required for confirmation. In a few cases, the posterior area may feel fuller than the unaffected side. An unusually prominent coracoid process may be felt, and a slight hollow may be felt above the humerus. Signs of taut tissues on the posterior aspect of the humeral head and lax tissues on the anterior aspect are often found. Evaluate the integrity of the pectoralis major.

Adjustment.   Correction can be made in the same doctor-patient position as for the alternative adjustment procedure of an in-

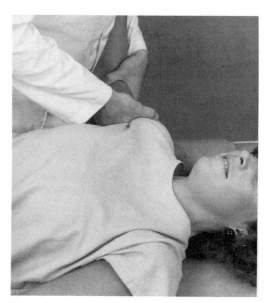

Figure 22.19.   Adjustment of subluxated inferior humerus.

ferior humeral subluxation by applying humeral traction first laterally towards yourself and then anteriorly towards the ceiling. A slow steady lateral pull should be concluded with an anterior tug to stretch the contracted tissues and "reset" the humeral head in its normal position. Follow with standard therapy for acute or chronic sprain, depending upon the history.

Alternative Adjustment Procedure. The patient is placed prone with the involved extremity at his side. The doctor stands on the side of involvement facing the patient's shoulder. A pisiform contact is made on the patient's posterior proximal humerus, as far cephally as possible, with the doctor's medial hand. The doctor's lateral hand stabilizes his contact hand. Pressure is made toward the flow, followed by a short thrust (Fig. 22.20).

Internal Humerus Subluxation

Background. This type of malposition is frequently associated with a fixation that restricts external rotation of the humerus. Rotator cuff tendinitis and inferior humerus subluxation may be associated.

Adjustment. The patient is placed supine on the adjusting table and the doctor stands facing the patient's shoulder on the side of involvement. The patient's elbow is

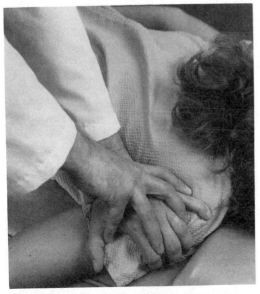

Figure 22.20. The alternative adjustment procedure of subluxated posterior humerus.

flexed and the arm is allowed to rotate externally somewhat by its own weight. The doctor's contact hand grasps the patient's proximal humerus firmly, just below the acromion process, and the other (lateral) hand slides under the patient to stabilize the patient's scapula. It is helpful if a thumb contact can also be made with the clavicle. A deep, but not severe, rotary thrust is made, and the line of correction is directed to produce external rotation of the humerus.

External Humerus Subluxation

Background. This type of subluxation is often related to restricted internal rotation of the humerus. Supraspinous tendinitis, bicipital tendinitis, tendon displacement from the bicipital groove, and inferior humerus subluxation are common complications.

Adjustment. The patient is placed prone on the adjusting table and the doctor stands facing the patient's shoulder on the side of involvement. The patient's elbow is flexed and the supinated hand is placed under the patient so that the palm comfortably rests against the patient's chest and the back of the hand is in contact with the table. This "sling position" will allow some internal rotation tension that will assist the forthcoming adjustment. The doctor's indifferent hand cups the shoulder so that the heel of the stabilizing hand holds the patient's clavicle while the fingers stabilize the patient's scapula. The doctor's contact hand firmly grasps the humerus just below the acromion process. A deep, but not severe, rotary thrust is made that is directerd to produce internal rotation of the humerus.

Dislocations

Falls and collisions causing shoulder dislocation are frequent in contact athletics, representing about 50% of all major joint dislocations and the most common dislocation area of the body. Incidence is highest in high-jumping, pole vaulting, gymnastics, horseback riding, and water polo. The typical mechanism is an extension force against an abducted arm that is externally rotated.

Most dislocations are anterior dislocations of the glenohumeral joint (85%), followed by acromioclavicular dislocations (10%), sternoclavicular dislocations (3%), and posterior dislocations (2%). True dislocations must be differentiated from pseudo-subluxations where the humerus is displaced inferiorly by hemarthrosis. Poor muscle tone is usually related in the occasional athlete.

The glenoid cavity covers only a small part of the head of the humerus. In extreme degrees of abduction, extension, and flexion, any force transmitted through the humeral shaft is applied obliquely in the body surface and directly on the capsule of the joint, through which the head of the bone is then forced. In fracture dislocations, the humeral fracture is invariably displaced with the articular surface outside the joint.

Apprehension Test. If chronic shoulder dislocation is suspected, begin to slowly and gently abduct and externally rotate the patient's arm with the elbow flexed toward a point where the shoulder might easily dislocate. If shoulder dislocation exists, the patient will become quite apprehensive, symptoms may be reproduced, and the maneuver is resisted as you attempt further motion.

Dugas' Test. The patient places his hand on his opposite shoulder and attempts to touch his chest wall with his elbow and then raise his elbow to chin level. If it is impossible to touch the chest with the elbow or to raise the elbow to chin level, it is a positive sign of a dislocated shoulder (see Fig. 22.21).

Calloway's Sign. The circumference of the proximal arm of a seated patient is measured at the shoulder tip when the patient's

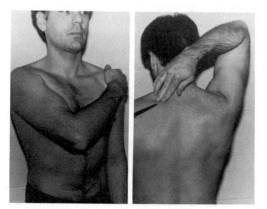

Figure 22.21. *Left*, Dugas' test to evaluate the integrity of the shoulder. *Right*, Apley's scratch test to evaluate humeral abduction and external rotation.

arm is laterally abducted. This measurement is compared to that of the noninvolved side. An increase in the circumference on the affected side suggests a dislocated shoulder.

Bryant's Sign. A posttraumatic ipsilateral lowering of the axillary folds (anterior and posterior pillars of the armpit), but level shoulders, is indicative of dislocation of the glenohumeral articulation.

Hamilton's Ruler Sign. Normally a straight edge (eg, a yardstick) held against the lateral aspect of the arm cannot be placed simlutaneously on the tip of the acromion process and the lateral epicondyle. If these two points do touch the straight edge, it signifies a dislocated shoulder.

Varieties

In primary dislocation, symptoms may be severe even if the soft-tissues and capsule are not greatly damaged. Heroic on-field reductions should be avoided. Four types may be classified according to the direction in which the humeral head leaves the socket, and these can be subclassed according to the point at which the head of the humerus comes to rest or according to limb position.

1. Anterior Dislocations. Subcoracoid (most common), intracoracoid, and subclavicular types may be found. The typical mechanism involves a combination of abduction, extension, and external rotation of the shoulder. The common means are (a) a fall on the outstretched arm where the trauma drives the humeral head forward against the anterior capsule; (b) abduction with the humerus in internal rotation or forward flexion with the humerus in external rotation, limited by the acromial arch—if forceful elevation is applied when this point of impingement is reached, the arch is used as a fulcrum to dislocate the proximmal head anterior and inferior; and (c) a fall or blow to the lateral shoulder from the rear.

In *subcoracoid luxation*, the head of the humerus lies under the coracoid process, either in contact with it or at a finger's breadth distance at most below it. The head may be displaced inward until three-fourths of its diameter lies to the medial side of the process or be simply balanced on the anterior edge of the glenoid fossa. The humeral axis passes to the medial side of the fossa. The elbow hangs away from the side, the lateral deltoid bulge is flat, and the acromion is prominent. The glenoid cavity is empty. Palpation reveals the absence of the usual bony resistance below the lateral aspect of the acromion and the presence of abnormal resistance below the coracoid process or in the axilla. Voluntary movement is lost, and assisted abduction is strongly resisted by the patient. Dugas' test is positive. The arm can be passively adducted but not to the degree that the elbow can touch the chest with the fingers resting on the opposite shoulder. Measurement in abduction shows shortening.

In *intracoracoid dislocations*, the humeral head is displaced further medially. The symptoms and signs are those of the subcoracoid type except that the head of the humerus is felt further displaced and the shoulder is more flattened. The arm may be fixed in horizontal abduction. Severe capsule laceration is usually involved which allows for the greater displacement.

Complications of Anterior Dislocations. When the humerus dislocates anteriorly, its posterolateral margin is often forced against the rim of the glenoid to produce a compression fracture (Hill-Sachs deformity). The malpositioned humerus frequently tears the cartilaginous labrum and capsule from the glenoid rim (Bankhart lesion) with an avulsed fragment of bone. If there is fracture of the anatomical neck, the humeral head will not participate in passive movement of the shaft, and crepitus can usually be felt. Fracture of the greater tuberosity, tears of the rotator cuff, and recurrent dislocation are common complications. Anterior fracture dislocations are usually related with displacement of the greater tuberosity, but the capsule is not displaced. Any anterior luxation can do great harm to the brachial artery, vein, or nerves. Circulation msut always be checked before reduction is attempted.

2. Inferior Dislocations. Subglenoid and luxatio erecta types are infrequently seen in which the humeral head lies below the glenoid fossa. The typical cause is forcible abduction followed by rotation or impulsion. The mechanism of injury is usually a leverage force on an abducted arm such as in an arm tackle. There is severe pain and disability. The arm is fixed at about 45° in abduction. A hollowness will be found at the joint space, with the humeral head inferior to its normal position and often palable within the axilla. The deltoid is flattened and extremely spastic. In *subglenoid* luxation, the symptoms are those of subcoracoid flattening, but abduction and flattening of the shoulder are more marked. The upper part of the greater tuberosity is usually torn. In rare instances of *luxatio erecta*, forcible elevation of the arm causes the head of the humerus to be displaced far downward so that the extremity remains in an erect position.

3. Posterior Dislocations. This is often a diagnostic challenge in the young well-muscled athlete because all joint motions may be unrestricted, yet disability is acute. Two types are seen which differ only in the extent of displacement; ie, subacromial and subspinous types. The cause is direct pressure lateral and posterior, or pressure has been exerted in the same direction along a flexed, adducted, and internally rotated humerus. It is sometimes produced during a convulsive attack. The patient's arm is abducted and rotated internally, and the elbow is directed slightly forward. The shoulder is flat in front and full behind, where the head of the humerus may be felt. The coracoid is prominent. The head of the humerus lies on the outer edge of the glenoid fossa or further posterior under the scapular spine or on the infraspinatus. These features are not as obvious as those of anterior dislocation. Passive abduction and external rotation motions are restricted. In severe cases, the lateral side of the capsule is usually torn, and there may be associated cuff tear or an avulsion fracture of the greater tuberosity resulting in persistent pain. The internal and external scapular muscles are usually quite lacerated or contain fragments of the torn tuberosities.

4. Superior Dislocations. A supraglenoid luxation is very rare except in sports. A routine A-P view may show narrowing of the space between the head of the humerus and the acromion, indicating a tear. In many cases, arthrography must be recommended. Take care not to confuse the growth plate of the proximal humerus with that of a fracture line.

Roentgenographic Considerations

Careful evaluation of the glenohumeral articulation is necessary to judge alignment congruity. An axillary (bird's eye) view to clearly expose the glenohumeral relationship is often quite helpful. A tangential view of the scapula may be helpful to elicit a fracture of the coracoid process or glenoid margin or to find evidence of defects in the humeral articular margin following chronic dislocation. In approximately 20% of cases of shoulder dislocation, fractures of the glenoid are related. Lesser tuberosity fractures are often related to a posterior dislocation of the shoulder. Vigorous contractions of the triceps muscle, as seen in throwing, may produce avulsion injuries to the inferior aspect of the glenoid. Roentgenography is required to analyze possible complications prior to any considered reduction.

Subcoracoid Dislocation Reduction Techniques

Before any reduction technique is utilized, the integrity of the circumflex nerve should be established by checking the dermatome (C5) with a pin or pinwheel, and signs of possible fracture should be sought. As a rule, early reduction of a shoulder dislocation may not require an anesthetic except in the highly apprehensive patient. Reassurance, warmth, and a quiet area help to augment relaxation. Occurrence and reduction should always be confirmed by x-ray.

• *Kocher's method* is to (1) apply gentle downward traction to the flexed elbow, and press it closely to the patient's side; (2) most carefully, ease the arm into full possible external rotation by moving the patient's arm away from the trunk (a sudden motion may fracture the humerus); (3) while maintaining the external rotation, carry the elbow well anterior and superior as to gently adduct the elbow across the patient's chest; then (4) reduction can be felt (and often heard) when adduction is complete. The arm is then rotated internally so that the patient's hand rests on his opposite shoulder. The elbow is simultaneously lowered. If this method fails, the classic method may

be attempted. Keep in mind, however, that failure in reduction may indicate a complicating fracture which would make further attempts contraindicated (see Fig. 22.22).

• *The classic (Hippocratic) method* is for the sitting doctor to place a shoeless foot in the supine patient's axilla for counterpressure and apply straight axial traction with both hands on the patient's arm. The gentle pull is towards the inferior and slightly lateral, *never* upward as there is danger of lacerating vessels. After a long steady pull (never a jerk), the muscles may yield and allow the head of the humerus to slip back into the socket as the arm is slowly internally rotated. If successful, relief is immediate. During traction, some doctors attempt to push the humeral head into the socket with the ball of the stockinged foot. If replacement is not complete, remove your foot from the patient's axilla, and flex the patient's elbow. Stabilize the elbow with one hand while applying gentle pressure downward on the forearm to cause slight internal rotation of the humeral head to complete the reduction. Place the flexed arm over the patient's chest and instruct him to hold it there until the joint can be secured with tape.

Note: Muscle spasm may be difficult to

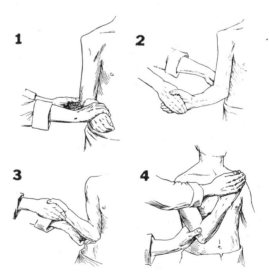

Figure 22.22. Kocher's method of reducing an anterior dislocated humerus. The four phases are (1) elbow flexion, (2) external rotation, (3) adduction, and (4) internal rotation.

overcome in the highly musculatured ath-lete. Regardless, never use severe leverage against the chest as it will undoubtedly break a rib if the thorax is used as a fulcrum. However, some are skilled at applying forceful adduction over a closed padded fist in the axilla.

• *Stimson's method*, a gentle alternative, is to place the patient prone on a cot or table with the affected limb hanging towards the floor. Fix a 10-lb weight to the wrist with tape. Frequently, this gentle continuous traction will reduce the dislocation within 20 minutes. It works best with the patient not presenting highly developed muscula-ture.

Techniques for long-duration dislocation requiring anesthesia are orthopedic proce-dures rather than emergency sports-related techniques.

Intracoracoid or Subclavicular Dislocation Reduction Technique

Outward traction usually has no difficulty in reduction unless the subscapularis or torn capsule intervenes. If this is the case, sur-gery is the only recourse. *Angelvin's method* is to place the hand of the dislocated extrem-ity about your neck. With your hands, direct the head of the humerus in intracoracoid luxation by applying extension, counterex-tension, and lateral traction as need be. In subclavicular dislocation, the same forces applied more energetically force the head of the humerus into the socket.

Inferior Dislocation Reduction Techniques

In subglenoid dislocation, treatment is by moderate abduction with direct pressure. This is a most difficult type of dislocation to reduce without anesthesia, and usually re-quires an orthopedist. To reduce mild to moderate displacements, the patient is placed supine and the doctor sits perpendic-ular to the affected side. If possible, place the patient's flexed elbow in your axilla for stabilization. The head of humerus must be first pulled laterally towards you and then cephally in one smooth movement. Coun-terpressure is applied by the doctor's knee against a pillow placed in the patient's lower axilla. Any degree of luxatio erecta is re-duced by upward traction until the head of the humerus slips into place.

Posterior and Superior Dislocation Reduction Techniques

In uncomplicated cases of posterior luxa-tion, reduction can usually be accomplished by inferior and lateral traction and direct pressure forward. In variably, this must be conducted under anesthesia by an or-thopedic surgeon. Unreduced dislocations exhibit an unusual amount of disability. When viewed from the lateral, the posterior area may appear fuller than the unaffected side. An unusually prominent coracoid process may be felt, and a hollow may be felt above the humerus. Avulsion of the subscapularis makes recurrence probable. Superior dislocation may be reduced by di-rect inferior traction via the classic method.

Management of Shoulder Dislocations

Some feel that, if possible, reduction should be made within 10 minutes after injury when local numbness is present and severe spasm has not occurred. A firm gentle manipulation will usually result in reduction. If not, avoid persistent attempts and refer to an orthopedist. Other authori-ties feel that prior x-rays should always be taken before attempting reduction to avoid possible problems associated with a frac-ture. There is always a great danger of forc-ing a bone clip into the joint which would require surgery. Thus, a decision must be made to either offer immediate relief with some risk by making one good attempt or leaving the patient in severe pain until films can be taken, processed, and analyzed. The longer reduction is delayed, the greater the muscle spasm which makes reduction dif-ficult.

Following reduction, a sling should be used to rest the joint and a harness em-ployed to restrict shoulder abduction. Such a sling should have a controlling swath around the thorax to stabilize the joint such as that incorporated within a modified Vel-peau bandage. Local soreness will subside within a few days as the soft tissues heal. Cold can be applied initially to reduce pain and swelling, followed by the usual treat-ment for severe sprain. The typical athlete is overly anxious to have the sling removed. Professional opinion differs as to the length of immobilization. Some feel prolonged im-

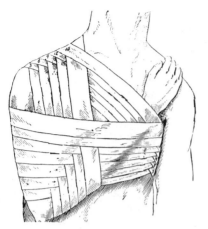

Figure 22.23. A modified Velpeau bandage. This sling-and-swathe bandage is frequently utilized for humeral head or acromioclavicular dislocations, fractures of the neck of the humerus or acromion, scapula fractures, and elbow fractures. The elbow of the affected arm is brought somewhat anterior and medial, with the fingertips resting upon the outer extremity of the opposite clavicle. Felt pads should be placed on pressure points. The turns are a combination of (1) slow spirals on the thorax and involved extremity, and (2) turns which represent combinations of the anterior and posterior triangles of the third bandage. Powder applied under the arm and in the axilla helps to avoid maceration between weekly changings of the bandage. In most all shoulder injuries, the straps should be applied with an upward pull. The exception to this is in acromioclavicular separation where tension is downward.

mobilization over 3 weeks produces more harm (atrophy) than good, while many others feel that at least 6 weeks are necessary to avoid recurring problems. Regardless, the shoulder should be allowed to heal solidly before progressive exercises are initiated. However, the fingers and wrist should be actively exercised early during immobilization.

The older patient is more prone to later stiffness problems than recurrence problems. Mild circumduction exercises may be initiated after about 4 days and progessive range-of-motion regimens after 2 weeks. Full external rotation and abduction should be avoided for 6 weeks in older patients, 9 weeks in younger patients. Isometric exercises of all involved muscle groups are always recommended while the shoulder is immobilized.

Recurring Dislocations

Several factors influence recurrent dislocation. The younger the patinet in glenoidrim fracture, the size of the capsular deformity (Hill-Sachs deformity), and the range of normal lateral motion all increase the chances for recurrent dislocation. If the humeral head is driven directly forward during injury, the cartilaginous labrum glenoidale is torn from its anterior attachment, which leaves a potential cavity into which the head can repeatedly slip. Another cause is too early mobilization following a primary dislocation. Incidence is highest in males 20–40 years of age. In the nonathlete, recurrences appear in over 90% of patients under the age of 20 after a primary dislocation. This rate drops to about 12% in patients over 40 years old. However, proper treatment can reduce this rate in any age group.

Recurring dislocations, almost always of the subcoracoid type, are a different problem from that of a primary dislocation. Posterior dislocations are usually not as painful and may be of the snapping variety. The dislocating force is usually mild and reduction is easy in comparison. Pain is severe and unrelieved until reduction is made. After reduction, symptoms disappear in 1–2 days whereupon progressive exercises can be initiated. Prolonged immobilization is ill-advised.

In some cases of a permanently loose joint surgical fixation may be the only solution—an orthopedic decision. Regardless, the decision should be based on what is in the athlete's long-term best interests and not what procedure will return him to competition the fastest. Sports which may subject the shoulder to constant severe stress must also be put into the prognosis puzzle.

The Lax Joint

Repeated subluxations without clinical dislocation often produce a loose joint. The history will reveal frequent episodes of mild trauma, each incorporating a period of pain and limited motion, followed by an audible "click" as the head of the humerus slips painfully back into the fossa. After reduction, examination reveals little except residual tenderness and a lax capsule.

Lax Capsule Test. To determine a lax capsule, have the patient clasp his fingers behind his head and laterally abduct his elbows. Palpate high in the axilla over the glenohumeral capsule while applying posterior force on the patient's flexed elbow. While laxity of the anterior capsule can always be demonstrated by this maneuver, care must be taken not to dislocate the humerus within its loose capsule. If episodes are frequent, some form of external support should be provided and the patient should be advised of the risks involved in repeated subluxation.

Fractures

Fractures of the proximal humerus are not common in athletics; they are most common clinically in mature women with a degree of osteoporosis.

Background. The mechanism is usually a fall on the outstretched pronated upper extremity. About 85% of these fractures are simple, usually involving the surgical neck and greater tuberosity of the humerus. A scapula fracture may be associated. In any case within athletics, early mobilization, without compromising long-term effects, is a necessity.

Roentgenographic Considerations. Fragments are usually displaced less than 1 centimeter, are angulated less than 45°, and are held in place by an intact rotator cuff and periosteum. Displacement of the greater tuberosity of more than 1 centimeter indicates a torn rotator cuff. Fractures through the surgical neck, frequently associated with brachial plexus injuries, are usually displaced anteriorly and medially due to the pull of the pectoralis major. Fractures through the head or anatomic neck of the humerus are rare, but they do have a high incidence of avascular necrosis.

As in the elbow joint, the epiphyseal lines

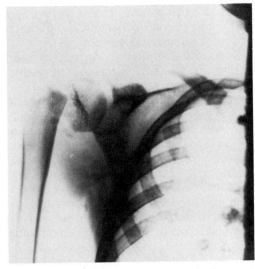

Figure 22.25. Positive x-ray print of a fracture-dislocation of the humeral epiphysis; right shoulder, male, age 12.

in the shoulder make interpretation difficult unless contralateral views are taken. Note that the epiphysis for the lateral end of the acromion process does not unite until about 20 years of age. In young baseball pitchers, the upper humeral epiphysis may be damaged from throwing overuse (Little League shoulder.

In the area of the subacromial or subdeltoid bursae, calcification may simulate a fracture of the greater tuberosity. A calcification shadow appears more dense and irregular than that of bone and is not trabeculated.

Tendinitis and Tenosynovitis

Tendon inflammation is not as common in the shoulder as it is in the elbow and wrist. However, because tendons are relatively avascular, they are subject to chronic trauma, microtears, slow repair, and aging degeneration in the shoulder. Overuse is the common cause, both within and outside of sports. The initial inflammatory reparative process is often associated with the deposition of calcium salts which may evade an overlying bursa. Abduction is quite painful against resistance in tendinitis.

Supraspinatus Tendinitis

Inflammation of paratendonous supraspinatus tissues is often a part of subdeltoid

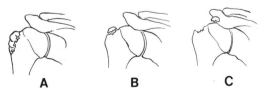

A   B   C

Figure 22.24. Three types of fracture of the greater tuberosity of the humerus: *a*, comminuted fracture due to direct blow on shoulder; *b*, avulsion fracture without displacement; *c*, avulsion fracture with upward displacement.

or subacromial bursitis. This is frequently a part of rotator cuff injury and a complication of severe supraspinatus strain.

Signs and Symptoms. An ache is present on rest which is aggravated by abduction. Pain may be referred as far distal as the deltoid insertion. The distinguishing feature is that pain is restricted to movement only within a certain point of the arc (painful arc syndrome). This is because the acromion proces affects the tendon area only during part of its excursion. Point tenderness will be found over the site of inflammation. The patient will complain that it is painful to sleep on the affected side. Treatment is similar to that of bicipital tendinitis.

Bicipital Tendinitis

The synovia of the bicipital groove is a common site of chronic peritendonous inflammation. It is frequently a complication of bicipital rupture (long head) or subluxation of the tendon from the groove.

Signs and Symptoms. Pain is aggravated on abduction and extension, and tenderness is localized over the inflamed tendon. Symptoms mimic supraspinatus tendinitis, but the pain is referred distally in the area of the biceps insertion to the radius. Tenderness is found along the anterior shoulder in the bicipital groove. Pain is increased if the patient abducts, flexes, and internally rotates the shoulder. When the patient flexes his arm and supinates his wrist against resistance, a positive sign is pain within the anterior medial upper humerus area.

Management. Check for lower cervical, 1st rib, and upper dorsal subluxations. A trigger point is frequently found over the scapula. Supraspinatus and infraspinatus muscle spasms are often associated. In the acute stage, cold rather than heat is indicated. Ultrasound combined with pulsating high-voltage galvanism is especially beneficial in degenerative tendinitis. Apply strapping for 3–5 days. An arm sling should be used for relieving the tendon of weight for 7–10 days from injury. Progressive exercises such as circumduction, lateral finger-wall walking, and front finger-wall walking may begin at home as soon as symptoms subside. Generally treat as a severe sprain.

Bursitis and Calcifications

The shoulder tendons are wide bands of collagen fibers. If stress roughens a tendon, its tensile strength decreases. This leads to fibrinoid degeneration in and between the collagen fibers and later fibrosis. With necrosis, the local tissues become alkaline which induces precipitation of calcium salts (see Fig. 22.26).

Subdeltoid Bursitis

Of the 140 bursae of the body, none receive the attention in sports as much as the subdeltoid bursa.

Background. Anterior, middle, or posterior deltoid strain can easily be associated with acute subdeltoid bursitis, but the clinical picture is quite different. Degenerative changes in the rotator cuff (floor of the subdeltoid bursa) lead to calcific deposits resulting in acute inflammation of the bursa. When a calcium deposit breaks into a bursa, it absorbs water which enlarges the bursal space, resulting in increased pressure. This causes severe pain and some warmth and redness of the overlying skin.

Signs and Symptoms. The patient presents acute, severe, deep-seated local pain and weakness with shoulder movement in any plane, but especially on abduction. The entire bursa and peritendinous tissues will be swollen and readily palpable. This welling prevents the greater tuberosity from sliding under the acromion during abduc-

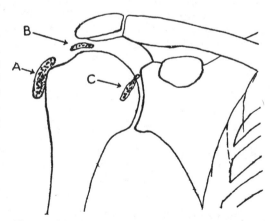

Figure 22.26. Location of the larger bursae about the shoulder which may be calcified: *A*, subdeltoid; *B*, subcrominal; *C*, coracobrachial.

tion. Dysfunction of the rotator, bicipital, and subscapularis tendons (which pass through the bursa) will be demonstrated. The initial attacks are localized in the vicinity of the greater tubercle. The chronic stage is characterized by subdeltoid tenderness, restricted motion in abduction and external rotation, and associated capsular contraction and adhesions. Keep in mind that bursitis is rarely a primary condition.

Management. A common pitfall is overtreatment of bursitis. When acute, treat with cold, pressure, and complete rest in an arm sling for 2–3 days. In severe cases where strapping is necessary, apply the direction of pull in the direction that affords the greatest relief to the bursa involved. When symptoms subside, a most gradual program of active exercise, traction, positive galvanism, and diathermy can usually begin in 4–7 days with careful monitoring. Most cases will respond well to ultrasound, swimming, vitamin C, E, manganese glycerophosphate, and acid calcium to diffuse the calcareous deposit. It is common to find an ipsilateral sacroiliac subluxation associated as well as C2, C3, and C5 subluxations. A good stretching and mobilization exercise is to have the patient flex the trunk and swing the arm anterior and posterior holding an iron or weight for three or four bouts daily. Reduce activity on the first signs of recurring local symptoms. Referral for aspiration and steroids may be necessary in stubborn cases, but the results of immediate injections in acute athletic injuries are not as good as that of more conservative care.

Rotator Cuff Calcifications

An example of calcification in tendons is commonly found in the supraspinatus tendon near its insertion to the greater tuberosity of the humerus. In the well-developed athlete, symptoms from calcification may not appear for many months after injury. Deposits may appear in shoulder tendons, ligaments, or aponeuroses, and especially within the rotator cuff. They may be chronic, silent, or extremely acute. Spontaneous absorption may occur relatively fast.

Background. A hypovascular area has been identified in the area of the supraspinatus tendon. This is referred to as the "critical zone," and it occurs between the anastomosis of the vascular supply from the humeral tuberosity and the longitudinally directed vessels arriving from the muscle's belly. Tullos and Bennett report that this relatively avascular area of the supraspinous corresponds to the most common site of rotator cuff tendinitis, calcification, and spontaneous rupture.

Two other "critical zones" of hypovascular phenomena are found at the insertion of the infraspinatus tendon and at the intracapsular aspect of the biceps tendon. These areas of avascularity seem to expand with age, enhancing the potential for tendon rupture. Other factors can be added to this. For example, prolonged abduction such as seen in the common side-lying sleeping posture also produces compression or impingement under the acromion process or coracoacromial ligament. In the early stages, this leads to an inflammatory response and scar tissue development. Later, reports Brewer, the avascularity leads to a breakdown of the tendon and encourages rotator cuff rupture in the middle-aged athlete.

Signs and Symptoms. Symptoms appear suddenly. Pain is usually severe and aggravated by shoulder movement, but the pain is less severe and movements more tolerated than in supraspinatus tendinitis. Tenderness is localized over the bursa. A painful arc syndrome may be noted, similar to that seen in supraspinatus tendinitis. It is viewed in roentgenography as a large dense opacity above the outer head of the humerus and most frequently related to middle age with no definite history of trauma. It is occasionally seen in the young athlete. Associated bursitis may be present, which is responsible for acute symptoms.

Adjunctive Management. Therapy often includes iontophoresis of .25 g methacholine in 100 cc of water. Ionization is also frequently helpful with a cloth soaked with magnesium sulphate (4 oz/qt of water) over the deposit. The negative pad is on the cloth over the deposit; the positive pad is placed on the arm. Once pain subsides, ultrasound should follow for a few visits.

Subacromial Bursitis

A painful, faltering abduction arc is also

characteristic of subacromial bursitis. To differentiate, palpate the coracoid process under the pectoralis major. It is easily found by circumducting the humerus and is normally tender. Once the process is isolated, slide your finger slightly lateral and superior until it reaches a portion of the subacromial bursa. If the same palpation pressure here causes greater tenderness than at the process, it is a positive sign of subacromial bursitis. Still holding pressure, abduct the patient's arm above the horizontal. An inflamed bursa is exposed to palpation when the arm is relaxed but not when the arm is abducted beyond a right angle (Dawbarn's test).

Subacromial Button Sign. The examiner stands behind the seated patient, cups a palm over the involved shoulder, and applies finger pressure over the subacromial bursa. If this produces pain or unusual tenderness, subacromial bursitis is suggested.

Dawbarn's Test. With the patient seated, the examiner stands behind the patient and deeply palpates the area just below the acromion process to determine symptoms of focal tenderness or referred pain. Then, while still maintaining this palpatory pressure to patient tolerance, the examiner grasps the wrist of the patient with the other hand and brings the arm to the lateral extended position so that it is abducted to about 100°. If subacromial bursitis exists, the pain elicited on initial palpation should decrease substantially when the arm is raised because the deltoid will cover the spot below the acromion during abduction. If the pain remains unaltered or is increased by this abduction maneuver, subacromial bursitis can usually be ruled out.

Triceps Brachii Calcification

Repetitive stretching of the posterior elements of the shoulder in baseball pitchers frequently causes an inflammation of the posterior capsule tissues of the shoulder. This may result in an osteotendinous calcification at the infraglenoid area where the long head of the triceps originates. Once calcification forms, the pitching follow-through is most painful to accomplish. Adjunctive management is similar to that of supraspinatus calcification.

Other Painful Shoulder Syndromes

Excessive postinjury immobilization leads to muscle atrophy and loss of capsular elasticity, a predisposing factor to capsulitis and periarthritis. Lack of joint movement fosters retention of metabolites, edema, venous stasis, and ischemia leading to fibrous adhesions and trigger-point development.

Capsulitis

Shoulder capsulitis is often the result of a sprain attended by a spontaneously reduced subluxation or of prolonged overuse. Joint pain is aggravated by movement. Tenderness and other symptoms are generalized within the whole joint area rather than being localized. Motion limitation may be considerable in adhesive capsulitis (frozen shoulder) where the head of the humerus is "glued" to the glenoid cavity.

Frozen Shoulder (Periarthritis)

Frozen shoulder (Duplay's syndrome) is often a challenge because it is usually near the terminal stage when the patient is first seen. Usually a combination of several chronic, diffuse, degenerative shoulder disorders are involved. Roentgenography is often negative with the exception of an obliterated joint space. Loss of scapulohumeral rhythm is a characteristic feature. This is readily noted when viewed from the posterior. During the early stage, shoulder motion stiffens at the extreme ranges of abduction and internal rotation. Differentiation must be made from the early stage of capsulitis.

Signs and Symptoms. Humeral motion restriction is exhibited in all planes, but adduction and rotation are especially affected. Scapulothoracic motion will be normal. Atrophy is readily noted and proportionate to the chronicity of the condition. Tenderness is diffuse throughout the upper arm with the possible exception of the posterior and medial aspects. The capsule becomes thick and contracted, which contributes to motion limitation. The rotator cuff also becomes thick and inelastic. The tendon becomes cemented within the groove. In time, all adhesions and soft tissues thicken and become tightly fixed, binding capsule to bone. As the joint cavity "dries," the head of the humerus is pulled tightly against the glenoid fossa. Arm use aggravates the condition, thus symptoms are more acute at night after a day's activity. Rest offers relief, thus improvement is seen in the morning. The accessory muscles overwork in an attempt to compensate for primary shoulder muscle deficiency, causing aching posterior shoulder and neck muscles. A superiorly subluxated 1st rib is a common contributing factor.

Management. Unless the instigating factor is removed, a meaningless course of treatments results with progressing deterioration. Rugged "shotgun" manipulation under anesthesia as practiced by some overly enthusiastic surgeons is strongly contraindicated. Specific conservative adjustments, progressive passive manipulation with and without traction and countertraction, graduated pendulum stretching exercises, circumduction manipulations against patient resistance, sinewave stimulation to the shoulder muscles, ultrasound, and heat will provide a high percentage of relief even in severe cases. In most cases, adhesions must be released of the humerus, clavicle, and scapula in several planes if movement is restricted. As in any case of capsulitis, early care and prevention is the best therapy.

Traumatic Arthritis

True osteoarthritis of the shoulder is seen more in literature than in actual practice. Usually, it is a periarthritis where degenerative changes occur within the soft tissues. Differentiation must be made from supraspinatus rupture, subdeltoid bursitis, and inflammation of other bursae about the shoulder.

Signs and Symptoms. Characteristic symptoms are pain, tenderness on pressure, and swelling (rarely). Passive motion is comparatively painless, but active motion induces severe pain.

Management. When effusion and swelling persist, cold and immobilization are advised. The lower cervical area and shoulder girdle should be checked for chronic subluxations and trigger points. In mild cases, heat, ultrasound, and massage may be sufficient adjuncts.

NERVE INJURIES

Contusion of the axillary nerve or brachial plexus is often seen in sports. Occasionally, scapular "winging" is found. If nerve damage is suspected, a thorough neurologic assessment should be conducted.

Contusion of the Axillary Nerve

Contusions of the axillary (circumflex) nerve commonly result from blows suffered along the nerve's course between the coracoid and head of the humerus. It is not an infrequent complication of the common anterior dislocation of the shoulder (10%).

Signs and Symptoms. The major sign in severe cases is loss of abduction from inadequate deltoid function. An area of anesthesia about the size of a silver dollar will be exhibited on the lateral aspect of the arm at the distal insertion of the deltoid: an important sign. In minor contusions, numbness and tingling may occur over the sensory area of the axillary nerve in the upper deltoid area only during strenuous activity. Weakness may be difficult to determine, but swelling and tenderness can usually be found high and deep within the posterior axilla.

Management. Treat as any nerve contusion. Ice massage is helpful initially. Rest the deltoid by using an arm sling. Measures to reduce spasm and intrinsic muscle swelling will relieve tenderness and paresthesias. Initiate progressive exercises when local symptoms subside. Electrical stimulation is helpful in strengthening the muscle. In severe contusions, fibrous tissue and neuroma usually form which require surgical care.

Brachial Plexus Injury

The branches of the brachial plexus of the shoulder lie just anterior to the glenohumeral joint. The axillary nerve is just below the joint. In brachial plexus trauma, the entire plexus or any of its fibers may be injured. These injuries may be divided into three general types: total-arm palsies, upper-arm palsies (most common), and lower-arm palsies. Motor involvement is the main feature, sensory loss being oscured by overlapping innervation.

Background. Stretching requires special

mention. As the roots of the plexus are relatively fixed at their origin in the spinal cord, any sudden or severe traction of the upper extremity may avulse roots from the cord or stretch the plexus to the point of tearing. During avulsion, the spinal cord itself is damaged and contralateral cord symptoms are found. If the lesion is due to stretching, contusion, or partial tearing, the prognosis is good and complete recovery may usually be anticipated.

Management. Treatment measures include support in the functional position, initial cold followed by massage, electric stimulation, progressive exercises, and acupuncture. Suture is required in complete tears, and some improvement can be hoped for. The prognosis is usually hopeless in avulsion from the cord. Fortunately, most injuries are a neurapraxia, and full recovery can be anticipated in time.

Scapular "Winging"

Injury to the long thoracic nerve of Bell (C5-7) can result in paralysis of the serratus anterior muscle. This is a purely motor nerve without sensory fibers. Its winding course under the brachial plexus varies considerably from person to person making localization difficult.

Signs and Symptoms. Rarely seen outside of athletics, this disorder features vague pains referred to the shoulder, a degree of abduction weakness, and visible scapula rotation when the arm is abducted laterally against resistance. Early diagnosis is important, yet there is rarely a complaint until marked atrophy has occurred. Seek the slightest sign of winging while the hands "wall walk" or while doing demanding pushups. Winging in the well-developed

athlete is often disguised by heavy trapezius, latissimus, and rhomboid muscles.

Scapular winging is often associated in postural faults, which refer pain to the shoulder but not the joint itself, as a result of imbalanced function of the suspensory muscles of the shoulder girdle. A functional dorsal kyposis may be found with alterations in scapulohumeral rhythm. A primary subluxation, which may have been present since childhood, may be found near the cervicothoracic transition or the apex of the thoracic curve. Secondary (sometimes primary) costovertebral fixations may also be found.

Management. Treat as a peripheral nerve contusion. Discontinue strenuous work until symptoms subside. This is an absolute which will probably meet patient resistance. Check for lower cervical subluxations and scapula fixations and trigger points. Faradic stimulation of the nerve 3–5 times a week during the early stage of rehabilitation is necessary to prevent atrophy while regeneration is in progress. Later, progressive exercises can be initiated, eg, shoulder shrugging against resistance, overhead weights and springs, and pushups.

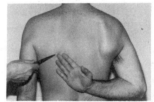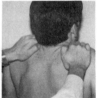

Figure 22.27. *Left,* evaluating internal rotation and adduction of the shoulder. *Right,* testing the spinal accessory nerve. The patient shrugs the shoulders against the examiner's resistance.

CHAPTER 23

Elbow, Wrist, and Hand Injuries

This chapter discusses traumatic-related disorders of the elbow, forearm, wrist, hand, and fingers. As in all traumatic injuries, the sooner the patient is examined after injury, the more accurate the diagnosis. Swelling, spasm, tenderness, and motion limitations rapidly cloud the picture.

INJURIES OF THE DISTAL ARM AND ELBOW

The highest incidence of elbow injury is in tennis, golf, Little League baseball, and occasionally in javelin throwing. Most forearm injuries are the result of direct blows or falls. Commonly seen are avulsion-type injuries of the elbow as a result of acute or chronic strain at a site of tendon or ligament attachment.

Physical Approach

Parkes divides common sports injuries involving the elbow into three categories according to their prevalence: (1) musculotendinous, (2) articular, and (3) neurovascular. Most injuries are the result of either a sudden unguarded or repetitive overload on the joint mechanism. This is especially true if the joint is weak or inflexible. An outline of common sports injuries about the elbow is shown in Table 23.1.

A review of pertinent neurologic, orthopedic, and peripheral vascular maneuvers, reflexes, and tests relative to the elbow and forearm is shown in Table 23.2.

Roentgenologic Considerations

As a consequence of avulsion injury, bone fragments may be seen in the area of the epicondyles or olecranon process, and epicondyle spurs may point to chronic stress. Standard projections are A-P, lateral, and oblique views. An intra-articular bone fragment may sometimes be only elicited by tomography, and comparative views of the sound limb are frequently necessary.

Soft Tissues. Displacement of fat pads is often found at the elbow after injury. It can occur in any injury that distends the joint capsule. A pad appears as a thin strip of radiolucent fat density. The anterior fat pad is normally seen on lateral views, but the posterior humeral pad is hidden by the epicondyles' posterior extensions. However, the posterior pad will become visible at the posterior edge of the humerus on lateral views if effusion causes displacement of the pad. The most important complication is ischemia of the forearm, which may cause an irreversible contracture deformity.

Growth Centers. Normal ossification of distal humeral epiphyses is not an even process, especially during the periods of rapid growth and development; thus knowledge of secondary ossification centers of the elbow is necessary in dealing with children or teenagers. One or more bony centers may remain uneven in density and irregular on the margins, especially the trochlea and olecranon epiphyses. Because of this irregularity, careful differentiation must be made between osteochondrosis and epiphysitis. The trochlear center is irregularly mineralized and always develops from several small foci. The lateral epicondyle does not fuse directly with the humerus as the medial epicondyle does; rather, it fuses first with the neighboring epiphyseal ossification center, the capitellum; then the fused mass joins the end of the shaft of the humerus. After injury, the position of various centers must be evaluated for possible displacement, laceration, and incarceration into the joint.

Pitching Injuries. Avulsion and displacement of the medial epicondyle may complicate supracondylar fracture, or they may occur in association with soft-tissue trauma alone. Biceps spasm after 5 minutes of pitching strongly suggests an avulsion. Finger numbness following pitching suggests a scalenus anticus syndrome from a cervical or 1st rib condition. Avulsion and displacement of the epicondyle are common

Table 23.1.
Common Sports-Related Elbow Injuries

Syndrome	Typical Clinical Picture
MUSCULOTENDINOUS INJURIES	
Lateral Aspect Extensor carpi radialis brevis strain, tendinitis Lateral epicondylitis Lateral epicondyle spur or adjacent calcium deposition Posteromedial radial head subluxation Lateral olecranon subluxation	Pain on gripping, point tenderness at the attachment of the common extensor tendon. Pain is aggravated by resisted hyperextension of the wrist or passive wrist flexion with the elbow extended. Some swelling is usually present.
Anterior Aspect Biceps-brachialis strain, tendinitis, rupture Anterior olecranon subluxation Superior ulna subluxation Avulsion at radial tuberosity	Anterior elbow pain aggravated by use, point tenderness over the insertion of the biceps tendon. Pain is increased by resisted elbow flexion, forearm supination, and passive elbow extension. Antecubital swelling is usually present.
Medial Aspect Strain, tendinitis, or rupture of wrist flexors and forearm pronators Medial epicondylitis, with or without avulsion Medial olecranon subluxation	Pain on throwing, forearm tennis shot, or gripping. Point tenderness at attachment of common tendon to medial epicondyle. Pain is aggravated by resisted wrist flexion or passive wrist extension when the elbow is extended.
Posterior Aspect Triceps strain, tendinitis Olecranon avulsion (uncommon) Bursitis Posterior olecranon subluxation	Pain on repetitive extension (eg, throwing, tennis, weight lifting, gymnastics). Point tenderness at or just above the insertion of the triceps on the olecranon process. Pain is aggravated by resisted extension or passive flexion of the elbow.
ARTICULAR INJURIES	
Lateral Compartment Traumatic damage to radial head, capitellum, or both Osteochondral fractures Compression osteochondritis of capitellum (youth) Osteochondritis of radial head Superior ulnar subluxation Loose body formation	Lateral elbow pain on throwing, gymnastics, racquet sports, sometimes associated with joint clicking, catching, grinding. Tenderness and swelling over radiocapitellar joint. Grating on forced forearm supination and pronation (often), and reduced range of elbow extension.
Medial Compartment Capsular tear Calcium deposition Coronoid process spur Ulnar nerve entrapment	Medial elbow pain and swelling aggravated by valgus stress (eg, throwing, weight lifting), point tenderness below medial epicondyle near humeral-ulnar joint, and possible sensitive ulnar nerve. Pain is aggravated by passive wrist extension or active flexion.
Posterior Compartment Olecranon tip spur Olecranon hypertrophy Loose body formation Olecranon fatigue fracture Posterior olecranon subluxation	Posterior pain on elbow extension, often with a catching or locking sensation; point tenderness in the olecranon fossa; reduced range of extension.

Table 23.1—*Continued*

Syndrome	Typical Clinical Picture
NEUROVASCULAR INJURIES	
Ulnar Nerve Entrapment Cubital tunnel syndrome	Paresthesiae and weakened motor power in 4th and 5th fingers, point tenderness in cubital tunnel.
Pronator Teres Syndrome Median nerve entrapment	Anterior elbow pain, usually radiating into thumb, index finger, and middle finger. Forearm cramps (sometimes), and tenderness over pronator teres. Pain is aggravated by resisted forearm pronation and passive supination. Possible thumb abduction weakness and sensory loss in the 1st, 2nd, and 3rd digits.
Musculocutaneous Nerve Entrapment	Weak elbow flexion, absent biceps reflex, biceps and brachialis atrophy, and numbness/tingling and numbness along the radial-volar aspect of the forearm.
Radial Nerve Entrapment (Uncommon)	Elbow pain along the lateral extensor muscle group. Tenderness along the radial nerve anteriorly about the radial head, but not over the lateral epicondyle as in tennis elbow. Pain is aggravated by passive forearm supination and pronation and forced extension of the wrist and 3rd finger. Weakness and stiffness of the extensor-supinator muscles are usually exhibited.
Brachial Artery Impingement Supracondylar fracture Posterior or posterolateral dislocation	Signs of vascular insufficiency; eg, progressively increasing pain, pain on passive extension of the fingers, median nerve paresthesia.

between 7 and 17 years of age and vary from slight epicondylar separation to complete avulsion and displacement into the elbow joint.

It has been estimated that two of every three professional baseball pitchers have an elbow abnormality. Arm and forearm hypertrophy is typical. Hypertrophy of the humerus is invariably demonstrated in roentgenography, and traction spurs and loose bodies of bone within the elbow joint are frequent. Most loose bodies are found in the olecranon fossa, near the epicondyle, and near the tip of the coronoid process—where ulnar nerve irritation is likely. In 50% of professional pitchers, flexion contracture of the elbow is present. In addition to pitching, outfield throwing and batting mishaps account for similar injuries.

Contusions and Strains

Traumatic Inflammation of the Elbow. There may be an injury to the upper radioulnar articulation by sudden overpro-

nation or oversupination followed by pain over the articulation with limitation of rotation. Trigger points are commonly found just below the horizontal midline of the antecubital fossa over the proximal radius and ulna. When the joint proper is involved, motion is limited chiefly in extension and may persist indefinitely. An associated injury to the brachialis anticus muscle with contracture is common. In children, a strip of periosteum may be torn from the anterior humerus, followed by bone formation and blocked joint motion. Local myositis ossificans may also develop in the tendon of the brachialis anticus. Some cases will be complicated by ulnar neuropraxia.

Management. During the early stage, rest in a sling for 3–4 days is required for the acute symptoms to subside. Thereafter, physical therapy with passive and progressive active exercises are recommended. Diathermy is especially helpful in absorption of joint effusion. Rarely is joint aspiration necessary.

Table 23.2.
Review of Neurologic, Orthopedic, and Peripheral Vascular Maneuvers, Reflexes, Signs, or Tests Relative to the Elbow and Forearm

Biernacki's sign
Bikele's test
Brachioradialis reflex
Cogwheel sign
Cozen's test
Elbow abduction stress test
Elbow adduction stress test
Elbow extension stress test
Elbow flexion stress test
Elbow pronation stress test
Elbow supination stress test
Erb's sign
Light touch/pain tests
Medial epicondyle test
Mill's test
Muscle strength grading
Periosteoradial reflex
Periosteoulnar reflex
Kaplan's test
Radial reflex
Range of motion tests
Strumpell's pronation sign
Tinel's elbow test
Tinel's sign
Triceps reflex
Ulnar reflex

Distal Bicipital Strain. Strains of the bicipital attachment to the ulna are not common. They occur in elbow hyperextension injuries and in overenthusiastic weight-lifting efforts. The course of the tendon will be tender on palpation. Management consists of rest in a sling for a few days along with standard sprain therapy.

Elbow Sprains

Intra-articular or extra-articular injuries to the elbow without fracture are not uncommon and are peculiarly resistant to treatment. There may be a primary or secondary injury to the upper radioulnar articulation by sudden overpronation or oversupination, followed by pain over the articulation and limited rotation. Overlooking radial-head dislocation is a common orthopedic pitfall.

Differentiation

Forced joint movement beyond full extension, abduction, or adduction causes rup-

tures within the capsular apparatus and its contained reinforcing ligaments from their attachment to the humerus, radius, and ulna. The capsule is tender and frequently distended with blood. Movement in the direction of injury aggravates the pain, and there is some restriction at extreme ranges.

1. Hyperextension Sprain. Hyperextension sprains strongly mimic posterior dislocation of the elbow. Swelling and tenderness will be found at the joint capsule posteriorly, bicipital tendon, olecranon fossa, lateral and medial collateral ligaments, and attachments of the flexors and extensors at the medial condyle. Pain is relieved by flexion and increased on attempted extension. If the joint proper is involved, extension is chiefly limited, and it may persist for weeks or years.

2. Hyperabduction Sprain. Tenderness is found below the lateral epicondyle, indicating sprain of the ulnar collateral ligament. Pain is increased by forcing the elbow into valgus stress.

3. Hyperadduction Sprain. Tenderness is exhibited below the medial epicondyle, indicating sprain of the radial collateral lig-

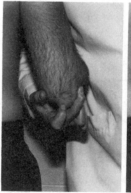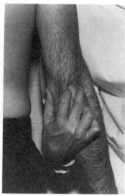

Figure 23.1. Check general bony relationships of the elbow by placing your thumb on the lateral epicondyle, index finger on the olecranon, and middle finger on the medial epicondyle. When the patient's elbow is fully extended, the tips of all three fingers should be level. During 90° flexion, the tips of the three fingers form an inverted triangle. This will offer a general appraisal of alignment. *Left,* the olecranon and the medial and lateral epicondyles form a triangle when the elbow is flexed at a right angle. *Right,* when the elbow is extended, the points at the olecranon and epicondyles lie in a straight line.

ament. Pain is increased by forcing the elbow into varus stress.

Elbow Stability Tests. To judge stability of medial and lateral collateral ligaments of the elbow, hold the patient's wrist with one hand and cup your stabilizing hand under the patient's distal humerus. As the patient is directed to slightly flex his elbow, (1) push medially with your active hand and laterally with your stabilizing hand, then (2) push laterally with your active hand and medially with your stabilizing hand. With your stabilizing hand, note any joint gapping during either the valgus or varus stress maneuver (Fig. 23.2).

Other Elbow Stress Tests. Besides elbow abduction and adduction, stability and range of motion should also be tested in extension, flexion, pronation, and supination. These motions should be carefully attempted when the elbow joint is as relaxed as possible. Pain or motion restriction will be found if contractures, acute tendinitis, and/or acute joint pathology are present. If negative, the tests should be repeated against patient resistance. Pain or instability will then be found if sprain, acute or chronic tendinitis, and/or chronic joint pathology are present.

Management

During the acute hyperemic stage, structural alignment, cold, firm compression, rest in a sling, positive galvanism, ultrasound, vitamin C, manganese glycerophosphate, rest and possibly elevation are indicated. Swelling and joint limitation usually subside in 2–4 days. After 48 hours, passive congestion may be managed by contrast baths, light massage, gentle passive manipulation, sinusoidal stimulation, ultrasound, and a mild range of motion exercise can be initiated. Great care must be taken throughout management that treatment (eg, vigorous manipulation) does not induce further reaction. Injuries of the proximal radial articulation and annular ligament, key components in pronation and supination, are often frustrating to manage.

During the stage of consolidation, local moderate heat, moderate active exercise, moderate range of motion manipulation, and ultrasound are beneficial. In the stage of fibroblastic activity, deep heat, deep massage, vigorous active exercise with and without weights, negative galvanism, ultrasound, and active joint manipulation speed recovery and inhibit postinjury effects. An elbow "cinch-strap" is a helpful but annoying support during competitive activity to prevent overextension. When myositis ossificans becomes a complication, surgical removal of the bony mass may be required.

Tennis Elbow

"Tennis elbow" is a painful condition of traumatic origins which occurs about the external epicondyle of the humerus. The term incorporates a group of conditions, especially epicondylitis or radiohumeral bursitis. It is caused by repeated violent elbow extension combined with sharp twisting supination or pronation of the wrist against resistance. The result is severe contraction of the extensor-supinator muscles of the forearm. The clinical picture is one of synovitis, subperiosteal hematoma, fibrositis, or partial rupture of the fibrous origin of muscles and ligaments at the affected epicondyle, with some associated periostitis. Radial nerve entrapment may be involved. If the medial epicondyle is sore, the flexor-pronator muscles and medial ligaments are affected. The lateral epicondyle area is affected seven times more often than the medial epicondyle.

Bowerman reports that strain of the lateral epicondylar area is actually more common in golf than in tennis. In fact, the disorder commonly referred to as "tennis elbow" is a misnomer in that it has a higher

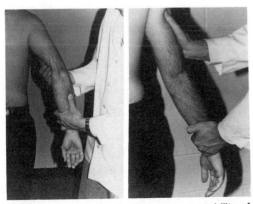

Figure 23.2. Testing for ligamentous stability of the elbow joint.

incidence in golf, badminton, squash, rowing, manual labor, and even violin playing than tennis. It is not uncommon in bowlers and professional chess players.

Roentgenographic Considerations. X-ray features in the elbow may include soft-tissue calcification at the margin of the lateral joint, lateral epicondyle and capitellum erosion and fragmentation, and spur development at the coronoid process of the ulna. A medial slope deformity of the lateral condyle of the humerus is frequently related. Strenuous unilateral use of the active upper extremity (eg, tennis) often leads to hypertrophy of muscle and bone in the forearm and hands as compared to the nondominant side in young players. Increased radial length and width is frequently found.

Typical Signs. Hasemeir describes the typical symptomatic picture as pain over the outer or inner side of the elbow, distal to the affected epicondyle. Pain may be severe and radiate when the patient extends his arm. The pain is usually sharp and lancinating on exertion, but it may be dull, aching, and constant. Squeezing an object with the fingertips is usually painful (writer's cramp). Tenderness, heat, and swelling are found over the affected epicondyle, and limited passive movement on extension may be found. This is the result of microscopic and macroscopic tears at the common origin of the extensor and flexor muscle groups—occurring as a consequence to overstress of tendon fibers. The supinator has its tendinous origin just behind the common extensor tendon. Grip strength as well as supination and pronation strength are affected.

Cozen's Test. With the patient's forearm stabilized, instruct him to make a fist and extend his wrist. Grip the elbow with your stabilizing hand and grip the top of the patient's fist with your active hand and attempt to force the wrist into flexion against resistance. A sign of tennis elbow is a severe sudden pain at the lateral epicondyle area (Fig. 23.3).

Mill's Test. The patient is instructed to make a fist, flex forearm, fully flex fingers and wrist, pronate forearm, and then attempt to extend forearm against resistance. This stretches the extensor and supinator muscles attaching to the lateral epicondyle.

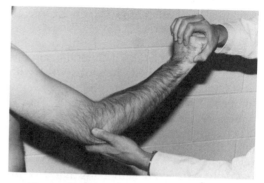

Figure 23.3. Cozen's tennis elbow test.

Pain at the elbow during this maneuver is an indication of radiohumeral epicondylitis.

Kaplan's Test. This is a two-phase test. (1) The seated patient is given a hand dynamometer and instructed to extend the involved upper limb straight forward and squeeze the instrument as hard as possible. Induced pain and grip strength are noted. (2) The test is then repeated as before except that this time the examiner firmly encircles the patient's forearm with both hands (placed about 1–2 inches below the antecubital crease). Induced pain and grip strength are noted. If the second phase of the test shows increased reduced pain and increased grip strength when the muscles of the proximal forearm are compressed, lateral epicondylitis is indicated.

Management. For adjustment procedure, see posteromedial subluxation of the radial head. Seek signs of possibly associated cervical, upper dorsal, and 1st rib subluxations. Rest with sling, cold packs, immobilization of wrist and elbow, diathermy, and ultrasound are the common adjunctives utilized. Treatment is similar to that of sprain. Underwater ultrasound is recommended by many. Return to activity immediately upon fading of symptoms invites recurrence. Squeezing a rubber ball helps in recuperation. Graduated restoration to painless function under competitive conditions is vital before full activity is resumed. Strengthening of the wrist extensors is important.

Vapocoolant Technique in Grade I and II Strains and Sprains. Place the patient in the sitting position with the elbow slightly flexed and abducted. Isolate trigger areas and site of major pain in the arm, elbow, and forearm, and spray sites. At the same time, ask the patient to extend his elbow and then slowly return it to the relaxed position. Repeat the spraying and active movement three or four times. Have the patient indicate with his finger the major source of pain. As the pain shifts position, spray the affected area. Once relief has been obtained in flexion-extension, add forearm pronation and supination in extension, spraying painful sites as necessary between movements. Have the patient attempt movements against resistance, and spray the painful area if necessary. Once relief is obtained, correct any subluxations isolated, apply an ace bandage or "tennis elbow" support, and instruct the patient in home exercises: 1–2 minutes each half hour during waking hours. Begin resistance and stretching exercises as soon as logical.

Variations

Golfer's Elbow. A severe opposite strain at the origin of the flexor pronator muscles at the medial epicondyle and strain of the medial ligament is sometimes called "golfer's elbow." Subperiosteal hematoma and periostitis are often involved. Poor warmup is usually the underlying cause in golf (or bowling), but taking a divot too deep during chipping is the initiating factor. Treatment is the same as that for tennis elbow, but the adjustment is reversed. That is, the wrist and fingers are extended and the forearm supinated while the elbow is fully extended.

Medial Epicondyle Test. On the side of involvement, the patient is instructed to flex the elbow about 90° and supinate the hand. If severe pain arises over the medial epicondyle when the patient in this position attempts to extend the elbow against resistance, medial epicondylitis (golfer's elbow) is suggested.

Baseball Elbow. This is the same condition in chronic form seen with baseball pitchers caused by elbow extension and snapping pronation or supination as the pitcher throws a "slider" or "breaking curve." Degenerative changes are more common on the medial epicondyle, thus indicating pronator strain. It can be considered an elbow "whiplash" injury where the olecranon im-

pinges the fossa at the distal humerus. Stress fracture or traumatic epiphysitis is often associated in adolescents. Loose bodies from cartilage flaking, trochlea osteophytes, medial ligament ossicles, and olecranon chips are frequently related.

Javelin Elbow. When the javelin is thrown, the olecranon pivots medially in the trochlea and its tip is forced against the edge of the fossa during the extreme forearm pronation and elbow extension. This may result in repeated sprain from amateur "round house" throws, complicated by fracture fragments, calcification, and spur development along the course of the medial collateral ligament of the elbow. Transient ulnar nerve paralysis and "Little League" symptoms are early indications. In some cases, a "golfer's elbow" syndrome is seen from flexor-origin strain.

Olecranon Bursitis

Mobility of the upper extremity is provided by this a fluid-filled bursa which is exposed when the elbow is fixed on a firm surface. It is subject to direct impact hemorrhage, abrasion, contusion, laceration, and puncture, as well as to common indirect mechanisms, all of which may cause chronic inflammation, thickening of synovium, and formation of excessive fluid. The mecha-

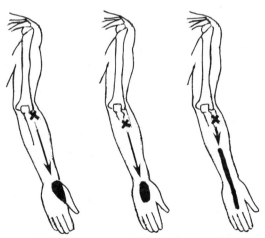

Figure 23.4. Posterior-aspect upper extremity trigger points; *X*, common sites. *Blackened areas* indicate typical areas of referred pain. *Left* diagram, supinators; *middle*, extensor carpi radialis; *right*, middle finger extensor.

nism of injury is usually one of repetitive direct injury, constant friction of extensor tendons as in tennis elbow, and/or repetitious local injuries with synovial irritation. Local pain, tenderness, swelling, and movement restrictions are exhibited. Incidence is high in basketball and indoor racket sports from falls on a hard floor. Secondary infection readily converts the inflammation into an abscess.

Management. Treat with cold, compression, and elevation for 1–2 days. Refer for aspiration if necessary, but crisscross taping in elbow extension usually brings quick relief. In mild-moderate cases, an elastic ankle support can be worn with the "heel" opening placed on the antecubital fossa. Recurrent swelling is common, and protective elbow padding is necessary long after symptoms subside.

Subluxations

Most subluxations in the elbow area will offer dramatic relief upon correction. Generally, correction is made with a quick, short thrust to minimize the pain (and time) of relocation. It is essential that the patient's muscles be relaxed or correction will be inhibited and extremely painful. Naturally, quick thrusts are contraindicated in arthritic and sclerotic conditions or if adhesions are advanced.

Posterior-Medial Radial Head Subluxation

This "pulled elbow" injury results from the radial head being jerked from the annular ligament, presenting symptoms of pain and tenderness in the area of the radial head. It was once called "Nursemaid's elbow," frequently found after young children were quickly lifted up by their extended forearm. Motion is severely limited in pronation and supination, but flexion and extension are normal. The arm is held in a pronated position and pain is fairly localized at the elbow. X-ray films are negative. Incidence is high in judo, especially with the young. This type subluxation is commonly associated with tennis elbow or wrist trauma, lateral elbow pain, and restricted anterior-lateral radial-head motion.

Adjustment. When manipulation is indicated, the physician holds the affected elbow with one hand in such a manner that his thumb rests on the back of the head of the radius. With the other hand, the doctor holds the patient's hand and moves the arm into a position of slight flexion of the elbow, full forearm pronation, and full flexion of the wrist. This manipulation (Mills' movement) consists in *fully* extending the elbow while maintaining pronation and flexion of the wrist. The movement is made gently, but quite sharply; thus, it is essential that the patient's muscles be relaxed. The manipulation causes no pain to a normal elbow, but there is sharp pain when a tennis elbow is "freed" that is quickly followed by relief. Evaluate the integrity of the pronator quadratus, biceps brachii, brachioradialis, wrist extensors, and supinator. Treat as a severe sprain, and offer rest in a flexion sling for several days (see Fig. 23.5).

Alternative Adjustment Procedure. To re-establish the slipped radial head, grasp the hand of the seated patient and extend the wrist. Support the elbow firmly with your contact hand. Flex the elbow to a right angle. Maintain axial compression along the radius, and firmly alternate forearm supination and pronation in a "screwing" manner until the head of the radius slips back into position. A click can usually be felt and heard on replacement.

Medial Olecranon Subluxation

Subluxation of the olecranon medially is often seen in association with ulna nerve paresthesias, wrist or elbow trauma, medial

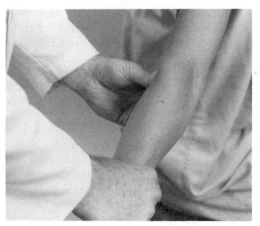

Figure 23.5. Position for adjusting radial head subluxated posterior-medial.

elbow pain, triceps dyskinesia, decreased distance between olecranon and medial epicondyle, and restricted lateral olecranon joint motion.

Adjustment. Face cephally on the affected side of the supine patient. The patient's arm is moderately abducted, and the elbow is extended. Your medial semi-extended contact hand is cupped on the medial aspect of the olecranon, while your stabilizing hand grasps the back of the patient's forearm. The elbow is brought into full extension, and a short thrust is made from the medial to the lateral with the contact hand while the stabilizing hand applies lateral to medial pressure. Evaluate the integrity of the lateral and medial triceps (see Fig. 23.6).

Alternative Adjustment Procedure. Doctor and patient positions are as above. Abduct the arm and extend the patient's elbow. Firmly grasp the medial olecranon with the 1st and 2nd fingers of your contact hand, and stabilize the patient's distal forearm with your other hand. A short, brisk, pronating, medial to lateral pull and elbow extension is made with your contact hand as your stabilizing hand supinates the lower forearm.

Lateral Olecranon Subluxation

This type of subluxation is related to elbow or wrist trauma, lateral elbow pain, triceps dyskinesia, decreased distance between olecranon and lateral epicondyle, and restricted medial olecranon motion.

Adjustment. Face caudally on the affected side of the prone patient. Abduct the arm, extend the elbow, and internally rotate the extremity. Make a soft pisiform contact with your medial hand on the lateral aspect of the olecranon, and stabilize the patient's lower forearm with your other hand. A short, brisk, thrust is made caudally to shift the olecranon medially as your stabilizing hand pronates the lower forearm. Evaluate the integrity of the lateral and medial triceps (see Fig. 23.7).

Anterior Olecranon Subluxation

Subluxation of the olecranon anteriorly is seen in relation to hyperextension sprains and restricted posterior olecranon motion.

Adjustment. Stand on the affected side and obliquely face the sitting patient. Moderately abduct the arm, and flex the elbow. Place your contact hand on the dorsal aspect of the patient's distal forearm. Cup your stabilizing hand deep within the antecubital fossa, and wrap your thumb around the forearm. Make a short, brisk thrust with

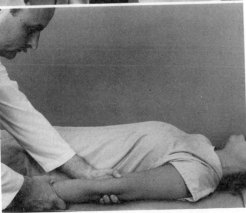

Figure 23.6. *Top*, position for adjusting an olecranon subluxated medially. *Bottom*, position for alternative adjustment.

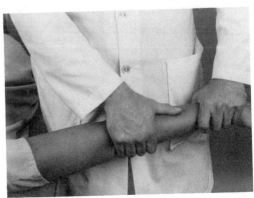

Figure 23.7. Position for adjusting an olecranon subluxated laterally.

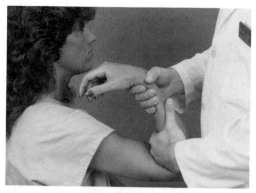

Figure 23.8. Position for adjusting an anteriorly subluxated olecranon.

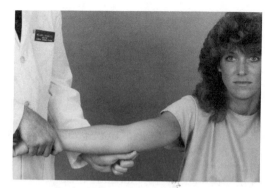

Figure 23.9. Position for adjusting a posteriorly subluxated olecranon.

your contact hand towards the patient's shoulder, using your stabilizing hand as a fulcrum to bring the olecranon out of its depressed position. Evaluate the integrity of the biceps brachii, brachialis, brachioradialis, and triceps (see Fig. 23.8).

Posterior Olecranon Subluxation

This type of subluxation is associated with elbow or wrist trauma, epicondyle and bursa tenderness, triceps dyskinesia, and restricted anterior olecranon movement.

Adjustment. Stand on the affected side of the sitting patient so that you are facing caudally. Abduct the patient's arm, extend the elbow, and slightly externally rotate the forearm. Cup the patient's elbow with your medial stabilizing hand, and place your thumb and index finger against the epicondyles for leverage. With your contact hand, grasp the volar aspect of the patient's lower forearm. A short, brisk thrust is made towards the floor on the distal forearm as your stabilizing fingers apply counterpressure upward. Evaluate the integrity of the triceps and biceps (see Fig. 23.9).

Superior Ulna Subluxation

Subluxation of the ulna superiorly is related to elbow or wrist trauma. It is often a consequence of a falling person catching himself with an outstretched hand, resulting in the ulna being jammed upward against the humerus.

Adjustment. The patient sits next to a narrow table, leans forward to slightly forward-abduct his arm, and extends his fore-

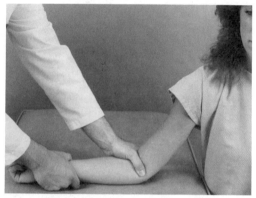

Figure 23.10. Position for adjusting a superiorly subluxated ulna.

arm horizontal to the table's surface. The elbow should never be fully extended as this will subject the tip of the olecranon process to injury. Stand on the opposite side of the table and face the patient. With your contact hand, grasp the ulnar aspect of the patient's lower forearm and slightly rotate it externally. Cup your other hand against the patient's lower anterior humerus and extend your elbow to stabilize the patient's arm. Apply traction with your contact hand, and then make a short, quick pull to bring the ulna towards your body. Evaluate the integrity of the triceps and wrist flexors and extensors (see Fig. 23.10).

Alternative Adjustment Procedure. Stand on the affected side of the supine patient. Abduct his arm, and flex his elbow. Grasp the patient's lower forearm with both hands, with emphasis on the ulnar aspect, and place your knee in the patient's antecubital fossa for stabilizing. Traction is applied, followed by a strong upward pull.

Fractures and Dislocations

The radial head at the elbow transmits the force of a fall on the hand to the shoulder, thus explaining why the radial head is a common site of fracture in the elbow area. Subtle impaction fractures of the distal humerus and radial head are not uncommon and often can only be witnessed on x-ray film after a week or two. Acute signs are local swelling, tenderness about the radial head, and severe pain increased on pronation or supination. Severe displacement is not typical.

Olecranon fractures result from a fall on the elbow or excessive triceps action. Displacement may be severe because of the strong pull of the triceps. Olecranon stress fractures are seen in overuse throwing injuries (eg, baseball, javelin).

Assessment

If obvious deformity and crepitus are not present, check range of motion, and determine radial pulse. Assess sensation by light touch and distal motion function by having the patient appose thumb and forefinger. Elbow fractures and dislocations should be reduced by an orthopedist; splint in "as is" position, sling, and refer. Delay in referral can easily result in massive heterotopic bone formation. Myositis ossificans, nerve damage, brachial arterial compression, contractures, abnormal carrying angle, and joint stiffness may complicate recovery from any severe elbow injury. Poorly reduced supracondylar fractures, resulting in cubitis valgus, readily lead to ulnar neuritis.

Roentgenologic Considerations

Elbow dislocations are usually the result of excessive hyperextension where the olecranon and radial head are displaced posteriorly. Severe soft-tissue damage is associated, usually resulting in subperiosteal hematoma. Comminuted or marginal fracture fragments from the radial head are frequently related with elbow dislocations. In uncomplicated cases, gentle forward traction on the forearm with the humerus stabilized can be conducted to ease pain prior to referral. Roentgenography is required to analyze possible complications prior to considering even simple dislocation reduction.

Especially within the adolescent player, trochlea, capitellum, and epicondyle growth centers may be enlarged, fragmented, displaced, or prematurely fused. Epiphyseal lines cause the most errors in interpretation of this area. Epiphyseal cartilage may be lacerated and the ossification centers displaced, sometimes into the articular cavity.

The most common fracture is a line running from the anterior to the posterior surface of the humeral shaft (supracondylar) with the proximal fragment shifted anteriorly. Fractures in the area of the elbow usually involve the joint. In the order of frequency, the most common fractures are supracondylar, fractures of the humerus, olecranon, head of the radius, and coronoid process. A fracture line between the condyles (intercondylar) or through one or both of the condyles (diacondylar) may be seen. Fracture of the ulnar shaft with dislocation of the radial head (Monteggia injury) and fracture of the radial head may also be presented.

Nerve Compression Injuries

Radial Nerve Compression at the Elbow

This nerve compression syndrome features pain and disturbed sensation in the area of distribution of the superficial branch, thus frequently confused with De Quervain's disease. If the deep branch is involved, pain is at or below the lateral epicondyle.

Examination. On palpation, the nerve trunk is tender near the origin of the extensor muscles, and active extension of the fingers initiates or aggravates pain. If the elbow is extended and the 3rd finger is actively extended against resistance, pain is especially increased because the extensor carpi radialis inserts at the base of the 3rd metacarpal.

Management. If conservative therapy fails to afford relief, exploratory surgery is indicated.

Musculospiral Contusion

The course of the radial nerve in the musculospiral groove along the lateral aspect of the distal-third humerus is relatively superficial and not infrequently receives a contusion. The clinical picture ("dead arm") is one of sudden radiating pain throughout the distal radial distribution and extensor paralysis. Damage is rarely permanent, and symptoms usually ease within a few minutes.

Management. Local ice massage and nerve-contusion management will usually be adequate. If symptoms persist, neurologic consultation is necessary.

Ulnar Nerve Compression at the Elbow

This nerve compression disorder is often called cubital tunnel syndrome or tardy ulnar nerve palsy. It is the result of trauma or compression of the ulnar nerve at the elbow when the medial ligament ruptures during elbow dislocation. It may also be involved if the medial epicondyle becomes fractured. This consequence is disability and pain along the ulnar aspect of the forearm and hand. Early signs are inability to separate the fingers and disturbed sensation of the 4th and 5th digits. Interosseous atrophy is usually evident, and light pressure on the cubital tunnel initiates or aggravates pain. Nerve conduction studies help to confirm the diagnosis.

Management. The cause is often repetitive trauma, and response to conservative therapy is poor unless the source of irritation can be removed. Surgery may stop progressive neuropathy, but it does not guarantee return of normal neurologic function.

Miscellaneous Pathologic Signs

Tinel's Elbow Test. The groove between the olecranon process and the medial epicondyle is tapped with the pointed end of a reflex hammer. A hypersensitive response is seen in ulnar neuritis or neuroma.

Strumpell's Pronation Sign. The patient is asked to extend the elbows, project the arms forward, and supinate the hands. If the patient is unable to keep an affected limb from drifting into pronation during active flexion or elevation of the arms from this position, it is said to be a sign (pathologic reflex) of an upper motor lesion (eg, hemiplegia).

Biernacki's Sign. Deep pressure over the ulnar nerve behind the elbow normally causes pain, even in a patient with a high pain threshold. A lack of response suggests a lesion of the fibers carrying deep pressure impulses or a lesion in the posterior columns of the spinal cord. Some authorities feel this sign is pathognomonic of tabes dorsalis.

Cogwheel Sign. If during passive elbow flexion and extension, the muscles feel taut (lead pipe rigidity) and the motion is felt like a series of irregular and jerky catches and releases (cogwheel motion), a lesion in the extrapyramidal system of the basal ganglia is indicated (eg, paralysis agitans).

Erb's Sign. If application of a galvanic current to a nerve or muscle motor point produces a tonic muscle contraction (tetanic reaction) rather than the normal single "make and break" response, hyperexcitability of the peripheral nerve is indicated (eg, as in tetany).

INJURIES OF THE FOREARM AND WRIST

Restriction in pronation suggests pathology at the elbow, at the radioulnar articulation of the wrist, or within the forearm. Restriction in supination is associated with a disorder of the elbow or radioulnar articulation at the wrist. Thickened tissues may cause compression symptoms, and nerve injury is often secondary to epicondylar fracture or severe trauma. The wrist extensors on the lateral aspect are often associated with tennis elbow. A palpable nontender ganglion may be found on either the dorsal or volar aspect of the wrist, felt as a pea-sized or slightly larger jelly-like cyst. Note any atrophy of the thenar (eg, median nerve compression) or hypothenar eminence (eg, ulnar nerve compression).

Tenderness. Tenderness over the medial collateral ligament, rising from the medial epicondyle, is a sign of valgus sprain. Muscle tenderness in the wrist flexor-extensor group is characteristic of flexor-pronator strain (eg, tennis, screwdriving motions). Tenderness in the first tunnel on the radial side is a common site for stenosing tenosynovitis associated with a positive Finkelstein's sign. Check for rupture of the tendon in the third tunnel, often resulting from a healed Colle's fracture defect at the dorsal radial tubercle or arthritis causing tendon wearing. Tenderness in the 5th or 6th tunnel is characteristic of synovitis, dorsal carpal subluxation, dislocation of the ulnar head, or rheumatoid arthritis. Check the easily fractured scaphoid by sliding it out from under the radial styloid with ulnar deviation of the wrist. Radial deviate the wrist and check the triquetrum, a common site of fracture. Pain, tenderness, and swelling about the ulnar styloid process suggest a Colle's fracture or a local pathology such as arthritic erosion.

Biomechanical Considerations of the Wrist

Trauma of the wrist should never be taken lightly. An improperly diagnosed and treated case can readily lead to severe arthritis. Good management rests on a thorough knowledge of the underlying anatomy of the carpal bones and fibrocartilage complex.

The wrist complex is far more than eight bones arranged in two horizontal rows between the forearm and hand. Three vertical columns must also be considered. The wrist is essentially a biaxial joint that is capable of motion in two planes: (1) radial and ulnar deviation and (2) palmar flexion and extension. The patterns of movement between the two horizontal carpal rows are reciprocal to each other. In radial deviation (about 15°), the distal row moves toward the radius, while the proximal row moves toward the ulnar. In ulnar deviation (about 35°), these movements are reversed; ie, the distal row moves ulnarly, while the proximal row moves radially.

The most important ligaments of the wrist are the volar and intercapsular groups. The weaker dorsal ligaments are arranged in laminar bands. As the proximal carpal row lacks tendon support, the integrity of the volar ligament intracapsular supporting system is vital.

Etiology

The most common wrist injuries seen in treating the athlete are shown in Table 23.3.

Physical Approach

A review of pertinent neurologic, orthopedic, and peripheral vascular maneuvers, reflexes, and tests relative to the wrist is shown in Table 23.4.

Table 23.3.
Common Sports-Related Injuries and Related Disorders of the Wrist and Distal Forearm

Anterior carpal subluxation
Approximated distal radius and ulnar
Arterial obtruction
Avascular necrosis of the lunate (Kienbock's disease)
Carpal tunnel syndrome
Entrapment syndromes
Hamate hook fracture
Inferior radius subluxation
Lunate dislocation
Metacarpal base posterior subluxation
Perilunar dislocation
Pisiform fracture
Posterior carpal subluxation
Scaphoid fracture
Scaphoid nonunion
Scaphoid rotary subluxation (scaphoidlunate dissociation)
Tenosynovitis
Trans-scaphoid perilunar dislocation
Wrist sprain

Table 23.4.
Review of Neurologic, Orthopedic, and Peripheral Vascular Maneuvers, Reflexes, Signs, or Tests Relative to the Wrist

Allen's test
Bracelet test
Extension stress test
Finkelstein's test
Finsterer's test
Flexion stress test
Froment's adduction test
Froment's cone sign
Light touch/pain tests
Maisonneuve's sign
Muscle strength grading
Phalen's test
Radial stress test
Range of motion tests
RUM tests
Tinel's sign
Tinel's wrist test
Ulnar stress test
Ulnar tunnel triad
Wrist drop test
Wrist tourniquet test

Contusions, Strains, and Related Conditions

Forearm Contusions. In many contact sports, the lateral forearm is a favorite weapon. Contusions, abrasions, lacerations, and bone bruises are common, but fractures are not. Forearm bruises are quite painful and exhibit functional weakness, but they respond quickly to standard care. Precautions against myositis ossificans should always be made. Treat with cold, compression, and elevation regardless of initial appearance. Swelling in the athlete is often hidden within well-developed forearm muscles. Rest in a sling for 1–2 days, diathermy, ultrasound, and massage are helpful. Protective padding should be applied during competitive activity for 2–3 weeks. Subperiosteal hematoma responds well to diathermy and ultrasound.

Traumatic Inflammation of the Wrist. Traumatic arthritis of the wrist is often associated with severe sprain, fracture, and dislocation of the carpals, especially scaphoid fracture and lunate dislocation. The symptoms are typical of tenosynovitis in other joints. Cold should be applied initially, followed by strapping or a leather wrist corset worn for several weeks until pain and swelling subside.

Forearm Strains. These usually affect the flexors. Simple strains such as from overenthusiastic weight lifting respond quickly to rest and routine strain management, but chronic strain (eg, crew) can develop into a frustrating problem if the athlete insists on continuing the sport. Avulsion at the bicipital tubercle and stress fracture of the olecranon are sometimes associated.

Brachialis Calcification. Following brachialis strain, a local myositis ossificans may develop in the brachialis anticus tendon. This is usually the result of recurrent bruising and bleeding, preventable by proper padding. Management is similar to that of supraspinatus calcification. This should be followed by passive and active exercises to return joint mobility to normal.

Contractures. After cerebral lesions involving the arm center and in almost any spinal or peripheral nerve lesion which involves one set of muscles and spares another, healthy muscles contract (or overact) and permanent deformities result. In trauma-related hysteria, similar contractures occur. Contractures have in themselves little or no diagnostic value but indicate a late and stubborn stage of whatever lesion is present.

Unilateral Wasting. Rapid atrophy occurs in all types of neuritis, as well as in poliomyelitis and progressive muscular atrophy. In the latter, it occurs without complete paralysis, though the wasted muscles are, of course, weak. Progressive muscular atrophy usually begins in the muscles at the base of the thumb and between it and the index finger. Less often, the process begins in the deltoid. In either case, the rest of the arm muscles are involved later. In the atrophies just mentioned, a lack of the trophic or nourishing functions are assumed to explain the trophic wasting. From this, we can distinguish atrophy due simply to disuse of the muscles without nerve lesions. Slow atrophy of disuse occurs in the arm in hemiplegia, infantile or adult and in other cerebral lesions involving the arm center or the fibers leading down from it. Cervical rib syndrome disorders occasionally lead to wasting as well as pain in the corresponding arm. The atrophy often seen in hysterical cases is probably due to disuse and is similar to that occurring in an arm that has been splinted after fracture or dislocation (see Fig. 23.11).

Wrist Sprain

Wrist sprain (eg, jammed wrist) is very common in many sports and may be associated with fractures and dislocations of the carpals, elbow, or shoulder girdle. Consequently, all severe wrist-joint injuries should include roentgenography of the elbow and shoulder.

Examination. The symptoms are the same as in any other extremity joint sprain and may be associated with tenosynovitis. Severe wrist sprains are invariably accompanied by carpal and/or radial subluxations. On the dorsal aspect of the wrist, the scaphoid is the common carpal problem; on the ventral aspect, it is the lunate, hamate, and pisiform. Extension sprain with radial deviation is characterized by tenderness along the ulnar-metacarpal collateral ligament. Dorsiflexion sprain features tenderness along the volar aspect of the wrist and distal radius. In either case, pain is short of fracture and crepitus is absent. Palpation of the anterior wrist is greatly hampered by

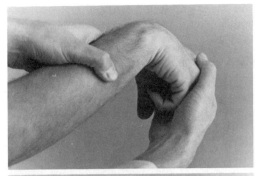

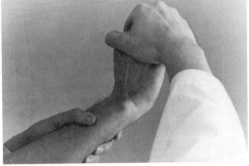

Figure 23.11. *Top*, testing strength of wrist extension against resistance; *bottom*, of wrist flexion.

the tendon bulk of the area and useless on either aspect after swelling has taken place. Scaphoid fracture, a dangerous situation, is often mistaken as a sprain.

Flexion/Extension Stress Tests. The examiner moves the wrist firmly into flexion and extension. If pain is induced, wrist fracture, subluxation, sprain, acute tendinitis, or pathology are suggested. If negative, the movements are repeated against patient resistance. Induced pain then indicates wrist strain, rupture, acute or chronic tendinitis, or pathology.

Radial/Ulnar Stress Tests. The examiner moves the wrist firmly into radial and ulnar deviation (abduction and adduction). If pain is induced, sprain, acute tendinitis, joint pathology, fracture, or subluxation are suggested. If negative, the movements are repeated against patient resistance. Induced pain then indicates acute or chronic tendinitis, strain, rupture, or joint pathology.

Management. Quick on-field examination can usually eliminate fracture in a few minutes before swelling takes place, and proper support can allow the player to con-

tinue competition. Never apply tape completely around the anterior wrist. During the acute stage, structural alignment, cold, compression, strapping, positive galvanism, rest, and possibly elevation are indicated. After 48 hours, passive congestion may be managed by contrast baths, light massage, gentle passive manipulation, sinusoidal stimulation, ultrasound, and a mild range of exercise initiated. Vitamin C and manganese glycerophosphate are advisable throughout treatment of most any sprain. During consolidation, local moderate heat, active exercise, mobilization, and ultrasound are beneficial. In the stage of fibroblastic activity, deep heat and massage, vigorous active exercise, ultrasound, and active joint manipulation speed recovery and inhibit postinjury effects.

Kienboeck's Disease. This disorder is a slowly progressive osteitis of the lunate, sometimes following wrist injuries. The condition is caused by interference with the blood supply from partial dislocation with spontaneous replacement of the bone. This is a rarefaction-type osteitis similar to that of Kummell's disease, with symptoms of pain on use. Prolonged immobilization and treatment for severe sprain are indicated. In rare cases, excision of the bone may be necessary.

Finsterer's Test. This is a two-phase test for Kienbock's disease. (1) If when clenching the fist firmly the normal prominence of the 3rd knuckle is not produced, the test is initially positive. (2) If percussion of the 3rd metacarpal just distal to the dorsal aspect of the midpoint of the wrist elicits abnormal tenderness, the test is confirmed.

Tenosynovitis

The forearm's extensor muscles are often affected in racket sport players, oarsmen, and canoeists. The clinical picture is one of pain along the dorsal forearm, crepitus along the extensor tendons, swelling (palable and visible), and possible hypertrophy of the thumb's extensors and abductors.

Management. Treat as a severe strain with rest, anterior crisscross strapping with the elbow almost flexed to a right angle, and antiinflammatory measures. A proximal radial or ulnar subluxation is sometimes involved. Fasciectomy and paratendon excision may be necessary in stubborn cases.

Arterial Obstruction

Allen's Test   The sitting patient elevates his arm and is instructed to make a tight fist to express blood from his palm. The examiner occludes radial and ulnar arteries proximal to the wrist by finger pressure. The patient then lowers the hand and relaxes the fist, and the examiner releases the arteries one at a time. Some examiners prefer to test the radial and ulnar arteries individually in two tests. The sign is negative if the pale skin of the palm flushes immediately when the artery is released. The sign is positive if the skin of the palm remains blanched for more than 3 seconds. The patient should not hyperextend the palm as this will constrict skin capillaries and render a false positive sign. This test, which should be performed before Wright's test, is significant in vascular occlusion at or distal to the wrist of the artery tested.

Edema

The four most common causes of arm edema are (1) thrombosis of the axillary or brachial vein, usually from heart disease; (2) pressure of masses; (3) inflammation, usually with evidence of lymphangitis spreading up the arm from a septic wound on the hand; and (4) deep axillary abscess: an insidious painful septic focus may burrow so deeply in the axilla that edema of the arm, as well as pain, is produced. Leukocytosis and slight fever accompany it. The diagnosis is easily made provided we are aware of the existence of this uncommon but distinct clinical entity which is increasing in prevalence with the sale of powerfully astringent underarm deodorants. The cause of edema is usually brought out by the general physical examination of the heart, local lesions, urinalysis, etc. The arm should be investigated for vessel changes and for the evidence given by their pulsations as to the efficiency of the heart.

Subluxations

As in any adjustive procedure, fracture, dislocations, and arthritis must be ruled out. Heat is frequently necessary prior to correction to afford maximum patient relaxation and rapid physiologic response to correction. Bilateral x-ray films are helpful in diagnosis.

Separated Distal Radius and Ulna

This type of subluxation is commonly seen in association with carpal tunnel syndrome, chronic wrist pain, and wrist trauma.

Adjustment.   Stand on the side of involvement and face the standing or sitting patient. Grasp the patient's wrist with both hands so that your overlapping thumbs are crossed against the lateral aspect of the distal radius and your interlaced fingers cup the medial aspect of the ulna. Apply a strong squeeze with your hands to approximate the distal radius and ulnar while simultaneously making a quick downward thrust with your thumbs by extending your elbows. Evaluate the integrity of the pronator quadratus (Fig. 23.12).

Approximated Distal Radius and Ulna

Approximated distal radius and ulna are often seen in chronic wrist pain or following wrist and hand trauma.

Adjustment.   Stand on the side of involvement, and face the standing or sitting patient. Grasp the patient's wrist with both hands so that your overlapping thumbs cross between the dorsal aspects of the distal radius and ulna and your interlaced fingers cup the volar aspect of the lower forearm. Apply a strong thumb thrust inward by extending your elbows while simultaneously using your fingers to separate the distal radius and ulna (Fig. 23.13).

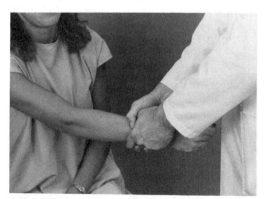

Figure 23.12.   Adjusting separated distal radius and ulna.

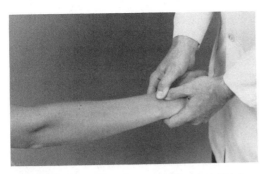

Figure 23.13. Adjusting approximated distal radius and ulna.

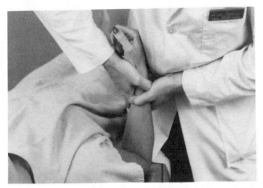

Figure 23.14. Position for adjusting a radius subluxated inferiorly.

Inferior Radius Subluxation

An inferiorly subluxated radius is often a consequence of wrist sprain from a fall on the outstretched hand.

Adjustment. Stand on the side of involvement and face the supine patient. Moderately flex the patient's elbow, and be sure that it is firm against a padded table. Grasp the wrist so that your thumbs overlap near the styloid process of the lateral distal radius and your fingers cup the medial aspect of the distal ulna. Apply thumb pressure against the radius, towards the patient's elbow, and then make a short, quick, forward thrust with moderate body weight. Evaluate the brachioradialis, biceps brachii, and pronator teres (Fig. 23.14).

Anterior Carpal Subluxation

Subluxation of a carpal anteriorly is related to carpal tunnel syndrome, chronic wrist pain, extension sprain, and restricted posterior wrist flexion. The lunate is the most common carpal involved.

Adjustment. Stand on the side of in-

volvement and face the standing or sitting patient. Grasp the patient's wrist with both hands so that a double index-finger contact is made under the volar aspect of the carpal involved, with the rest of your fingers supporting the other carpals. Lift the patient's forearm slightly, flex the wrist a few degrees, and place traction on the wrist. Relax the joints with mild sideward movements. The correction is made by holding firm contact pressure with your index fingers and snapping the wrist quickly into extension. Never forcibly flex the wrist as this will cause sprain. With athletes having highly developed forearms (eg, tennis pros), it may be necessary to place your knee in the patient's antecubital fossa for counterpressure. Evaluate the radius, pronator quadratus, and the extensor carpi radialis longus and brevis (Fig. 23.15, *Top*).

Alternative Adjustment Procedure. Turn the involved wrist palm up. Make overlapping thumb contact on the involved carpal and support the patient's dorsal hand with your fingers. Apply traction, slightly

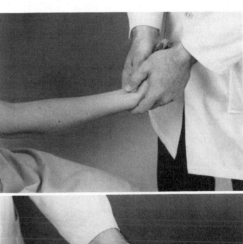

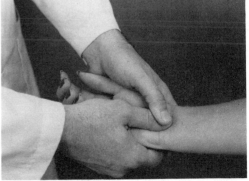

Figure 23.15. Positions for adjusting an anterior carpal subluxation.

flex the wrist, and make firm posteriorly-directed thumb pressure while rolling the wrist through alternated rotation, extension, flexion, and lateral flexion by describing a wide figure 8 (Fig. 23.15, *Bottom*).

Posterior Carpal Subluxation

This type of subluxation is frequently associated with wrist trauma, chronic pain upon motion, carpal tunnel syndrome, and restricted wrist extension.

Adjustment. Stand on the side of involvement and face the standing or sitting patient. Grasp the patient's pronated wrist with both hands so that an overlapping thumb contact is made on the involved carpal, with the rest of your fingers supporting the volar aspect of the wrist. Apply traction to the wrist, make a quick downward thumb thrust by extending your elbows while simultaneously extending the patient's wrist a few degrees. Again, it may be necessary to apply counterpressure with your knee within the patient's antecubital fossa. Evaluate the pronator quadratus and the flexor carpi radialis and ulnaris (Fig. 23.16).

Alternative Adjustment Procedure. This is the reverse of the alternative adjustment procedure for an anterior carpal, varied by turning the involved wrist palm down and taking thumb contact on the dorsal aspect of the carpal.

Metacarpal Base Posterior Subluxation

A metacarpal base subluxated posteriorly is associated with pain especially increased by wrist flexion, excessive wrist flexion

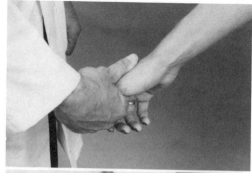
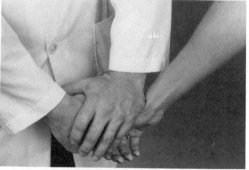

Figure 23.17. Position for adjusting a posterior metacarpal base of the thumb. *Top*, the contact thumb rests on the proximal end of the metacarpal; *Bottom*, a pisiform contact is placed over the contact thumb prior to thrust.

sprain, wrist ganglion, and restricted wrist extension.

Adjustment. Stand on the side of involvement of the sitting patient. The patient's wrist should be resting on a firm pillow. Grasp the patient's involved digit with your contact hand so that your thumb rests on the proximal head of the metacarpal and your fingers wrap around the involved finger for stability. With your other hand, take a pisiform contact on top of the distal phalanx of your contact thumb. Apply moderate distal traction with your contact fingers and make a short, quick thrust downward by fully extending your elbows. As the thrust is made, the patient's wrist will dorsiflex. Evaluate the muscles of the wrist and hand.

Fractures and Dislocations

Uncomplicated low-forearm fractures and dislocations should be aided somewhat on-field by steady axial traction. Assess motor and sensory function of the hand, and

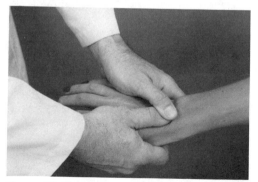

Figure 23.16. Position for adjusting a posterior carpal subluxation.

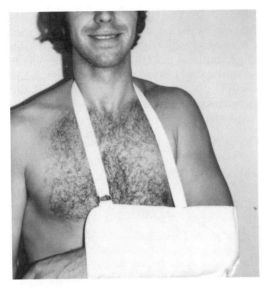

Figure 23.18. Typical forearm sling.

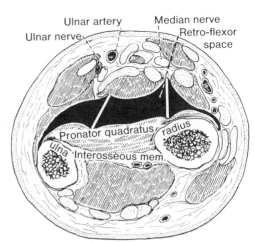

Figure 23.19. Cross-section of forearm just proximal to wrist. Retroflexor space lying above pronator quadratus and interosseous membrane and beneath the flexor muscles and tendons invaded by an infectious process following rupture of the radial or ulnar bursae.

note circulation by capillary filling of the fingernails with finger pressure. Pad, splint in the position of function, and refer (see Fig. 23.18). Roentgenography is required to analyze possible complications prior to considered reduction.

Injuries at the Proximal Forearm and Shafts

P-A and lateral x-rays views are standard, but several degrees of obliquity may be necessary. Comparison should be made with views of the contralateral (uninjured) arm.

Fractures of the bones in the forearm usually involve both bones. Sometimes, however, these bones do not fracture at the same level. The bulk of forearm bone injuries are from falls or direct blows. When a midarm blow fractures the radius or ulna, both ends of each bone must be evaluated for possibly associated subluxation, dislocation, and rotational abnormality. Dislocation of the proximal radius accompanies midulna fracture in Monteggia injury, while midradius fracture is accompanied by distal ulnar subluxation in the Galeazzi fracture. The ulna is usually displaced posteriorly when the distal ulna is subluxated. In radial or ulnar fractures, ulnar rotational abnormalities may be a complication. Malposition of the bicipital tubercle proximally and the ulnar styloid distally are helpful clues to rotational abnormalities.

Injuries at the Distal Forearm

In cases where a fracture of the distal radius is difficult to view on film, careful inspection of the pronator muscle fat pad should be made just proximal to the wrist. It may be the only radiologic sign present. This fat pad, which separates the pronator quadratus muscle and tendons of the flexor digitorum profundus, is normally viewed on lateral films of the wrist. Blurring, bowing, or obliteration of the fat pad may be seen as a consequence of injury or disease of the radius or volar soft tissues.

Fracture of the distal radius (Colle's) is the first consideration in wrist injuries, but the close relationship of both forearm and wrist bones and all articulations must be carefully evaluated. The joint spaces between the carpal bones are normally uniform. Epiphyseal fractures and fractures through the growth plate with or without shifting are not uncommon in youth. The typical deformity in this injury is a compression of the posterior margin of the radius, resulting in a backward tilting of the anterior surface as viewed in the lateral view. The articular margin of the radius will be disturbed, and the distal radius may be fragmented and impacted. Old fractures are differentiated from recent ones by the presence of rarefaction and the absence of a distinct fracture line.

On the lateral view, the radiocarpal articulation should be carefully evaluated. The radial longitudinal axis normally extends through the lunate's midpoint. On the P-A view, disruption of the distal radio-ulnar articulation is seen as joint widening or narrowing. During an impacted fracture of the radius, bone fragments are frequently telescoped and both styloid processes are seen at the same but more distal level; ie, the radial styloid is normally seen 1-cm distal to the ulnar styloid process.

Maisonneuve's Sign. Normal extension of the wrist rarely exceeds 75°. Marked hyperextension (near 90°) is a sign of Colle's fracture.

Carpal Fracture-Dislocations

Any carpal may be a potential fracture or dislocation site. In order of frequency, the bones usually involved are the scaphoid, lunate, and capitate—all of which may be associated with injuries of the radius or ulna. Of the carpals, the lunate is the most frequently dislocated; the scaphoid is the most frequently fractured. The scaphoid is the most lateral of the four bones in the proximal row of carpals; the lunate, second from thumb side.

Even slight tenderness in the anatomic snuffbox about the scaphoid and swelling obliterating the space between the thumb's extensor tendons suggest the danger of scaphoid fracture which may not appear on

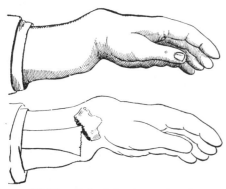

Figure 23.20. Colles' fracture, showing characteristic deformity (silver-fork deformity) at the wrist as the result of backward displacement of the lower fragment.

film for 10–14 days. Axially directed percussion on the knuckle of the patient's index finger when his fist is closed will usually elicit scaphoid pain if fractured. Bone necrosis and nonunion are always a danger as the bone is poorly nourished in a third of the population. Scaphoid fracture has a high incidence in ice hockey.

Boxer's Wrist (Lunate Injury)

This dislocation-fracture may be seen in any athlete from a fall on the outstretched hand, but it is most common in boxers whose hands are carelessly wrapped. Damage to the median nerve is a complication. The clinical picture is one of anterior wrist swelling, with stiff and semiflexed fingers. Carpal dislocations, especially lunate or paralunate, are frequently missed during evaluation. These are often associated with a trans-scaphoid fracture and necrosis.

The lunate usually dislocates posteriorly or anteriorly, disrupting its relationship with the neighboring carpals and the distal radius. Anterior displacement is the common mechanism, where the bone rests deep in the annular ligament and may affect the median nerve. The lunate is loosely stabilized by an anterior and posterior ligament which contains small nutritive blood vessels. A torn ligament thus interferes with the lunate's nutrition, resulting in necrosis. On a P-A view, the lunate's normal quadrilateral shape becomes triangular, and the third metacarpal and capitate usually move proximally. With paralunate dislocation, the lunate keeps normal alignment with the radius but the distal carpals become displaced from their normal position with associated changes in intercarpal joint spaces.

Golfer's Wrist

If a full golf swing hits the ground or a hard object other than the ball, an isolated fracture of the wrist may result. The mechanism appears to be one of violent contraction of the flexor carpi ulnaris insertion through the pisiform-hamate ligament. Roentgenography may show a fracture of the hamate.

General Nerve Injuries and Disorders

RUM Tests. Quick RUM (radial, ulnar, medial nerve) neurologic tests are as follows:

• *Radial nerve:* Have patient extend wrist. Nerve pathology causes wrist drop. The radial nerve supplies sensory fibers to the dorsum of the hand on the radial aspect, especially at the web between the thumb and index finger.

• *Ulnar nerve:* Have patient hold a piece of paper by opposing thumb and index finger (Froment's adduction test). The examiner tries to pull the piece of paper away while the patient resists. If the patient cannot hold on to the slip, the weakness suggests ulnar nerve pathology. The ulnar nerve supplies sensory fibers to the ulnar aspect of the hand, both dorsal and palmar surfaces, and the ring and little fingers.

• *Median nerve:* The median nerve is tested by asking the patient to touch each finger with the thumb. Remember that the median nerve is under the transverse carpal ligament. The median nerve supplies sensory fibers to the radial aspect of the palm and the palmar surfaces of the thumb and first two fingers, but it is purest on the palmar surface of the tip of the index finger.

Referred Pain. Cervical osteoarthritis or rheumatoid arthritis of the wrist may refer pain to the elbow, as can shoulder pathology. Symptoms may be referred to the wrist or hand from the cervical spine, shoulder, or elbow such as from cervical disc disorders, osteoarthritis, brachial plexus syndromes, shoulder and elbow entrapments.

Hysterical and Traumatic Neuroses. The history and mode of onset, the frequent association of sensory symptoms which do not fit the distribution of any peripheral nerve, spinal segment, or cortical area, the normal reflexes, and the electrical reactions distinguish most cases of this type, but sometimes diagnosis is most difficult.

Tinel's Sign. As a differential diagnostic aid between complete and incomplete peripheral nerve interruption, one might apply Tinel's test. Normally, percussion of a nerve above or below a point of complete severance elicits no subjective sensations. In cases of partial severance or in cases of compression of this given peripheral nerve where some conduction is preserved, percussion distal to the involvement will elicit a tingling paresthesia below the point of tapping. This represents a positive Tinel's sign. This sign, if positive, is also indicative of nerve regen-

eration if it is elicited over a nerve which had previously been negative on percussion. In this respect, it may have prognostic as well as diagnostic value.

Radial Nerve Injury and Wrist Drop

In addition to causes such as wounds and lacerations, the radial nerve may be damaged by fracture of the middle third of the humerus, external pressure from a crutch in the axilla, or the arm hanging over a bench, table, or the like during unconsciousness. The outstanding symptom is "wrist drop." The thumb cannot be abducted (policis longus and brevis paralysis), finger flexion is impaired, and the wrist cannot be extended. When the nerve is actually severed or "caught," surgery is required.

Wrist Drop Test. The two opposing palms are placed together with the hands in dorsiflexion. On separation, failure to maintain dorsiflexion indicates a positive test and is significant of radial nerve impairment.

Median Nerve Injury and Entrapment

The median nerve is commonly injured in laceration of the anterior wrist. Consequently, sensation and motion of the fingers should be carefully studied. It is difficult to lacerate any of the flexors of the medial anterior wrist without damaging the median nerve. When injured, the characteristic "flat hand" deformity results.

Median nerve paresthesias may have their cause in the spine but just as commonly from interference in the thoracic outlet, the shoulder, the elbow, or at the wrist. Correction must be directed to where the interference is located and not where it "should" be.

Carpal Tunnel Syndrome. This is a nerve compression syndrome featuring median nerve entrapment at the carpal tunnel resulting in symptoms in the hand and fingers, often extending up the arm to the elbow. The cause may be either an increase of structural volume within the tunnel or any condition that tends to narrow the tunnel. The history will often indicate an old scaphoid fracture, perilunar dislocation, or tendinitis at the wrist. Frequently, the history tells of a fall stopped abruptly by the palm of the hand when the wrist was sharply dorsiflexed or of overstress in people who strongly manipulate their wrists (eg, javelin, tennis, hockey, batting, or with chiropractors, bakers, hairdressers, waiters). A syndrome may also be produced by radial or ulnar arterial impairment since these arteries also pass beneath the transverse carpal ligament. Such symptoms may be aggravated by pressure of a sphygmomanometer cuff during blood pressure evaluation.

Signs and Symptoms. There is a history of pain, numbness, and tingling, which worsen at night and with wrist compression in the first two or three digits and/or the area proximal to the wrist. Weakness is exhibited by a history of dropping light objects and difficulty in holding a pen or pencil while writing. Venous engorgement and a bulge may be seen of the flexor mass in the distal wrist, which are characteristic of tenosynovitis or hypertrophied muscles. The first sign is swelling at the volar wrist. Later, thenar atrophy and sensation impairment of the thumb, forefinger, middle finger, and medial half of the ring finger exhibit. In many cases, there is distinct difficulty in pronating or supinating the forearm. Compression or percussion of the carpal ligament usually initiates or increases pain. Electromyogram and nerve conduction studies offer confirmative data for a diagnosis. Misdiagnosis is sometimes seen by attributing a unilateral or bilateral syndrome to slight arthritic changes of the midcervical vertebrae.

Phalen's Test. Have the patient place both flexed wrists into opposition and apply slight pressure for 30–45 seconds. A positive sign of carpal tunnel syndrome is the production of symptoms (eg, pain, tingling) (Fig. 23.21).

Tinel's Wrist Test. With the patient's elbow flexed and the hand supinated, the volar surface of the wrist is tapped with the broad end of a triangular reflex hammer. If this induces pain in all fingers of the involved hand except the little finger, carpal tunnel syndrome is indicated.

Wrist Tourniquet Test. A sphygmomanometer cuff is wrapped around the involved wrist of a seated patient. The cuff is inflated to a point just above the patient's systolic blood pressure level and maintained for 1–2 minutes. If an exacerbation of pain

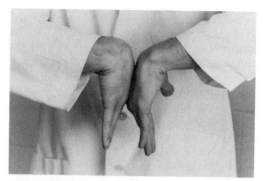

Figure 23.21. Phalen's test to elicit signs of carpal tunnel syndrome.

is exhibited, carpal tunnel syndrome is indicated.

Ochsner's Clasping Test. The patient is instructed to clasp the hands together and interlock the fingers. If the index finger on the involved side fails to flex, median nerve paralysis is indicated—with the lesion at or above the level where the nerve to the flexor digitorum superficialis branches.

Wartenburg's Oriental Prayer Sign. The patient is instructed to fully extend the adducted fingers and the thumb of each hand so that the palms are flat and then to move both hands so that the thumbs and index fingers touch. In median nerve palsy, the thumbs will not touch because of paralysis of the abductor pollicis brevis.

Management. The cause for the syndrome must be determined. During this investigation, anti-inflammatory therapy and a cock-up wrist splint for immobilization may be applied. Invariably, the subluxation is one of joint spread at the distal radial-ulnar articulation. If pain originates or extends to the elbow, a subluxation of the proximal radius may also be involved. Following corrective adjustment, it is well to apply a leather wrist strap over a felt pad for about 2 weeks; an elastic wrist band is contraindicated. Underwater ultrasound, pulsating diathermy, acupuncture, and B complex have been found helpful. Referral for surgery is indicated if neurologic symptoms fail to respond or increase after a trial of conservative therapy.

Ulnar Nerve Injury and Claw Hand

This nerve is more commonly injured

than any other nerve of the upper extremity with the exception of the radial nerve. The injuries are usually at the inner side of the elbow where it is quite vulnerable in its superficial position along the elbow's posteromedial aspect. Most injuries can be prevented with proper elbow padding. When damaged, a characteristic "claw hand" results, with sensory loss of the medial side of the hand.

Ulnar Compression at the Wrist. This compression syndrome features ulnar nerve entrapment, usually in the canal of Guyon. Entrapment may be of the superficial or the deep branch of the ulnar nerve, but the superficial branch is rarely affected by itself. The pisiform-hamate tunnel syndrome is similar to but less frequently seen than that of carpal tunnel syndrome.

Signs and Symptoms. Entrapment of the deep branch produces a motor loss exhibited by a weak pinch, weak little finger and thumb abduction, inability to actively flex the metacarpophalangeal joints, and interosseous atrophy. Compression of the superficial branch features burning sensations in the 4th and 5th digits. Palpation of the pisiform-hamate tunnel initiates or aggravates pain. In roentgenography, a hamate fracture or pisiform dislocation may be found in tangential views.

Froment's Cone Sign. In paralysis of the ulnar nerve, there is an inability to approximate the tips of fingers to the thumb to form a cone (*cone sign*) or make an "O" with the thumb and index finger.

The Ulnar Tunnel Triad. If inspection and palpation over the ulnar tunnel in the wrist determines the three signs of (1) tenderness, (2) clawing of the ring finger, and (3) hypothenar wasting, ulnar compression in the tunnel of Guyon is indicated.

Management. The cause for the syndrome must be determined. During this investigation, anti-inflammatory therapy and immobilization may be applied. Goodheart states that subluxation of the hamate or pisiform towards the wrist and in the direction of the hand's dorsal aspect is a common finding. This is usually the result of a sharp blow to the pisiform area when the wrist is dorsiflexed. A double-thumb contact on the subluxated carpal with a thrust directed distally is usually sufficient for correction. In most cases, the mechanical correction should be supported by placing a piece of felt over the affected carpal and being strapped for about 2 weeks. Adjunctive therapy is similar to that for carpal tunnel syndrome. Referral for exploratory surgery is indicated if neurologic symptoms fail to respond or increase after a trial of conservative therapy.

Rheumatoid Arthritis

Bracelet Test. The examiner surrounds the patient's wrist with the thumb and forefinger and applies mild–moderate compression to the distal ends of the radius and ulna. If acute pain arises in the wrist and/or radiates to the forearm or hand, rheumatoid arthritis should be suspected.

INJURIES OF THE HAND AND FINGERS

The hand, being the least protected and most active part of the upper extremity, is easily hurt. From a structural standpoint, the hand is made for grasping, not for hitting. Bilateral grip strength is best tested with a dynamometer and pinch strength by a pinch meter if objective records are necessary.

Etiology and Physical Approach

The most common hand/finger injuries seen in treating the athlete are shown in Table 23.5. A review of pertinent neurologic, orthopedic, and peripheral vascular manuevers, reflexes, and tests relative to the hand and fingers is shown in Table 23.6.

Contusions and Lacerations

Palm damage tends to injure skin, vessels, tendons, and nerves. Injuries of the dorsal hand tend to damage only skin, tendons, and infrequently bones. Highly painful compression injuries can severely damage all structures.

Abrasions and Bruises of the Hand

All cuts should be quickly cleaned and examined for deep injury. Use cold, compression, and elevation as necessary to reduce edema. Take care to avoid serious hand infection from careless management of small lacerations. The hand is particularly

Table 23.5.
Common Sports-Related Injuries and Related Disorders of the Hand and Fingers

Abrasions
Carpometacarpal joint sprain
Carpometacarpal subluxation
Contusions
Extensor pollicis longus rupture
Extensor tendon central slip
Flexor tendon rupture
Interphalangeal joint sprain
Interphalangeal subluxation
Joint fixations
Lacerations
Metacarpal fracture/dislocation
Metacarpophalangeal joint sprain
Metacarpophalangeal subluxation
Phalanx fracture/dislocation
Subluxation of extensor tendon over metacarpophalangeal joint
Terminal extensor tendon strain or avulsion
Thumb fracture/dislocation

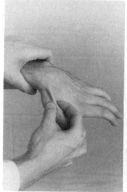
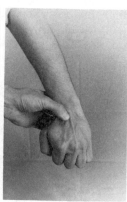

Figure 23.22. *Left*, when the thumb is extended, palpation of the tendons of the abductor pollicis longus and brevis are more prominent. *Right*, when the fist is clenched, palpation of the extensor carpi radialis longus and brevis is enhanced.

Table 23.6.
Review of Neurologic, Orthopedic, and Peripheral Vascular Maneuvers, Reflexes, Signs, or Tests Relative to the Hand and Fingers

Bunnel-Littler's test
Extensor digitorum communis test
Finkelstein's test
Flexor digitorum profundus test
Flexor digitorum superficialis test
Froment's cone sign
Kleist's hooking sign
Klippel-Weil's test
Light touch/pain tests
Muscle strength grading
Ochsner's clasping test
Palmomental reflex
Pollicus longus tests
Range of motion tests
Wartenburg's prayer sign

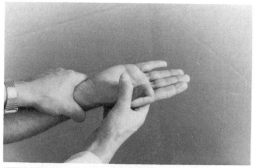

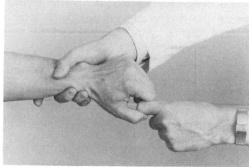

Figure 23.23. *Top*, testing strength of thumb abduction. *Bottom*, testing pinch strength.

vulnerable to infection with venous and lymphatic extension. Contusions of the dorsal aspect of the hand usually come from being stepped on when down. Cleats, sticks, and skate blades, obviously, increase the severity of the injury. Palmar bruises are often seen over the metacarpal heads in the glove hand of the hockey goalie, baseball player, or handball enthusiast.

Hamate Bruise. Sometimes a bone bruise is seen situated deep in the proximal hypothenar eminence in the hamate-pisiform area. This affliction is common to sports requiring a hand-held object such as a hockey stick, ski pole, bat, or racket due to impact on the hamate prominence. It may

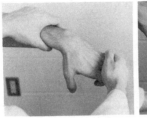
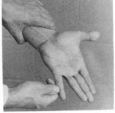

Figure 23.24. *Left*, muscle test for finger extension. *Right*, muscle test for finger abduction.

Dorsal aspect   Palmar aspect

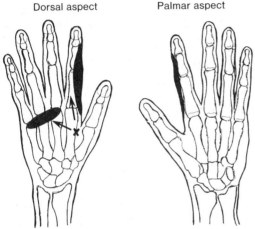

Figure 23.25. First interosseous trigger point; *X*, common site. *Blackened areas* indicate typical sites of referred pain.

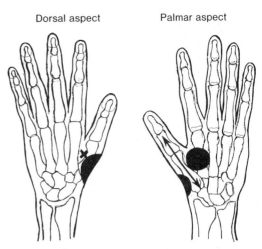

Figure 23.26. Adductor pollicis trigger point; *X*, common site. *Blackened areas* indicate typical sites of referred pain.

flexion of the 3rd finger is typical. An entrapment syndrome may be produced as infiltrative scar tissue clamps the extensor tendon. In minor injuries, transient swelling and painful metacarpophalangeal joints will be seen. Occasionally, hand and wrist fractures will be presented. Remarkably, a large number of hands severely abused by such a severe form of hand conditioning show no visible soft-tissue calcification or damage to the metacrapal heads.

Handlebar Palsy. An overuse injury experienced by bicyclists is occasionally seen which is a neuropathy secondary to injury of the deep palmar branches of the ulnar nerve (handlebar palsy). The trauma results from prolonged severe pressure on the handlebars during long races. The clinical picture is one of muscle weakness and wasting in the intrinsic muscles of the hands without sensory impairment. This disorder is sometimes seen in factor workers from the constant pressure of industrial tools and thus may not be sports related.

Boxer's Knuckle. Two conditions are involved here which may be separate or superimposed: (1) After trauma, a bursa may form over a metacarpal head and become chronically inflamed. (2) Distraction of the metacarpal ligament may result in boxers who have their hands taped in full extension when the intermetacarpal ligaments are relatively slack. As the hand is flexed, the

also be seen from a fall when the outstretched hand strikes an irregular surface. Chronic aggravation results in deep swelling, carpal-tunnel-like vascular symptoms, and distal neuralgia. Initial treatment must be quick to minimize bleeding and swelling through cold, compression, elevation, and rest. Padding, often specially designed, must be worn as long as tenderness persists. During recovery, corrective manipulation, local heat, ultrasound, and massage may be applied to relieve related soreness; however, rest and careful padding is the priority therapy.

Karate Lump. It is not uncommon for karate enthusiasts to scarify their hands and feet by striking a straw-covered pliable post (makiwara) in several years of practice. The result can be scar-tissue development over the injured part, most commonly witnessed at the dorsal aspect of the 3rd and 4th metacarpophalangeal joints. Severe pain on ligaments tighten and the fingers are forced into apposition, which tend to cause ligamentous distraction if any material becomes inserted between the fingers.

Aneurysms of the Hand. In sports where the hand is used as a bat (eg, handball, karate) or struck or crushed, aneurysms and thrombosis of the palm may occur. The two common sites are at the hook of the hamate and at the base of the thenar eminence where branches of the radial and ulnar arteries are relatively unprotected from injury.

Cut Tendons

Flexor Digitorum Profundus Test. This test is based on the fact that flexor digitorum profundus tendons work only in unison. Stabilize the metacarpophalangeal and interphalangeal joints in extension. Have the patient flex the finger being tested at the distal interphalangeal joint. If the patient cannot do this, the sign is positive and indicates a cut tendon or denervated muscle.

Flexor Digitorum Superficialis Test. To test the integrity of the flexor digitorum superficialis tendon, hold all of the patient's fingers in extension except for the finger being tested. Have the patient flex the tested

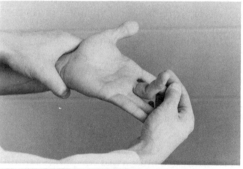

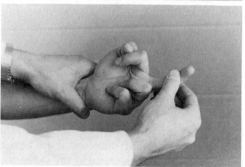

Figure 23.27. Testing the integrity of the flexor digitorum profundus tendon.

finger at the proximal interphalangeal joint. If the patient cannot do this, the sign is positive for a cut or absent tendon.

Strains, Sprains, and Related Disorders

Severe finger sprains with or without avulsed fragments are frequently treated in sports care. In acute sprain, the ligament tears and allows the bone ends to subluxate and disrupt the integrity of the joint structure. Local pain, tenderness, swelling, and motion restriction are exhibited. A previously torn ligament may predispose a joint to recurring luxation because of laxity of the stabilizers.

The Sprained Thumb

A severe injury can occur to the inner thumb ligaments from a fall on a thumb directed outward or when caught in an opponent's uniform. This often results in a complete tear which requires surgery. The thumb is also often jammed, and the medial or lateral ligaments sprained, when hitting with the closed fist.

Pollicus Longus Tests. The examiner stabilizes the proximal phalanx of the patient's thumb, and the patient is instructed to flex and extend the distal phalanx. Inability to flex the phalanx indicates an injury to the tendon of the flexor pollicus longus. Inability to extend the phalanx indicates an injury to the tendon of the extensor pollicus longus.

Management. Treat as a severe sprain, and strap with a figure-8 bandage using half-inch tape. As soon as the acute stage passes, advise several hot soaks a day to "flood" the thenar muscles and help prevent joint stiffness or a "glass thumb." Squeezing a rubber ball helps to strengthen grip during recuperation.

Bowler's Thumb. Ulnovolar neuroma (bowler's thumb) is the result of trauma to the digital nerve from the edge of the thumb hole in the ball. After repeated bowling, fibrous proliferation and enlargement of the 3rd and 2nd fingers are frequently seen. Callus formation may be evident on roentgenography.

Skier's Thumb. In skiing, a rupture to the ulnar collateral ligament of the thumb may occur during a fall on a slope when the leather loop at the handle of the ski pole is wrapped around the thumb (skier's thumb). This injury can be avoided if a pole is used without a loop at the handle.

Metacarpophalangeal and Interphalangeal Sprains

The mechanism of metacarpophalangeal injury is one of sudden hyperextension or a severe lateral force. Subluxation, pain, and disability are often severe, and recovery is slow until ligaments tighten to prevent recurring subluxation.

The interphalangeal joints are easily sprained, torn, and dislocated. This is due to their thin capsule, delicate collateral ligaments, and slender articulations. Associated subluxations are often left untreated by the unaware, resulting in long-term disability and possible permanent deformity.

A twisted finger causes painful tears of the collateral ligaments. Capsulitis is a common complication. Immobilize in moderate flexion, and treat as a severe sprain. Graduated exercises may begin in about 10 days.

Extensor Digitorum Communis Test. The patient is instructed to first make a fist, and then to extend all fingers. Inability to extend any finger indicates an injury to that particular tendon of the extensor digitorum communis.

Mallet (Baseball) Finger

In sports, a hard object may strike a finger resulting in an extensor digitorum tendon injury where the tendon avulses from its insertion at the posterior base of the terminal phalanx. The jammed distal phalanx assumes a position of about 70°. It appears "dropped" and is rigidly flexed, with active distal interphalangeal extension severely limited. In such an injury, small bone fragments may be seen at the distal interphalangeal joint's posterior aspect on roentgenography. Both phalangeal fractures and extensor tendon abnormalities may produce mallet finger.

Unexpectedly, few such injuries are caused by a baseball. Most are the result of a finger striking the ground or a hard object. In fact, the incidence of such injuries in baseball is far below those seen in basketball, volleyball, football, and soccer.

Management. If there is no crepitus and the range of joint motion is normal, a simple strapping of the splinted injured finger with its neighbor may be sufficient for stability. Treat as a severe sprain, and apply a molded splint. There is no need for manipulation, but a slight "milking" action helps prior to strapping to disperse stagnant fluids. Inspect weekly, and retape as is necessary for the degree of healing that has taken place. Operative repair seldom gives better results.

Ganglion

A ganglion is a cystic swelling occurring in association with a joint or tendon sheath, apparently formed by a defense mechanism when the wrist is repeatedly twisted and strained. It has a fibrous outer coat and an inner synovial layer containing a thick gelatinous fluid. A common site is in the wrist or hand; they are rarely found in the ankle or foot. A firm localized swelling and possible weakened grip strength are found. Aching or sometimes pain from pressure on adjacent structures is typically exhibited.

Suppurative Tenosynovitis

If pus collects within the sheath of a palm tendon, four characteristic features (Karavel's cardinal points) are witnessed: (1) the finger is carried in slight flexion for comfort; (2) the finger is swollen in its entire circumference in contrast to swelling from a localized infection; (3) pain is increased during involved finger extension; and (4) marked pain is felt along the course of the inflammed tendon sheath.

De Quervain's Disease

This is a painful stenosing tenosynovitis due to the relative narrowness of the common tendon sheaths of the abductor pollicis brevis and longis. Tendon thickening occurs on the dorsum of the hand at the base of the thumb. Repetitive wrist and thumb overstress may produce pain along the distal radius which is increased by thumb motion. Chronic irritation causes the thumb's extension tendons to become inflamed as they pass through the narrow tunnel on the lateral wrist. Incidence is highest in racket sports, table tennis, golf, and bowling, and sometimes results from clipping hedges or piano playing.

Finkelstein's Test. The patient is asked to make a fist with his thumb tucked inside

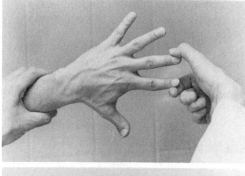

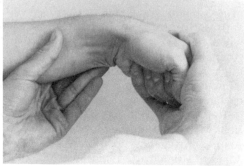

Figure 23.28. *Top,* testing the strength of the intrinsic muscles of the hand by the patient attempting to maintain the fingers spread against resistance. *Bottom,* Finkelstein's test.

his palm (Fig. 23.28, *Bottom*). The examiner stabilizes the patient's distal forearm with one hand and ulnar deviates the wrist with his other hand. Sharp pain in the area of the first wrist tunnel (radial side) strongly points toward stenosing tenosynovitis (De Quervain's disease), where inflammation of the synovial lining narrows the tunnel opening and causes pain on tendon movement.

Management. Treat as a severe sprain, and provide rest with splinting. If conservative management fails, refer for pain relief, steroids, and possible surgical release. Surgery is required to free the binding if conservative measures fail.

Trigger Finger

This is an entrapment syndrome produced by scar tissue compressing an extensor tendon, often a consequence of De Quervain's disease. Its incidence is high in fencing. Squeezing action by the constricted sheath tends to develop a pea-like mass distal to the thickening. It is most often seen in the thumb, but several fingers may rarely

be affected. Simple surgery remedies the situation.

Contractures

Bunnel-Littler or Retinacular Test. Hold the metacarpophalangeal joint in slight extension and try to flex the proximal interphalangeal joint of any finger being tested. If the joint cannot be flexed in this position, it is a positive sign that the intrinsic muscles are tight or capsule contractures exist. To distinguish between intrinsic muscle tightness and capsule contractures, let the involved metacarpophalangeal joint flex slightly, relaxing the intrinsics, and move the proximal interphalangeal joint into flexion. Full flexion of the joint shows tight intrinsics; limited flexion indicates probable contracture of the interphalangeal joint capsule.

Fusiform Effusion

A palpable fusiform effusion at the prox-

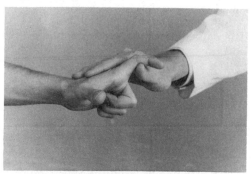

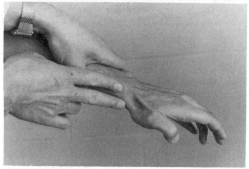

Figure 23.29. *Top,* the Bunnel-Littler test to evaluate the tightness of the hand intrinsics. Examiner attempts to flex the proximal interphalangeal joint with the metacarpophalangeal joint extended a few degrees. Inability to flex the joint points to either tight intrinsics or joint-capsule contracture. *Bottom,* the abductor pollicis longus and the extensor pollicis brevis tendons define the radial border of the carpal snuffbox.

imal interphalangeal finger joints may be centered on the joint and symmetrical on both sides. Even if signs of osseous change are not evident in x-ray films, a rheumatic diathesis exists.

Fractures and Dislocations

All contact sports have a high incidence of metacarpal fractures, but severe displacement is not common.

Finger Fractures

The incidence of metacarpophalangeal thumb joint fracture-dislocation is highest in wrestling and skiing. A fracture of a proximal phalanx tends to displace anteriorly in an angular fashion because of lumbrical pull. A rotated phalanx, often noted by a nail's relationship with its neighbors, is an indication of fracture. Fracture symptoms mimic severe sprain plus abnormal bone or joint contour. Crepitus is not always exhibited in finger fractures.

Finger Dislocations

Many finger dislocations often spontaneously reduce themselves. Dislocation of

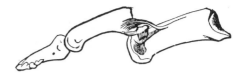

Figure 23.31. Complex metacarpophalangeal dislocation of the thumb by forceful flexion (with the permission of the Associated Chiropractic Academic Press).

the proximal interphalangeal joint usually entails severe injury of the collateral ligaments and is likely to heal with an instable, swollen, stiff joint.

Examination. During on-field evaluation, judge bone length of a suspected fracture or dislocation by comparing with the uninjured hand. Check by applying axial and leverage pressure to patient tolerance. Keep in mind that incomplete and impacted fractures may be present, yet associated tendon, nerve, and vascular damage are quite rare in sports. Comparative x-ray views of the sound limb are frequently helpful. Depending upon one's expertise, roentgenography may or may not be required to analyze possible complications prior to considered reduction.

Management. These conditions are extremely painful; thus, care must be taken to assure that one attempt at correction is sufficient. Do not use prior traction as in many other adjustments; the pain is too great. For good control and to avoid slippage, place the patient's phalanx, distal to the injured joint, high between your index and middle finger, then gently close your hand into a fist with your thumb over your index finger. Stabilize the patient's hand with your free hand.

Simple dislocations may be reduced by increasing the deformity and using leverage to slip the distal articulation into normal position. In metacarpophalangeal dislocations, hyperextend the phalanx and apply pressure and traction at its base to quickly slip it over the metacarpal head. This is much better than straight axial traction. If the displacement is superior-medial or superior-lateral, your pull and pressure must be varied accordingly.

Follow correction immediately with a finger splint that is strapped to an adjoining finger. Treat as a severe sprain, and apply a molded splint for 4–6 weeks. Note that the

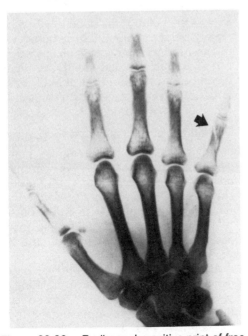

Figure 23.30. Radiograph positive print of fractured 5th finger; right hand, female, age 32 (with the permission of the Palmer College of Chiropractic).

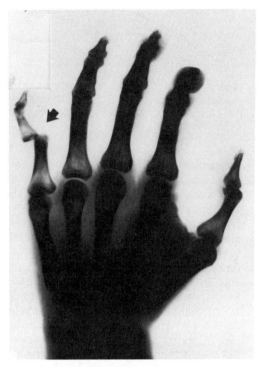

Figure 23.32. Radiograph positive print of dislocated finger; left hand, male, age 31 (with the permission of the Palmer College of Chiropractic).

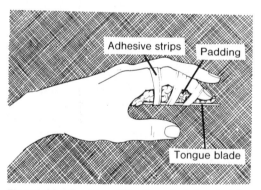

Figure 23.33. Immobilization of dislocated finger.

index finger's metacarpophalangeal joint is extremely resistant to closed reduction and often requires surgery.

Thumb Dislocations

Dislocations often occur between the 1st metacarpal and carpal joint, often difficult to detect, or between the 1st metacarpal and phalangeal joint. Reduction and general management is the same as for finger dislocations.

Fistfighter's Dislocation-Fracture. A fracture of the 4th and/or 5th metacarpal, especially at the neck, is often referred to as a "fighter's" dislocation-fracture. The bone's head and neck are often pushed into the palm. This is most often seen in the bareknuckled fighter or during riots rather than with the gloved boxer who more commonly presents a fracture at the proximal third of the 1st metacarpal.

Miscellaneous Pathologic Signs

Kleist's Hooking Sign. The patient is instructed to place both supinated hands forward, with the elbows moderately flexed. The examiner grasps the fingers and gently moves them into extension. If the patient's fingers react into flexion rather than passively going into extension, this is a pathologic reflex that is thought by several authorities to indicate a frontal or thalamic lesion.

Klippel-Weil's Test. The examiner quickly pries open the flexed fingers of the spastic limb. A reflex response of automatic thumb flexion and adduction indicates a pyramidal tract lesion.

Palmomental Reflex. The examiner strokes the palm of the patient with a moderately blunt instrument. In pyramidal tract disease, the ipsilateral mentalis muscle will often contract so that the lower lip will protrude and raise and the skin of the chin wrinkles so that a facial expression of contempt or scorn is produced.

Injuries of the Nails and Fingertips

Finger nailbed injuries are quite common. The degree of injury may vary from nail splits to painful complete nail avulsion at the base with tears in the nailbed. The nailbed is contiguous with the periosteum of the underlying bone. Bleeding may be associated with phalanx fracture or a crush injury.

Management. In uncomplicated avulsions, apply cold to reduce bleeding and swelling. An avulsed nail should be repositioned and a light pressure bandage applied to keep it from snagging clothing or other objects until it painlessly separates by itself. Care must be taken not to bandage the distal end so tightly as to restrict drainage.

CHAPTER 24

Thoracic and Abdominal Injuries

This chapter discusses intrathoracic, rib, sternal, dorsal spine, abdominal, and perineal injuries seen in athletics. Even minor injuries to the thoracic cage and abdomen require close monitoring because severe symptoms may not arise for a day or two after injury.

CHEST INJURIES

Injuries to the chest occur in sports in spite of well-developed musculature and protective equipment. Successful management requires early diagnosis and intelligent care. In those sports where chest injury can be anticipated, oxygen support should be available.

Posttraumatic Assessment

Anterior chest and abdominal injuries can be life-threatening. Thus, the priority concern is to assure that there is normal breathing and circulation and that steps be taken to minimize shock. In regard to the thoracic spine, potential cord injury takes priority consideration. As in any musculoskeletal disorder, evaluation should include muscle strength grading, joint ranges of motion, sensory perception, appropriate tendon reflexes, and other pertinent clinical tests when indicated. A review of various neurologic and orthopedic signs and tests relative to the thorax is shown in Table 24.1.

Roentgenologic Considerations

Careful attention must be given to position and exposure. P-A and lateral views are standard, but full-chest views often fail to show a fracture site, making focal views necessary. The overlap of posterior and anterior midline structures should be carefully evaluated for signs of rotation on the P-A view. Inspiration can be evaluated by counting the number of ribs above the hemidiaphragm.

Heart Shadows. A large stroke volume is achieved in some athletes, particularly endurance-related competitors, without alterations in heart muscle contraction force. This gain is made at the expense of some expansion of volume at the end of diastole and more complete ventricular emptying. Thus, an athlete's enlarged heart shadow on an x-ray film must be distinguished from the dilated heart shadow associated with heart disease.

Soft-Tissue Signs. Hematoma and pneumothorax can be associated with most any type of rib fracture and should always be anticipated. In absence of pleural adhesions, air normally rises to the apex in pneumothorax, and this is often associated with a mediastinal shift contralaterally. When this occurs, a severe life-threatening tension pneumothorax results which may compromise both lungs unless a chest catheter is surgically inserted. Signs of hemorrhage or rupture should be sought. Mediastinal or lower neck hemorrhage can sometimes be seen as displacement of the trachea from its normal midline or slightly right of the midline position.

Air. Bronchial or tracheal rupture may show signs of air leakage along the mediastinal tissue planes, seen as vertical lucent streaks adjacent to mediastinal shadows. A gastric air bubble displaced medially may point to a splenic hematoma.

Rib Displacement and Ruptures. Blunt trauma may cause superior or anterior dislocation of the lower ribs, and lower rib fractures may be associated with diaphragmatic, splenic, or hepatic rupture. In diaphragmatic rupture, the hemidiaphragm takes on an abnormal contour which sometimes can be seen on the standard P-A full-chest view. In addition, gastric herniation through the ruptured diaphragm and hemothorax may be evident. Most diaphragmatic ruptures occur on the left side as the liver offers considerable protection during a blunt blow on the right.

Table 24.1.
Review of Neurologic and Orthopedic Maneuvers, Reflexes, Signs, or Tests Relative to Musculoskeletal Thoracic Syndromes

Adams' test
Abdominal reflex
Barkman's reflex
Brudzinski's test
Beevor's sign
Chest expansion test
Comolli's sign
Forestier's bowstring sign
Lewin's supine test
Light touch/pain tests
Muscle strength grading
Naffziger's test
Obliquus reflex
Pectoralis flexibility test
Pitres' chest sign
Range of motion tests
Schepelmann's sign
Soto-Hall's test
Spinal percussion test
Sternal compression test
Thomas' sign
Trousseau's line test

Superficial Injuries

Chest Wall Contusions

Chest wall contusions usually result from blows, falls, jamming, and allied causes. A solar-plexus inhibition of respiration is likely to be associated causing temporary shock and cyanosis. Hemoptysis is a suspicious sign of pulmonary contusion if bleeding from nose, mouth, and throat injury can be ruled out.

The Female Breast.   If mammary trauma has occurred, conduct thorough inspection and palpation. Check for consistency, elasticity, tenderness, retractions, and lumps. Tenderness suggests an underlying inflammation; malignant lesions are seldom tender. A palpable mass within breast tissue is a significant sign of an abnormality; however, while nodularity, thickening, and hardness are important signs, they should not be considered as masses. When inspection and palpation of the breasts are completed, transilluminate the breasts as a final check. If the female breast is involved in contusion, cold, support, and rest are indicated. Massage and heat are contraindi-

cated. Hematoma and fat necrosis are always a consideration, and both will present a palpable mass.

Muscle Strains and Tears

Muscle trauma and tears commonly affect the pectorals (especially disabling), serratus, intercostals, and latissimus dorsi at rib junctures. Pectoral strain is fairly unique to athletics (eg, pushups, shotput). Symptoms often mimic rib fracture, thus care should be taken to rule out fracture. Pain and tenderness may be at either the humeral tendon's attachment or origin at the lateral sternum and 1st-5th ribs. Pectoralis major tears from overly enthusiastic effort are often visible and palpable in the area of the anterior axillary fold. Pectoralis minor tears most often result from falling forward on the elbows. A firm swelling may be palpable about 2 inches below the coracoid process and is associated with a deep ache.

Management.   Strains and slight tears can be treated with rest and cold packs for 48 hours, followed by the usual physiotherapeutic measures and support. Disability subsides in several days and normal strength returns in another week if initial swelling is not severe. Graduated exercises should be initiated with careful monitoring.

Deep Injuries

Severe chest injuries in sports can include esophageal injury, tracheal or bronchial rupture, fractures of the ribs and sternum, rupture of the diaphragm, cardiopulmonary contusion, injury of the great vessels, pneumothorax, mediastinal emphysema, and numerous types of strains, sprains, and subluxations. The priority concerns are oxygen exchange, possible hemorrhage, and shock.

Obstructed Trachea or Bronchus. When this occurs, it is usually the result of the poor habit of chewing gum or tobacco during active participation to avoid a dry mouth. Another more obvious cause is a relaxed tongue during asphyxia of a supine victim.

Chest Wounds.   Chest wounds may occur in any variety of combinations. As any of them may be followed by disturbances of the pulmonary and cardiac functions which can prove fatal if not corrected, the only safe plan is to regard all chest wounds as potentially serious, however small the wound may be and however good the patient's condition may appear at first examination.

Concussions and Compressions. A nonpenetrating wound implies that trauma has not passed through the chest wall to directly damage the pleura or thoracic contents. However, while direct trauma may be confined to the chest wall, injury may indirectly involve any tissue or organ within the thoracic cavity by concussion or compression. A wound showing only slight external damage may produce serious damage within. For example, direct blows may produce a contusion on the surface of the lung. Transient hemoptysis and a roentgenographic area of consolidation may be the only signs. There may be temporary shock with small hemorrhages in the lung and the expectoration of blood. Sudden heart failure is always a danger.

Cardiac Contusion. Blows to the chest may result in hidden contusions of the heart or great vessels which may be asymptomatic initially. Developing precordial pain and possible arrhythmias should be evaluated by ECG.

Aortic Injury. Shearing-blunt injury has been shown to cause traumatic aneurysm and a fracture rupture of the aorta. This is most common in vehicular sports. Rupture usually occurs at the aortic isthmus where the arch is relatively fixed by the ligamentum arteriosum, but it sometimes occurs at the aortic root (supravalvular portion). Both sites shows relative fixation and a weak tensile strength. Roentgenography may be the first clue, with signs appearing in the mediastinal shadows and widening of the aortic outline especially at the descending arch. Symptoms are those of pressure and then hemorrhage and shock. Death occurs in 25–35% of subjects within 24 hours.

Vena Cava Injury and Traumatic Chylothorax. Symptoms and signs mimic aortic injury, but to a slightly lessened degree. Traumatic rupture of the thoracic duct is rare. A latent period of 3–4 days precedes rapid accumulation of fluid and emaciation. Aspiration helps to relieve pulmonary compression, yet mortality is high.

Injury of the Diaphragm. Potential in-

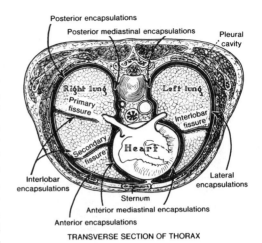

TRANSVERSE SECTION OF THORAX

CORONAL SECTION OF THORAX

Figure 24.1. Sections of thorax showing pleural reflections and anatomic location of various types of pleural collections.

volvement of the diaphragm is always a consideration in thoracic or abdominal injuries. A large opening leads to early or late diaphragmatic hernia, seen especially on the left. The symptomatic picture varies on what viscera pass through the hernial opening and whether adhesions from an old injury are present. There are usually signs of air and fluid in the chest with neck and shoulder pain due to irritation of phrenic nerve fibers. Dyspnea, shock, vomiting, and disturbed heart function are typical.

Pulmonary Contusion

Orringer reports that blunt chest injury

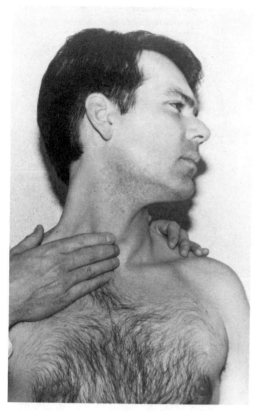

Figure 24.2. Palpating the suprasternal notch. The middle finger is placed deeply within the sternal notch to palpate for thrills and bulgings of the arch of the aorta.

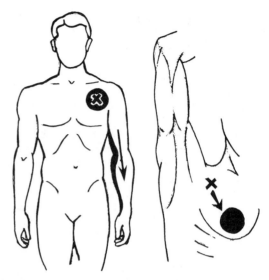

Figure 24.3. *Left*, pectoralis minor trigger point; *X*, common site. *Blackened areas* indicate typical sites of referred pain. *Right*, pectoralis major.

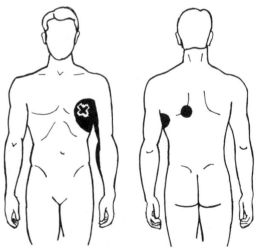

Figure 24.4. Serratus anterior trigger point; *X*, common site. *Blackened areas* indicate typical sites of referred pain.

commonly leads to pulmonary contusion, which is characterized by covert edema, reflex bronchorrhea, hemorrhage within the lung, and progressing atelectasis. This is especially true in high-velocity accidents that produce a compression-decompression injury to the chest. Physical findings in mild–moderate cases generally include a rapid respiratory and pulse rate, wet rales, and a copious cough that may be blood stained. In severe cases, hypoxia, respiratory acidosis, secondary pleurisy, and deteriorating respiratory insufficiency may lead to death in spite of heroic efforts.

Pitres' Chest Sign. The axis of the sternum is marked on the chest wall with a skin pencil, and a string is then stretched between the center of the sternal notch and the symphysis pubis. This line normally coincides with the line of the sternal axis. If this does not occur, as in cases of monola-

teral pleurisy, the angle that it forms with the sternal line indicates the degree of pleural effusion in the thorax.

Pneumothorax

Pneumothorax presents a quantity of air between the visceral and parietal layers of the pleura. Normally there is no actual space between the layers, but when air comes between them, a true space is created. If

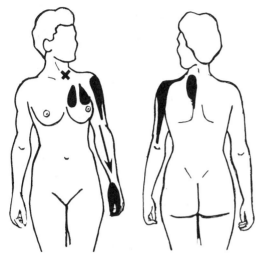

Figure 24.5. Scalene trigger point; X, common site. *Blackened areas* indicate typical sites of referred pain.

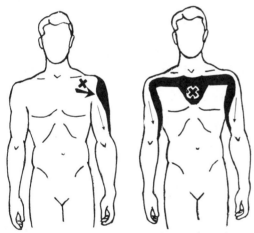

Figure 24.6. *Left*, deltoid trigger point; X, common site. *Blackened areas* indicate typical sites of referred pain. *Right*, sternalis trigger point.

enough space is created, the affected lung collapses. In athletics, it is usually the effect of a fractured clavicle or rib. In vehicular accidents especially, a bronchial tube may be ruptured at the tracheal junction from a severe suprasternal blow producing a major pneumothorax. Three types are of importance: open, tension, and spontaneous pneumothorax.

Open Pneumothorax

An open pneumothorax occurs in wounds of the chest wall that permits air to enter and leave the pleural space during respiration. A distinct sucking sound is heard at the open site as air passes through bloody froth into and out of the wound. The lung on the affected side falls away from the chest wall. During inspiration, air is drawn from this lung into the opposite lung, and the mediastinum is displaced toward the uninjured side. During expiration, air is blown from the lung on the sound side into the other lung, and the mediastinum is displaced toward the injured side. These phenomena are called paradoxical respiration because the lung on the injured side deflates on inspiration and inflates on expiration. In paradoxical respiration, the quantity of air which reaches the lungs from the atmosphere is less than normal. The air in the lungs contains an excess of carbon dioxide and a diminished proportion of oxygen because it is being rebreathed repeatedly.

Signs and Symptoms. As breathing difficulties increase, mediastinal movements become more violent, and venous return to the heart is impeded. Cardiac output is diminished, and a worsening cycle of hypoxia ensues. Signs of profuse shock become evident.

Tension Pneumothorax

In tension pneumothorax, as in the open type, air is sucked into the chest cavity through a wound in the chest wall. But in this type of pneumothorax, air does not escape through the wound because structures in or near the wound obstruct it partially or wholly to prevent air escape. Through this valve-like action in the wound, an increasing amount of air is built up on the injured side. The injured lung becomes compressed, and the mediastinum shifts to the uninjured side where it compresses the uninjured lung. It does not return to its normal position in the midline.

Signs and Symptoms. Symptoms may develop slowly. Breathing becomes difficult, air seepage causes compression of the lungs and heart, and each inspiration compresses the vital structures of the thorax more and more. Sputum and cough products may be bloody. Cyanosis becomes acute, hypoxia increases, and death from cardiac compression or anoxia may soon follow.

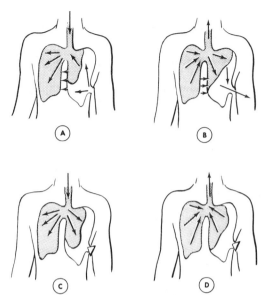

Figure 24.7. Schematic showing the effect open pneumothorax has on respiration. In *A* and *B*, note mediastinal shift with paradoxical respiration. In *C* and *D*, note effect which sealing the wound has on respiration.

Emergency Care

Make the wound airtight by sealing a sterile pressure dressing with several wide overlapping strips applied during forced exhalation. A dressing impregnated with vaseline or some other type of nonirritating lubricant is preferred to a dry dressing. If adhesive tape is not available, apply the dressing over a piece of sheet plastic or foil, cover the dressing, and bind securely with a belt. Assure an open airway and prevent or treat shock, but not in the head-low position. Having the patient lie on the affected side usually offers the best position for pain relief.

Spontaneous Pneumothorax

A person may develop a spontaneous pneumothorax during strenuous exercise or sea diving. The precipitating cause is usually a blister-like lesion of a lung's surface which ruptures and produces a major air leak. This "blep" or emphysematous bulla may be of congenital origin or follow previous infection. Symptoms may be dramatic or develop slowly as tension develops. Surgical correction is necessary. About 30% of the cases experience a recurrence.

RIB AND STERNAL INJURIES
Contusions and Sprains

Rib Contusions. Impacts on the free ends of the floating ribs painfully involve related muscles. Pain and disability are severe and often beyond the control of conservative measures. Both movement and breathing aggravate and prolong disability, even during bed rest. Concomitant kidney damage must be ruled out. Competitive activity should not be resumed until gradual exercises include vigorous running and twisting motions without discomfort.

Costosternal Sprains and Separations. Rib cartilages may be ruptured at the costosternal junctions which are often impossible to view during roentgenography. Symptoms frequently mimic a gallbladder disorder or gastric ulcer. Management is the same as that for rib fracture, but pain is usually not as severe. A shoulder dislocation may be associated. A rib belt often corrects pain in a few days, but healing may take several weeks because of the relative avascularity of cartilage. If conservative strapping and sprain therapy do not afford relief, excision may be required to remove a cartilage fragment.

Costosternal Subluxation-Fixations

Articular fixations at the costosternal articulations can produce hypermobility in the related thoracic vertebrae. This is usually manifested as an increased spread of the spinous processes on full flexion. However, if a costosternal area is in a state of fixation and the corresponding anterior longitudinal ligament is in a state of shortening, the local area will be forced into an exaggerated state of kyphosis even in the erect position. In addition, the hinge joint between the manubrium and the body of the sternum is normally active in forced breathing and extreme A-P movements. Fixation at this joint will restrict these motions. Such fixations are frequently mobilized spontaneously during an upper dorsal adjustment directed anteriorly of a prone patient.

Anterior Rib Pit Fixations

Anterior rib fixations resulting in decreased chest excursion can be determined by motion palpation of the thoracic cage during deep inspiration with the patient either standing or supine. Traction the skin of the lateral thorax towards the midline with broad bilateral palmar contacts and place your thumbs near the sternum on the rib being examined. As the patient inhales deeply, note if both thumbs move equally. Thumb motion restricted unilaterally suggests the side of fixation. Once identified, a general rib mobilization technique with and without traction on the ipsilateral iliac crest or shoulder can then be applied on the angles of the ribs involved to loosen restrictions.

Anterior Rib Pit Subluxation

This condition features a vague dull or sharp pain over the parasternal area at the costosternal junction. Some anterior intercostal neuralgia may be involved. One or more of the upper three ribs are most frequently involved.

Adjustment. Stand about perpendicular to the supine patient on the opposite side of the subluxation. With your cephalad hand, take a pisiform contact over the anteriorly subluxated rib slightly lateral to the sternum. Place your caudal stabilizing hand under the patient's scapula so that upward traction can be made during correction. Apply medial and slightly inferior traction with your stabilizing hand while your contact hand makes a light pushing-type thrust at the end of patient expiration, laterally and slightly superior to follow the curve of the rib. It frequently helps to have the patient internally rotate his ipsilateral humerus during the adjustment.

Alternative Adjustment Procedure. This is a slight adaptation of the adjustment for an anterior medial clavicular subluxation (which see) where contact is made on the medial rib angle rather than the medial clavicle.

Intercostal Fixations

Palpation should reveal opening posteriorly during flexion, anteriorly during extension, on the convex side during lateral bending, and on the side opposite to the direction of vertebral body rotation. If the intercostal muscles are in a state of hypertonicity, the ribs will abnormally appose and the thoracic cage will exhibit an area of lateral flattening that restricts mobility on contralateral bending. The patient will assume a somewhat "hunched" posture in the neutral position, depending upon the extent of fixation. The fixations are best determined laterally near the rib angles.

Rib Fractures

Most rib fractures are highly painful even if slight because movements cause constant grating of highly innervated fracture endings. Both displaced fractures and stress cracks may be found. A fracture may communicate with the skin or the pleura and other thoracic contents. Cellular emphysema is always a common complication but often disappears spontaneously. The longest and most prominent ribs (5th–9th) are those most fractured. The upper ribs are better protected; the lower ribs are more mobile and more susceptible.

Signs and Symptoms

Diagnosis must frequently be made without the classic signs. The history, pain, and point tenderness are the best clues. If present, pain is felt most sharply on inspiration or coughing. Localized tenderness is usually evident, the break can sometimes be felt with the fingers, and crepitus may be exhibited. However, crepitus is absent if the fracture is incomplete or if fragments override. Because ribs are highly mobile, preternatural mobility has little value. Broken ribs make excellent knives; if the lung is punctured, the patient may cough up bright, red, frothy blood. Roentgenographic evidence may be obvious or nonconclusive. If a case presents no evidence on film, but pain, disability, and dyspnea persist for a few days and a localized periostitis is apparent, treat as a fracture.

Roentgenographic Considerations. Rib fractures are usually obvious but may be missed within overlapping axillary shadows. Fracture of the costal cartilage may be invisible unless partially calcified. Breaks run obliquely or irregularly where calcification has not yet occurred. In seeking signs of rib fracture, one should not overlook careful evaluation of the costospinal junction (often associated with costovertebral subluxation) or the costosternal junction. Except for the very high or low ribs, ruptured costotransverse ligaments from a severe blow may lead to superior subluxation of the ribs. Numerous injuries occur in wrestling, but few show radiographic evidence. One common injury visible on film is that of rib fracture.

Golfer's Fractures. Some rib fractures are peculiar to certain sports. For example, novice golfers who complain of pain and discomfort in the upper back near the shoulder may present "golfer's fractures." This injury usually involves multiple mid ribs (4th–7th) in the posterior. Right-handed golfers exhibit left-sided fractures, and vice versa.

Management

Due to respiratory and cardiac movements, fractured ribs are difficult and dangerous to immobilize. Strapping must be limited to one side and not cover the entire cage as encircling will restrict compensatory diaphragmatic and accessory muscle action. Shave the mature skin, cover the nipple with a gauze pad, and paint the area with benzoin. Each strap must be applied after forced expiration in an oblique fashion, anchored high behind and low in front to follow rib curve, for several inches above and below the fracture. Straps should be changed once a week for 3–4 weeks. Injuries to top ribs require a sling to immobilize the ipsilateral shoulder. In multiple rib injury below the 4th rib, the canvas rib belt with adjustable buckles and shoulder support has proved its merit. Activity can be resumed with padding in 3–4 weeks if there is no separation, but separated ends require termination of participation for the season as a safeguard against visceral puncture.

Hemothorax. Rib fractures may cut intercostal vessels, and quick surgery is necessary. There will be signs of fluid in the pleural space. With hyperresonance and breath sounds above the fluid level plus a contralaterally shifted trachea, an even more serious hemopneumothorax may be present.

Fat-Embolism Syndrome. This syndrome usually occurs within 3 days after fracture. It is a limited pulmonary state of tachycardia, dyspnea, petechial hemorrhages, and disturbances of consciousness. A platelet count below 150,000, urine fat,

and increased serum lipase are typical. Roentgenography may show patchy pulmonary infiltrates. For emergency care, provide respiratory support, treat for shock, and refer for hospitalization. Oxygen support and corticosteroids may be necessary to assist ventilation and diminish the inflammatory pulmonary changes.

Sternal Injuries

Any injury strong enough to fracture the sternum is likely to produce severe damage to underlying parts with cardiac tamponade and/or arrhythmias that will demand priority. A flail sternum, which may require ventilatory assistance and intubation, features paradoxical movement of the sternum inward with inspiration and outward with expiration. Developing tension pneumothorax is a possibility.

Slight sternal fractures or those of the costal cartilages are most difficult to view on roentgenography except with elaborate techniques. The tenderness from a sternal bone bruise even without major damage lingers for an abnormally long time. Xiphisternal sprains are sometimes seen which are also persistently annoying and difficult to treat because of irritation from rectus activity. In rare instances, especially in somersaulting gymnastics, the manubrium may be ruptured from its attachments.

Pectoralis Flexibility Test. With the patient placed supine and the hands clasped behind the head, the elbows are allowed to slowly lower laterally toward the table. If the elbows do not approximate the tabletop, shortening (eg, spasm, inflexibility, contracture) of the pectoralis group is indicated.

DORSAL SPINE INJURIES

Assessment follows the same procedures used for the cervical spine; ie, inspection, palpation, and percussion if indicated. Observe function during gait and other movements for carriage, deformities, and functional deficiencies.

Biomechanical Considerations

It would be an error to consider the thoracic spine biomechanically apart from the rib cage. The attached ribs, although individually quite flexible, offer increased stiffness and strength to the vertebral segments, and the thoracic spine's moment of inertia is increased by the rib cage that also increases the area's stiffness against torques and bending moments. The stiffness property of the thoracic spine is decreased at least in half in all loading directions once the ribs are removed.

Spinal movements in the thorax are relatively limited as compared to the cervical area, especially in the upper regions, due to the restrictions imposed by the costovertebral and costotransverse articulations, the direction and shape of the articular facets, the relatively thin discs, and the tension of the ligamentum flava. Movement of the thoracic spine cannot occur in any direction without the involved vertebrae somewhat carrying their attached ribs with them.

Several unique factors should be considered in regard to stability of the thoracic spine. The major points are that it (1) is stiffer, (2) is less mobile, (3) has a smaller vertebral canal, (4) has a high incidence of cord damage associated with structural damage, (5) exhibits less vascularity for the cord, (6) has restricting costal articulations, (7) has an increased moment of inertia because of the added thoracic cage, (8) has an anatomic curvature directed posteriorly, (9) tends to be clinically unstable during flexion, (10) has relatively thin discs, (11) is a common site for bursting anterior centrum fractures (lower region only), (12) has the nuclei more centered within the anuli, (13) has thicker yellow ligaments, (14) has thinner and looser apophyseal capsules, (15) has thinner and weaker interspinous ligaments, (16) has a great resistance to extension, (17) possesses coupling variants from top to bottom, and (18) is the major source of supply of sympathetic fibers.

Common Mechanisms of Injury

Knowledge of the mechanism of injury focuses attention on the tissues most likely to be injured:

1. Anterior compression injuries commonly occur during flexion as this position affords maximum protection to the face and vital organs. The normal thoracic kyphosis places the spine in flexion during the neutral position; thus even axial forces produce greater forces anteriorly than posteriorly.

The most severe bending moment is at the apex of the kyphosis. When the thorax is flexed, compression forces distributed anteriorly are four times stronger than those distributed to the posterior elements. The nucleus serves as a fulcrum when forces are not centered.

2. The vertebral arch and posterior ligament complex are usually injured in severe hyperflexion that stretches the posterior elements or in vertical loading. This usually occurs secondary to anterior injury. A degree of torsion is also frequently involved. Roaf showed that it is almost impossible to tear the posterior ligament complex in pure flexion or the anterior longitudinal ligament in pure extension but quite easy to do either if torsion or horizontal shear are added. The most severe forces occur at the thoracolumbar transition.

3. Isolated fractures are sometimes seen in the posterior elements. Fractures of the upper thoracic spinous processes are usually the result of shoveling, severe cervical hyperextension, or a direct blow. They most frequently occur at the thoracocervical area. Fractures of the lower transverse processes are frequently associated with a direct blow from the posterior or to the flank where a violent contraction of the quadratus lumborum occurs. An isolated fracture of an articular process is usually the result of severe lateral flexion with rotation about the long axis of the spine so that leverage is exerted against the jammed processes. Isolated fractures of the vertebral arch are extremely rare.

Scoliosis

Scoliosis is classified into three major types (nonstructural, transient structural, and structural), and each has its subdivisions according to its major etiology. Only the nonstructural and transient types are significant in athletics, with the exception of traumatic structural scoliosis which may have a vertebral origin (eg, fracture, subluxation/fixation, surgery) or extravertebral origin (eg, burns, surgery).

Adams' Test. If the patient has an S or C scoliosis, note if the scoliosis straightens when the spine is flexed forward. If it does, it is a negative sign and evidence of a functional scoliosis. A positive sign is noted when the scoliosis is not improved, thus evidence of a pathologic scoliosis.

Basic Biomechanics of Thoracic Scoliosis

Scoliosis is an obvious mechanical disorder when gross, but there are always many biologic influences operating as well as purely mechanical forces. When relatively straight, the spine behaves much like a column. When deformed, it becomes subject to bending loads and behaves more like a bending beam than it does a column. In either case, however, and unlike engineered columns of uniform size and homogeneous materials, the effects of spinal loading on a biped are much more complex to understand or to predict via the laws of physics.

When a postural distortion is recognized, several clinical questions arise. For example, how severe is the distortion? Is it affecting function? Is the distortion stabilized or progressing? What was the initial cause or causes: acquired, congenital, pathologic, or a combination of factors? Can it be corrected? If so, how? How much correction can be expected? How long will it take? How much patient cooperation will be necessary? The first step in answering these questions is a holistic postural evaluation.

Scoliosis frequently begins in the midthoracic area. In lateral flexion of a healthy spine, the upper thoracic vertebral bodies are normally coupled to rotate toward the concavity, the lower bodies rotate toward the convexity, and the transitional midthoracic vertebrae tend to be fixed by the rotary forces above and below. However, there is frequently a normal physiologic curve to the right in the midthoracic area, attributed to the aorta. If this curve becomes exaggerated, there is a tendency for lumbar-like coupling in the midthoracic vertebrae in which rotation is to the *convexity*. This can initiate a series of adverse biomechanical events. The involved epiphyses, end plates, anuli, nuclei, and apophyseal joints are put under asymmetrical loading, the lateral paravertebral muscles and ligaments become imbalanced, and the effect is progression to distinct scoliosis.

White feels that the determining factor of this biomechanical syndrome is when the focal midthoracic vertebra rotates (ie, clinically subluxates) towards convexity rather than to the concavity of the lateral physiologic curve. The axial rotation of idiopathic scoliosis appears to invariably be into the convexity of the lateral curve. The precipitating cause is usually subluxated facets from intrinsic trauma (eg, unilateral muscular stress) whereafter the motion unit becomes fixed, but it could also occur from reflex, vascular, lymphatic, or chemical irregularities or from myotonic malfunction.

Lovett's Principles

An understanding of Lovett's principles and the basic types of lumbar scolioses offers insight into distortion analysis. Lovett's basic principle states that if the base of a weight-bearing segmented column such as the spine is caused to tilt (eg, unilateral anteroinferior sacral base subluxation), the center of weight bearing will shift toward the high side of the base because it is the shortest distance between the point of weight origin and weight reception. The involved segments will then seek to escape the load by shifting and rotating to the opposite side.

Lovett Positive Scoliosis. In a Lovett positive scoliosis, the axis of vertebral rotation in the lumbar area is posterior to the articulating processes. When the segments are asymmetrically loaded, the bodies of the involved segments normally deviate farther from the midline than their spinous processes. If a Lovett positive scoliosis occurs that is far more than that demanded by the base inferiority, the condition is referred to as an *excessive Lovett positive*. This state is usually attributed to an iliopsoas spasm on the side of concavity that accentuates the curve beyond the norm.

Lovett Negative Scoliosis. If a lumbar scoliosis shows that the spinous processes have deviated from the midline farther than the vertebral bodies, the condition is said to be atypical (negative). A negative scoliosis is indicative of marked muscle involvement. The common causes of this muscle involvement are: (1) muscle spasm associated with facet irritation (eg, jamming, instability); (2) disturbed or incompatible movement dynamics (eg, subluxation, fixation); (3) local unilateral muscle contraction as the result of noxious viscerosomatic reflexes (eg, viscera pathology); (4) antalgic splinting, resulting in scoliotic deviations whose transverse planes are almost completely horizontal. If left uncorrected, such antalgic curves will eventually produce a secondary sacroiliac distortion that will compromise normal lumbopelvic dynamics.

Illi describes three basic types of Lovett negative scolioses:

1. A scoliotic state where there is very little rotation of the vertebral segments, as shown by the midline position of the spinous processes. In the lumbar spine, it frequently indicates unilateral shortening (ie, spasm, hypertonicity, or contracture) of the iliopsoas on the side of convexity or of the contralateral multifidi.

2. A scoliotic state where the lumbar spinous processes have distinctly deviated farther from the midline than the vertebral bodies. This is indicative of acute muscle contraction, usually involving the multifidi and/or rotatores on the side of convexity.

3. A scoliotic state where the spine is fairly axially aligned when a compensatory scoliotic deviation should be expected because of an inferior-base. This abnormal state may be in the thoracic-lumbar relationship, lumbar-pelvic relationship, or both. Janse gives the example of a right lumbar scoliosis where there is failure of a left compensatory dorsal scoliosis to develop because of hypertonicity of the deep right thoracic musculature resulting from chronic reflex irritation arising from an inflamed gallbladder or some other viscerosomatic reflex. A scoliosis is sometimes seen where the degree of lumbar deviation is far less than that which would be expected by the degree of pelvic tilt. The usual cause for this is antalgic lumbar splinting, but a viscerosomatic reflex (eg, iliocecal syndrome, ovarian cyst) should not be overlooked.

Thoracic Strains

Upper Dorsal Strain

This upper trapezius strain syndrome, often labeled cervical fibrositis, is found in patients who have a forward head and round upper back. The compensatory head position is associated with a slumped and rounded upper back resulting in fixated hyperextension of the cervical spine.

Signs and Symptoms. Undue compression posteriorly on the facets of the vertebrae is characteristic. The clinical picture is one of posterior neck pain, stretch-weakness of anterior neck flexors, and tenderness of the upper dorsal transverse processes. Tension of the neck extensors, including the upper trapezius and cervical spine erectors, causes a constant fatigue and ache in the back of the neck. The patient frequently flexes the neck in an attempt to gain relief. The apparent impingement of the suboccipital nerves as they emerge through the fascial and muscular features at the base of the skull may account for associated occipital headaches.

Scapulocostal Syndrome

In this myofascial-periostitis, the trigger area is at the site of the attachment of the levator scapula muscle to the upper medial angle of the scapula. The mechanism is postural and tension traction of the attachment site.

Signs and Symptoms. Pain is located in the upper interscapular area and assumed to be between the medial border of the blade and the underlying rib cage. The onset is insidious. Discomfort may radiate to the (1) neck and occiput, (2) upper triceps and deltoid insertions, (3) around the chest to the anterior, or (4) medial forearm and/or the hands and fingers where numbness and tingling are sites of complaint. The course is chronic and characterized by remissions and exacerbations.

Comolli's Sign. Shortly after trauma to the upper posterior thorax, a triangular swelling may develop in the region of the involved scapula due to an accumulation of blood anteriorly and posteriorly to the scapula. For anatomic reasons, the blood cannot escape; hence, a cushion-like swelling develops more or less corresponding to the outline of the scapula and may persist for several days. This sign, which can be confused with an intramuscular hematoma (eg, rhomboideus major, infraspinatus, trapezius) is especially helpful in the physical diagnosis of fracture of the surgical neck and body of the scapula.

Middle and Lower Dorsal Strain

A painful upper-back condition results from gradual and continuous tension on the middle and lower trapezius muscle (a stretch-weakness condition). The chief problem is one of excessive tension on the posterior muscles. There is also a problem of undue compression on the anterior surfaces of the bodies of the dorsal spine with an increased kyphotic curvature and a depression of the rib cage. Common causes are habitual posture of forward (round) shoulders and rounded upper back, over-development of the anterior shoulder girdle muscles with shortening, or heavy breasts that are not adequately supported. Reflex vasoconstriction in the muscles may prevent normal adaptation to use.

Signs and Symptoms. This state of chronic muscle strain is rarely associated with an acute onset, but the symptoms may reach a point of severe pain after sports activity. The clinical picture is characterized by soreness and fatigue, progressing to a burning sensation within the course of the middle and lower trapezius. Traction of the muscle on bony attachments may cause complaints of an isolated sore spot. Because of this, palpation may elicit pain or acute tenderness in the region of the dorsolumbar attachment of the lower trapezius.

Dorsal Spine Sprains

Acute traumatic spondylitis may follow contusions or wrenching of the spinal column. As in sprains of other joints, the symptoms are pain, tenderness, and reflex muscular rigidity which limits function. Symptoms may appear immediately after injury or not become apparent for a few hours or days. Diagnosis is based upon history, physical findings, and x-ray to exclude fracture and destructive lesions.

Management. During the acute hyperemic stage, structural alignment, cold, strapping or bracing, positive galvanism, ultrasound, and rest are indicated. After 48 hours, passive congestion may be managed by light massage, gentle passive manipulation, sinusoidal stimulation, ultrasound, and a mild range of motion exercise initiated. During the stage of consolidation, local moderate heat, moderate active exercise, motorized alternating traction, moderate range of motion manipulation, and ultrasound are beneficial. In the stage of fibroblastic activity, deep heat, deep massage, vigorous active exercise, motorized alternating traction, negative galvanism, ultrasound, and active joint manipulation speed recovery and inhibit postinjury effects.

Vertebral Subluxation-Fixation. Dorsal vertebral subluxations and/or fixations are attended the same as in general practice, but the athletic subluxation is more commonly associated with acute symptoms of paravertebral strain and sprain. Leverage adjustive technics on the medial transverse processes are preferred to pisiform recoil corrections with a spinous process contact. Because of the athlete's heavy musculature, heat prior to correction is necessary, as a rule, to relieve spasm unless acute symptoms make this contraindicated.

Thoracic Disc Herniation. Thoracic disc herniation is the least common of any spinal region. It occurs predominantly in males over 50 years of age, most likely occurring in the T11–T12 area. The clinical picture is one of relative pain, usually unilateral in chronic cases or bilateral in acute cases, with girdle-like distribution. Pain may radiate to the abdomen, flank, or groin. Spastic paraparesis with sensory complaints may be involved. Bowel and bladder incontinence and impotence are rarely associated. Motion restriction and tenderness on percussion may be the only local physical signs. Hyperactive tendon reflexes in the lower extremity and a positive Babinski are sometimes seen. Differentiation must be made from intercostal neuralgia, ankylosing spondylitis, metastatic or intramedullary spinal cord tumors, neurofibroma, disc-space infection, or viscerosomatic reflexes.

Costovertebral and Costotransverse Subluxations

These subluxations are featured by misalignment of the costal processes in relation to the vertebral bodies and transverse processes independent of vertebral motor-unit subluxation (ie, primary) or misalignment of the costal processes in relation to the vertebral bodies and transverse processes as a result of vertebral motor-unit subluxation (ie, secondary). They present painful, difficult and/or restricted respiratory movements of the ribs, shearing stress to the capsular ligaments and synovia, induction of a vertebral motor unit subluxation and/

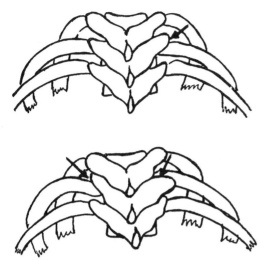

Figure 24.8. *Top*, site of a primary costoverte-bral-costotransverse subluxation. *Bottom*, site of secondary costovertebral-costotransverse subluxation.

or contribute to the chronicity of a subluxation, induction of spinal curvatures and/or contribute to the chronicity of curvatures present, and irritation of the sympathetic ganglia and rami communicantes. Vague terms such as pleurodynia or intercostal fibrositis are often used in medical literature.

Signs and Symptoms

The unilateral pain, which may be either stabbing or dull and usually episodic, may be expressed centrally and/or intercostally. The onset is usually rapid following a fall, push, misstep, stretch, sneeze, or cough. Transient but sharp neuralgia, angina, or dyspnea may be reported. Tenderness, intercostal spasm, and resistance are found at the rib angle and/or near the vertebral or sternal attachments. Midrib subluxation frequently presents pain radiating down the lateral arm to mimic a scapulocostal syndrome. Symptoms are frequently aggravated during deep inspiration when the trunk is flexed. Compressing the rib cage increases pain in fracture and sprain but not in intercostal strain. Springing the ribs P-A of the prone and relaxed patient to create stress at the vertebral connections aggravates symptoms and causes an immediate apprehensive muscle-guarding response in

sprain and subluxation. Overreaction makes one suspicious of a hidden fatigue fracture.

Unilateral asymmetry may be palpated inferior to the axilla by noting that one rib is unusually medial to the one above or below, indicating some type of detraction mechanism is involved. Maurer points out that, in the nonscoliotic thoracic spine, detraction from the marginal line usually implies the existence of rotation alterations of the vertebral body to which the rib is attached (subluxation), flexion alteration of the same, or alteration of the costovertebral or costotransverse articulation. Detraction would obviously involve numerous soft-tissue changes also.

To determine the exact site and direction of subluxation, Schoenholtz recommends that the patient be examined seated. Stand behind and ask the patient to laterally flex away from the painful side while lifting the ipsilateral arm over the head to open the ribs. As this is done, place your fingertips under the lower border of the suspected rib and push upward, then on the superior border and exert downward pressure. Pain will be increased in the direction of subluxation.

Superior First Rib Head Subluxation

Of all rib head subluxations, those of the short, acutely curved 1st rib are the most common. The next in incidence are the 2nd, 5th, and 6th ribs, respectively, according to Schultz. Palpation is aided if the patient's scapula is adducted.

The 1st rib is frequently subluxated superiorly when lower cervical compression tests are positive (eg, scalenus anticus syndrome), in cervicobrachial neuralgias, and in various neurovascular shoulder girdle, arm, and hand syndromes. Superior subluxation obviously narrows the costoclavicular space and places traction on the neurovascular bundle. It can also be the primary or a contributing factor in torticollis, herpes zoster, and vague anginal or breast aches. The 1st rib has no transverse articulation, only a small round articular facet with the body of T1. A superior 1st rib subluxation is frequently associated with quadratus lumborum muscle weakness and/or levator costorum and scaleni muscle spasm. The displacement mechanism is usually initiated by pushing with the elbows locked.

Adjustment. With the patient supine, stand on the ipsilateral side of the involved rib, facing caudally. With your lateral hand, take an open-web contact near the involved rib's crest that is high on your lateral index finger, with your thumb anterior and your fingers posterior to the patient's chest. The point of contact is about 4–5 inches lateral to T1 spinous. Your stabilizing palm is cupped over the patient's contralateral ear with the fingers supporting the occiput. To relax the ipsilateral neck muscles, raise the patient's neck several inches with your stabilizing fingers and let the occiput extend into your palm. Rotate the patient's head 20–30° away from the subluxation, and make a moderate thrust inferiorly and slightly posteromedially towards T4.

Alternative Adjustment Procedure. With the patient prone, stand on the ipsilateral side of the involved rib facing the patient's contralateral shoulder. With your lateral hand, take an open-web contact on the rib's crest that is high on your lateral index finger as above. Your lateral elbow will be flexed and pointing superior-lateral as you lean over the patient. A palm contact is made with your stabilizing hand on the patient's lateral occiput above the ear on the opposite side of involvement. With your stabilizing hand, slightly extend the patient's head and rotate it away from the involved rib. Apply slight lateral flexion to relax the ipsilateral muscles, and make a thrust with your contact hand that is directed inferomedial towards T4.

Inferior Second-Seventh Rib Head Subluxation

Palpation will reveal increased intercostal space above and decreased space below the rib which has subluxated inferiorly to its vertebra. Inferoextension displacements are infrequent in comparison to superoflexion subluxations, taking much greater force to correct. They are more common at the lower ribs, with local pain which often radiates to the abdomen and splinting lateral flexion on the contralateral side.

Adjustment. With the patient prone, stand on the ipsilateral side of the involved rib, facing cephally. With your lateral hand, take a thumb-ball contact just below the inferior border of the subluxated rib between the rib's tubercle and angle. Your contact-hand fingers will overlap the scapula. With your medial stabilizing hand, take a soft pisiform contact over your contact thumb. Apply traction superiorly to tighten the overlying tissues and to bring your contact thumb directly on the inferior border of the involved rib. Ask the patient to take a deep breath and to exhale deeply. At the end of expiration, make a short, moderate, recoil anterosuperior thrust by quickly extending your elbows.

Superior Second-Seventh Rib Head Subluxation

Palpation reveals increased intercostal space below and decreased space above the rib which has subluxated superiorly to its vertebra.

Adjustment. This is essentially the opposite of a rib listed as inferior. With the patient prone, stand above the ipsilateral side of the involved rib, facing caudally. With your lateral hand, a thumb contact is made slightly above the superior border of the involved rib at the rib's angle. With your medial stabilizing hand, make a pisiform contact over your contact thumb. Apply traction inferiorly to tighten the overlying tissues and to bring your contact thumb directly onto the rib's superior edge. At the end of patient expiration, make a short, moderate, recoil thrust directed anteroinferiorly.

Costovertebral Fixations

The articulation between the rib head and vertebral body or between the rib tubercle and the transverse process is a common site of fixation, commonly due to serratus and/or levator costarum hypertonicity. Gillet believes this type of fixation is contributed to by capsular shortening that allows enough torsion for unrestricted breathing during nondemanding activities. Associated adhesion-type bands could very easily irritate an entrapped sympathetic ganglia during normal motion. Costovertebral fixations are rarely complete. They usually tend to restrict mobility in one or more directions but not in all directions.

Posterior Rib Head Fixations

Posterior rib fixations resulting in decreased chest excursion can be determined by motion palpation of the thoracic cage during deep inspiration with the patient either standing or prone. Traction the skin of the lateral thorax towards the spine with broad bilateral palmar contacts and place your thumbs near the dorsal midline on the rib being examined. As the patient inhales deeply, note if both thumbs move equally. Thumb motion restricted unilaterally suggests the side of fixation. Once identified, a general rib-mobilization technique with and without traction on the ipsilateral iliac crest or shoulder can then be applied on the angles of the rib or ribs involved to loosen restrictions. This should be followed by a regimen of heat and graduated stretching exercises.

"Bucket-Handle" Complications

Costovertebral and costotransverse subluxations, and less frequently costosternal subluxations, are frequently complicated by reflex spasms in the thoracic cage. Hypertonicity of the scalene group, levator costarum, cervical longissimus, cervical and thoracic iliocostalis, and/or serratus posterior superior tends to raise and displace the upper ribs superiorly. On the other hand, hypertonicity of the thoracic longissimus, lumbar iliocostalis, and/or serratus posterior inferior tends to depress and displace the lower ribs inferiorly. Such attending hypertonicities or weakness of the antagonists should be corrected prior to structural adjustment, or the structural adjustment will not hold.

Vertebral Fractures

Dorsal fractures most frequently occur at the T12–L1 level, next in the midthoracic region. Most dorsal spine fractures are compression fractures with collapse of a vertebral body. They are rare in sports except for vehicular accidents. Midthoracic fractures generally result from falls on the pelvis or when the head is severely forced between the knees. Fortunately, neurologic damage and severe disability are rare. Adequate management can usually be provided by bed rest followed by extension exercises to strengthen the muscles. A light brace or corset should be worn when the patient is ambulated.

Nonsports-related fracture of the thorax may also occur during convulsions. Fractures resulting from seizures usually occur in the T5–T8 region.

Soto-Hall Test. This test is primarily employed when fracture of a vertebra is suspected. The patient is placed on his back without pillows. Place one hand on the sternum of the patient, and exert a slight pressure to prevent flexion at either the lumbar or thoracic regions of the spine. Your other hand is placed under the patient's occiput, then the head is slowly flexed toward the chest. Flexion of the head and neck upon the chest progressively produces a pull on the posterior spinous ligaments from above, and when the spinous process of the injured vertebra is reached, an acute local pain is experienced by the patient.

Spinal Percussion Test. With the seated patient in the forward flexed position, the examiner percusses the spinous process of the involved area. Induced pain suggests intervertebral sprain, fracture, acute subluxation, IVD lesion, or dislocation. If negative, the paravertebral soft tissues (about 1–2 inches lateral) are percussed. Induced pain suggests strain, radiculitis, transverse process fracture, or a costovertebral lesion.

Roentgenographic Considerations

Fracture lines are difficult to recognize within vertebral bodies. They are usually the result of considerable violence such as sudden extreme flexion, heavy crushing injuries, or extreme muscular exertion. Abnormalities in outlines and relations with neighboring vertebrae are the usual findings, especially in the lateral view.

There are two general types, compression fractures and comminuted fractures:

1. Compression fractures vary from a single slight irregularity in the anterior or lateral margins of the body similar to a longbone torus fracture, to a complete collapse of a portion of the vertebral body. Milder forms are usually asymptomatic, but there may be persistent local tenderness. Chronic vertebral compression forces such as in trampolining or horseback riding are usually diagnosed without difficulty except for the

active adolescent with endplate irregularities. Vertebral margin irregularities usually point to old trauma or infection.

2. Comminuted fractures are the result of greater trauma in which the vertebra is severely shattered either by direct violence or by another vertebra impacting it.

In comparison to vertebral body fractures, fractures of the neural arch including the articular processes are more disabling because of the nerve irritation increased by motion. Demonstration of a definite break is often most difficult in the thoracic region, but callus formation offers indirect evidence. Unlike vertebral bodies, the posterior aspects readily form callus which becomes calcified in a few weeks. Severe acute traumatic subluxation may call attention to a subtle fracture.

Fractures of the transverse processes are usually multiple among adjacent vertebrae, but single processes may be broken by a blow from a sharp object. A slight callus can be expected, and fibrous union sometimes develops. The black lines formed by muscle shadows crossing transverse processes should not be confused with fracture. Muscle lines are smooth, are straight, and extend beyond the bony margins.

Traumatic lesions are sometimes difficult to distinguish from infectious lesions. Traumatic lesions usually show a substantial portion of the intervening disc still present, while the disc commonly disappears or thins greatly in infection. The infectious process is frequently accompanied by a paravertebral abscess.

Ankylosis

Chest Expansion Test. With the patient standing, chest measurements are taken around the circumference of the thorax near the nipple level; first after the patient inhales and then after the patient exhales completely. A 2-inch difference (possibly less in females) is a negative sign. A positive sign is indicated by no or very little difference in measurements—a suspicion of osteoarthritic ankylosis or ankylosing spondylitis. Roentgenography offers confirmatory evidence.

Forestier's Bowstring Sign. The patient in the upright position is asked to bend laterally, first to one side and then to the other. Normally, the contralateral paravertebral muscles will bulge because of the normal coupling rotation of the lumbar spine (exhibited by the spinous processes pointing to the ipsilateral side of lateral flexion). However, in ankylosing spondylitis (Marie-Strumpell's disease) or a state of extensive spinal fixation, the musculature will appear to bulge greater on the side of the curve's concavity.

Lewin's Supine Test. This test is identical to Chapman's test, except that Lewin believes a positive sign is indicative of an ankylosing dorsolumbar lesion. The patient is placed supine, and the examiner fixes the patient's extended knees firmly against the table top. The patient is then instructed to attempt to sit up without utilizing the hands. Inability to do so constitutes a positive sign.

Pathologic Considerations

Scheuermann's Disease. Osteochondrosis of the vertebral plates is commonly associated with backache and round shoulders in adolescents. It can be asymptomatic and is unlikely to be associated with sports injury except when activity results in a superimposed injury. This growth disturbance of the vertebral epiphyseal ring results in deformity of the vertebral end plate with formation of Schmorl's nodes, vertebral body wedging, and a smooth kyphosis. Tight hamstrings are often associated. Unless symptoms and signs are severe, corrective adjustments and therapeutic exercises will allow continued sports participation.

Spinal Meningitis. Two physical tests are helpful in supporting a suspicion of meningitis. (1) *Brudzinski's Test*: A positive sign is elicited when the patient's head is passively flexed toward the chest and this is followed by involuntary flexion of the lower limbs. Such a reaction is indicative of meningeal irritation. In such cases, the neck is rigid and painful to flexion and, in most cases, also to rotation. This test is unreliable in children before 2 years of age. (2) *Trousseau's Line Test*: This sign of meningitis consists of a bright red line produced where the finger is drawn across the trunk or forehead.

Spinal Tumors. A test can be performed by having the patient sit or recline while you hold digital pressure over the jugular veins from 30–45 seconds (*Naffziger's test*).

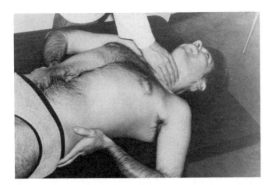

Figure 24.9. Naffziger's jugular compression test.

See Figure 24.9. The patient is then instructed to cough deeply. Pain following the distribution of a nerve may indicate nerve root compression. Though more commonly used for low back involvements, thoracic and cervical root compression may also be aggravated. Local pain in the spine does not positively indicate nerve compression; it may indicate the site of a strain, sprain, or another lesion. The sign is almost always positive in the presence of cord tumors, particularly spinal meningiomas. The resulting increased spinal fluid pressure above the tumor causes the growth to compress or pull upon sensory structures to produce radicular pain. The test is contraindicated in geriatrics and extreme care should be taken with anyone suspected of having atherosclerosis. In all cases, the patient should be alerted that jugular pressure may result in vertigo.

ABDOMINAL INJURIES

After abdominal injury, thorough inspection, light and deep palpation, percussion succussion, and auscultation should be conducted in an unhurried fashion (see Table 24.2).

Miscellaneous Reflexes and Signs

Abdominal Reflexes. Contractions above the navel on sharp downard friction of the abdominal wall indicate normal activity of the spinal cord from the 8th to the 12th thoracic nerves. An absent reflex could indicate the following defective arc: upper-quadrant reflex absent, T5–T8; midquadrant reflex absent, T9–T11; lower quadrant reflex

Table 24.2
Review of Some Clinical Maneuvers, Reflexes, Signs, or Tests Relative to Abdominal Injuries and Posttraumatic Disorders

Barkman's reflex
Beevor's sign
Chapman's test
Cope's test
Epigastric reflex
Glenard's test
Light touch/pain tests
Murphy's biliary tract sign
Murphy's punch test
Muscle strength grading
Obliquus reflex
Pende's reflex

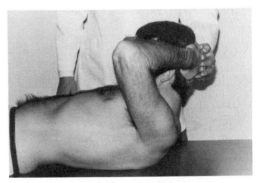

Figure 24.10. Evaluating the presence of Beevor's sign.

absent, T11–T12; all sites diminished or absent, suspect of upper motor neuron involvement. Abdominal reflexes are normally diminished or absent in the obese and the elderly.

Epigastric Reflex. This contraction of the abdominal muscles is caused by stimulating the skin of the epigastrium or over the 5th and 6th intercostal spaces near the axilla.

Beevor's Sign. Examiner notes position of umbilicus when patient tenses his abdominal muscles as in trying to rise from a supine position with the hands behind the head. Movement of the umbilicus upward is significant of paralysis or weakness of lower abdominal muscles, rectus abdominis; if umbilicus moves right, weakness of left abdominal muscles; if umbilicus moves left, weakness of the right abdominal muscles (Fig. 24.10). A positive sign is indicative of thoracic neurometric segments T8–T10 such as in spinal cord injury or lesion, vertebral tumor, compression fracture, and disc protrusions.

Briquet's Syndrome. An hysterical diaphragmatic paralysis that results in dyspnea and aphonia.

Murphy's Gallbladder Sign. Inability to take a deep breath when the palpating fingers are pressed deeply beneath the right costal arch, below the hepatic margin is a sign of gallbladder disorder (eg, biliary tract inflammation).

Barkman's Reflex. This normal sign features homolateral contraction of the rectus abdominis muscle when the skin just below the nipple is stimulated. It is often used to test the integrity of the T4–T5 (approximately) segmental levels.

Obliquus Reflex. Stimulation of the skin below the inguinal ligament may normally contract a part of the homolateral obliquus externus abdominus. Its presence confirms the integrity of the ilioinguinal nerve and the T12–L1 (approximately) level of the spinal cord.

Chapman's Test. With the patient in the supine position, the examiner stabilizes the patient's legs and asks the patient to attempt to flex the trunk to the sitting position without using the hands. This test, which requires strong contraction of the abdominals, is positive for abdominal weakness if the patient is unable to sit upright, but abdominal pain is not produced. If abdominal pain is produced during the attempt, an inflammatory abdominal lesion should be suspected.

Cope's Test. With the patient supine, the examiner stands at the side of the patient. The hip and knee are flexed, and the doctor places the cephalad hand on the patient's knee and the caudad hand grasps the patient's foot or ankle. The hip is then internally rotated, which causes a stretch to the homolateral ileopsoas group. A positive sign is seen if pain is perceived in the lower quadrant on the side being tested, indicating an inflammatory condition within the lower abdomen or pelvis (eg, psoas abscess, appendicitis, oophorosalpingitis, etc).

Glenard's Test. This test is based on the presumption that a pendulous abdomen with low hanging viscera produces distress of the lower abdomen. The symptom is found most commonly in patients with visceroptosis. To perform the test, the examiner stands behind the patient and reaches around and elevates the pendulous abdomen. The test is considered positive if this procedure offers relief to the patient's symptoms.

Pende's Reflex. In subjects who are distinctly sympathicotonic, stroking of the skin (especially of the abdomen) may produce a "goose flesh" response; ie, a pilomotor reflex.

Roentgenologic Considerations

Evidence of either splenic or hepatic injury is most difficult to witness on standard films, and more sophisticated procedures are frequently required (eg, ultrasonic studies, arteriography). The right psoas muscle shadow is normally visualized in 69% of standard abdominal films; the left psoas, 75% of subjects. Severe retroperitoneal hemorrhage or ascites may be indicated by an obscured psoas muscle margin and displacements of bowel gas. Occasionally, splenic rupture will obscure the left psoas shadow and present a large splenic shadow. Sometimes soft-tissue masses may be viewed.

The Abdominal Wall

Except for catcher and umpire chest protectors in baseball and that of the hockey goalie, the abdominal area is fairly unprotected in most sports. While padding would greatly reduce risk, the bulk necessary would greatly hamper typical performance.

Abrasions, Contusions, and Strains

Abrasions. These are caused by tangential forces with excoriation of the superficial layers of skin. They are often highly contaminated. Clean with soap and water to help avoid infection. Apply antiseptics and a sterile dressing to enhance healing.

Contusions. Exudation in and around the involved tissues are usually due to a rather strong force. A temporary shock may be present, associated with transient vomiting, localized pain, tenderness, and swelling. Ecchymosis often appears later, and sometimes a hematoma forms from ruptured vessels. Treat by resting the part, applying cold packs for 24 hours, and follow with heat, massage, and other appropriate physiotherapy measures. A small hematoma can be controlled by pressure and natural absorption; others must be referred for aspiration or evacuation. Minor contusions readily respond to cold packs, but severe muscular injury can be a major problem.

Strains. Unless a muscle is weakened by prior injury, it usually takes severe force to rupture an abdominal muscle. Symptoms of stress are pain, localized swelling, tenderness at the point of torn muscle or tendinous fibers, with ecchymosis occurring later. Motion increases pain. If a rupture has occurred, there is usually depression and hematoma at the site. Local support by strapping in a position of relaxation and cold packs for 24–28 hours are advised. These should be followed by heat, massage, and other appropriate physiotherapeutic measures.

Rectus Abdominis Rupture. Although tearing of the abdominis muscle is rare, diagnosis must be rapid to avoid secondary lesions from hematoma. The common site

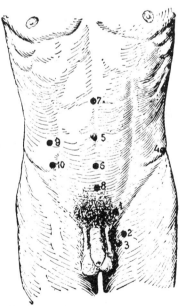

Figure 24.11. Typical locations of hernia of anterior abdominal wall: *1,* inguinal; *2,* femoral; *3,* obturator; *4,* lumbar; *5,* umbilical; *6 to 8,* hernia of linea albae (hypogastric); *7,* epigastric; *8,* supravesicular; *9 and 10,* lateral ventral hernia, spigelian line.

is at the right-inferior aspect. Because of its sheath of strong transverse bands, bleeding easily pools; and because of its extension from the lower ribs to the pubis, difficult breathing (thoracic) and coughing spells are usually exhibited. These signs are followed by severe "stomach ache," rigidity, and inability to forward flex the trunk when supine. A torn inferior epigastric artery may be involved, characterized by shock and a large tender hematoma. In adolescents, avulsion from the anterior-superior iliac spine may be involved. Traction stress exhibits localized tenderness at the pubic attachment; later roentgenography will show bony sclerosis. When bleeding is suspected, apply ice packs to the area and refer immediately for surgical attention.

Stitches

Crippling but temporary abdominal stitches are acute unilateral (usually on the right) pains on inspiration in the area of the lower ribs and upper abdominal quandrant. They are not a state of asphyxiation but are associated with windedness. Disability arises by the fact that air hunger is combined with increased pain on deep inspiration. Fortunately, the "spell" usually subsides in 3–5 minutes. Attacks commonly occur during running, especially downhill. Running on a full stomach appears to be an aggravating factor.

Etiology. The exact causative mechanism is not known, but one important factor appears to be tension on the ligament of Trietz which connects the pylorus portion of the stomach with the diaphragm. This ligament is associated with skeletal muscle tissue and cerebrospinal nerve endings which evidently are involved in some type of reflex irritation. If mild jogging or horseback riding initiates an attack, a peritoneal irritation such as a subclinical chronic appendix inflammation should be suspected. If this be the case, recurrence is common.

Management. Rest of abdominal movement relieves the condition, especially if the player is placed supine with knees flexed and arms raised. If a runner is near the finish of a race, he may finish by running with the trunk flexed. It is an awkward position, but it may allow one to complete the course.

Solar Plexus Impaction

The large celiac plexus of nerves and ganglia located in the peritoneal cavity at the level of L1 contains two large ganglionic masses and a dense network of fibers surrounding the roots of the celiac and superior mesenteric arteries. It supplies nerves to the abdominal viscera and is indirectly associated with the respiratory mechanism. Thus, a strong blow to the abdominal area can inhibit breathing (winding), resulting in unconsciousness. An abdominal blow overstimulates the autonomic fibers of the plexus, especially the parasympathetic fibers, and causes delayed venous return to the inferior vena cava.

Signs and Symptoms.   The picture is one of neurologic shock: faintness, prostration, dyspnea, clammy skin, and pallor. Air hunger often leads to panic. Fortunately, symptoms subside spontaneously in 1–2 minutes. Then, deep abdominal injury should be ruled out. A far more serious condition to be considered is an associated splenic or hepatic rupture producing hemorrhage within the abdominal cavity.

First Aid.   In unconsciousness from an abdominal blow, place the player on his back, moisten the face with a cool damp cloth or sponge, loosen clothing around the waist and thorax, and encourage the player to relax and to breathe slowly and rhythmically. The knees may be carefully flexed, but forceful spinal flexion or leg pumping are contraindicated because an anterior vertebral injury may have been incurred with the forceful flexion from the abdominal blow. The player should not be allowed to return to play until all signs are normal for at least 10–15 minutes. Delayed hemorrhage is always a risk. Rest alone will usually allow the temporary bradycardia and bronchospasm to subside. If unconsciousness is prolonged or if possible rupture may exist, seek surgical consultation immediately. The greater the delay in diagnosis, the greater the incidence of fatality.

Visceral Injuries

Any solid or hollow abdominal organ may be involved in abdominal trauma, but the spleen and kidneys appear to be the most vulnerable to injury. Typical signs in any visceral injury are shifting dullness, ab-

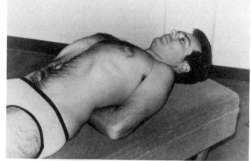

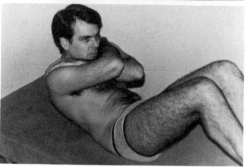

Figure 24.12.   *Top*, evaluating active spinal extension strength in the supine position. *Bottom*, evaluating active abdominal muscle strength in flexion.

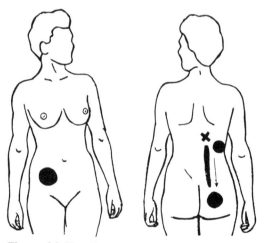

Figure 24.13.   Iliocostalis trigger point; *X*, common site. *Blackened areas* indicate typical sites of referred pain.

sent peristalsis, along with hypotension and a fast pulse rate to suggest hemorrhage.

Ruptured Spleen

Several examples of sports deaths have been attributed to blunt trauma to the ab-

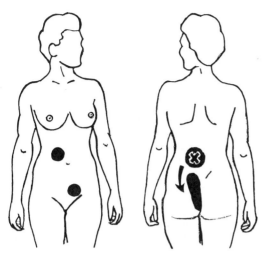

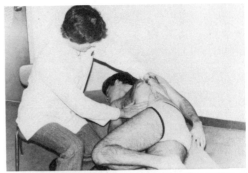

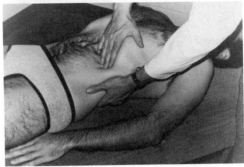

Figure 24.14. Multifidus trigger point; *X*, common site. *Blackened areas* indicate typical sites of referred pain.

Figure 24.15. Position of hands in palpating the spleen.

dominal area. The most common fatality is that of rupture of the spleen, as well as intrasplenic or subsplenic hematoma and retroperitoneal hemorrhage. Laceration may result from rib fracture, especially that of the 9th or 10th which lie directly behind the spleen. Rupture of the splenic capsule produces severe hemorrhage, often from what is considered minor trauma. It may even rupture spontaneously following infectious mononucleosis.

Tenderness in the upper-left quadrant may be the only sign present (Fig. 24.15). A falling hematocrit is typical. Pain is aggravated by breathing. Increasing hemorrhage causes diaphragmatic irritation referring pain to the left shoulder and root of the neck, along with generalized abdominal pain, rigidity, shifting dullness, and shock. Hypotension occurs late. Immediate surgical intervention is required to reduce mortality; if not, mortality ranges from 80–100%. If rupture is not complete, a splenic hematoma may develop that may lead to delayed bleeding. This may not occur until 2 weeks after injury.

Renal Damage

Kidney injury has the second highest rate of injury in abdominal blunt trauma. The mechanism is usually a loin blow. The extent of damage may be minor bruising or a serious rupture. The most constant feature is hemorrhage, either perirenal or into the urinary tract, or both. There is usually local pain radiating to the genitals, vomiting, shock, tenderness, and muscle spasm in the costovertebral angle. Bleeding does not invade the peritoneal cavity unless the fascial barrier is broken. Predisposing hydronephrosis requires only moderate trauma for severe consequences.

Studies show that albuminuria, casts, and microscopic hematuria occur in football during conditioning exercises and increase during contact practice. About 16% of players show gross hematuria after regular play, with normal values returning in a few days. Basketball, hockey, and boxing also have a high incidence of transient renal signs and symptoms, often leading to permanent structural damage. Exertion proteinuria and myoglobinuria appear to be related to intensity and duration of effort. The latter condition may lead to tubular necrosis.

Murphy's Kidney Test. With the patient in a relaxed position, the examiner places a thumb under the posterior aspect (superior flank area) of the 12th rib on the involved side and makes a few deep jabs

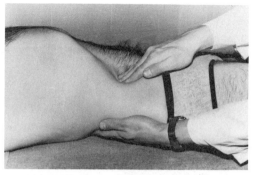

Figure 24.16. Palpation of the kidney.

(Fig. 24.16). If this produces a lancinating pain that radiates toward the anterior or into the groin, a renal infection or some other inflammatory condition (eg, abscess) under the retroperitoneal fascia is indicated.

Enteric Rupture

Intestine damage, sometimes multiple, is usually the result of an anterior crushing injury against the spine that causes a sudden pressure increase of gas or fluid in loops of intestine. Frequently, no trace of injury to the skin will be seen, yet early diagnosis is vital. Common sites are at the fixtures of the duodenum (often fatal because of lack of symptoms) and the ileocecal junction. Diverticula may result when the small in-

testine is driven through adjacent structures. The clinical picture is often delayed until peristalsis becomes active, producing leakage into the peritoneal cavity. Nonconstant vomiting often occurs. Shock is usually mild in the early stages. Vague abdominal pain, rigidity, and flank fluid may not develop for 8–12 hours after trauma. Bowel sounds will then be absent. Considerable hemorrhage and infection are associated with colon rupture.

Lacerated Liver

Liver injury is not common, yet the possibility cannot be ignored. The liver easily ruptures and tears with fragmentations, frequently involving the gallbladder and/or ducts. Fortunately, most injuries are limited to a small laceration and hematoma. Tangential forces are usually the traumatic mechanism involved. Usually the dome of the right lobe is affected, referring pain to the right shoulder and upper-right quadrant which is aggravated by breathing. When liver damage is present, the danger of hemorrhage with consequent sepsis is great. Fortunately, most hepatic vessels are low pressure ones from the portal circulation which can often be controlled by pressure. Acute hemorrhage will show evidence of internal bleeding and shock. Rapid death may occur.

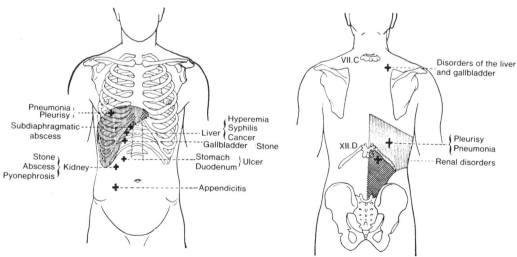

Figure 24.17. *Left*, points of anterior tenderness in right hypochondrium with their respective common causes and modes of radiation. *Right*, points of posterior tenderness associated with right hypochondriac tenderness with their causes.

Pancreas Rupture

Although the pancreas is quite protected, blunt injuries in sports have been reported (1–2%) with serious consequences. Injury is likely due to crushing forces against the spine. Symptoms may be dramatic or subtle. There may be epigastric tenderness and pain, often radiating to the back or left scapula, moderate shock, mild muscle resistance, and signs of hemorrhage. A raised serum amylase is usually diagnostic, but surgical exploration is necessary for confirmation.

Gallbladder Injury and Hemobilia

Blows or compression forces to the lower-right chest may be responsible for rupture of a distended gallbladder from the liver so that it lies free in the abdominal cavity or laceration of the organ's wall where gall leaks into the abdominal cavity (bile peritonitis). Diagnosis is extremely difficult, but a mild jaundice sign may appear in the sclera.

While incidence is small, blunt abdominal trauma is the most common cause of hemobilia (hemorrhage into the biliary tracts), usually resulting in melena, occult bleeding, or hematemesis. The origin of the bleeding may be from the liver, pancreas, gallbladder, or bile ducts.

Urinary Tract Injuries

Bladder Rupture. This rarely occurs in organized sports due to the absolute necessity of urinating before any practice or competitive event.

Urethra Injury. The urethra is rarely injured outside of contact sports, gymnastics, or cycling where astride blows injure the perineum. Damage often follows coccygeal injury. A perineal swelling between the scrotum and anus and possible slight urethral bleeding which may or may not be associated with micturition are suspicious signs of a ruptured urethra. After healing, a resulting stricture easily leads to chronic bladder and renal disorders if not treated adequately.

Chemical Epididymitis. A ruptured urethra from a blow where the spermatic cord enters the urethra may result in urine leaking into the scrotum and produce a chemical epididymitis. A swollen testicle and pain increased on micturition are presented.

Open Wounds

Patients with deep abdominal wounds, viewed as a group, stand a poor chance of recovery in emergency situations. Most abdominal wounds are grossly contaminated by the contents of the gastrointestinal or urinary tracts. Abdominal wounds require prompt surgery to stop hemorrhage. The immediate attention given is of a more supportive than treatment nature. With good supportive care, some patients will stabilize on their own and live to survive surgery.

Emergency Care in Abdominal Wounds. The priority is to dress the wound and treat for shock while waiting for transportation to a hospital. Cover the wound with one or more sterile dry dressings to prevent further contamination, but do not touch or try to push protruding organs or tissue into the wound. However, if it is necessary to move an exposed intestine onto the abdomen in order to cover the wound adequately, then do so. Secure the dressing in place with dressing tails and additional bandage. Since internal bleeding cannot be controlled by pressure and excessive pressure can cause further injury, do not bandage the wound tightly. Leave the patient on his back, but turn his head to one side since he will probably vomit. Watch him closely to prevent choking. If the patient is on a litter, raise the foot of the litter 6 inches. Keep him comfortably warm. Permit nothing by mouth, but occasionally moisten his lips with a wet cloth to help alleviate thirst.

Hernia

Any player with a demonstrable hernia invites intestinal strangulation when participating in stenuous activity or scuba diving (intra-abdominal pressure increase). True "traumatic" hernia is rare. It is associated with a direct blow and accompanied by evidence of actual tearing of tissues. Most hernias seen will be "hernias of effort" where the hernia appears after heavy lifting, falling, slipping, or any cause which increases intraabdominal pressure.

PERINEAL AREA INJURY

Rectal examination is essential in the presence of bowel symptoms, bleeding, and low back pain. Overt symptoms of constipation, diarrhea, pelvic disease, low back pain, female complaints, urinary symptoms, and suspected carcinoma should be referred by the team doctor to the family doctor for evaluation.

Superficial Disorders

The Skin

Contusions and Lacerations. These are rare, usually occurring from kicks or impaling a hurdle or some other obstacle.

Pruritus Ani. This is a common complaint among athletes. Excessive sweating and poor hygiene are factors. It is characterized by intensely itchy eczematous-type lesions. Management consists of absolute cleanliness and attempts to keep the area dry. Topical corticosteroids and antifungal or antibacterial lotions may be necessary. In some cases, a sacral or coccygeal reflex may be involved where a "notch" contact immediately relieves intense itching.

Cyclists Saddle Neuropathy. Paresthesia of the pudendal nerve is a compression neuropathy seen in bicyclists. It is produced by pressure on the perineum by the narrow seats of racing bicycles. In the male, scrotal and penile hypesthesia may be the complaint.

Pudendal Neuritis. Priapism sometimes occurs in racing cyclists from a poorly fitting saddle which irritates the pudendal nerve. A persistently painful erection is the only major feature.

Saddle Sores. Bicyclists may exhibit a paniculitis leading to localized areas of fat necrosis from excessive friction between saddle and perineal skin. Rest and release of edema pressure by puncture offers quick relief. If left unattended, ulceration and secondary infection result.

The Anal Canal

Lacerations are rare. Most complaints will be from a strangulated hemorrhoid which can be easily managed by warm soaks, ointments, and neurotherapy to relax the sphincter. If not, galvanism, surgery, injections, or cauterization should be advised.

Uncomplicated pilonidal sinus and chronic fissures can be referred for surgical attention between seasons.

Male Genital Injuries

Traumatic Testicular Injuries

Contusion. Testicular contusions are common in most sports. Even if damage is slight, there is often shock-like pallor, agonizing pain, nausea, and lower abdominal symptoms.

Torsion. A severe twisting motion may result in torsion (90–360°) of the testicles and their related cords, muscles, and vessels. Incidence is highest between 13–25 years of age. The circulatory blockage causes immediate pain. Testicular infarction can develop within a few hours, leading to gangrene. If the rotation cannot be reduced manually, surgery is necessary. The direction of rotation can be judged by the direction which relieves pain. Recurrence in varying degrees is common and may require surgical fixation.

Displacement or Rupture. A most rare traumatic luxation may occur where one or both testes are jammed up into the abdominal cavity, exhibiting an empty, contracted scrotum, with a tender mass near the internal inguinal ring. A knee kick to the groin is the common cause. Adhesions rapidly form to hold the dislodged testes in malposition. Predisposition comes from an extreme testicular mobility related to muscular effort. A direct blow may lead to rupture, laceration, hematoma, or a large painful hematocele. If the epididymis is ruptured from a testicle by force, a hematoma develops which may result in a fibrotic scar leading to sterility.

Hydrocele. Both hydrocele and varicocele are incurred by atheletes from a scrotal blow. A straw-colored fluid forms between the testicle and the tunica vaginalis in hydrocele. Both hydrocele of the cord and hernia give an impulse on coughing, but hydrocele usually shows a distinct limit above. On pulling the cord, the swelling moves too. The mass is painless, irreducible, and does not increase size during coughing. Large indirect hernias may protrude into the scrotum and become mistaken for a hydrocele, but transillumination will differentiate.

Cystic hydroceles of the tunica vaginalis transilluminate readily, with an area of normal scrotum above. Tumor of the testis is painless.

Varicocele. Varicosity of the spermatic cord (varicoceles) is usually on the left in mature males. The veins descend to and involve the pampiniform plexus to present an aching upper scrotal sac that is soft, elastic, and purple. The sac feels like a bag of worms. There is not true impulse on coughing, and the mass disappears for the most part when the patient assumes a reclining position.

Management. Severe injury requires immediate surgical exploration. Minor injuries can be treated with cool packs, rest, and a firm supporter while resolution gradually occurs. A scrotal cup should be worn for protection for several months during competition. It may take months to absorb scrotal extravasation.

Infection

Epididymitis, the major scrotal inflammatory process, is differentiated from a scrotal tumor by concomitant infection of the urinary tract, inflammation of the spermatic cord, prostate infection, and systemic toxic signs. The scrotum is normally cool, but it is warm in inflammatory processes. Orchitis will swell the entire organ. Dermatophytosis produces marked erythema in the groin and scrotum with sharply raised borders covered with pinpoint vesicles. Moniliasis is characterized by a zone of dry, flaking erythema and pruritis.

Female Genital Injuries

Contusions

Contusions are usually the result of vaulting injuries or saddle "bumps." Cold packs will prevent hemorrhage and reduce swelling. Forceful vaginal douching can occur in waterskiers when protective rubber panties are not worn. Severe consequences can result.

Traumatic Abortion

This condition is rare. Several studies have indicated that pregnancy is helped rather than hindered by moderate exercise. Most authorities feel that when spontaneous abortion follows a well-demarcated sports event, it is either a matter of coincidence or the abortion was already predetermined and the excitement or strain simply advanced its expulsion by a few hours or days.

CHAPTER 25

Lumbar Spine, Pelvic, and Hip Injuries

The lumbar spine, sacrum, ilia, pubic bones, and hips work as a functional unit. Any disorder of one part immediately affects the function of the other parts. A wide assortment of muscle, tendon, ligament, bone, nerve, and vascular injuries in this area are witnessed during athletic care.

LUMBAR SPINE INJURIES

Low back disability, amounting to up to 25% of all athletic injuries, rapidly demotivates athletic participation. For biomechanical reasons, the incidence of injury is two times higher in taller athletes than in shorter players. The mechanism of injury is usually intrinsic rather than extrinsic. The cause can often be through overbending, a steady lift, or a sudden release—all of which primarily involve the musculature. Intervertebral disc conditions are more often, but not exclusively, attributed to extrinsic blows and wrenches. An accurate and complete history is vital to offer the best management and counsel.

Initial Assessment

The first step in the examination process is knowing the mechanism of injury if possible. With this knowledge, evaluation can be rapid and accurate. A player injured on the field should never be moved until emergency assessment is completed. Once severe injury has been evaluated, transfer to a back board can be made and further evaluation conducted at the aid station.

Tenderness. Tenderness is frequently found at the apices of spinal curves and rotations and not infrequently where one curve merges with another. Tenderness about spinous or transverse processes is usually of low intensity and suggests articular strain. Tenderness noted at the points of nerve exit from the spine and continuing in the pathway of the peripheral division of the nerves is a valuable aid in spinal analysis; however, the lack of tenderness is not a clear indication of lack of spinal dysfunction. Tenderness is a subjective symptom influenced by many individual structural, functional, and psychologic factors which often makes it an unreliable sign. Always evaluate the presence and symmetry of lower-extremity pulses.

Range of Motion

The range of lumbar spine motion is determined by the disc's resistance to distortion, disc thickness, and the angle and size of the articular surfaces. While motion is potentially greater than that of the thoracic spine because of lack of rib restriction; facet facing and heavy ligaments check the range of motion. Most significant to movements in the lumbar spine is the fact that all movements are to some degree three dimensional; ie, when the lumbar spine bends laterally, it tends to rotate posteriorly on the side of convexity and assume a hyperlordotic tendency.

The transitional lumbosacral area of L5-S1 constitutes a rather unique "universal joint"; eg, when the sacrum rotates anterior-inferior on one side within the ilia, L5 tends to rotate in the opposite direction, thus effecting a mechanical accommodation with the lumbar spine above assuming a posterior rotation on the side of the unilateral anterior-inferiority. It also tends to assume an anteroflexion position, thus effecting the three-dimensional movements of the lumbar spine. In view of the intricacy of the lumbosacral junction, anomalies such as asymmetrical facets have a strong influence on normal movements in this area.

If lumbar active motions are normal, there is no need to test passively. A patient may be observed, however, who replaces normal lumbar motion by exaggerated hip motion, or vice versa. In such a situation, range of motion of the restricted lumbar on hip joints should be passively tested.

During flexion of the lumbar spine, the anterior longitudinal ligaments relax and the supraspinal and interspinal ligaments stretch. Flexion will not normally result in a kyphosis of the lumbar area as flexion may in the cervical area. While a number of disorders result in decreased flexion, paraspinal muscle spasm is the first suspicion. The degree of extension is controlled by stretching of the anterior longitudinal ligament and rectus abdominis muscles, relaxation of the posterior ligaments, and the integrity of the intrinsic muscles of the back.

Evaluating Neurologic Levels of the Lower Extremities

A sensory and motor neurologic assessment should be made as soon as possible. Determine tonus (flaccidity, rigidity, spasticity) by passive movements. Then test voluntary power of each suspected group of muscles against resistance, and compare the force bilaterally. Test cremasteric (L1-L2), patellar (L2-L4), gluteal (L4-S1), Achilles (L5-S2), plantar (S1-S2), and anal (S5-Cx1) reflexes. Note patellar or ankle clonus. Test coordination and sensation by gait, heel-to-knee and foot-to-buttock tests, and Romberg's station test.

Trigger Points

Trigger points for the lumbosacral and sacroiliac articular complexes are commonly located (1) alongside the T12 spinous process, (2) alongside the L5 spinous process, (3) over the greater sciatic notch through the gluteal muscles, (4) over the crest of the ilium, (5) over the belly of the tensor fascia lata muscle, (6) in the ischiorectal fossa apex, and (7) at the sciatic outlet onto the back of the thigh from under the gluteus maximus.

Distortion Patterns

A unique feature of a spinal and pelvic distortion or subluxation is the fact that the segment or segments can be carried into the deviation of the distortion pattern much more readily than out of the gravitational pattern of the deviation.

The transition points of the spinal curvatures (ie, the atlanto-occipital, cervicobrachial, thoracolumbar, and lumbosacral points) serve as mobile differentials about which flexion, extension, circumflexion, circumduction, and compensatory scoliotic deviations should occur. If these areas are kept mobile, the adaptive, compensatory, and ordinary motor functions of the spine are enhanced.

Contusions and Strains

Fortunately, most injuries seen will involve uncomplicated contusions and subluxations of the spinal area and adjacent free ribs that are relatively easy to manage. However, severe contusion of the lumbodorsal fascia is occasionally seen which frequently leads to an extensive painful hematoma. When severe injury does occur, the type widely varies from sport to sport. In some cases, a silent condition such as a spina bifida occulta may only be brought to light through strenuous athletic activity.

Load Considerations

The importance of spinal loads is underscored with weight lifters, bowlers, oarsmen from lifting the shell, and lordotic long-distance runners. It has been estimated that when an object is held 14 inches away from the spine, the load on the lumbosacral disc is 15 times the weight lifted. Lifting a 100-lb weight at arms' length theoretically places a 1,500-lb load on the lumbosacral disc. This load, of course, must be dissipated, otherwise the L5 vertebra would crush. The load is dissipated through the paraspinal muscles and, importantly, by the abdominal cavity which acts as a hydraulic chamber absorbing and diminishing the load applied. These observations on spine loading emphasize the vulnerability of the spine to the mechanical stresses placed upon it, especially in people with poor muscle tone. Bony compression of the emerging nerve roots arises as a result of subarticular entrapment, pendicular kinking, or foraminal impingement due to vertebral subluxation.

Muscle Spasms

General spasm of the spinal muscles guarding motion in the vertebral joints can be viewed by watching body attitude (eg, stiff carriage) and by efforts to bend the spine forward, backward, and to the sides. If the examiner is familiar with the average range of motility in each direction and at different ages, this test is usually easy and rapid.

Management

The benefits of articular adjustments are well known within the profession. To relieve muscle spasm, heat is helpful, but cold and vapocoolant sprays have sometimes shown to be more effective. The effects of traction are often dramatic but sometimes short-lived if a herniated disc is involved. A predisposing ankle or arch weakness may be present which requires special stabilization.

Passive Stretch. Mild passive stretch is an excellent method of reducing spasm in the long muscles, but heavy passive stretch destroys the beneficial reflexes. For example, hypertonic erector muscles of the spine can be simply relaxed by placing the patient prone on a split head-piece adjusting table and tilting the abdominal and pelvic section upward to flex the spine. The weight of the structures above and below the midpoint of the flexed spine offer a mild stretching effect, both cephally and caudally. The muscles should relax within 2–3 minutes. Thumb pressure, placed on a trigger area, is then directed towards the muscle's attachment and held for a few moments until relaxation is complete. Psoas or quadriceps spasm can be relaxed with Bragard's test by holding the straight leg for a minute or two in extension and dorsiflexing the foot.

Vapocoolant Techniques in Acute Low Back Muscle Spasms. Place the patient in the lateral recumbent position with the involved side up and the knees slightly flexed. Isolate trigger areas and site of major pain and spray sites. At the same time, ask the patient to pull his knees up toward his chest and then slowly return them to the relaxed position. Repeat the spraying and active movement three or four times. Have the patient indicate with his finger the major source of pain. As the pain shifts position, spray the affected area. Once relief is obtained, have the patient turn to the other side if the condition is bilateral, and repeat the procedure. Once relief has been obtained in flexion-extension, add rotation

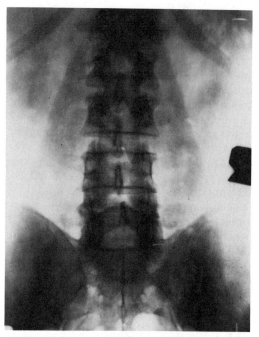

Figure 25.1. While roller skating, a 61-year-old male suffered a minor fall and a crash into a wall which injured his lower back. He had been interested in hockey and roller skating most of his life. A low-back injury from a skating fall also occurred 20 years previously. At this time, pain also radiated into the right leg. Lasegue's and Bragard's signs were positive at 45°. Bechterew's and the well-leg-raising test were negative for lumbar disc injury. X-ray examination of the lumbosacral spine demonstrated a first-degree spondylolisthesis of L4-L5 with narrowing of the L5-S1 disc interspace. A midlumbar scoliosis was present with the convexity to the right and rotary subluxations were noted in the lower lumbar region. Chiropractic case management consisted of adjustments to reduce the vertebral subluxations, intermittent motorized lumbar traction, electronic muscle stimulation to the lumbar spine and along the course of the right leg, and ultrasonic therapy for the relief of pain. After the patient steadily improved, it was recommended that he pursue monthly follow-up visits and periodic spinal examinations (with the permission of the New York Chiropractic College).

and lateral flexion, spraying painful sites as necessary between movements. Have the patient attempt to walk, and spray the painful area if necessary. If possible, have the patient bend forward with his heels on the floor. Once relief is obtained, correct any subluxations isolated, support the area, and

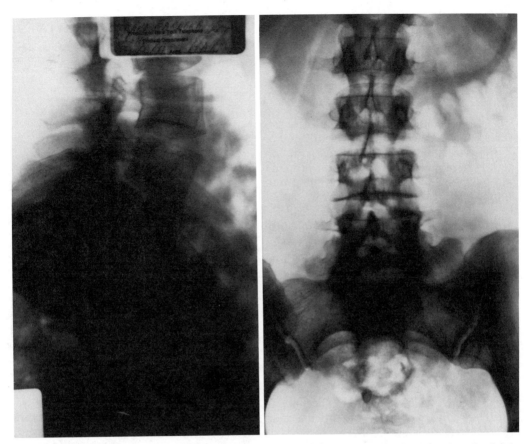

Figure 25.2. A female, age 26, presented severe pain in the lower back radiating into the left leg following an accident playing volley ball. She had originally injured her lower back playing volley ball at the age of 15. At that time she collided with another player and was thrown to the ground. Since that time she had developed recurrent low-back pains. However, no episode had taken place for more than 5 years prior to the current attack. To relieve pain in lower back and left leg, the patient stood in the antalgic position to the right. The straight-leg-raising test and Bragard's sign were positive at 50°. In the prone position, Ely's test was positive on the left side. Pain, tenderness, and sensory defects were noted along the sciatic nerve distribution which referred to the L5-S1 nerve root. The x-ray examination revealed a flattening of the lumbar lordosis, decreased disc interspace between L5-S1, and a decrease in the normal Ferguson's angle. There was a right rotation of L3 on L4, L4 on L5, and L5 on S1. There was an area of lucency on the posterosuperior aspect of the sacrum suggestive of a previous fracture. The patient responded favorably to lumbar traction. Electronic muscle stimulation seemed to create proper muscle tone along the lower back and leg. Ultrasound was instrumental in reducing pain, and the patient responded favorably to chiropractic adjustments. It was recommended that the case be followed on a periodic visit basis to guard against exacerbation of the problem (with the permission of the New York Chiropractic College).

instruct the patient in home exercises for 1–2 minutes each half hour during the waking hours. Advise the patient to avoid remaining in any one position for too long. Begin resistance, stretching, and weight-bearing exercises as soon as acute symptoms subside.

Adjuncts. Other methods may prove helpful. Peripheral inhibitory afferent impulses can be generated to partially close the presynaptic gate by acupressure, acupuncture, or transcutaneous nerve stimulation. Isotonic exercises are useful in improving circulation and inducing the stretch reflex when supine to reduce exteroceptive influences on the central nervous system.

An acid-base imbalance from muscle hypoxia and acidosis may be prevented by supplemental alkalinization. In chronic cases, relaxation training and biofeedback therapy are helpful.

Facet Syndromes

The subluxation of lumbar facet structures, states Howe, is a part of all lumbar dyskinesias and must be present if a motion unit is deranged. In a three-point articular arrangement, such as at each vertebral motion unit, no disrelationship can exist that does not derange two of the three articulations. Thus, determination of the integrity or subluxation of the facets in any given motion unit is important in assessing that unit's status.

Roentgenographic Considerations

An evaluation of the alignment of the articular processes comprising a facet joint may be difficult from the A-P or P-A view alone when the plane of the facet facing is other than sagittal or semisaggital. In this case, oblique views of the lumbosacral area are of great value in determining facet alignment since the joint plane and articular surfaces can nearly always be visualized.

When one cannot visually identify disrelationships of the facet articular structures, Howe suggests use of Hadley's S curve. This is made by tracing a line along the undersurface of the transverse process at the superior and bringing it down the inferior articular surface. This line is joined by a line drawn upward from the base of the superior articular process of the inferior vertebra from the lower edge of its articular surface. These lines should join to form a smooth S. If the S is broken, subluxation is present. This A-P procedure can be used on an oblique view. See Figure 25.3.

Differentiation

To help differentiate the low back and sciatic neuralgia of a facet syndrome from that of a disc that is protruding:

1. With the patient standing with feet moderately apart, the doctor from behind the patient firmly wraps his arms around the patient's pelvis and firms his lateral thigh against the back of the patients' pelvis. The patient is asked to bend forward. If it is

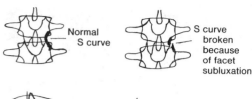
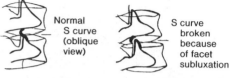

Figure 25.3. Determination of lumbosacral facet subluxations (with the permission of the ACA Council on Roentgenology).

a facet involvement, the patient will feel relief. If it is a disc that is stressed, symptoms will be aggravated.

2. In facet involvement, the patient seeks to find relief by sitting with feet elevated and resting upon a stool, chair, or desk. In disc involvement, the patient keeps knees flexed and sits sideways in his chair and moves first to one side and then to the other for relief. If lumbosacral and sacroiliac pain migrates from one to the other side, it is suspected to be associated with arthritic changes.

Management

The associated pain, accentuated by hyperextension of the trunk, results when an inferior apophyseal facet becomes displaced upward so that it impinges on the IVF contents of the inferior vertebral notch (eg, nerve root) of the superior vertebra. Cryotherapy and other forms of pain control are advisable during the acute stage for 48 hours. Considerable relief will be achieved by placing the patient prone with a roll under the lower abdomen to flex the lumbar spine while applying manual traction techniques. This should be followed by corrective adjustments to relieve associated fixations and abnormal biomechanics, traction, and other physiotherapy modalities. A regimen of therapeutic exercises and shoe inserts designed to improve postural balance and lessen gait shock are helpful during recuperation.

Acute Lumbosacral Sprain

These sprains are of frequent appearance.

Heavy loads or severe blows may rupture some associated ligaments and/or subluxate the joint. Pain may be local or referred. Symptoms are usually relieved by rest and aggravated by activity. Care must be taken to differentiate from a sacroiliac or hip lesion. Localized tenderness and various clinical tests are helpful in differentiation.

Various neurologic and orthopedic procedures relative to lumbosacral syndromes are listed in Table 25.1.

Management. During the acute hyperemic stage, structural alignment, cold, compression support, ultrasound, and rest are indicated. After 48 hours, passive congestion may be managed by gentle passive manipulation, sinusoidal stimulation, ultrasound, and a mild range of motion exercise initiated. During consolidation, local moderate heat, moderate active exercise, motorized alternating traction, moderate range of motion manipulation, and ultrasound are beneficial. In the stage of fibroblastic activity, deep heat, deep massage, vigorous active exercise, motorized alternating traction, negative galvanism, ultrasound, and active joint manipulation speed recovery and inhibit postinjury effects. Vitamin C and manganese are helpful throughout treatment to speed healing.

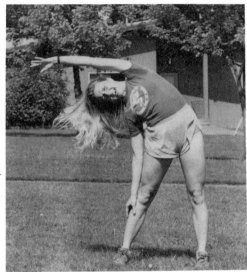

Figure 25.4. Conditioning reduces low-back strains. Dr. Margaret Karg demonstrates lateral spinal flexion stretching (with the permission of the ACA Council of Women Chiropractors, photo by Paul M. Everson).

Acute Lumbosacral Angle Syndrome

In this condition, Olsen states that the

Table 25.1.
Review of Neurologic and Orthopedic Maneuvers, Reflexes, Signs, or Tests Relative to Lumbosacral Syndromes

Achilles' reflex	Ely's heel-to-buttock test	Milgram's test
Adams' sign	Fajersztajn's test	Minor's sign
Adductor reflex	Gaenslen's test	Muscle strength grading
Anal reflex	Giegel's reflex	Nachlas' test
Babinski's plantar reflex	Gluteal reflex	Naffziger's test
Babinski's sciatic sign	Goldthwait's test	Neri's bowing sign
Barre's sign	Gower's sign	Neri's test
Bechterew's test	Hamstring reflex	O'Connell's test
Beery's sign	Heel walk test	Patella reflex
Belt test	Hyperextension tests	Pitres' sign
Bonnet's sign	Jandrassik's maneuver	Range of motion tests
Bowstring sign	Kemp's test	Romberg's station test
Bragard's test	Kernig's sign	Sicard's sign
Buckling sign	Laseque's differential sign	Smith-Peterson's test
Cremasteric reflex	Laseque's SLR test	Spinal percussion test
Dejerine's triad	Lewin's punch test	Toe walk test
Demianoff's sign	Light touch/pain tests	Turyn's sign
Deyerle-May's test	Lindner's sign	Vanzetti's sign
Double leg raise test		Westphal's sign
Duchenne's sign		Yeoman's test

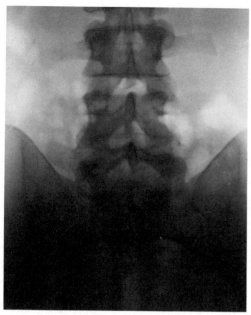

Figure 25.5. A male executive, age 36, presented an acute sciatic neuritis of sudden onset during a tennis match. A sudden "crack" was experienced with searing pain radiating down the back of the left leg. A positive Lasegue's straight-leg-raising sign, a positive Goldthwait's test at 35°, a positive left Bragard's sign, and bilaterally weak hamstrings and glutei maximus were exhibited. Neurologic and roentgenographic examinations were unremarkable except for a slight rotational misalignment of L5 in the A-P view. The patient appeared to be in excruciating pain. A decision was made to manipulate immediately. Adjustments were made to the cervicals and thoracics, and then the patient was given a lumbar roll with the pain side up. An audible release was heard, and the patient reported immediate relief. Follow-up visits at 2 days, 1 week, 2 weeks, and a month demonstrated no pain return nor further audible releases (with the permission of the New York Chiropractic College).

acute syndrome of L5 on S1 is twofold: (1) There is bursal involvement due to an overriding of the facets which stretches the bursa. (2) There is a narrowing of the intervertebral foramen (IVF) causing a telescoping from the superior to the inferior of the facet joints. Radiologically, the type of bursitis cannot be defined. Orthopedically, the problem is described as the facet-pain syndrome.

Cartilage is found between all articular surfaces, and undue stress during weight bearing on the facets can cause injury to the cartilage that will progress with degenerative changes. The degeneration may cause L5 to slip forward (degenerative disc disease), portray decreased disc space (discogenic disease), or exhibit decreased space with eburnation (discopathy). Sacralization is the only time when it is normal to have a decreased disc space, unless the disc is underdeveloped (hypoplasia). Along with the facet syndrome, there may also be an increased lordosis of the lumbar spine.

The facet syndrome can occur with (1) the anteriorly based sacrum with a normal lordosis, (2) the anteriorly based sacrum with an accentuated lordosis, (3) the anteriorly based sacrum with a "sway back", or (4) a normally based sacral angle and the "sway back" type of individual.

Evaluation is made by drawing a line through the superior border of the sacral base and through the inferior border of L5. If these lines cross within the IVF or anterior to it, this indicates a facet syndrome. Olsen recommends the use of *Fergurson's angle*, where the body of L3 is Xed and a line is dropped perpendicular from the center of the vertebral body. This line normally falls over the sacral prominatory or the anterior edge of the sacrum and reveals normal lumbosacral weight bearing (Ferguson's line of gravity). The L5 disc spacing is seen normally as symmetrical with the one above, and the actual weight bearing is on the nucleus pulposus.

A persistent notochord may be seen where the disc is normal but embedded into the body of the vertebra. This is seen in a postural facet syndrome where the anterior disc space is wide at the expense of narrowed disc space posteriorly and the body of the vertebra has rocked on the nucleus. It is not pathologic. For example, a normal vertebra presents decreased disc space posteriorly with the lines crossing in the IVF. There is normal disc space anteriorly, but in order for this to happen, there is a herniation. The disc is normal, but the symmetry of the disc interspace is broken.

Lumbosacral Instability

Lumbosacral instability is a mechanical aberration of the spine which renders it more susceptible to fatigue and/or subsequent trauma by reason of the variance from the optimal structural weight-bearing capabilities. Hariman states that between 50% and 80% of the general population exhibit some degree of the factors which predispose to instability whether by reason of anomalous development of articular relationships or altered relationships due to trauma or disease consequences. It is the most common finding of lumbosacral roentgenography and often brought to light after an athletic strain.

Disturbance of the physiologic response of the spinal motor unit is the primary finding with the sequela of "stress response syndrome" which may take the form of any degree between sclerosis of a tendon to and including an ankylosing hypertrophic osteophytosis or arthrosis. Frequent trauma to the articular structures as a result of excessive motility results in repetitive microtrauma. The scope of involvement and the tissue response are determined by the type and severity of the instability.

Signs and Symptoms. Unusual early fatigue is a constant symptom, and this leads to strain, sprain, and subsequent disc pathologies. Symptom susceptibility increases with the age of the individual. Postural evaluation is especially important in the physical diagnosis of the sequelae as well as to an extraspinal causation (eg, anatomic short leg).

Roentgenographic Considerations. Roentgen diagnosis is one of the sure means of delineating the type and severity of the underlying productive agent of the condition of instability. There is no characteristic finding except the recognition of the various anomalies and pathologies present. Care should be taken to include the entire pelvis in this determination as, for instance, a sacroiliac arthrosis may lead to instability.

Management. This condition often requires supportive therapies such as heel lifts and/or orthopedic belts in addition to specific adjustive therapy directed toward stabilization of the motion unit. Hariman feels the prognosis is excellent with adjustive and supportive management. High doses of vitamin C with calcium and magnesium have also proved helpful in disc conditions. Efforts and counsel should be directed to minimize the production of future microtrauma.

Loss of stability and compensation due to injury in the future may be expected to reproduce symptoms in an exaggerated form.

Pertinent Procedures in Lumbosacral Syndromes

Giegel's (Inguinal) Reflex. With the patient supine, the skin of the upper thigh is stimulated from the midline toward the groin. A normal response is an abdominal contraction at the upper edge of Poupart's ligament. This reflex (L1–L2) is essentially the female counterpart of the cremasteric reflex in the male.

Adductor Reflex. With the patient supine and the thigh moderately abducted, a normal response is seen when the tendon of the adductor magnus is tapped and a contraction of the adductor muscles occurs. This reflex reaction tests the integrity of the obturator nerve and L2–L4 segments of the spinal cord, as does the patellar reflex.

Hamstring Reflex. The patient is placed supine with the knees flexed and the thighs moderately abducted. The tendons of the semitendinosus and semimembranosus are hooked by the examiner's index finger and the finger is percussed. Normally, a palpable contraction of the hamstrings occurs. An exaggerated response indicates an upper motor neuron lesion above L4, and it may be associated with a reflex flexion of the knee (Stookey response). An absent response signifies a lower motor neuron lesion affecting the L4–S1 segments, as do absent Achilles and plantar reflexes.

Heel Walk Test. A patient should normally be able to walk several steps on the heels with the forefoot dorsiflexed. With the exception of a localized heel disorder (eg, calcaneal spur) or contracted calf muscles, an inability to do this because of low back pain or weakness can suggest an L5 lesion.

Toe Walk Test. Walking for several steps on the base of the toes with the heels raised will normally produce no discomfort to the patient. With the exception of a localized forefoot disorder (eg, plantar wart, neuroma) or an anterior leg syndrome (eg, shin splints), an inability to do this because of low back pain or weakness can suggest an S1–S2 lesion.

Double Leg Raise Test. This is a two-phase test: (1) The patient is placed supine, and a straight-leg-raising (SLR) test is performed on each limb: first on one side, and then on the other. (2) The SLR test is then performed on both limbs simultaneously; ie, a bilateral SLR test. If pain occurs at a lower angle when both legs are raised together than when performing the monolateral SLR maneuver, the test is considered positive for a lumbosacral area lesion.

O'Connell's Test. This test is conducted similar to that of the double leg raise test except that both limbs are flexed on the trunk to an angle just below the patient's pain threshold. Then the limb on the opposite side of involvement is lowered. If this exacerbates the pain, the test is positive for sciatic neuritis.

Nachlas' Test. The patient is placed in the prone position. The examiner flexes the knee on the thigh to a right angle, then, with pressure against the anterior surface of the ankle, the heel is slowly directed straight toward the homolateral buttock. The contralateral ilium should be stabilized by the examiner's other hand. If a sharp pain is elicited in the ipsilateral buttock or sacral area, a sacroiliac disorder should be suspected. If the pain occurs in the lower back area or is sciatic-like in nature, a lower lumbar disorder (especially L3–L4) is indicated. If pain occurs in the upper lumbar area, groin, or anterior thigh, quadriceps spasticity/contracture or a femoral nerve lesion should be suspected.

Gower's Maneuver. The patient uses the hands on the thighs in progressive short steps upward to extend the trunk to the erect position when arising from a sitting or forward flexed position. This sign is positive in cases of severe muscular degeneration (eg, muscular dystrophy) of the lumbopelvic extensors or a bilateral low back disorder (eg, spondylolisthesis).

Hyperextension Tests. These two tests help in localizing the origin of low back pain. (1) The patient is placed prone. With one hand the doctor stabilizes the contralateral ilium, while the other hand is used to extend the patient's thigh on the hip with the knee slightly flexed. If pain radiates down the front of the thigh during this extension, inflamed L3–L4 nerve roots should be suspected, if acute spasm of the

quadriceps or hip pathology have been ruled out. (2) With the patient remaining in the relaxed prone position, the examiner stabilizes the patient's lower legs and instructs the patient to attempt to extend the spine by lifting the head and shoulders as high as possible from the table by extending the elbows bilaterally. If localized pain occurs, the patient is then asked to place a finger on the focal point.

Also see Adam's sign, Bechterew's test, Beery's sign, Forestier's bowstring sign, Bragard's test, Fajersztajn's test, Goldthwait's test, Gower's maneuver, Hibb's test, Kemp's test, Kernig's sign, Lasegue's SLR test, Minor's sign, Naffziger's test, Neri's bowing sign, Neri's test, Smith-Peterson's test, and Westphal's sign.

Basic Neurologic Aspects of Lumbar Subluxation Syndromes

Disturbances of nerve function associated with subluxation syndromes manifest as abnormalities in sensory interpretations and/or motor activities. These disturbances may be through one of two primary mechanisms: direct nerve or nerve root disorders, or of a reflex nature.

Nerve Root Insults

When direct nerve root involvement occurs on the posterior root of a specific neuromere, it manifests as an increase or decrease in awareness over the dermatome; ie, the superficial skin area supplied by this segment. Typical examples might include forminal occlusion or irritating factors exhibited clinically as hyperesthesia, particularly on the (1) anterolateral aspects of the leg, medial foot, and great toe, when involvement occurs between L4–L5; and (2) posterolateral aspect of the lower leg and lateral foot and toes when involvement occurs between L5–S1. In other instances, this nerve root involvement may cause hypertonicity and the sensation of deep pain in the musculature supplied by the neuromere; for example, L4 and L5 involvements, with deep pain or cramping sensations in the buttock, posterior thigh and calf, or anterior tibial musculature. In addition, direct pressure over the nerve root or distribution may be particularly painful.

Reflexes. Nerve root insults from subluxations may also be evident as disturbances in motor reflexes and/or muscular strength. Examples of these reflexes include the deep tendon reflexes such as seen in reduced patella and Achilles tendon reflexes when involvement occurs between L4–L5. These reflexes should also be compared bilaterally to judge whether hyporeflexia is unilateral; unilateral hyperreflexia is pathognomonic of an upper motor neuron lesion.

Atrophy. Prolonged and/or severe nerve root irritation may also cause evidence of trophic changes in the tissues supplied. This may be characterized by obvious atrophy which would be rare in athletics. Such a sign is particularly objective when the circumference of an involved limb is measured at the greatest girth in the initial stage and this value is compared to measurements taken in later stages.

Kemp's Test. While in a sitting position, the patient is supported by the examiner who reaches around the patient's shoulders and upper chest from behind. The patient is directed to lean forward to one side and then around to eventually bend obliquely backward by placing his palm on his buttock and sliding it down the back of his thigh and leg as far as possible. The maneuver is similar to that used in cervical compression. If this compression causes or aggravates a pattern of radicular pain in the thigh and leg, it is a positive sign and indicates nerve

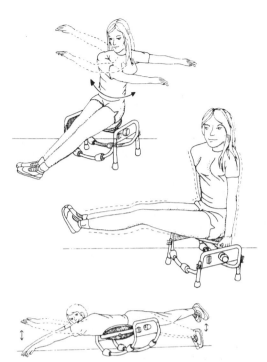

Figure 25.7. Use of Adapto-Disc in the development of balance, coordination, and agility (with the permission of the Widen Tool & Stamping, Inc).

root compression. It may also indicate a strain or sprain and thus be present when the patient leans obliquely forward or at any point in motion.

Since the elderly weekend athlete is less prone to an actual herniation of a disc due to lessened elasticity involved in the aging process, other reasons for nerve root compression are usually the cause. Degenerative joint disease, exostoses, inflammatory or fibrotic residues, narrowing from disc degeneration, tumors—all must be evaluated.

Clinical Signs

Note the comparative height of the iliac crests. If chronic sciatic neuralgia is on the high iliac crest side, degenerative disc weakening with posterolateral protrusion should be suspected. If occuring on the side of the low iliac crest, one must consider the possibility of a sacroiliac slip and lumbosacral torsion as the causative factor. There is a lessening or lack of the deep tendon reflexes of the lower extremity in sciatica (*Babinski's*

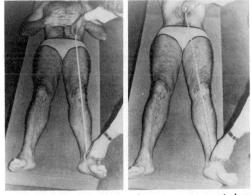

Figure 25.6. To determine an apparent leg length discrepancy, measurement is made from a fixed point such as the ASIS (*left*) to a fixed point or from a nonfixed point such as the navel (*right*) to a fixed point.

sciatica sign). When the patient's great toe on the affected side is flexed, pain will often be experienced in the gluteal region (*Turyn's sign*). Also in sciatica, the pelvis tends to maintain a horizontal position despite any induced degree of scoliosis (*Vanzetti's sign*), unlike other conditions in which scoliosis occurs where the pelvis is tilted.

Lasegue's Straight-Leg-Raising Test. The patient lies supine with legs extended. The examiner places one hand under the heel of the affected side and the other hand is placed on the knee to prevent the knee from bending. With the limb extended, the examiner flexes the thigh on the pelvis keeping the knee straight. Normally, the patient will be able to have the limb extended to almost 90° without pain. If this maneuver is markedly limited by pain, the test is positive and suggests sciatica from lumbosacral or sacroiliac lesions, subluxation syndrome, hamstring tightness, disc lesions, spondylolisthesis adhesions, or IVF occlusion. A second method of using this sign is to have the patient attempt to touch the floor with the fingers while the knees are held in extension during the standing position. Under these conditions, the knee of the affected side will flex, the heel slightly elevate, and the body elevate more or less to the painful side. Many reports confirm that when Lasegue's sign is positive, the pupils will dilate, blood pressure will rise, and the pulse will become more rapid. These phenomena are not present in the malingerer or psychoneurotic individual. See Figure 25.8.

Bragard's Test. If Lasegue's test is positive at a given point, the leg is lowered below this point and dorsiflexion of the foot is induced. The sign is negative if pain is not increased. A positive sign is a finding in sciatic neuritis, spinal cord tumors, intervertebral disc (IVD) lesions, and spinal nerve irritations. A negative sign points to muscular involvement such as tight hamstrings. Bragard's test helps to differentiate the pain of sciatic involvement from that of sacroiliac involvement. The sacroiliac articulation is not stressed by the Bragard maneuver, nor is the lumbosacral joint.

Fajersztajn's Test. When straight leg raising and dorsiflexion of the foot are performed on the asymptomatic side of a sciatic

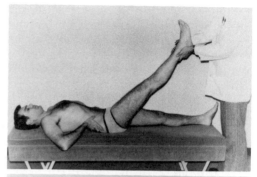
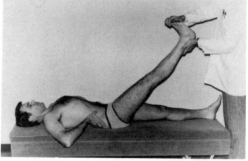

Figure 25.8. *Top*, Lasegue's straight-leg-raising test. *Bottom*, Bragard's test.'

patient and this causes pain on the symptomatic side, there is a positive Fajersztajn's sign, which is particularly indicative of a sciatic nerve root involvement such as a disc syndrome, dural root sleeve adhesions, or some other space-occupying lesion. This is sometimes called the cross-leg straight-leg-raising test

Demianoff's Test. This is a variant of Lasegue's test used in lumbago and funiculitis with the intent of differentiating between lumbago and sciatica. When the affected limb is first extended and then flexed at the hip, the corresponding half of the body becomes lowered and with it the muscle fibers fixed to the lumbosacral segment. This act, which stretches the muscles, induces sharp lumbar pain. Lasegue's sign is thus negative as pain is caused by stretching the affected muscles at the posterior portion of the pelvis rather than stretching the sciatic nerve. To accomplish with the patient supine, the pelvis is fixed by the examiner's hand firmly placed on the anterior superior iliac spine, and the other hand elevates the leg on the same side. No pain results when the leg is raised to a 80° angle. When lumbago and sciatica are coexistent, Demianoff's sign is negative on the affected side but positive on the opposite side unless the pelvis is fixed. Demianoff's sign is also negative in bilateral sciatica with lumbago. The fixation of the pelvis prevents stretching the sciatic nerve, and any undue pain experienced is usually associated with ischiotrochanteric groove adhesions. This sign has been found to be valuable in determining local lesions of muscles, upper lumbar nerve roots, and funicular sciatica.

Belt Test. The standing male patient bends forward with the examiner holding the patient's belt at the back. If bending over without support is more painful than with support, it indicates a sacroiliac lesion. Conversely, if bending over with support is more painful than without support, it is indicative of lumbosacral or lumbar involvement.

Deyerle-May Test. This test is often helpful in differentiating the various etiologies of sciatic pain and particularly designed to differentiate between pain from pressure on the nerve or its roots and pain due to other mechanisms in the lower back. Compression or tractional pressure on muscles, ligaments, tendons, or bursae may cause reflex pain that often mimics actual direct nerve irritation. Usually, reflex pain does not follow the pattern of a specific nerve root, is more vague, does not cause sensory disturbances in the skin, comes and goes, but may be very intense. The procedure, in the sitting position, is to instruct the patient to sit very still and brace himself in the chair with his hands. The painful leg is passively extended until it causes pain, then lowered just below this point. The leg is then held by the examiner's knees and deep palpation is applied to the sciatic nerve high in the popliteal space which has been made taut by the maneuver. Severe pain indicates definite sciatic irritation or a root compression syndrome as opposed to other causes of back and leg pain such as the stretching of strained muscles and tendons or the movements of sprained articulations.

Minor's Sign. A patient with sciatica will arise from the seated position in a particular supporting position. If the chair has arms, both will be grasped and the trunk will be flexed forward. When arising, the elbows extend to push the trunk forward and upward, the hand on the uninvolved side will then be placed on the thigh, the other hand will be placed on the hip of the involved side, and the knee on the involved side will remain flexed to relieve the tension on the sciatic nerve. The knee on the uninvolved side is then extended to support the majority of body weight.

Buckling Sign. With the patient supine, the examiner slowly raises the involved lower limb (flexes it on the trunk) with the unsupported knee extended. A patient with radiculitis will automatically flex the knee to relieve the tension from the sciatic nerve.

Lindner's Sign. The patient is placed supine. A positive sign is found when conducting Brudzinski's test (progressive occiput, cervical, and upper thoracic flexion), if the patient's ipsilateral sciatic pain is reproduced or aggravated. It is indicative of lower lumbar radiculitis, as contrasted to the sharp but diffuse pain experienced in meningitis.

Sicard's Sign. A patient with sciatic-like symptoms is placed in the supine position. The limb on the involved side is raised with the knee extended to the point of pain, then it is lowered about 5°, and the examiner firmly dorsiflexes the large toe. Because this will increase tension forces on the sciatic nerve, pain will be reproduced in the posterior leg and/or thigh in cases of sciatic neuritis.

Lewin's Punch Test. This test, which should be reserved for the young and muscular, is conducted with the patient in the relaxed standing position. If local pathology has been ruled out, a positive sign of lower lumbar radiculitis is seen when a sharp blow to the ipsilateral buttock over the area of the belly of the piriformis elicits a sharp pain, but a similar blow to the contralateral buttock does not elicit pain.

Bonnet's Sign. A patient with sciatica is placed supine. The examiner lifts the involved limb slightly, adducts and internally rotates the thigh while maintaining the knee extended, and then continues to flex the thigh on the trunk to patient tolerance as in a SLR test. If this maneuver exaggerates the patient's pain or the pain response is sooner than that seen in Lasegue's SLR test, sciatic neuritis, psoas irritation, or a hip lesion is indicated.

Lasegue's Differential Sign. This test is used to rule out hip disease. A patient with sciatic symptoms is placed supine. If pain is elicited on flexing the thigh on the trunk with the knee extended but it is not produced when the thigh is flexed on the trunk with the knee relaxed (flexed), coxa pathology can be ruled out.

Management

As direct trauma to the nerve is so rare, careful evaluation of lumbar, sacral, and sacroiliac subluxations and fixations must be made, as well as lower back, pelvic, and hip musculature and trigger points. Corrective osseous adjustments, muscle techniques, and reflex techniques should be applied when indicated. Local heat and corrective muscle rehabilitation speed recovery when applied in the appropriate stage. Of all nerves in the body, the sciatic is one of the slowest to regenerate. The feet, upper cervical area, thoracolumbar junction, and overall posture should be evaluated for signs of predisposing defects in biomechanics.

Spinal Cord Injuries

Any trace of sensory abnormality, objective or subjective, should immediately raise suspicion of injury to the spinal cord or cauda equina. Injuries to the lumbosacral cord or its tail occur from vertebral fractures, dislocations, or penetrating wounds in severe accidents. In other rare instances, the cord may be damaged from violent falls with trunk flexion. The T12–L1 and L5–S1 areas are damaged from violent falls with trunk flexion. The T12–L1 and L5–S1 areas are the common sites of injury, especially those of crushing fractures with cord compression. Neurologic symptoms develop rapidly, but the lower the injury, the fewer the roots that will be involved. More common than these rare occurrences are cord tractions, concussions, and less frequent contusions.

Traction of the Spinal Cord. A scoliotic deviation must always be attended by a commensurate vertebral body rotation to the convex side. If this does not occur, it is atypical and most likely pain producing. If the vertebral bodies were not subject to the law of rotation during bending, the spine would have to lengthen during bending and its contents (ie, cord, cauda equina, and their coverings) would be subjected to considerable stretch. Thus, in a case of scoliotic deviation in the lumbar area without body rotation towards the convex side, seek signs indicating undue tension within the vertebral canal. It should also be noted that atlanto-occipital, atlanto-axial, and coccyx disrelation with partial fixation place a degree of traction upon the cord, dura, and dural sleeves in flexion-extension and lateral bending efforts.

Concussion of the Spinal Cord. Immediate signs are usually not manifested in mild or moderate injuries; but weeks later, lower extremity weakness and stiffness may be experienced. It takes time for the nerve fibers to degenerate. Deep reflexes become exaggerated, and originally mild sensory, bladder, and rectal disturbances progress. The picture is cloudy, often mimiking a number of cord diseases (eg, sclerosis, atrophy, syringomyelia). Life is rarely threatened, but full recovery is doubtful.

Contusions of the Spinal Cord. Cord concussion usually complicates cord contusion. If laceration occurs, shock is rapid. Deep reflexes, sensation, and sphincter control are lost. The paralysis is flaccid. Obviously, a prognosis cannot be made until the shock is survived.

Kernig's Test. The supine patient is asked to place both hands behind his head and forcibly flex his head toward his chest. Pain in either the neck, lower back, or down the lower extremities indicates meningeal irritation, nerve root involvement, or irritation of the dural coverings of the nerve root. A variation of this test is also attributed to Kernig: The examiner flexes the thigh at a right angle with the torso and holds it there with one hand. With the other hand, the ankle is grasped and an attempt is made to extend the leg at the knee. If pain or resistance is encountered as the leg extends, the sign is positive, provided there is no joint stiffness or sacroiliac disorder.

Milgram's Test. Ask the supine patient to keep his knees straight and lift both legs off the table about 2 inches and to hold this position for as long as possible. The test stretches the anterior abdominal and iliosoas muscles and increases intrathecal pressure. Intrathecal pressure can be ruled out if the patient can hold this position for 30 seconds without pain. If this position cannot be held or if pain is experienced during the test, a positive sign is offered indicating intrathecal pathology, herniated disc, or pressure upon the cord from some source.

Intervertebral Disc Syndrome

It is generally agreed that a true diagnosis of disc herniation with or without fragmentation of the nucleus pulposus can only be made on surgical intervention. Thus the term "intervertebral disc syndrome" is generally used when conservative diagnostic means are used exclusively. There is considerable dogmatism associated with both diagnosis and management.

Classes

In a *Grade I* syndrome, the patient has intermittent pain and spasm with local tenderness. There is very little or no root compression. Paresthesia and/or radiculitis may extend to the ischium.

In a *Grade II* syndrome, some nerve root compression exists along with pain, sensory disturbance, and occasionally some atrophy. Paresthesia and/or radiculitis may extend to the knee.

In a *Grade III* syndrome, there is marked demonstrable muscle weakness, pronounced atrophy, and intractable radicular pain. Paresthesia and/or radiculitis may extend to the ankle or foot.

Beyond these three grades, we find frank herniation. In rupture, there is a complete

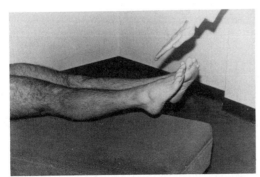

Figure 25.9. Milgram's test (with the permission of the Associated Chiropractic Academic Press).

extrusion of the nucleus through the anulus into the canal or IVF. All above symptoms are found in herniation, and, in addition, pain is worse at night and not generally relieved by most conservative therapies.

The IVD syndrome usually has a traumatic origin and occurs more commonly between the ages of 20 and 60. There may be a history of low back complaints with evidence of organic or structural disease. Most protrusions seen in athletes occur at the L4–L5 or L5–S1 level, involving the L4, L5, or S1 roots. A unilateral sciatic pain following a specific dermatome segmentation and not remissive except by a possible position of relief is often presented. There is usually a C scoliosis away from the side of pain, splinting, and a flattening of the lumbar spine. Laseque's, Kemp's and Naffziger's tests are positive. There may be diminished tendon reflexes of the involved segment and possible weakness and/or atrophy of the musculature innervated.

Lasegue's Rebound Test. At the conclusion of a positive sign during the straight-leg-raising test, the examiner may permit the leg to drop to a pillow without warning. If this rebound test causes a marked increase in pain and muscle spasm, then a disc involvement is suspect.

Other Clinical Signs

A number of helpful neurologic and orthopedic procedures have been developed to aid the diagnosis and differentiation of IVD lesions. See Table 25.2.

Bechterew's Test. The patient in the seated position is asked to extend first one knee with the leg straight forward (parallel to the floor). If this is performed, the patient is asked to extend the other knee likewise. If this can be performed, the patient is asked to extend both limbs simultaneously. If the patient is unable to perform any of these tests because of sciatic pain or able only by leaning far backward to relieve the tension on the sciatic nerve, a lumbar disc disorder or acute lumbosacral sprain should be suspected.

Dejerine's Sign. If sneezing, coughing, and straining at the stool (Dejerine's triad) or some other Valsalva maneuver produces or increases a severe low back or radiating sciatic pain, a positive Dejerine's sign is

Table 25.2.
Review of Neurologic and Orthopedic Maneuvers, Reflexes, Signs, or Tests Relative to Intervertebral Disc Syndromes

Adams' sign	Goldthwait's test	Milgram's test
Astrom's suspension test	Gower's sign	Minor's sign
Babinski's sciatic sign	Hyperextension tests	Muscle strength grading
Bechterew's test	Kemp's test	Naffziger's test
Beery's sign	Kernig's sign	Neri's bowing sign
Bowstring sign	Laseque's rebound	Range of motion tests
Bragard's test	test	Tendon reflexes
Dejerine's sign	Laseque's SLR test	Turyn's sign
Deyerle-May's test	Lewin's supine test	Vanzetti's sign
Fajersztajn's test	Light touch/pain tests	

present. This is indicative of some disorder that is aggravated by increased intrathecal pressure (eg, IVD lesion, cord, tumor, etc).

Astrom's Suspension Test. This is a confirmatory test for sciatic neuritis and/or lumbar traction therapy. The patient is asked to step on a low stool, grasp a horizontal bar, and hang suspended for several seconds. In most cases, the traction effect produced will be sufficient enough to retract a protruding disc, separated the articular facets, open the IVFs, and, thus, relieve the patient's discomfort. A variation of this test is for the examiner to conduct a spinal percussion test while the patient is suspended.

Also see Beery's sign, Goldthwait's test, Neri's bowing sign, Lewin's supine test, Brudzinski's test, and Naffziger's test.

Roentgenographic Considerations

Normally, as a major adaptive change to the carrying of weight, there is a flattening of the lumbar lordosis and a mild rotation of the sacrum into a more vertical position. The maximum adaptation occurs at the lumbosacral junction with only minor adjustments at the higher levels. The L5 disc assumes a more nearly horizontal position with widening posteriorly and compression anteriorly, which results in a decrease in the downward sliding force applied at the S1 level. These reflections by Olsen go on to state that the usual manifestation of disordered function of any part of the motor unit is weakness. He quotes DeJarnette's 1967 notes that "The position of the sacral base is often compensatory to keep severe situations from becoming worse through weight bearing."

When an IVD leaves its normal anatomic position, routine radiographic examination without contrast medium may present diagnostic characteristics such as narrowing of the intervertebral space (most typical), retrolisthesis of the vertebral body superior to the herniated disc, posterior osteophytes on the side of the direction of the herniated disc or apophyseal arthrosis, and sclerosis of the vertebral plates as a result of stress on "denuded" bone (frequent). Malformations as asymmetric transitional lumbosacral vertebra and spina bifida are seen more frequently with herniated disc than in cases in which such anomalies do not exist. Scoliosis is more common in the L4–L5 disc than in the L5–S1 disc.

Three functional views should be taken in the erect position: A–P neutral and right and left maximum lateral flexion. Points to especially evaluate are asymmetry and unilateral elevation of disc spaces, limited and impaired mobility on the affected side, blocked mobility contralaterally one segment above the L5–S1 level, and slight rotation of the L4 or L5 vertebral body toward the side of collapse. Abnormal findings suggesting a fixed prolapse in these functional views include flattening of the lumbar curve, posterior shifting of one or more lumbar vertebral bodies, impaired mobility on forward flexion so that the disc space does not change as compared to the findings in the neutral position, and impaired mobility on dorsiflexion.

Management

The cause of pain may vary from a mild bulge to a severe protrusion to frank prolapse and rupture of the IVD into the vertebral canal. While physical signs are helpful, but not conclusive, in determining the extent of damage, subjective symptoms are often misleading.

Cryotherapy and other forms of pain control are advisable during the acute stage for 48 hours. Some relief will be achieved by placing the patient prone with a small roll under the lower abdomen to flex the lumbar spine while applying manual traction techniques. This should be followed by corrective adjustments to correct attending fixations and abnormal biomechanics, traction, and other physiotherapy modalities. A regimen of therapeutic exercises to improve torso strength, a temporary lumbopelvic support, and shoe inserts designed to improve postural balance and lessen gait shock are extremely helpful during recuperation.

Spondylolisthesis

The anterior or posterior sliding of one vertebral body on another (spondylolisthesis) can result from either traumatic pars defects or degenerative disease of the facets. There is a separation of the pars interarticularis which allows the vertebral body to slip forward, carrying with it a portion of the neural arch. Davis points out that many authorities consider the condition as congenital, while others are of the opinion that trauma in early childhood is more often responsible. Regardless, when witnessed in an adult, the lesion dates from childhood rather than from some recent injury. Rehberger states it occurs in 4–6% of people, but is present in about 25% of people complaining of constant backache.

Background

An increase in the S1 sagittal diameter in spondylolisthesis occurs during teen maturation. Displacement tends to increase before the age of 30, but this trend sharply decreases thereafter unless there is an unusual cause such as chronic fatigue coupled with an unusual prolonged posture.

Predisposing spinal instability is frequently related to a degenerated disc at the spondylolisthetic level. Quite often the lesion is asymptomatic during the first 2 decades of life. Dimpling of the skin above the level of the spondylolisthesis may be ob-

served or extra skin folds may be seen because of the altered spinal alignment. When the condition does become symptomatic, the pain is usually recurrent and increases in severity with subsequent episodes. Low back pain often develops after insignificant injury or strain, with recurrent pain gradually increasing in intensity. Weakness, fatigue, stiffness, unilateral or bilateral sciatic pain, and extreme tenderness in the area of the spinous process of L5 are associated. Pain usually subsides in the supine position.

Roentgenographic Considerations

Disc tone is best analyzed through neutral, flexion, and extension views. As with spondylolysis, the most common site of spondylolisthesis is in the lower spine, but it has been reported in all areas of the lumbar spine and the cervical area. The typical situation is slippage of L5 on the sacral base (75% to 80%), but it is occasionally seen at the L4 segment.

Spondylolisthesis is graded by dividing the sacral base or the superior end plate of L5 into four equal parts when viewed in the lateral film: the *Meyerding method*. The part occupied by the posterior-inferior tip of the vertebra above indicates the degree of forward slip. In suspected cases where no obvious gross slippage has occurred, the *Meschan method* is used on the lateral projection. A line is drawn across the posterior, superior, and inferior tip of the L5 vertebral body. A second line is drawn from the posterior-superior tip of the sacrum to the posterior-inferior tip of L4. Normally, these lines should overlap or nearly so. If they are parallel or form an angular wedge at the superior, it indicates an anterior movement of L5. If the angle formed is greater than 2° or if the lines are parallel and separated more than 3 mm, a spondylolisthesis is present. To determine the degree of instability, flexion and extension studies in the lateral projection are utilized. The degree of angulation formed in flexion is subtracted from the degree of angulation formed in extension, as the maximum degree of slippage is seen during extension. The result of these two measurements offers the degree of instability present. See Figure 25.10.

Oblique views show a defect in the isthmus or pars interarticularis where the neural

MESCHAN'S LINING METHOD
IN RADIOGRAPHIC
DIAGNOSIS

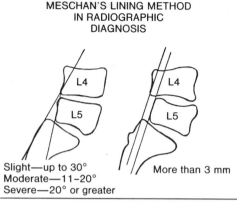

Slight—up to 30°
Moderate—11–20°
Severe—20° or greater

More than 3 mm

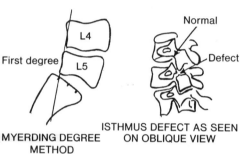

First degree

Normal

Defect

MYERDING DEGREE
METHOD

ISTHMUS DEFECT AS SEEN
ON OBLIQUE VIEW

Figure 25.10. *Top,* The Meschan lining method. *Bottom, left,* Myerding degree method; *right,* isthmus defect seen on oblique view (with the permission of the ACA Council on Roentgenology).

arch is visualized as a picture of a terrier's head. The pedicle and transverse process form the head of the dog, and the dog's ears are formed by the superior articular process, the neck by the pars interarticularis, the body by the lamina, and front legs by the inferior articular process. When the defect appears as a collar on the dog, a spondylolysis is present. If the terrier is decapitated, a spondylolisthesis is present.

Other roentgenographic findings include an unusual lumbar lordosis with increased lumbosacral angle and overriding of facets adjacent to the defect which is usually visible on the A–P view. In time, the overriding apophyseal joints indicate osteoarthritic changes. The amphiarthroidial joint between the vertebral bodies frequently shows narrowing, spurring, and associated osteoarthritic changes. A lumbar kyphosis is rarely seen, indicating the possible of a herniated disc.

Management

Symptoms progress from mild stiffness and low-back spasm after working or lifting in the forward flexion position to a sharp pain upon mild hyperextension of the trunk. Pain elicited by spinal percussion exhibits late, but depression of the spinous process is an early physical sign.

Cryotherapy and other forms of pain control are advisable during the acute stage (eg, 48 hours). Considerable relief will be achieved by placing the patient prone with a small roll under the lower abdomen to flex the lumbar spine while applying manual traction techniques. This should be followed by corrective adjustments to release attending fixations, improve abnormal biomechanics, and help reduce the separation. Traction and other physiotherapy modalities are helpful adjuncts. A regimen of mild stretching exercises, with emphasis on flexion, is extremely helpful during recuperation. Sole lifts or lowered heels may be necessary if the sacral angle is abnormally wide. Lifting should be prohibited until the patient is unsymptomatic for several weeks, and then initiated only with caution.

Lumbar Spondylolysis

Spondylolysis is similar to spondylolisthesis in that there is also a defect in the pars interarticularis, but there is no anterior slipping of the vertebral body. Disc narrowing and facet sclerosis are frequently associated. It is a degenerative condition of early middle life, more common to males and often associated with athletic or occupational stress. The most common site of spondylolysis is in the lower spine.

In describing spondylolysis, Davis reminds us that the term "pre-spondylolisthesis" is a misnomer as it indicates that spondylolisthesis will occur. This term is also inaccurate to describe an exaggeration of the sacral base angle. It is true that spondylolysis will contribute to spinal instability much the same as an exaggerated sacral base angle, but it is not true that spondylolisthesis will result in either condition. Degenerative arthropathy of the apophyseal joints will most likely result from the stress and strain placed upon the facets. The defective arrangement will also predispose the individual to spinal fatigue. The condition is also referred to as hypertrophic osteoarthritis, which is a misnomer as there is no inflammatory involvement present. The appropriate nomenclature is *discogenic spondylolysis*.

Incidence. There is a high incidence of trauma and strenuous physical activity in the history of spondylolysis. Incidence in sports is particularly high in fast bowlers, affecting the contralateral side of the active arm. It is common in the obese, robust, endomorphic individual such as heavy boxers and professional wrestlers. It is not uncommon in oarsmen. A large number of college and professional football interior linemen present lowback pain with abnormalities present on radiographs. A large percentage of such cases show a degree of spondylolysis or spondylolisthesis, usually with normal neurologic signs. Because of chronic lumbar stress, weight lifting is also commonly associated with an increased incidence in spondylolysis and disc herniation at the lower lumbar area. Rarely, vertebral-body fracture is associated.

Roentgenographic Considerations. Turner describes the process as primary change in the IVD with progressive loss of turgor and elasticity contributing to softening and weakening of the disc margin. Marginal spurring, lipping, and the consequence of osteophytic formation ensues. The sacroiliac areas are not usually involved. Narrowing of one or more IVD spaces may develop when the disc space together with changes in the curvature of the spine appear narrowed. The clinical picture, associated with spondylosis deformans, is usually referred to the area of structural deformity that results in compromise of contour and diameter of the related IVF. Oblique views, along with standard A–P and lateral views, are helpful in showing defects or fractures of the pars interarticularis. Not infrequently, cephalad-angled views or tomograms are necessary.

Management. Mild and moderate cases respond well to chiropractic anterior lumbar techniques. Adjunctive care includes low back traction in selected cases, positive galvanism, ultrasound, and alternating contractile currents to improve muscle tone.

Immobilization using a lumbosacral support helps in the more advanced cases. Once the disorder becomes asymptomatic, corrective exercises should be recommended to maintain optimal muscle tone.

Prognosis. Prognosis is good in first- and second-degree types with minimal neurologic symptoms. Prognosis is good in cases of minimal changes but poor in cases of gross changes where the patient is usually left with a residual rigidity and stiffness in the lower spine. If conservative measures fail, surgical fusion and removal of the neural arch are recommended.

Subluxations, Fractures, and Dislocations

Subluxations are discussed throughout this chapter, but a few general points should be made here. The apices of curvatures and rotations are logical points for spinal listings since they are frequently the location of maximum vertebral stress. Subluxations may occur at other points in curves and rotations, particularly at the beginning point of a primary defect in balance such as in the lower lumbar and upper cervical sections. Subluxations also frequently occur at the point where a primary curve merges into its compensatory curve. A posterior L3 is rare when the apex of the lumbar curve is too high or too low, but common at L4, L5, or the sacral base. When the apex of the lumbar curve is too low, a posterior subluxation will most likely be found in the upper lumbar area.

Roentgenographic Considerations

As in other areas of the body, x-ray views of the spine must be chosen according to the part being examined and the injury situation. And as with the cervical spine, careful evaluation must be made of the vertebral structures, the IVDs and paraspinal soft tissues. The L5–S1 and sacroiliac joints, the pelvis, and its contents deserve careful scrutiny. Acute injuries to the supporting soft tissues about a vertebra are rarely demonstrable. Their presence is suggested when the normal relations of bony structures are disturbed. However, when ligament lesions heal, hypertrophic spurs and sometimes bridges may develop locally on the margins of the bones affected.

The lower back and pelvis are the most common sites for avulsion-type injuries. Severe, sudden muscle contraction can produce fragmented osseous tears near sites of origin and insertion. Avulsions in the lumbar area often occur with transverse-process fragmentation at the site of psoas insertion. Although the transverse processes of the lumbar spine are quite sturdy, multiple fractures are seen in some football injuries. Lumbar transverse-process fractures are sometimes not evident or are poorly visualized in roentgenography unless markedly displaced or angulated due to overlying gas and/or soft-tissue shadows which obscure detail. Howe suggests a cleansing enema or other means of clearing overlying soft-tissue shadows whenever all bony processes are not well visualized. Transverse-process fractures are frequently asymptomatic, or nearly so, and lack the symptoms to encourage a most careful examination.

Miscellaneous Pathologic Signs

Romberg's Station Test. During this test, the examiner must stand close to the patient in the event the patient loses balance. The patient is asked to stand in a relaxed position and to close the eyes. If this cannot be accomplished without falling or severe swaying that requires the feet to be moved to regain balance, a positive sign is established that rules out cerebellar to labyrinthine disease. A positive sign is seen in locomotor ataxis associated with marked alcoholic neuritis, spinocerebellar tract disease, and in pernicious anemia when the columns of Goll and Burdach are affected. While a patient with cerebellar or labyrinthine disease may have difficulty standing, the position is usually taken equally well with or without visual support.

Neri's Test. The patient is placed supine with the knees extended. The examiner flexes the involved thigh on the trunk to approximately 45° while keeping the knee extended, as in a SLR test. Normally, the contralateral limb will remain fairly flat against the table. In organic hemiplegia, however, the opposite limb will flex at the knee.

Barre's Sign. The patient is placed in the prone position by the examiner with the knees passively flexed at right angles to the thigh. If the patient cannot actively hold this position with either or both limbs, it is a positive sign of pyramidal tract disease.

INJURIES OF THE PELVIS

In evaluating the athletic injury, inspection and palpation offer the most significant signs. Common pelvic landmarks are the anterior superior iliac spine (ASIS), posterior superior iliac spine (PSIS), and the anterior inferior iliac spine (AIIS).

Clinical Signs

A listing of neurologic and orthopedic manuevers, reflexes, signs, and tests relative to the pelvis and sacroiliac joints is shown in Table 25.3.

Buttock Sign. A lower extremity of a supine patient is passively flexed at the hip with the knee extended as in an SLR test. If the flexion of the limb on the trunk is restricted by local or radiating buttock pain (rather than pain in the hip or lower back), it is significant of a inflammatory pelvic lesion such as ischiorectal abscess, osteomyelitis of or near the hip joint, coxa bursitis, sacroiliac septic arthritis, or an advanced pelvic neoplasm.

Also see adductor reflex, anal reflex, cremasteric reflex, Ely's heel-to-buttock test, Hibb's test, and Nachlas' test.

Physiologic or Anatomic Short Leg

Upon fully extending the legs (supine position) in pelvic mechanical pathologies, the one on the side of involvement will be retracted ¼–½ inch more than the one on the opposite side because the posterior innominate rotation causes the acetabulum to be carried superior and anterior, the superior position producing the retraction of the limb. However, upon bringing the extremities upward to an extended position of right angles to the body, the short leg will measure the longest because the acetabulum of the posterior innominate has been carried superior and anterior, and the anterior position now produces the added length.

Evidence of an anatomic short leg or an anteroinferior sacral subluxation, or both, also show that: (1) If a standing patient

Table 25.3.
Review of Neurologic and Orthopedic Maneuvers, Reflexes, Signs, or Tests Relative to the Pelvis and Sacroiliac Joints

Disorder	Procedures/Signs	
Pelvic Syndromes	Adductor reflex	Ludloff's sign
	Anal reflex	Patella reflex
	Buttock sign	Patrick's F-AB-ER-E test
	Cremasteric reflex	Piriformis myofascitis test
	Ely's heel-to-buttock test	Piriformis spasm test
	Hibb's test	Pitres' sign
	Light touch/pain tests	Trendelenburg's test
Sacroiliac Syndromes	Bechterew's test	Lewin's supine test
	Belt test	Light touch/pain tests
	Buttock sign	Mazion's step-flex test
	Demianoff's sign	Mennell's test
	Erichsen's pelvic rock test	Minor's sign
	Gaenslen's test	Nachlas' test
	Gillis' test	Neri's bowing sign
	Goldthwait's test	Patella reflex
	Hibb's test	Patrick's F-AB-ER-E test
	Hip abduction stress test	Range of motion tests
	Iliac compression test	Sacroiliac stretch test
	Laguerre's test	Smith-Peterson's test
	Lewin-Gaenslen's test	Yeoman's test

seeks to rest his back by shifting from one foot to the other, he will come to rest himself by hearing his weight on the side on which the leg is short, the sacrum has gravitated anterior and inferior, and the innominate in compensation has rotated posterior and superior. Using the dual weight scales, the patient usually carries the most weight on the side of the short leg and anteroinferior sacrum. (2) With the patient in the Adams position, the pelvis slants anteriorly and inferiorly and the lumbar spine gravitates into scoliotic deviation to the low sacral side, which establishes a state of reverse rotation between L5 and the sacrum.

Contusions and Strains

The majority of sports-related pelvic injuries treated will be those of a musculotendinous unit. Palpation and testing muscle action against resistance will usually quickly pinpoint the site of trauma.

Hip Pointer

This is a very common painful injury of the superior iliac crest seen in all sports. It is often difficult to heal. The easily irritated

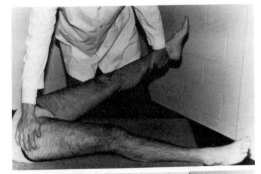

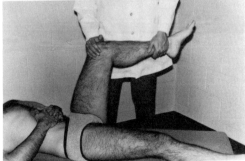

Figure 25.11. *Top,* seeking an iliopsoas sign; *bottom,* seeking an obturator sign. Both signs are also used to elicit signs of retroperitoneal irritation.

epiphysis of the iliac crest does not close until about 24 years of age and is easily injured by a shoulder, helmet, knee, or shoe blow. In addition, the picture is one of ilioinguinal and iliohypogastric nerve contusion, painful avulsion of the iliolumbar ligament from the ilium and/or sprain at its L4–L5 attachment, and crushing of the muscle bulge overlapping the crest.

Signs and Symptoms. Symptoms often mimic fracture; ie, acute, steadily increasing pain and severe progressing disability. On onset, a moderate injury will present tenderness below the iliac wing and at the overlapping muscle bulge but not on the crest itself, indicating a bone bruise with nerve contusion. An impact to the anterior spine may actually strip attachments along the crest. Thus, severe injury presents extreme tenderness throughout and above the crest, indicating torn attachments. The pain is agonizing, easily aggravated, and often requires hospitalization. If examination is delayed, bleeding, spasm, and swelling obscure localization of all initial diagnostic signs.

Management. Initial management requires direct cold packs to stop the bleeding, swelling, and spasm and careful strapping to tilt the trunk toward the ipsilateral pelvis to prevent further spasm. Disability and swelling must be monitored daily during the early stage. In minor strains with minimal swelling, cold may be discontinued after 24 hours. Active motion without heat may begin at this time. Ultrasound has been found especially helpful in resolution. Active motion with support and padding is beneficial, but heat is usually contraindicated. Activity may be resumed in 3–10 days depending upon the extent of injury. In severe strains with extensive swelling, cold must be continued for 72 hours. Activity may be resumed in 2–3 weeks if management is carefully controlled.

Groin Strains

These are often difficult to manage and often seen early in the season before full conditioning has occurred. They are common in hockey and from slips on muddy fields where severe hip abduction might occur. A wrenching-type disability arises slowly rather than suddenly as in a quickly torn muscle.

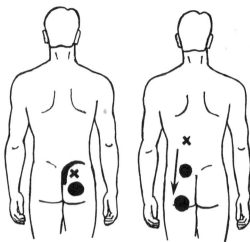

Figure 25.12. *Left*, gluteus medius trigger point; *X*, common site. *Blackened areas* indicate typical sites of referred pain. *Right*, longissimus dorsi trigger point.

Management. In spite of extensive ecchymosis, there is usually immediate relief after correcting attending sacroiliac and pubic subluxations if severe avulsion has not taken place. Cold, compression, pressure by an elastic figure-8 bandage to prevent hyperextension, and rest will rapidly control the swelling. Standard physiotherapy will relieve attending muscle spasm due to the irritation from the infammatory reaction. Carefully monitored graduated exercises must be initiated as soon as possible to avoid posttraumatic contractures that will produce recurrent disability. Return to full-scale activity can usually be expected within 7–10 days.

Sartorius Strains and Tears

This often mild but persistent disability is often seen with "squatting" football linemen and occasionally in oarsmen. Discomfort is aggravated by abduction, extension, and eased after warmup.

Piriformis Disorders

If the patient has deep gluteal pain, has sciatic neuralgia, and walks with the foot noticeably everted on the side of involvement, involvement of the piriformis should be suspected.

Spasm Test. To test for piriformis spasm, place the patient supine, lying on a firm flat table, grasp the patient's heels and firmly invert the feet. If one foot resists this effort and the act is attended by pain in the gluteal area, the piriformis should be suspected. Differentiation of piriformis spasm from other causes can be elicited by reproducing the pain on internal rotation of the femur when it is at a lower level than the original point of pain.

Strength Test. To determine piriformis strength, place the patient supine, fully flex the hip, and flex the knee to a right angle. Bring the foot being tested across the opposite leg, stabilize the knee with your other hand, and apply adduction pressure to the ankle against patient resistance (thigh abduction).

Myofascitis Test. To test for piriformis myofascitis, seat the patient on a table with hips and knees flexed. Apply resistance as the patient attempts to separate the knees. In piriformis myofascitis, pain and weakness will be noted on resisted abduction and external rotation of the thigh. Inflammation will be confirmed by rectal examination exhibiting tenderness over the lateral pelvic wall proximal to the ischial spine.

The Soccer Syndrome

In soccer, the common "scissors" kick frequently leads to instability of the sacroiliac and symphysis pubis joints. Groin pain is aggravated during full stride, jumping, and in the stretching motion of kicking with power. Also in soccer players and jockeys, a periosteal reaction may be noted at the origin of the adductor muscles (gracilis syndrome).

Roentgenographic Considerations. When pain in the area of the symphysis pubis is the complaint, views should be taken in the weight-bearing position, first with full weight on one limb and then the other to exhibit instability. Oval or semicircular lucency and avulsion sites may be exhibited at the pubic bone near the symphysis at the origin of the gracilis muscle and the adductors longus and brevis. In addition, symphysis widening, instability, frayed corners, fluffy margins, symphyseal osteoporosis, and muscle attachment periosteal reactions may be seen. Stress sclerosis of the iliac portions of the sacroiliac joints are often associated in these conditions.

Osteitis Pubis

This is a rare disability seen most often in runners, competitive walkers, and football players. It is frequently chronic and episodic. The picture is one of severe groin pain sometimes radiating to the hips, groin, or abdomen that is aggravated by hip rotation, abdominal flexion, and sometimes by iliac compression. Swelling and tenderness will be noted over the symphysis pubis. A slight epiphyseal slip may be a predisposing factor. Roentgenography may reveal an eroded symphysis with joint widening, tending to calcification in later stages. Fever, dysuria, leukocytosis, and an increased sedimentation rate are inconsistent associations. Differentiation must be made from ankylosing spondylitis, adductor-origin strain, and perineal disease.

Management. Rest, cold, diathermy, mild ultrasound, vitamin-mineral supplementation, and attention to lumbar subluxations are helpful in these often stubborn cases. Mobilization of frequently associated hip fixations is essential. Graduated return to activity must be carefully monitored to prevent recurrence of acute symptoms. If conservative measures fail, fusion of the symphysis may be advised, but postoperative results are not always good.

Gluteal Contusions and Strains

Contusions, especially to the ischial tuberosity and the well-developed athletic buttocks, are frequently seen. Incidence is high in hockey and field sports. Just walking may be aggravating, but pain is usually not severe. Swelling and bleeding may be extensive, but it is reduced quickly if cold is applied immediately. Recurrent bleeding is always a problem, but its likelihood is reduced if cold is continued for 3–4 days. Activity can be resumed with padding, but it is rarely adequate protection against reinjury. Full healing without reinjury will usually take place within a month.

Strain may be infrequently seen in the muscles which rotate the thigh and stabilize the hip such as the glutei, piriformis, gemilli, and quadratus femoris. Awkward slips are the typical injury mechanism, and dysfunction is extremely debilitating. Strains of the origin of the hamstring muscles, associated with lower buttock pain on exercise and

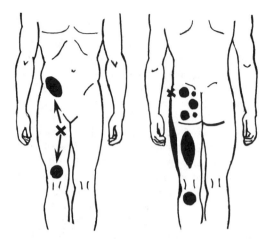

Figure 25.13. *Left,* adductor longus trigger point; *X,* common site. *Blackened areas* indicate typical sites of referred pain. *Right,* gluteus minimus trigger point.

ischial tenderness on forward flexion, are common among football players and sprinters. Sciatica tests will be negative. Heat, gentle passive stretching, and graduated active exercises should be incorporated into the standard strain management program.

Golfer's Strain. An unimpeded forceful, full golf swing may injure a golfer by causing an avulsion of the ischial apophysis.

Rider's Strain. An adductor strain is frequently suffered by horsemen, cyclists, fast bowlers, and runners. The complaint will be one of stiffness, tenderness, and pain during abduction that is high in the groin. In addition to regular strain therapy, treatment should include applying adductor tendon stretch up to patient tolerance

Sprains and Subluxations

Sacroiliac Sprain

These sprains are of frequent appearance, especially when weights are lifted. Heavy loads or severe blows may rupture some associated ligaments and slightly subluxate the joint.

Background. Pain may be local or referred. Symptoms are usually relieved by rest and aggravated by activity. The patient assumes the characteristic posture with a flattened lumbar area, trunk inclined away from the lesion, guarded gait, and limited spinal motions, especially spinal flexion due

to hamstring tension. Jarring the spine causes a sharp localized pain in the affected joint. In some cases, abnormal mobility may be found in thigh flexion or hyperextension. Care must be taken to differentiate from a sacral base or lumbar lesion. Localized tenderness and the classic clinical tests are helpful in differentiation.

Management. During the acute hyperemic stage, structural alignment, cold, compression support, acupressure, ultrasound, and rest are indicated. Vitamin C and manganese supplementation are helpful. The stages of passive congestion, consolidation, and fibrosis are treated as in other sprains.

Sacroiliac Subluxation

This is characterized by misalignment of the sacrum in relation to the ilia independent of bilateral innominate involvement (ie, primary) or misalignment of the sacrum in relation to the ilia as a result of bilateral innominate involvement (ie, secondary). These situations point toward (1) irritative microtrauma to the interarticular structures, (2) induction of a vertebral motion unit subluxation and/or are contributory to chronicity of subluxations, (3) induction of spinal curvatures and/or are contributory to the chronicity of curvatures present, and (4) biomechanical impropriety of the pelvis in static postural accommodation and in locomotion.

If the innominate is in posterior rotation subluxation, with the patient standing sup-

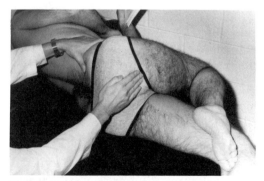

Figure 25.14. Palpation of the ischial bursa. Bursitis here can be easily confused with sciatic neuritis unless the precise source of pain can be identified.

porting himself with hands on the back of a chair, he carries his thigh forward, flexes his knee and carries it upward against his abdomen (and thus rotates the innominate further posteriorly) much more readily than extending the thigh backward and thus rotating the innominate anteriorly. With the patient supine and the pelvis fixed by the examiner, the patient will find it noticeably more difficult to straight raise the leg on the side of sacroiliac subluxation.

Differentiation. To differentiate sacroiliac from lumbosacral involvement: Have the patient supine on a firm flat table. A folded towel is placed transversely under the small of the patient's back. The doctor stabilizes the patient's pelvis by cupping his hands over the ASISs and exerting moderate pressure. The patient is instructed to raise both extremities simultaneously in a straight-leg manner. If the patient senses discomfort or an increase of discomfort in the low back or over the sacrum and gluteal area at about 25–50° leg raise and before the small of the back wedges against the towel, sacroiliac involvement is suspected. If, on the other hand, discomfort is experienced or augmented only after the legs have been raised beyond 50° and the small of the back wedges firmly against the towel, lumbosacral involvement should be suspected. Other tests are described below.

Clinical Tests

Gaenslen's Test. The patient is placed supine well to the side of the table with knees, thighs, and legs acutely flexed by the patient, who clasps his knees with both hands and pulls them toward his abdomen. This brings the lumbar spine firmly in contact with the table and fixes both the pelvis and lumbar spine. With the examiner standing at right angles to the patient, the patient is brought well to the side of the table and the examiner slowly hyperextends the opposite thigh by gradually increasing force by pressure of one hand on top of the knee while the examiner's other hand is on the flexed knee for support in fixing the lumbar spine and pelvis. Some examiners allow the hyperextended limb to fall from the table edge. The hyperextension of the hip exerts a rotating force on the corresponding half

of the pelvis. The pull is made on the ilium through the Y ligament and the muscles attached to the anterior iliac spine. The test is positive if the thigh is hyperextended and pain is felt in the sacroiliac area or referred down the thigh, providing that the opposite sacroiliac joint is normal and the sacrum moves as a unit with the side of the pelvis opposite to that being tested. Test bilaterally. If the sign is negative, a lumbosacral lesion is suspect. This test is usually contraindicated in the elderly. See Figure 25.15.

Erichsen's Pelvic Rock Test. With the patient supine, the examiner places his hands on the iliac crests with his thumbs on the ASISs and forcibly compresses the pelvis toward the midline. Pain experienced in the sacroiliac joint suggests a joint lesion which may be either traumatic or infectious in origin. See Figure 25.15.

Iliac Compression Test. Place patient in side-lying position with affected side up. The examiner places the forearm over the iliac crest and leans pressure downward for about 30 seconds. A positive sign of sacroiliac inflammation or strain is seen with an increase in pain; however, absence of pain does not necessarily rule out sacroiliac involvement. It is usually contraindicated in geriatrics and pediatrics. This is a variation of Erichsen's test.

Mennell's Test. The examiner places a thumb over the PSIS and exerts pressure, then slides the thumb outward and then inward. The sign is positive if tenderness is increased. When sliding outward, trigger

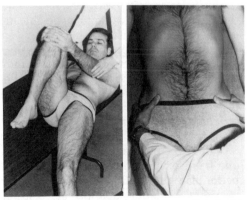

Figure 25.15. *Left,* Gaenslen's test. Pain in this position indicates a sacroiliac lesion. *Right,* pelvic rock test.

deposits in structures on the gluteal aspect of the PSIS may be noted. If when sliding inward tenderness is increased, sprain of the superior sacroiliac ligaments is indicated. Confirmation is positive when tenderness is increased when the examiner pulls the ASIS posterior while standing behind the patient or when the examiner pulls the PSIS forward while standing in front of the patient. This test is helpful in determining that tenderness is due to overstressed superior sacroiliac ligaments.

Yeoman's Test. Place the patient prone. With one hand, make firm pressure over the suspected sacroiliac joint, fixing the pelvis to the table. With the other hand, flex the patient's leg on the affected side to the limit and hyperextend the thigh by lifting the knee off the examining table. If pain is increased in the sacroiliac area, it is significant of a sacroiliac lesion because of the stress on the anterior sacroiliac ligaments. Normally, no pain will be felt on this maneuver.

Goldthwait's Test. The patient is placed supine. The examiner places one hand under the lumbar spine with each fingerpad pressed firmly against the interspinous spaces. The other hand of the examiner is used to slowly conduct a SLR test. If pain occurs or is aggravated before the lumbar processes open (0°–30°), a sacroiliac lesion should be suspected. Goldthwait felt that if pain occurred while the processes were opening at 30°–60°, a lumbosacral lesion was suggested; 60°–90°, an L1–L4 disc lesion.

Smith-Peterson's Test. If it is possible during Goldthwait's test to raise the limb on the unaffected side to a greater level without pain than on the involved side, a positive Smith-Peterson's sign is found, which confirms a sacroiliac lesion; ie, pain usually occurs at the same level for either leg when a lumbosacral lesion is present.

Sacroiliac Stretch Test. The patient is placed supine. The examiner, standing to face the patient, crosses his arms and places one hand on the contralateral anterior-superior iliac spine and the other hand on the ipsilateral anterior-superior iliac supine. Oblique (posterolateral) pressure is then applied to spread the anterior aspects of the ilia laterally. A positive sign of sacroiliac

sprain is a deep-seated pelvic pain that may radiate into the buttock or groin. While the iliac compression test is designed to stretch the posterior sacroiliac ligaments, this test stretches the ligaments on the anterior aspect of the joints.

Lewin-Gaenslen's Test. The patient is placed in the side-lying position with the underneath lower limb flexed acutely at the hip and knee. The examiner stabilizes the uppermost hip with one hand. With the other hand, the uppermost leg is grasped near the knee and the thigh is extended on the hip. Initiated or aggravated pain suggests a sacroiliac lesion.

Hip Abduction Stress Test. The patient is placed as in Lewin-Gaenslen's test. With the upper limb held straight and extended at the knee, the patient is instructed to attempt to abduct the upper limb while the examiner applies resistance. Pain initiated in the area of the uppermost sacroiliac joint or the hip joint suggests an inflammatory process of the respective joint.

Hibb's Test. The patient is placed in the prone position. The examiner stabilizes the uninvolved hip, flexes the patient's knee on the involved side toward the buttock, and then slowly adducts the leg, which internally rotates the femur. Pain initiated in the hip joint indicates a hip lesion; pain rising in the sacroiliac joint, but not the hip, points to a sacroiliac lesion.

Gillis' Test. With the patient prone and the examiner standing on the side of involvement, the examiner reaches over and stabilizes the uninvolved sacroiliac joint while the thigh on the involved side is extended at the hip. Pain initiated by this maneuver in the sacroiliac area of the involved side is a positive sign of an acute sacroiliac sprain/subluxation or sacroiliac disease.

Mazion's Step-Flex Test. A standing patient with low back pain is asked to take a large step forward, hold this position by keeping the toes in place, and then flex the trunk forward. According to Mazion, the initiation or aggravation of the patient's complaint on the contralateral limb (the one behind) exhibits a positive sign of an unilateral subluxated ilium in relation to the sacrum (ie, sacral base anteroinferior).

Also see Bechterew's test, belt test, buttock sign, Demianoff's sign, Gaenslen's test, hyperextension tests, Lewin's supine test, Minor's sign, Nachlas' test, Neri's bowing sign, and Yeoman's test.

Pubic Sprain and Subluxation

This frequently occurring condition is often mistaken for sacroiliac slip, although sacroiliac displacement may have occurred and been spontaneously reduced. Keep in mind that there is some degree of bone elasticity between the extreme A-P points of the pelvis except in the elderly. The disorder is also associated with lateral hip subluxations. In pure pubic subluxation, the only definite evidence will be found at the pubic symphysis—a fixed rotation of one innominate. The sacroiliac area will not be tender, but tenderness will be found over the painful pubis.

Management. The displaced pubis should be corrected. This should be followed by stretching of the sciatic nerve and by typical sprain therapy.

Adjustment. Place the patient in the lateral recumbent position, with the involved side up. If the pubis on the involved side is low, adjust as you would an anterior ilium or posterior ischium with an ischial contact. If the involved pubis is high, adjust as you would a posterior ilium or anterior ischium with an ilia contact. Direct contact on the pubic area is avoided because of the hypersensitivity of the area.

Coccyx Sprain and Subluxation

An irritating displacement is frequently overlooked. It is more common among women than men. The typical coccyx lies in the same curved plane as the sacrum when viewed during inspection. Slight displacements are never obvious on x-ray films. The direction of displacement is usually anterior, but it is rarely seen posterior. The cause is usually a fall in the sitting position. Ligamentous tears may be associated with subluxation and/or fracture. If a gluteus maximus is unilaterally weak, the coccyx will deviate contralaterally. Coccygodynia may be from mild to severe, and urogenital, rectal, sciatic-like complaints, and general nervousness may be associated. In traumatic situations, pain and local levator ani spasm may be pronounced and often episodic. Local tenderness is consistently present.

Keep in mind that the terminal of the spinal cord is attached to the cornua of the coccyx. As the segment moves anteriorly, the apex of the sacrum acts as a fulcrum. As the cornua rotates backward and downward, traction is made on the spinal cord. Thus, symptoms from the resulting cord tension need not be confined to the pelvic region alone (eg, occipital headaches, torticollis).

Adjustment. While many techniques can be described, the best method is the direct method with the index finger in the rectum and the thumb on the base of the coccyx. This adjustment can be done immediately after digital examination. If the patient has difficulty in relaxing the sphincter, have him perform Valsalva's maneuver. Take care not to injure the impar ganglion of the delicate rectal wall. Gentle steady pressure is made in the direction opposite to displacement for several seconds, relaxed for several seconds, and then reapplied. This cycle should continue for about three to six times. Pressure is all that is needed. A distinct thrust may break a partial ankylosis and cause more trouble than the condition itself. However, it sometimes helps to give light thrusts simultaneously on the apex of the sacrum with your free hand. After correction, evaluate integrity of the coccygeous muscles.

If upper lumbars or lower dorsals are also involved, do not adjust until after the coccygeal adjustment as the sympathetic stimulation will tend to activate probably spastic anal muscles.. However, L5 or the sacrum can be adjusted, for the parasympathetic supply from these areas tends to relax anal muscles.

Fractures and Dislocations

Note pelvic symmetry, deformity, and carefully palpate for bony crepitus about the ischium, rami, and hip areas. Rolling injuries are usually at fault in pelvic ring fractures such as seen in horseback riding accidents, ski falls against a hard surface, cycling and automobile accidents. Vascular, bladder, and perineal injuries are commonly associated.

Avulsions in Sports

Stress and avulsion fractures are far from uncommon, but the most typical injuries are associated with muscle, tendon, fascia, and cartilage injuries of the lower extremity. The most common sites of avulsion fractures in one 2-year study occurred at the ischial tuberosity at the hamstring origin, the ASIS at the sartorius origin, and the AIIS at the origin of the rectus femoris muscle. Incidence is highest in track and field sports. In sprinters, sudden severe pain in the area of the hip or buttock may be traced to an avulsion of the hamstring attachments at the ischial tuberosity. Roentgenography may indicate large crescent-shaped bone masses near the injured ischium. Most musculotendinous injuries in sprinters occur during the stride phase or at the transition point between stride to maximum finishing speed.

Fractures

While pelvic fractures are not common, they should never be taken lightly as they are reported to be the second most common cause of traumatic death—second only to head injuries. Pelvic fractures often cause severe internal bleeding difficult to halt even on surgery. Shock is present in 40% of the cases. The patient with pelvic fracture, unable to stand or walk, complains of pain in the pelvic region or back and, if the bladder or kidney is injured, passes blood in the urine. A pelvic girth injury is suggested by severe low back pain (especially in retroperitoneal bleeding), severe pain with compression of the iliac crests, and pubic tenderness.

Pelvic fractures, usually due to violent injuries, are frequently multiple and result in severe deformity. The most common area involved are those about the sacroiliac joints and the symphysis pubis. In fact, a fracture or dislocation of the pubis is frequently associated with separation of a sacroiliac joint or the neighboring sacrum or ilium.

Roentgenographic Considerations. Fractures of the ilium are visible as sharply defined lines of diminished density that are possibly stellate. Colon or rectal gas may mimic or obscure a pelvic fracture, but as these shadows are not constant, they can be ruled out on future examination. Another source of error are the blood-vessel grooves in the ilium, but their branching character and bilaterality help in identification. In examining the young, keep in mind that the pelvic epiphyses are among the last to unite: open until 20–25 years of age.

Emergency Procedure. Apply firm supporting bandages around the pelvis. Hold the legs together by a figure-8 bandage wound around the feet and ankles. Also secure the thighs with a bandage. A splint should be provided from armpit to foot. In pelvic fracture, there is often an urgent desire to urinate. If possible, this should be avoided to prevent possible extravasation from a ruptured urethra which would lead to perineal cellulitis.

Pelvic Falls

After pelvic injury, all related structures should be carefully evaluated. Direct buttock falls upon a hard surface (eg, ice or roller skating, skateboarding) often result in sacral fractures, dislocation of the coccyx, and lumbar subluxation. After pelvic or leg injury, hip dislocation is sometimes missed.

Howe points out that after falls or trauma to the back, particularly where the blow is applied to the bottom of the pelvis with force traveling up the spinal column, compression fractures of vertebral bodies frequently result. The most often missed of these occur at the T12-L1 junction, but they may possibly extend as high as T10. The reason they are often missed is that the pain is usually referred to the lumbosacral area, and there may be no spasm or even tenderness in the fracture area. If the x-ray beam is centered at the location of pain, the view may not extend high enough to include the lower thoracic area. A compression fracture is frequently not evident until several days later when deformity becomes more pronounced.

Pubic Stress Fractures

On rare occasions, the adductor muscle attachment area at the inferior pubic ramus may be the site of a stress factor. This usually occurs from a fall or a sudden foul-line stop while delivering a bowling ball in an unbalanced position. Avulsion of the inferior pubic ramus and rupture of the adduc-

Table 25.4.
Review of Neurologic and Orthopedic Maneuvers, Reflexes, Signs, or Tests Relative to the Hip Area

Adam's sign	Gauvain's sign	Muscle strength grading
Allis' hip sign	Hennequin's sign	Ober's test
Allis' knee sign	Hibb's test	Patrick's F-AB-ER-E test
Anvil test	Hyperextension tests	Piriformis myofascitis
Brudzinski's sign	Laguerre's test	test
Buttock sign	Langoria's sign	Piriformis spasm test
Ely's heel-to-buttock	Leg length tests	Range of motion tests
test	Light touch/pain tests	Thomas' test
Ely's sign	Ludloff's sign	Trendelenburg's test

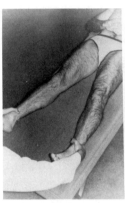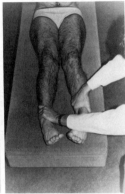

Figure 25.16. *Left,* testing strength of hip abduction (gluteus medius) against resistance. *Right,* testing adductor muscle strength against resistance.

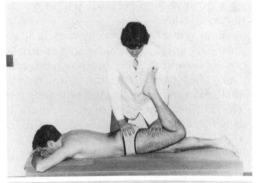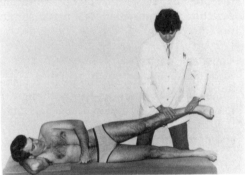

Figure 25.17. *Top,* testing strength of gluteus maximus against resistance. *Bottom,* testing hip abduction strength against resistance.

tor longus' origin may be associated, as well as laceration to scrotal vessels.

INJURIES OF THE HIP

Carefully palpate bony and soft tissues, and evaluate active and, if necessary, passive ranges of motion. See Table 25.4.

Trendelenburg's Hip Test. A patient suspected of hip involvement stands on one foot, on the side of involvement, and raises the other foot and leg in hip and knee flexion. If the hip and its muscles are normal, the iliac crest and sacral dimple will be slightly low on the standing side and high on the leg-elevated side. But, if there is hip joint involvement and muscle weakness, the iliac crest and sacral dimple will be markedly high on the standing side and low on the side the leg is elevated. A positive sign indicates the gluteus medius muscle on the supported side is either weak or nonfunctioning. The gait will exhibit a characteristic lurch to counteract the imbalance caused by the descended hip.

Contusions and Strains

General Muscle Spasm

Limitations of motion due to muscular spasm are seen with special frequency in joint disease and spinal dysarthrias, but may occur in almost any form of joint trouble, particularly the larger joints. In the hip joint, two forms of spasm are important: (1) that which is due to irritation of the psoas alone, and (2) that in which all muscles moving the joint are more or less contracted. General spasm of the hip muscles is tested via Patrick's test.

Patrick's F-AB-ER-E Test. This test is of particular value in that it indicates hip joint pathology. The patient lies supine, and the examiner grasps the ankle and the flexed knee. The thigh is flexed (F), abducted (AB), externally rotated (ER), and extended (E). Pain in the hip during the maneuvers, particularly on abduction and external rotation, is a positive sign of coxa pathology. See Figure 25.18.

Management. To relieve muscle spasm, heat is helpful, but cold and vapocoolant sprays have often shown to be more effective. Mild passive stretch is an excellent method of reducing spasm in the long muscles, but heavy passive stretch destroys the beneficial reflexes. Quadriceps spasm can usually be relaxed by passive hip and knee flexion. Peripheral inhibitory afferent impulses can be generated to partially close the presynaptic gate by acupressure, acupuncture, or transcutaneous nerve stimulation.

Iliopsoas Spasm

In pure psoas spasm, the thigh is usually somewhat flexed on the trunk, though this may be concealed by forward bending of the trunk. Very slight degrees of psoas spasm may be appreciable only when, with the patient lying prone, the examiner attempts hyperextension. In pure psoas spasm, other motions of the hip (rotation, adduction, abduction, and flexion) are not impeded. Keep in mind that in the normal erect posture only about 12% of the weight of the abdominal organs is borne by the suspensory ligaments; the majority of weight is supported by the inclined psoas and contained thereon by the abdominal wall.

Standard Tests. To test iliopsoas integrity, the seated patient is asked to raise each knee by hip flexion against resistance of the examiner's hand placed on the distal anterior thigh. Then test in the supine position. The ability to flex the thigh in the supine position but not in the seated position indicates an iliopsoas lesion. To further test, raise the leg to be tested of the supine patient to about 45°, keeping the knee extended. The patient is asked to resist a downward and slightly lateral pressure when the examiner exerts pressure against the lower anteromedial leg.

Ely's Heel-to-Buttock Test. To support iliopsoas spasm suspicions, place the patient prone with toes hanging over the edge of the table, legs relaxed. One or the other heel is approximated to the opposite buttock. After flexion of the knee, pain in the hip will make it impossible to carry out the test if there is any irritation of the psoas muscle or its sheath. The buttock will tend to rise on the involved side. However, a positive Ely's sign can also be an indication of a lumbar lesion or a contracture of the tensor fascia lata.

Thomas' Test. This is a test to determine excessive iliopsoas tension. Have the supine patient hold one flexed knee against his abdomen with his hands while the other limb is allowed to fully extend. The patient's lumbar spine should normally flatten. If the extended limb does not extend fully or if the patient rocks his chest forward or arches his back, a fixed flexion contracture of the hip is indicated, as from a shortened iliopsoas muscle. Iliopsoas hypertonicity can be confirmed by tension and pain during deep palpation of the abdomen below the umbilicus and lateral to the linea alba. Test bilaterally. The normal range of hip flexion is 120°. See Figure 25.19.

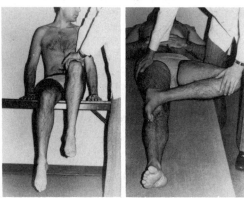

Figure 25.18. *Left,* evaluating muscle strength of psoas muscle in hip flexion against resistance. *Right,* Patricks' F-AB-ER-E test.

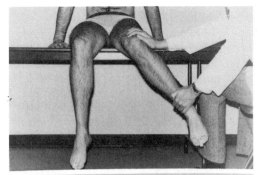

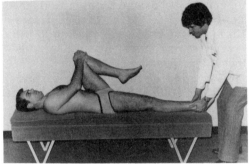

Figure 25.19. *Top*, testing strength and motion restriction for internal and external hip rotation in the sitting-fixed position. *Bottom*, Thomas' test.

Perthe's Disease

This is a state of osteochondrosis of the femoral capital epiphysis. The picture is one of ischemic necrosis followed by reconstitution, seen in children usually before the age of 10. It is more common in boys and usually is unilateral. There is an insidious limp, especially when fatigued, with some hip abduction limitation. Leg shortening is witnessed only in the late stages. Physical signs may be negative, while roentgenography is indicative; ie, increased epiphyseal density, wide joint space, dense femoral head fragments, followed by metaphyseal area cavitation and a fragmented epiphysis. During spontaneous resolution, bone texture normalizes, the shortened femoral neck widens, and the femoral head tends to mushroom. This cycle takes about 3 years to complete.

Trochanteric Bursitis

Uncommon contusions directly on the prominent greater trichanter undoubtedly result in a varying degree of bursitis that has a picture similar to that of the olecranon bursa. This bursa separates the gluteal attachments and the iliotibial band. Injury may also be the result of overuse. Incidence is higher in females than in males. The area will be warm, swollen, and tender. In stubborn cases, aspiration may be necessary. Care must be taken to seek signs of fracture such as crepitus and bony tenderness before swelling occurs. Situations of chronic bursitis are sometimes related to a mobile "snapping" tensor fascia lata tendon. This seems to be more common to the ectomorphic long-distance runner. Cold, support, rest, and later deep heat will usually resolve the situation without resorting to referral for steroids.

Causalgia Syndrome

This is a reflex sympathetic dystrophy characterized by pain, paresthesia, swelling, trigger points, burning feelings, heat or cold, redness or pallor. It consists chiefly of sympathetic phenomena following severe trauma involving one or more limbs and is often followed by organic changes such as bone atrophy and mottling resulting from persistently recurring nutrient artery spasms as well as skin and muscle atrophy. Joint immobility with or without pain, scleroderma, and contracture may occur. The syndrome is a vasomotor and sympathetic disorder wherein trophic disturbance in which any thermic, tractile, sensory, or even psychic stimulus may result in an explosive attack. It may involve either or both the lower or upper extremities.

Hip Sprain

The hip articulation is situated deeply beneath heavy muscles, fat, and fascia which protect the joint but often obscure physical signs. Fortunately, injury is rare in well-supervised sports.

Background. In the young, sprains of this joint frequently injure the upper femoral epiphysis; in adults, trauma more frequently causes injury to the muscles about the joint than to the hip joint itself.

Laguerre's Test. With the patient supine, the thigh and knee are flexed and the thigh is abducted and rotated outward. This forces the head of the femur against the anterior portion of the coxa capsule. Increased groin pain and spasm are positive signs of a lesion of the hip joint, iliopsoas muscle spasm, or a sacroiliac lesion. It differentiates from a lumbosacral disorder.

Signs and Symptoms. Motion is restricted and pain is often referred to the medial aspect of the knee. A limp is invariably present. Use Laguerre's, Ely's, Patrick's F-AB-ER-E, and Ober's tests to support your diagnosis. Thomas' sign is positive in hip contracture, Trendelenburg's hip sign is positive in hip dislocation, and Allis' knee sign is positive in hip fracture. In hip sprain, the mechanism is usually a twisting or wrenching motion. Occasionally, a stubborn case will show pus on aspiration.

Management. When symptoms of joint involvement are present, functional rest is indicated until signs of irritation disappear. Treat as any joint sprain depending upon the stage in progress. Strapping as well as crutches should be provided during the acute stage. The patient should be carefully monitored for a month or longer.

Subluxations and Fixations

Fixations

A lateral fixation of the hip joint is not an uncommon finding. On the involved side, internal rotation will be restricted and the psoas muscle will test weak.

Strength Test. Weakness in the psoas can be tested by having the supine patient lift the extended limb to 45°, externally rotate the foot, and resist the doctor's attempt to move the patient's foot laterally and towards the floor. The examiner should stand at the foot of the table so that his nonactive hand can stabilize the patient's contralateral pelvis.

Adjustment. Place the patient supine with the involved hip and knee flexed so that the foot rests flat upon the table without strain. Stand at the foot of the table, facing the patient. Interlock your fingers over the patient's flexed knee, and lean forward so that your sternum is almost above the knee. With your medial forearm, press the patient's leg laterally to internally rotate the femur about 25°. While holding this pressure, make a gentle thrust through the longitudinal axis of the femur. Check if the fixation has been freed by evaluating bilateral internal rotation of the hip and psoas strength.

Internally Rotated Femur

This subluxation is commonly associated with anterior pelvic tilting, external tibia rotation, and subtalar pronation. A degree of genu valgum and hip pain are presented.

Adjustment. Place the patient supine with flexed knees so that his buttocks are near the end of the table. Stand medially, facing perpendicular to the thigh of the involved hip. Contact the medial midshaft aspect of the thigh, while your stabilizing hand grasps the patient's calf. Externally rotate the femur, apply traction with your stabilizing hand, and make a gentle thrust with your contact hand, directed towards further external rotation. Follow by checking the integrity of the gluteus maximus, piriformis, guadratus femoris, obturators, psoas, iliacus, gemellus, and posterior fibers of the gluteus medius.

Externally Rotated Femur

This subluxation is related to internal tibia rotation and subtalar pronation. A degree of genu varum and hip pain are exhibited.

Adjustment. Place the patient supine. Stand lateral to the patient on the side of involvement, facing obliquely medial. Take contact on the superolateral aspect of the femur at midshaft with your cephalad hand, while your stabilizing hand is wrapped over the patient's leg so that your palm supports the patient's upper calf. Internally rotate the femur, apply caudal traction with your stabilizing hand, and make a gentle thrust with your contact hand that is directed towards further internal rotation. Follow by checking the integrity of the tensor fascia lata, gluteus minimus, adductor brevis, and anterior fibers of the gluteus medius.

Superior Femur Subluxation

This situation is usually seen when nagging hip pain complicates low back pain. A degree of fixed internal or external rotation is often involved.

Adjustment. Place the patient supine. Stand at the foot of the table, facing the patient, and grasp the lower leg of the involved limb just above the ankle. Stabilize the patient's contralateral foot against your knee. Apply traction, and make a gentle pull that takes into considerations any internal or external rotation involved.

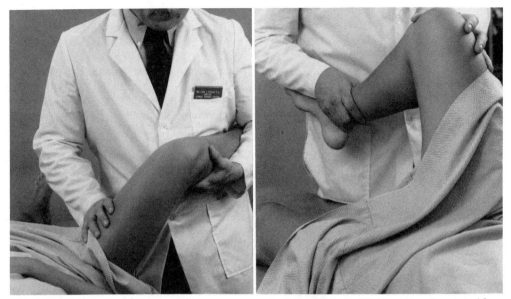

Figure 25.20. *Left*, position for adjusting an internally rotated femur. *Right*, externally rotated femur.

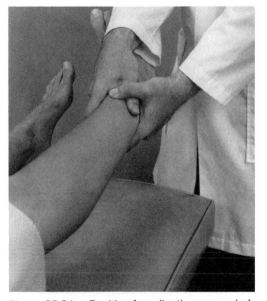

Figure 25.21. Position for adjusting a superiorly subluxated femur.

Anteriorly Subluxated Femur

This is a lesser degree of an anterior (obturator) dislocation. The cause is usually a severe fall or being forced backward against an obstacle or tackler. On the involved side, the patient exhibits hip pain and an externally rotated limb that is lengthened. The head of the femur lies near the obturator foramen.

Adjustment. Place the patient supine. Stand at the foot of the table, near the side of involvement, facing the patient. With your lateral hand, grasp the patient's posterior-distal leg just above the ankle. With your medial hand, reach across the patient's food and grasp his heel. Both hands will be on the lateral aspect of the patient's ankle area. Apply gentle traction and medial rotation to the limb. Adduct the patient's involved limb across his other leg, maintaining careful control. Constant traction, medial rotation, and adduction should reseat the displaced femoral head.

Posteriorly Subluxated Femur

When the femur is subluxated backward, the patient has difficulty in extending his thigh. Measurement indicates limb shortening. The mechanism of injury is usually a fall, long jump, or severe upper-thigh tackle from the anterior

Adjustment. Place the patient supine. Stand on the side of involvement, facing medially and centered at the patient's flexed knee. Bring the patient's knee laterally so that it is firm against your upper abdomen. With your cephalad hand, stabilize the patient's contralateral ilium. With your caudad contact hand, grasp the patient's ankle from the anterior. With your body weight, apply abduction to the flexed knee, while simultaneously applying superior pressure with your contact hand to increase hip flexion and carrying the patient's lower leg medially. This hip flexion, abduction, and external rotation should reseat the displaced femoral head.

Sciatic Displacement

This is a chronic postural disorder associated with pelvic tilt where weight balance is decidedly unilateral on the involved side. Acute trauma is rarely involved, but it may be in the patient's history. The patient presents hip pain, internal limb rotation, and a shortened limb. The head of the femur is found near the lesser sciatic notch.

Adjustment. Place the patient supine. This maneuver is essentially the opposite of adjusting an anteriorly subluxated femur. Stand at the foot of the table near the side of involvement. Face the patient. With your lateral hand, grasp the patient's posterodistal leg just above the ankle. With your medial hand, reach across the patient's foot and grasp his heel. Both hands will be on the lateral aspect of the patient's ankle area. Apply gentle traction and lateral rotation to the limb. Abduct the patient's involved limb. Constant traction, lateral rotation, and abduction should reseat the displaced femoral head.

Fractures and Dislocations

Any type of hip pain encourages careful physical and roentgenographic evaluation of the soft tissues on the lateral and medial aspects of the hip. A hip dislocation with or without fracture should be considered a major injury and referred immediately without attempts of reduction. Roentgenographs will never indicate all soft-tissue damage present. Severe pain on motion is typical in both hip dislocations and fractures.

Allis' Knee Sign. With the patient supine, knees flexed, and soles of feet flat on table, the examiner observes heights of knees superiorly from the foot of the table. If one knee is lower than the other, it is indicative of a unilateral hip dislocation or severe coxa disorder.

Langoria's Sign. Relaxation of the ex-tensor muscles of the thigh is an indication of intracapsular fracture of the femur.

Hennequin's Sign. The patient is placed supine with the knees extended. A positive sign is found if deep palpation just inferior to Poupart's ligament and lateral to the large inguinal vessels produces deep tenderness, pain, and crepitation—signs of femoral neck fracture.

Anvil Test. If a fracture of the leg or femur is suspected, the patient is placed supine and the examiner grasps the ankle of the involved side in one hand and strikes the patient's heel with the fist of the other hand, sending a shock wave up the extremity. The result may be localized pain that will help to locate the site of fracture or pathologic focus.

Gauvain's Sign. With the patient in the side-lying position, the examiner stabilizes the patient's uppermost iliac crest with the heel of the hand and with the fingerpads fixed against the patient's lower abdomen. With the patient's uppermost knee extended, the examiner grasps the patient's upper ankle with the other hand, moderately abducts the limb, and firmly rotates it internally and externally. With the patient's knee locked in extension, these rotary maneuvers will affect the entire limb, as far superiorly as the head of the femur. A positive sign is seen when a strong abdominal contraction occurs, indicating a somatosomatic reflex spasm that is usually attributed to hip pathology (eg, coxa tuberculosis).

Also see buttock sign, Ely's heel-to-buttock test, Hyperextension tests, Hibb's test, Ober's test, Nachlas' test, and Patrick's F-AB-ER-E test.

Roentgenographic Considerations

The most common hip injuries viewed are dislocations and fractures, both of which may lead to avascular necrosis of the femoral head. Femur fracture occurring above the intertrochanteric line are within the joint capsule. They heal, as a rule, without the formation of visible callus.

Shenton's line is frequently disturbed in hip fracture (Fig. 25.22). A gracefully arching line is drawn connecting the inferior margin of the superior pubic ramus with the medial margin of the neck of the femur. With minimal hip displacement, normal

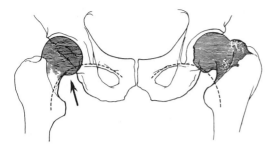

Figure 25.22. In roentgenographic analysis of possible fracture of the proximal femur, Shenton's line is represented by the dotted line drawn at the right hip along the medial margin of the femoral neck which smoothly arches to connect with the inferior margin of the superior pubic ramus. Note on the left that the points of reference are altered due to fracture of the femoral neck, causing the femoral head and fragment of the upper femoral neck to protrude into the arch to cross Shenton's line.

landmarks will be altered when compared bilaterally.

Prognosis. The possibility of nonunion and of absorption of the femur neck must be kept in mind when forming a prognosis in hip fracture. The vitality of the femur head can be inferred from its density; ie, a viable head becomes decalcified to the same degree as surrounding bone. If it is dead, density will be equal to or greater than that of a healthy bone.

Impactions. Following an impaction injury, it is often difficult to locate a fracture of the margin of the head of the femur. It is shown by slight contour changes and unusual densities. Comparative views, oblique and stereoscopic views, tomography, or arthrography are frequently necessary to identify small fracture fragments.

Avulsions. The trochanteric areas should be checked for possible injury of the gluteal insertion at the greater trochanter or avulsion of the iliopsoas insertion at the lesser trochanter. Any type of hip pain encourages careful evaluation of the soft-tissue structures in the area of the obturator internus.

Epiphyseal Slippage. It is common for athletes in later years to exhibit degenerative disease of the hip, suggesting evidence of an old slipped capital femoral epiphysis. Even in minimal slip of this epiphysis, a chronic "tilt deformity" may result which

exhibits the femoral head sitting eccentrically on the neck in a drooped or tipped position. When swelling and ecchymosis appear at the base of Scarpa's triangle and the patient is unable to raise the thigh while in the sitting position, traumatic separation at the epiphysis of the lesser trochanter is indicated (Ludloff's sign).

Evidence is clear that there is an association of certain forms of degenerative hip disease, often with osteophytic flanges on the femoral head, secondary to a rearranged femoral-acetabular articulation. Thus, recognition during the early years is most helpful. Slippage of the femoral capital epiphysis often occurs 1–2 years earlier in females because the most rapid growth in that area comes earlier.

Necrosis of the Femur Head

Recognize the possibility of postischemic changes in the head of the femur during roentgenography of a hip or pelvic fracture. Subcondral collapse, related sclerosis, and irregularity on the weight-bearing anterolateral and superior femoral head are characteristic of ischemic necrosis. Aseptic necrosis may result from hip dislocation without fracture. Hip necrosis is best shown in the "frogleg" abduction, lateral, and partially flexed-hip A-P views.

Care should be taken not to confuse a radiodense femoral head with that of necrosis. After bone or vascular injury, bone ischemia may exist without roentgenographic evidence. Most of the density noted on films following bony ischemia is attributed to the reparative sclerosis of new bone laid upon the necrotic trabeculae (ie, creeping substitution). In addition to this, the relative increased density can be contributed by osteoporosis in the nonischemic zone or by a situation of minute trabecular collapse which attenuates the x-ray beam.

Fractures of the Proximal Femur

Femoral neck fractures are rare in the young; usually a degree of osteoporosis is predisposing. However, in contact athletics, a stress fracture of the femoral neck may become a complete fracture following later torsional stress. In anterior dislocations, a shear fracture of the superior aspect of the femoral head is usually associated. The limb will usually be externally rotated without leg shortening. In posterior dislocations, the inferior aspect of the head may be fractured. Severe trauma may result in comminuted femoral head fractures. Relaxation of the fascia between the crest of the ilium and the greater trochanter is a sign of fracture of the neck of the femur (Allis' hip sign).

Dislocations

Posterior Dislocations. The most common luxation is posterior dislocation of the femoral head, exhibiting thigh adduction and internal rotation at the hip and leg shortening on the affected side. When dislocation takes place, the head of the femur may be driven into the posterior or central acetabulum creating acetabular comminution fragments. But posterior displacement may also be seen without fracture, with a single major posterior acetabular fragment or with femoral head fracture. The cause is usually a force against the flexed knee with the hip in flexion and slight adduction. Complications include sciatic nerve stretching causing foot drop and numbness of the lateral calf.

Anterior Dislocations. Anterior dislocation is relatively rare because Bigelow's ligament offers considerable protection. The limb will be externally rotated and abducted, without leg shortening. Obturator, iliac, and pubic displacement may be seen, as well as that associated with femoral head fractures. In athletics, these usually occur from a blow to the back while squatting, a fall where forced abduction occurs (eg, valuting), or forced abduction of the extended hip.

Central Dislocations. These may be seen with displacement towards the inner wall only, the partial dome fractures or with central displacement with comminution of the dome. This type of dislocation-fracture commonly results from a severe force to the lateral trochanter and pelvis directed through the femoral head (eg, baseball slide). Occasionally, they are produced by a force on the long axis of the femur when the hip is abducted.

CHAPTER 26

Thigh and Knee Injuries

This chapter discusses injuries to the thigh, knee, patella, and associated disorders. In some sports the incidence of injury to these areas is as high as 60%. A variety of bruises, strains, sprains, inflammations, subluxations, dislocations, and fractures will be witnessed in sports care.

THE THIGH

Sports injuries and related disorders of the thigh include contusions, abrasions, strains, contractures, vascular abnormalities, and rarely femoral fractures. Pain can be referred from above (eg, lumbar spine, hip) or from below (eg, knee, ankle, foot). Minor mat, court, or grass abrasions of the thigh are seen in sports that do not require protection. These are usually easily managed if precaution is taken against secondary infection. Lacerations are rarely seen outside of vehicular and cycle sports, but muscle contusions and strains are often seen.

A review of neurologic and orthopedic signs and tests relative to the thigh is listed in Table 26.1.

Quadriceps Contusion

The most common bruise of the thigh is the result of an anterior blunt blow. The effect may be a minor but disabling "charley horse" if the muscles are contracted. A severe rupture of the rectus femoris or vastus intermedius may result, producing extensive intramuscular bleeding leading to myositis ossificans.

A quadriceps contusion can be one of the most crippling of all contusions seen in sports. Even when carefully fitted padding is provided, it is not always adequate for the impacts received. Hemorrhage may extend from knee to groin. If the mass tenses the overlying tensor fascia lata, signs of circulatory impairment will be noted in the toes, requiring immediate fasciotomy. Such "ballooning" of the thigh occurring many hours after injury is typical of a massive "charley horse." It often results from what was thought to be a trivial injury. The tendency for bleeding to recur may remain for a week after injury. The time for resorption of the mass extends from several weeks to months.

In the "low charley" contusion of the vastus medialis, a complication may occur with hemarthrosis of the knee joint which offers false signs of joint injury. In such cases, prolonged diagnosis allows fibrosis to become extensive. This may require many weeks to overcome.

Management. Bleeding is the first problem. Cold packs, a pressure bandage, and elevation should be started immediately. This therapy must be continued up to 60 hours if a mass can be felt and flexion is limited. Heat should not be applied for 5 days, and even then there is a risk for a few days. When bleeding has stopped and other signs subside, monitored walking can be begun that can slowly progress to jogging if symptoms do not return. Premature post-injury activity may easily lead to greater disability. Running should always be preceded by stretching exercises (eg, pulling heel towards buttocks).

Quadriceps Strains

Quadricep injuries are often a management problem as healing is especially slow. Poor warmup or overstrain early in the season is a common factor.

Signs and Symptoms. Symptoms may be exaggerated at either the hip or the knee and may not appear for several hours in mild strains. Pain is aggravated by movement, especially going downstairs. Swelling is usually mild, but spasm is always present to some degree depending upon the extent of injury. Quadriceps flexion will reveal a distinct degree of limitation. It is impossible to have a strong knee and weak quadriceps, and the quadriceps are the first to show atrophy after knee injury.

Fibrotic Masses. Fibrotic masses, as

Table 26.1.
Review of Neurologic and Orthopedic Maneuvers, Reflexes, Signs, or Tests Relative to the Thigh

Berry's sign	Light touch/pain tests	Patella reflex
Guilland's sign	Ludloff's sign	Phelp's test
Huntington's test	Nachlas' test	Quadriceps hyperthyroidism test
Kelly's test	Neri's bowing sign	Remark's sign
Langoria's sign	Neri's sign	Trendelenburg's vein test
Lewin's knee sign	Ober's test	Tripod sign

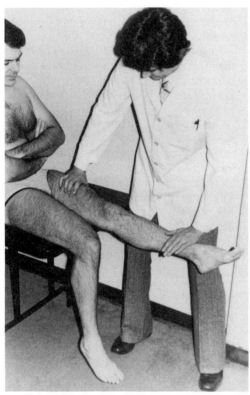

Figure 26.1. Quadriceps muscle test.

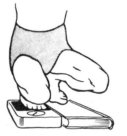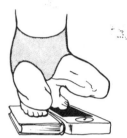

Figure 26.2. A simple test for evaluating lower extremity muscle strength in comparison to the contralateral side is by weight lifting on a scale. The patient stands on a bathroom scale with one foot while the other foot is on an equally high block or book. The patient then squats and raises himself, and the maximum weight is recorded. The feet are then reversed, and a comparative reading is made. This offers an indication of how much weight the injured side can tolerate.

well as bony lesions in muscles and connective tissue, often develop within the quadriceps (or hamstrings) after rupture of the muscle. They are palpable in the relaxed muscle, usually circumscribed, and often visible. They are most often seen in track sports. The mechanism is intrinsic, ie, one of uncoordinated forceful activity without a direct blow to the muscle.

Quadriceps Flexion Test. Resulting scars always limit the working length of all muscles in the group. Quadriceps contracture is simply tested by placing the patient prone, flexing the leg towards the buttocks to tolerance, and measuring the distance

from heel to buttock. Once the point of tolerance is measured, the lumbosacral spine will arch and the buttocks will rise to prevent further stretch. This test may prove a lesion too deep to palpate or to evaluate progress during therapy. Not even light jogging should be allowed until flexion exceeds 90°. All squatting activities must be avoided until full healing is demonstrated. Premature postinjury activity may easily tear a weakened muscle.

Management. Treat as any long, bulky muscle strain, keeping in mind that the quadriceps is the largest muscle group in the body. In comparison to moderate strains, mild tears (highly disabling) are much more difficult to manage. Bleeding is always a problem; heat should not be applied for 72 hours. Support strapping consists of criss-crossed strips up the anterior thigh. This will require 10–14 diagonal strips overlapped by a third. These are anchored by overlapping semicircular horizontal strips extending from the medial to the lateral aspects of the thigh. Any taping procedure for the quadriceps is helpful but never fully adequate.

Hamstring Strains

Strains of the posterior thigh are common, have myriad variations, are difficult to treat, and are difficult to prevent from recurring if a faulty biomechanical style persists. They are common in sports which require highly developed, explosive forward speed and motion such as in dash starts, broad jumpers, high jumpers, football running backs, and baseball outfielders. Because of their importance, it is not unusual for the experienced athlete to know more about his or her hamstrings than the attending doctor. Poor warmup is usually a factor in injury. A palpable, compensatory, fibrous thickening may be exhibited.

Background. Tears often involve the long head of the biceps, the semimembranous, or semitendinosus. Bicipital tendonitis is a frequent complication of distal bicipital strain. Care must be taken to differentiate bicipital strain from knee sprain of the lateral ligaments or lateral meniscus tear. Injury is usually the result of deficient reciprocal actions of opposing hamstrings and quadriceps, poor muscle flexibility, inadequate warmup, fatigue, or sudden violent contraction or stretching. Symptoms may be exaggerated at either the hip or the knee.

Signs and Symptoms. The picture is one of acute pain, generally at the origin of the short head of the biceps femoris, restricted motion, hamstring dyskinesia, loss of strength, discoordination, and an altered gate. Symptoms develop slowly with progressive disability. Bleeding is usually mild, but general spasm is common. Tenderness is found at the ischial origins and attachments at the musculotendinous junctions. Roentgenographs may show avulsion fracture at the fibular head. In contrast to a strain, a tear features a history of bursting pain during competition and a highly tender mass at the site of hemorrhage. The size of the mass varies from that of a walnut to a small melon and parallels the degree of spasm and weight-bearing disability. During recovery, a startling ecchymosis usually appears in the popliteal fossa and slowly extends downward. This sign often indi-

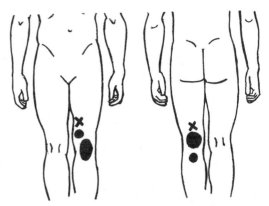

Figure 26.3. *Left,* vastus medialis trigger point; *X,* common site. *Blackened areas* indicate typical sites of referred pain. *Right,* biceps femoris trigger point.

cates at least 2 weeks of rehabilitation for full recovery.

Beery's Sign. This test is positive if a patient with a history of lower trunk discomfort and fatigue is fairly comfortable when sitting with the knees flexed but experiences discomfort in the standing position. Beery's sign is typically positive in spasticity or contractures of the posterior thigh and/or leg muscles.

Lewin's Knee Sign. If quick extension of a knee in the standing position produces pain and a sharp flexion response, hamstring spasm should be suspected.

Neri's Bowing Sign. The sign is positive when a patient can flex the trunk further without low back discomfort when the ipsilateral leg is flexed than when both knees are held in extension. A positive sign suggests hamstring spasm, contractures of the posterior thigh and/or leg muscles, sciatic neuritis, a lumbar IVD lesion, or a sacroiliac subluxation syndrome.

Quadriceps Hyperthryoidism Test. The patient sits well forward on the edge of a straight chair and attempts to hold his legs out at right angles to the trunk. A strong healthy person can usually hold this position for a minute or more, but a person with hyperthyroidism or taut hamstrings has difficulty holding this position for a few seconds.

Management. Treat as a strain of any large muscle group with emphasis on flexibility and strengthening exercises. Bleeding is always a problem, thus heat should not be applied for at least 3–4 days. Return to activity should not be forced, and any attempt by the player to "work out" the discomfort must be restricted. Reinjury readily leads to severe tear and scar formation. Once bleeding has stopped, walking is the first exercise, followed by "high knee" exercises and graduated jogging. To prevent a chronic problem, rehabilitation with emphasis on stretching exercises should continue until complete recovery. When returning to activity, speed running and hill running should be avoided until full strength and flexibility have returned. The optimal balance between quadricep and hamstring strength is in a ratio of 60:40. Management should also consider rehabilitation of the medial and lateral hamstrings as well as the gluteus maximus.

Hamstring Contractures. Tight, scarred hamstrings result from improperly treated strains and tears. They are a common factor of prolonged immobility. In some cases, the cause can be traced to overtraining that has produced a horizontal tear across the muscle's belly. Cryokinetic therapy is helpful, but recurring episodes are typical. A program of graduated activity must be undertaken even in off-seasons for prolonged rest encourages tightening and functional disability.

Adductor Strains

Painful groin strains may involve either the gracilis, adductor longus, or iliopsoas,

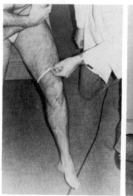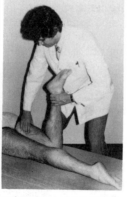

Figure 26.4. *Left*, evaluating the quadriceps for signs of possible atrophy. Circumference of the thigh is measured 3 inches above the medial tibial plateau edge. *Right*, hamstring muscle test.

but differentiation is usually not necessary in management. Bleeding is always a problem. Heat should not be applied for 72 hours. Healing is slow, often taking 2–3 months for full recovery.

Low strains, contusions, and bone bruises seen on the medial femoral epicondyle often mimic knee-joint injury. Such strains result from a fall on the adducted knee causing overadduction and avulsion stress to the adductor tendon that may lead to periosteal calcification (Pellegrini-Stieda disease). Fortunately, severe posttraumatic disability is rarely a factor.

Phelp's Test. The patient is placed in the prone position with both lower limbs extended in the relaxed position. The patient's thighs are abducted just short of the patient's threshold of pain, and then the examiner flexes the patient's knees to 90° angles with the thighs. If this flexion allows greater abduction of a thigh on the hip without undue discomfort, a contracture of the gracilis muscle is suggested.

Management. Treat as any strain; however, a first-aid analgesic pack is often required. This consists of spreading a balm such as menthyl salicylate over the site of injury about ½ in thick and covering it with an 8- x 10-inch or larger cotton pad. The analgesic pack is secured with tape and covered with an elastic bandage. In strapping, the final strips should be applied so that medial traction is maintained (ie, around the contralateral hip and posteriorly).

The Iliotibial Band Syndrome

The importance of this syndrome within athletics has been recently pointed out in a paper forwarded to us by Dr. John M. Nash of Texas Chiropractic College. It has also been described by Dr. R. H. Hazel, who feels it is limited to long-distance runners.

Functional Anatomy. The iliotibial band (ITB) is the distal extension of the thick lateral fascia of the thigh, and, as such, it serves in the capacity of a supplemental support of the knee on its lateral aspect. It arises proximally from the fascia lata and gluteus maximus and inserts distally into Gerdy's tubercle on the lateral tibial condyle.

When flexed, the knee essentially depends on muscular support rather than that of its ligamentous elements. This is performed laterally by the ITB and biceps femoris; medially by the combined action of the semitendinosis, semimembranosus, gracilis, and sartorius; anteriorly by the quadriceps femoris; and posteriorly by the action of the politeus.

Because the ITB crosses the knee joint, its effect on the knee varies according to the position of the hip. Evans, states Hazel, believes that this band greatly assists rest in the standing position.

Function During Gait. During the walking cycle, the knee is in full extension at the moment of heel strike–the only time in the cycle when this occurs. At all other phases of the cycle, the knee is in various degrees of flexion. When running on flat terrain, the knee does not accomplish full extension at heel strike. However, it is close enough that lateral stability is satisfactorily accomplished by the ligamentous straps. This situation changes, however, when running on hills, particularly during the up-hill aspect, where flexion of the knee reduces the support contributed by the ligaments and places more emphasis on dynamic muscle tissue.

Etiologic Considerations. With these factors in mind, we can now consider three factors that can and will alter the system sufficiently to produce symptoms:

1. The first factor occurs during semiflexion of the knee. During this action, as mentioned above, the dynamic muscle groups must perform the stabilization. Such a circumstance, when performed repetitively, can precipitate the formation of trigger points in the stressed tissues, especially when even slight biomechanical faults are associated. The ITB is victimized often since it has such a high connective tissue content. The resulting trigger points cause aberrant control of the leg during performance, and they also produce the pain that is experienced.

2. The second factor involves contracture and inelasticity of the hamstrings—a common finding in the entire populace and especially in the athlete. Hamstring shortening disallows full extension of the knee at heel strike, which precipitates the same negative situation that is seen in hill running.

3. The third factor is related to contracture of the triceps surae, which alters normal gait by causing push-off before the full stride is accomplished—thus producing the characteristic knee posture and semiflexion at heel strike. The result is the same as described in Factors 1 and 2.

Athletes, either serious or of the weekend variety, can fall victim to this problem when they alter their training suddenly, either by an increase in duration or intensity. A change in terrain or footwear can also be a causative or precipitative situation. Other contributing factors include novice runners with tibia vera and pronated ankles, excessive length in stride, and excessive wear on the outer sole of a running shoe.

Symptomatology and Examination. An afflicted individual will report pain during or immediately following a workout, but there is usually no sign of effusion. Tests for ligament or menisceal faults are negative, but palpation of the lateral distal thigh will invariably show evidence of single or multiple trigger-point development. The usual sites across the ITB, at or just above the joint line. Gerdy's tubercle will be surprisingly pain free.

Topographically, the ITB is palpated distally by locating the tendon of the biceps femoris, moving anteriorly into the groove that separates it from the ITB (see Fig. 26.5). When applicable to any other part of the muscular system, the location of the pain will identify the structural culprit.

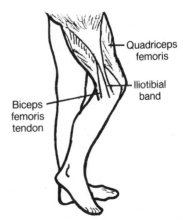

Figure 26.5. Schematic of the iliotibial band and its relationship with the quadriceps femoris and biceps femoris muscles.

Hazel recommends three tests that he feels are a must in the accurate diagnosis of a ITB syndrome. First, the sitting patient should flex and extend the involved leg while the examiner applies pressure to the lateral femoral epicondyle. Second, the patient is placed in the lateral recumbent position and instructed to rapidly abduct the leg (to about 20°) several times. This puts considerable tension on the tensor fascia lata and gluteus maximus. Third, just prior to examination, have the patient jog to (but not beyond) the point of pain. This will help localize the focal point of stressed tissues. Running beyond the threshold of pain will cause the pain to become diffuse, and point tenderness will be lost.

Management. Treat as an acute sprain. Initial cryotherapy and adequate rest are vital to rapid recovery. During the acute stage, Hazel suggests eight aspirin tablets a day (two every 4 hours) as a sufficient salicylate level to have an anti-inflammatory effect. Nash describes the treatment of associated trigger points to be transverse friction over the reactive points for 3–4 minutes on alternate days for 1–2 weeks, depending on the severity and the responsive nature of the patient. Each treatment should be followed by negative pole high-volt therapy, which may be preceded by an ice massage of 15–20 minutes for anesthetic purposes.

A regimen of bilateral passive and then active stretching exercises for the tensor fascia lata, quadriceps, and hamstrings should be prescribed, but exercises designed to strengthen the quadriceps should be avoided completely. Training should be modified according to the facts at hand, and consideration should be given to nontraumatic activities such as swimming or bicycling in the interim period. Ice massage should be applied to the involved area after each workout. When conservative measures fail, the alternative is surgical release of the ITB or removal of the lateral epicondyle.

Recurrence Prevention. To prevent recurrence, close evaluation of the entire situation must be made. This might include footwear, foot mechanics, knee mechanics, pelvic motion, and even the terrain on which the workout is performed. Walking upstairs can be especially aggravating, but walking on level ground appears to have no ill effects. Again, clinical success can only be achieved through careful analysis of *all* factors involved.

Iliotibial Band Contracture

Ober's Test. The patient is placed directly on his side with the unaffected side next to the table. The examiner places one hand on the pelvis to steady it and grasps the patient's ankle with the other hand, holding the knee flexed at a right angle. The thigh is abducted and extended on the coronal plane (see Fig. 26.6). In the presence of iliotibial band contracture, the leg will remain abducted and the degree of abduction will depend on the amount of contracture present.

Ober cells attention to the frequency of a negative roentgenogram in the presence of clinical signs and symptoms of irritation of the sacroiliac or lumbosacral joints, and he refers to the importance of the iliotibial band as a factor in the occurrence of lame backs, with or without associated sciatica. To differentiate, pain on extension and abduction points to sacroiliac lesion; pain when the knee is released suggests lumbosacral strain; and contraction of the iliotibial band is indicated when the thigh does not return to the table when it is released. Ely's test will help to pinpoint femoral nerve (L3–4) involvement; Lasegue's SLR test will differentiate lumbosacral from upper lumbar involvement.

Gait Clues

During the stance phase, note heel strike, foot flat, midstance, and toe push-off of each extremity. Failure of the knee to extend

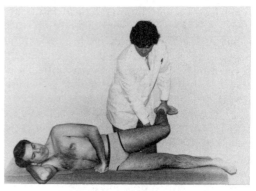

Figure 26.6.   Ober's test.

during heel strike is a sign of weak quadriceps or a flexion fusion of the knee. Weak quadriceps will display themselves in excessive flexion and poor knee stability during midstance. A midstance forward lurch of the hip is a typical indication of a weak gluteus medius, while a midstance backward lurch is a sign of a weak gluteus maximus.

During the swing phase, note acceleration, midswing, and deceleration of each extremity. If the patient must rotate the pelvis severely anterior to provide a thrust for the leg, the cause is most likely weak quadriceps. A harsh heel strike, usually associated with knee hyperextension, is a frequent sign of weak hamstrings.

Selected Disorders of the Thigh

Myositis Ossificans

Because of the thigh's massive muscular volume and its vulnerability to collision, especially in football, myositis ossificans may result. As the trauma may not be remembered, the mass can be mistaken for a neoplasm. Even early biopsy often confuses the disorder with osteosarcoma at certain stages.

X-ray findings vary according to duration. There is an early cloud of mineralized tissue varying to a bone mass with a definite cortical rim containing trabeculae. Sometimes following a direct blow, posttraumatic masses will be seen developing on the surface of the bone's shaft where the bone has formed a periosteal focus.

Epiphysitis and Osteomyelitis

Epiphysitis and osteomyelitis are more common than any other serious lesion of the thigh except fracture. The cases may be divided into acute septic and chronic cases. The acute cases begin with severe pain, tenderness, fever, chill, and leukocytosis. Later, induration and finally fluctuation appear; and the abscess, if left unattended, will break externally. General, sometimes fatal, septicemia may take place.

The diagnosis of the acute cases depends chiefly on excluding arthritis of any type. Careful examination with testing of joint motions will usually demonstrate that the pain and tenderness are in the bone and not

in the joint. The leukocyte count is but slightly elevated in most cases of arthritis but is decidedly high (20,000 or more) in most cases of acute osteomyelitis. The same is true of temperature. Monarticular arthritis, the only variety likely to be considered in such a diagnosis, is rare in youth, when most cases of acute osteomyelitis and epiphysitis occur. Whether the disease starts in the shaft of the bone or in the epiphysis is determined by the seat of pain, tenderness, and x-ray findings.

Meralgia Paresthetica

This syndrome, often referred to as lateral femoral cutaneous neuropathy, features a patch of anesthesia, paresthesia, or hyperesthesia, with or without pain, on the anterior surface of one or both thighs in the distribution of the lateral femoral cutaneous nerve.

Background. The lateral femoral cutaneous nerve arises from the posterior divisions of L1–L3, appears at the lateral border of the psoas, passes obliquely across the iliacus to the anterior superior iliac spine, and then travels under the inguinal ligament to enter the anterolateral aspect of the thigh.

Etiologic Considerations. Most authorities feel that the syndrome has its origin in some form of inflammatory process involving the lateral femoral cutaneous nerve or its roots. This focus of irritation may often be found (1) at the L1–L3 IVFs from subluxation encroachment or arthritic hyperplasia of (2) in the pelvis from repetitive trauma as seen in athletic injuries and late pregnancy. Nevertheless, pathology lying anywhere along the course of the nerve may be responsible, whether it be intraspinal, intersegmental, paraspinal, retroperitoneal, pelvic, or, rarely, abdominal.

Differential Diagnosis. The typical patient reports a sense of numbness or burning in the anterolateral aspect of the thigh, which is rarely painful until the late stages. Care must be taken to differentiate this syndrome from trochanteric or iliopectineal (iliopsoas) bursitis, both of which refer pain to the anterolateral thigh. It should also be kept in mind that pronation or supination of the ankle, genu varum, genu valgum, genu recurvatum, flexion contracture, etc, can cause or contribute to anterosuperior thigh pain.

Management. Associated lumbar subluxations should be freed immediately. In a privately distributed *Orthopedic Brief* of the ACA Council on Chiropractic Orthopedics, Aiken reports that low wattage ultrasound applied paraspinally at the L2 level for 3 minutes and at the area where the nerve leaves the pelvis for 2 minutes may be of value. High voltage stimulation in the area of L2 and again in the anterolateral aspect of the thigh may also assist recovery. Massage and muscle stripping of the involved thigh is recommended in the postgraduate notes of Northwestern College of Chiropractic, as is moist heat. Weight reduction should be recommended if obesity is a factor.

Varicosities

Trendelenburg's Vein Test. This simple test helps to decide which valves are incompetent when varicose veins appear with standing. Raise the affected leg of the patient in the supine position until the veins drain completely. Next, apply a tourniquet about the upper thigh and have the patient stand upright. The perforators are incompetent if the varicosites now fill partially from below, allowing blood to flow from the deep to the superficial system. However, if the veins remain collapsed upon standing, remove the tourniquet, whereupon rapid filling from above indicates that the saphenous valves are faulty.

Kelly's Test. To differentiate between saphenous varix and femoral hernia, compress the veins below the knee with one hand applied to the calf. With the other hand, squeeze sharply the inner side of the thigh just above the knee. The blood will be returned through the internal saphenous vein and will make the swelling in the groin quiver.

Phlebitis

Bruising of the inner leg or thigh may present superficial venous thrombophlebitis as a complication. Fortunately, the lesion is usually well localized and emboli are rare. Phlebitis with thrombosis of a vein, usually the saphenous, is a common cause for a swollen thigh and leg with pain and tenderness, especially over the inflamed vein where a cordy induration may be felt. Secondary bacterial infection is the usual cause, yet sometimes the cause cannot be found. Diagnosis depends on eliminating the presence of any other demonstrable cause.

Management. Rest, heat after the acute stage, and an elastic bandage are all that are usually required. Anticoagulants are considered by Williams and Sperryn to be unnecessary unless the thrombotic process is actively spreading.

Abscesses and Tumors

Psoas abscess or hip-joint abscess may burrow down so as to point high on the thigh. The evidence of disease in the hip or vertebrae is usually sufficient to make the diagnosis clear. Psoas abscess presents the ordinary signs of pus and is commonly associated with vertebral tuberculosis (dorsal or lumbar).

Sarcoma of the femur is the most common and largest tumor of the thigh. A hard, spindle-shaped growth encircles the femur. The lower end is the most common site, but any part of the bone may be affected. Osteoma occurs less often. It is much smaller and of slower growth. This last trait usually serves to distinguish it from sarcoma, but roentgenography is the deciding factor.

Metastatic cancer of the upper half of the femur may occur after cancer of the breast but rarely gives rise to symptoms unless spontaneous fracture occurs: an event which always should suggest cancer. Epithelioma of the thigh is seen infrequently; its traits are those of epithelioma elsewhere. Tuberculosis of the knee may simulate sarcoma of the lower end of the femur, but sarcoma grows more rapidly. Laboratory tests are essential to diagnosis.

Fractures

Adult diaphyseal fractures require more severe trauma than that in sports, outside of vehicular or parachuting accidents. Extensive soft-tissue, vascular, and possibly nerve damages are associated. Fat embolism is always a danger, and severe shock is typical. Diagnosis is usually not difficult, and immediate orthopedic care is required. Incidence of isolated shaft fracture is much higher in children and usually oblique from rotational stress. If fracture is suspected, great care must be made to avoid soft-tissue damage during movement. See Figure 26.7.

Neurologic Considerations

Sciatic Pain. Sciatic pain and tenderness more or less clearly confined to the distribution of the sciatic nerve can usually be traced to lumbar or sacroiliac subluxation, strain, or looseness; spondylitis; neuritis; prostatitis, prostatic abscess or neoplasm; or pelvic tumors or abscesses, including psoas abscess.

Hamstring Reflexes. Two hamstring reflexes have significance: (1) *Internal*: Place patient recumbent, knee slightly flexed, leg abducted and partially externally rotated. The examiner's fingers are placed on the medial aspect of the leg below the knee, over the muscles and tendons, and the fingers are percussed. A reflex supplied by L4-S2 results in increased flexion of the leg upon the thigh. (2) *External*: Similar to above, fingers are placed over the tendon of the biceps femoris muscle just above its insertion on the lateral side of the head of the fibula and lateral tibia condyle, and the fingers are percussed. A reflex supplied by L5-S3 results in flexion of the leg on the thigh and moderate external rotation of the leg.

Remark's Sign. This sign results when for any reason the conducting pathways of the spinal cord are interrupted. When the upper third of the anterior surface of the thigh is mildly stimulated by stroking, the reflex consists of extension of the knee with plantar flexion of the first three toes in which the foot may also participate plantarwise.

Huntington's Test. A patient with apparent lower limb paralysis is placed in the supine position so that the knees are flexed and the legs hang over the edge of a table at a right angle to the thighs. The patient is then instructed to cough. A brisk extension of the knee and flexion of the thigh on the hip in the involved limb signifies an upper motor lesion.

Tripod Sign. The patient is placed prone with the knees flexed over the edge of the table as in Huntington's test, and active and passive muscle strength and range of motion of knee extension are evaluated. If the patient must lean back (extend the trunk on the pelvis) and grasp the table to support body weight on the arms when the knees are bilaterally extended, hamstring spasm is indicated. This may be the result of any lower motor irritation located between the midthoracic area and the lower sacrum.

Guilland's Sign. With the patient supine and both limbs extended in the relaxed position, pinching the skin over a quadriceps muscle produces a quick flexion of the contralateral hip and knee. Several authorities view this sign as a positive indication of meningeal inflammation.

THE KNEE

Within football, knee injuries have the highest injury incidence (60%). Just because a player can walk off the field after injury is no sign that severe injury has not occurred. Skiing also has a high incidence of knee sprains, fractures (usually of the medial collateral ligament), and ankle injuries, but the incidence has lowered with the popularity of release-type bindings. The more common fracture in skiing has changed from that of the ankle to that of the lower third of the tibia.

A review of neurologic and orthopedic signs and tests relative to the knee is listed in Table 26.2.

Special Clinical Considerations

Injuries due to excessive stress appear especially on the short arm of the first-class-lever joint such as the elbow and knee. This can be witnessed with the mechanism of injury to the medial collateral ligament when the valgus knee is overstressed. During extension, a force (eg, body weight) is applied at the distance from the fulcum several times that occurring between the fulcum and the ligament.

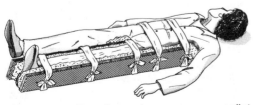

Figure 26.7. Boards used as emergency splint for fractured thigh.

Table 26.2.
Review of Neurologic and Orthopedic Maneuvers, Reflexes, Signs, or Tests Relative to the Knee

Anterior drawer sign	Knee effusion test	Patella apprehension sign
Apley's compression test	Knee hyperextension	Patella reflex
Apley's distraction test	stress test	Patella wobble sign
Bounce home test	Knee hyperflexion stress	Payr's sign
Childress' duck waddle test	test	Perkin's patella grinding test
Clarke's sign	Lachman's test	Posterior drawer sign
Collateral ligament stability	Lasegue's hysteria sign	Q-angle sign
tests	Lewin's knee sign	Range of motion tests
Dreyer's sign	Light touch/pain tests	Slocum's test
External rotation-recurvatum	Losee's test	Steinmann's signs
test	Lust's sign	Suprapatella reflex
Fouchet's test	McIntosch's test	Trendelenburg's vein test
Helfet's test	McMurray's tests	Westphal's sign
Hughston's jerk sign	Muscle strength grading	Wilson's sign

Inspection of the Knees for Balance

Genu Valgum. If there are more than a few centimeters between the knees when the subject is standing with the kneecaps straight ahead, a degree of genu valgum (knock knees) is present which may be more marked on one side than the other. There is (1) excessive internal rotation of the femur and external rotation restriction, (2) excessive external rotation of the tibia and internal rotation restriction, and (3) medial patella deviation due to femur rotation. This results in a short leg that causes pelvic imbalance if the condition is unilateral. Be aware, however, that people with a large degree of joint flexibility can hyperextend their knees along with femoral rotation which gives a false appearance of structural deformity.

Genu Varum. If the medial malleoli are touching and the knees are not, the space between the knees determines the degree of genu varum (bow legs). There is (1) excessive external rotation of the femur and internal rotation restriction, (2) excessive internal rotation of the tibia and external rotation restriction, and (3) lateral patella deviation due to femur rotation.

Genu Recurvatum. This mark of hyperextensibility is sometimes associated with a joint disorder involving A-P instability. Contact sports, high jumping, or any activity that may induce anterior leg trauma or strenuous "take offs" from a locked knee would be contraindicated.

Tibial Rotation and Torsion. If the kneecaps are facing straight ahead and the feet point distinctly outward, a positive sign exists of external rotation of the tibia on the femur and it is usually more pronounced on one side that the other. If the feet appear normally positioned but the patellae appear rolled medially inward, it is a positive sign of tibial torsion.

General Tests of Knee Integrity

Knee Hyperflexion Stress Test. With the patient in the supine position, the examiner places one hand on the involved knee and the other on the ipsilateral ankle. The knee is moderately flexed, the thigh is brought towards the patient's abdomen, and the patient's heel is slowly pushed toward the patient's buttock. Unless the patient is considerably obese, the normal knee can be flexed without pain so that it touches the buttock. If knee pain or severe discomfort is induced on this maneuver, a subtle localized knee lesion may be brought out.

Knee Hyperextension Stress Test. The patient is placed prone with the knees extended in the relaxed position. The examiner places a fist under the distal thigh of the involved side, flexes the knee to about 30° with the other hand, and then allows the leg to drop without assistance when the muscles are relaxed. Most knee lesions limit extension to some degree. Thus, if extension is limited or the rebound is abnormal during this "knee drop" test (as compared to the contralateral knee), some type of knee disorder should be suspected and may possibly be localized.

Q-Angle Sign. The patient is placed in the supine position with the knees extended in a relaxed position, and the quadriceps (Q) angle of the knee is measured. The Q-angle is formed by a line drawn along the long axis of the femur that is intersected by a line drawn through the center of the patella and the tibial tubercle. To make a recording, a goniometer is centered on its side over the patella with one arm aimed at the ipsilateral anterior-superior iliac spine and the other arm placed in line with the center of the patellar tendon. This angle is normally 10° in men and 15° in women. In external tibial rotation and/or genu varus, however, the Q-angle can be markedly increased; ie, the angle increases as the tibial tubercle is displaced laterally or when the distal femur and proximal tibia are angled toward the midline.

Roentgenologic Considerations

Lateral and A-P views are the standard views of the knee. Weight-bearing views, a tangential view of the patella, and a tunnel view of the intercondylar notch to show articular margin defects (eg, condylar compression fracture) are frequently helpful. Stress views of the knee, under local anesthesia, are beneficial in eliciting evidence of fracture or ligamentous ruptures by expressing abnormal hinging which are not evident on standard views. Anthrography is more helpful in the diagnosis of acute ligament or meniscus injury and synovial cysts than are standard views.

The most common type of soft-tissue injury in the knee area is the result of effusion at the suprapatellar joint space where adjacent fat pads are displaced. Lateral views are best for determining effusion if it can be viewed at all. The fatty tissue above the patella, anterior to the femur, and posterior to the quadriceps tendon near the superior aspect of the patella is somewhat lucent in the normal knee. If effusion exists, fatty areas are replaced by fluids matching the density of the thigh muscles, and normal signs become obliterated.

Knee effusion may be shown in the A-P view by soft-tissue density medial to the tibia below the joint line. This is usually attributed to paratibial synovial cysts progressing posteriorly and medially which may extend via bursae connections to the popliteal space or to the posterior aspect of the upper calf. Rarely is extension to the posterior thigh.

The residual epiphyseal cartilage of the distal femur should be of rather uniform thickness. No displacement of its margins should be noted. The articular margins of the femoral condyles are normally smooth, but fragmentations will be noted in osteochondritis dissecans and osteochondral fractures. Evidence of swelling at the site of insertion of the quadriceps tendon at the apophysis of the tibial tubercle suggests Osgood-Schlatter's disease.

Strong, sudden muscle contractions may also cause fracture avulsions in the lateral knee area. For example, small bone fragments may be found in an A-P view at the lateral edge of the proximal tibia upon iliotibial band injury.

In partial tendon tears, ossification may be found in the patellar tendon following hemorrhage. If joint dislocation has occurred, signs of ossification may be found in the soft tissues. After blunt trauma to a limb, soft tissues may show evidence of heterotopic bone formation. Such ossification involves not only the muscle tissue but also occurs within the fascial planes. The typical history is one of trauma, muscle pain and soreness, and hemorrhage into the soft tissues, with signs of poorly defined ossification developing in 2–5 weeks.

Contusions

Bruises. A blow to the prepatella bursa may quickly lead to a ballooning hemorrhage that may extend several inches above the patella, and that is quite alarming to the unexperienced physician. Careful examination must be made to differentiate the effects of contusion about the knee from a low quadriceps strain with suprapatellar bursal hemorrhage. Bone bruises are not difficult to differentiate as there is no effusion, motion restriction, joint instability, locking, ligament tenderness, or joint line tenderness.

Popliteal Aneurysm. When direct trauma affects major vessels and hematoma develops, aneurysmal dilation or a fistula may be produced as a complication. These occurrences are most frequently seen in the popliteal region following injury. Such lesions must be differentiated from a pulsating hematoma that is not a true aneurysm. A pulsating hematoma is fed by a ruptured arteriole and requires the skill of a vascular surgeon for correction. Discomfort behind the knee or upper calf on forced dorsiflexion of the foot is often a sign of thrombosis in the leg (Homan's sign).

Traumatic Synovitis

Even mild trauma can produce extensive knee swelling if the alar folds of the synovial fringes are pinched between the tibial and femoral condyles. Movement quickly becomes limited, maintained in about 20° flexion, pain is severe, and tenderness is acute. Swelling is less severe in complete rupture because the fluid is able to escape through the tear. Hemarthrosis does not demand aspiration unless disability is unusually severe. Cold, compression, and passive exercise will usually be sufficient.

Differentiation. Upper calf swelling and pain must be differentiated from and is often confused with thrombophlebitis. Long-standing posttraumatic effusion may be so great as to distend the semimembranosis-gastrocnemius bursal complex in the popliteal area to produce a Baker's cyst. Synovial cysts are frequent complications of knee injuries and meniscus tears, as they are in various arthritides (especially rheumatoid). A firm, mildly tender meniscus cyst may occur; it is usually on the anterolateral aspect of the knee and is nonfluctuating. Uncommon tears of the posterior capsule, characterized by extension instability, may produce painful swelling and bleeding into the popliteal fossa.

Knee Stability

Strong ligaments, a large joint capsule, and adjacent muscles and tendons offer stability to the normal knee joint. Severe sprain, especially that of hyperextension, readily leads to functional instability with chronic "giving way." Undoubtedly, a large degree of proprioception loss and loss of quadriceps power are involved. In partial ligamentous tears, sprain symptoms are more pronounced, but there is little or no instability involved. Complete tears exhibit marked laxity upon stress movements but may present little pain. Several clinical tests which have been devised to evaluate stability are described below.

External Rotation-Recurvatum Test

To test for external rotation-recurvatum, place the patient supine and grasp the heel with one hand and support the calf with the other hand. Allow the knee to pass from about 10° flexion into full extension. A positive test occurs when the knee assumes a position of slight recurvatum, the tibia rotates externally, and there is increased tibia vara. Such a sign indicates injury to the arcuate complex, lateral half of the posterior capsule, or a degree of injury to the posterior cruciate ligament.

Anterolateral Rotary Instability

McIntosh's Test. This is a test for anterolateral rotary instability of the knee joint. The patient is placed supine, the lower ex-

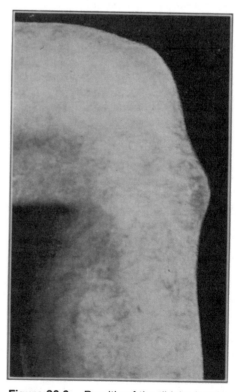

Figure 26.8. Bursitis of the tibial tubercle.

tremity is supported at the heel with one hand, and the other hand is placed laterally over the proximal tibia just distal to the patella. The caudad hand applies valgus stress and internally rotates the tibia as the knee is gradually moved from full extension into flexion. During flexion of the knee, the lateral tibial plateau can be felt to subluxate anteriorly in relation to the lateral condyle. Lateral crepitation may be felt, and a slight resistance to flexion may be perceived. When the knee is in about 35° of flexion, the iliotibial band tightens and passes behind the transverse axis of rotation. The tibial plateau is then suddenly reduced, often with a "clunking" sensation that can be both felt and heard.

Hughston's Jerk Sign. This is a modification of the McIntosh test for anterolateral rotary instability of the knee. With the patient supine, the foot is grasped with one hand while the other hand rests over the proximal lateral aspect of the leg just distal to the patella. The knee is flexed at 90°, and valgus stress is applied as the tibia is rotated internally. The knee is then gradually extended. The lateral tibial plateau is initially in a reduced position to the femoral condyle; however, as the knee is extended to about 35° of flexion, the lateral tibial plateau suddenly subluxates forward in relation to the femoral condyle with a jerking sensation. The lateral plateau slowly obtains its reduced position, which completes on full extension as the knee is extended.

Slocum's Test. This is another modification of the McIntosh test for anterolateral rotary instability of the knee. The patient is placed in the lateral recumbent position with the involved knee uppermost. The under extremity is flexed at 90° at both the hip and knee. The pelvis is rotated slightly posterior about 30°, and the weight of the extremity is supported by the inner aspect of the foot and heel. This position causes a valgus stress at the knee and a slight internal rotation of the leg. The examiner then grips the distal thigh with one hand and the proximal leg with the other hand and presses back of the fibula and femoral condyle with the thumbs. The knee is then gently pushed from extension into flexion and again, as the iliotibial tract passes behind the transverse axis of rotation at about 35°, the lateral tibial plateau, which has

subluxated forward, is reduced with a palpable "clunk" or "giving way" sensation.

Lachman's Test. With the patient supine, the examiner slightly flexes the involved knee (5°–10°), cups a palm against the proximal calf, and attempts to pull the tibia forward. Excessive anterior translation of tibia from the femur (anterior drawer sign) indicates incompetency of the anterior cruciate ligament.

Losee's Test. With the patient supine and the knee flexed, the examiner applies valgus stress to the tibia with one hand while the head of the fibula is pushed anterior with the other hand. If an anterior subluxation occurs at the lateral tibial plateau when the knee approaches full extension, anterolateral rotatory instability is indicated.

Anterior-Posterior Instability

Anterior Drawer Sign. The anterior and posterior cruciate ligaments provide A-P stability to the knee joint. These intracapsular ligaments originate from the tibia and insert onto the inner aspects of the femoral condyles. To examine A-P stability, place the patient supine and flex the knees to 90° so that the feet are flat on the table. The examiner should sit sideways so that his hip can keep the patient's feet from moving during the tests. The examiner positions his hands around the knee being examined similar to but lower than the bony palpation starting position; ie, thumbs pointing superiorly over the lateral and medial joint lines with fingers wrapped around the lateral and medial insertions of the hamstrings (Fig. 26.9). In this position, the examiner pulls the tibia forward. When a distinct sliding forward of the tibia from under the femur is noted, a torn anterior cruciate ligament is indicated. A positive sign is called an "anterior drawer sign." Slight anterior sliding, however, is often normal.

A positive anterior drawer sign should be confirmed by repeating the maneuver with the patient's leg internally rotated 30° and externally rotated 15°. The reason for this is that even if the anterior cruciate ligament is torn, external rotation should reduce forward movement of the tibia; if it doesn't, both anterior cruciate and posteriomedial joint capsule may be torn. Likewise, even if the anterior cruciate ligament is torn, inter-

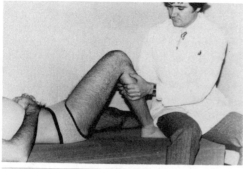
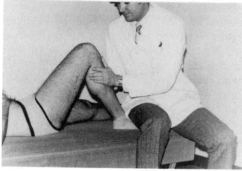

Figure 26.9. *Top,* testing for the anterior drawer sign. *Bottom,* testing for the posterior drawer sign.

nal rotation should reduce forward movement of the tibia; if it doesn't, both the anterior cruciate and the posterolateral joint capsule may be torn. The medial collateral ligaments may also be involved in loss of A-P stability.

Posterior Drawer Sign. The stability of the posterior cruciate ligament is tested in the same manner as the anterior cruciate except the tibia is pushed backward rather than pulled forward. Thus, it can be done in one continuous movement with the anterior drawer test. A distinct sliding backward of the tibia from under the femur is indicative of a torn posterior cruciate ligament. A positive sign is called a "posterior drawer sign" and is less common than the anterior sign.

Management. Injuries resulting in anterior or posterior instability may be treated conservatively if a complete rupture has not occurred. Initial cryotherapy and pressure support followed by a carefully supervised regimen of articular correction, massage, crutch walking, guarded weight bearing with the knee in 30° flexion, physiotherapy

to enhance circulation and promote healing, and quadriceps strengthening exercises are often successful in returning an athlete to competition in 3–6 weeks.

Posterolateral Rotary Instability

Posterolateral rotary instability is a posterior subluxation of the lateral tibial plateau in relation to the lateral femoral condyle accompanied by abnormal external tibial rotation. To test for posterolateral rotary instability, perform the external rotation-recurvatum and a posterior drawer test. Note excessive posterior sag of the lateral tibial plateau with external tibial rotation. This type of instability results from laxity of the arcuate complex, the lateral half of the posterior capsule, and a degree of failure of the posterior cruciate ligament.

Capsule Sprains

Because it is a strong joint yet relatively unstable (a clinical paradox), sprain of the knee may be complicated by derangement of the intra-articular structures; precautions must be taken to carefully examine for possible displacement of the cartilages and rupture of related stabilizing ligaments. Biomechanically, the knee is far more than a simple hinge joint.

Signs and Symptoms. As the knee is a superficial joint and also the largest joint in the body, symptoms after severe trauma are readily apparent. Any forced movement beyond the normal range of movement can produce symptoms and signs. Tenderness may be immediate, but effusion and stiffness are usually slow in development. Fluctuation and ballotement of the patella from joint distention may be present, and hemarthrosis may be associated. Pain and motion limitation are constant symptoms.

Management. After mild injuries, cold, corrective manipulation, and strapping may be sufficient. When effusion into the joint is quite severe, aspiration may rarely be necessary, followed by compression bandages. Physiotherapy should be employed daily, and a knee support is advisable until full functional power is achieved. During the acute hyperemic stage, structural alignment, cold, compression, positive galvanism, and possibly elevation are indicated. Ultrasound is especially effective. Hyaluronidase is helpful to reduce tissue swelling and edema if it is "driven in" with iontophoresis. Rest is usually contraindicated in mild or moderate sprains, but use of a cane may be helpful. Therapy must take into consideration rapid quadriceps atrophy, especially that of the vastus medialis.

After 72 hours, passive congestion may be managed by contrast baths, light massage, gentle passive manipulation, sinusoidal stimulation, ultrasound, and a mild range of motion exercise. During the stage of consolidation, local moderate heat, moderate active exercise, moderate range of motion manipulation, and ultrasound are beneficial. Supplementation with 140 mg of manganese glycerophosphate six times daily throughout care speeds healing. In the stage of fibroblastic activity, deep heat and massage, carefully monitored active exercise, negative galvanism, ultrasound, and active joint manipulation speed recovery and inhibit postinjury effects.

Vapocoolant Technique in Grade I Knee Sprains. Place the patient supine with a pillow under the knee. Spray the painful and tender areas, and gently assist and resist the patient in knee flexion-extension, with emphasis on extension and quadriceps setting. As the pain shifts position, spray the affected area. Have the patient attempt to walk, semisquat, and kneel; spray the painful area if necessary. If possible, have the patient stand on his toes and bend forward with his heels on the floor. Once relief is obtained strap the joint, and instruct the patient in home exercises, 1–2 minutes each half hour during the waking hours. Full weight bearing should be restricted until the quadriceps indicate good strength. Begin resistance, stretching, and weight-bearing exercises as soon as logical.

Collateral Ligament Injuries

Collateral ligament sprain presents the same symptoms of localized pain, tenderness, and swelling as does capsule sprain. Stress tests help in differentiation.

Background. Minor sprains usually have a history of a sudden or unexpected movement, especially when the knee is in valgus position from an internally rotated thigh, a pronated or flat foot, or abduction during foot strike in gait. These injuries are produced by a sudden rotational sprain such as during stumbling, misstepping off a curb or stair, or stepping into a hole or onto a small object. Such sprains are common to cross-country runners, joggers, and jumpers who land with the knee in a valgus position. Severe rupture of the lateral ligaments are produced by trauma where the internal lateral ligament is ruptured by overabduction of the leg or the external ligament is ruptured by overadduction. Excessive lateral motion during complete extension indicates laceration of lateral ligaments. The internal lateral ligament is impaired if abduction of the leg is excessive; the external ligament, if adduction is excessive.

Medial (Tibial) Collateral Ligament Sprain. An external twisting stress with the valgus knee in partial flexion produces partial tearing of the long anterior fibers. Complete rupture may occur from violent abduction while the knee is extended or in external rotation and abduction while the knee is partially flexed. Hematoma usually results, especially if the mechanism of injury is a severe blow. In minor sprains, effusion is slight and rapidly disappears wih rehabilitative activity.

Lateral (Fibular) Collateral Ligament Sprain. Ligament tears are caused by violent adduction, often associated with knee dislocation. The mechanism is usually one of partial flexion, varus position, and internal rotation stress. In minor lateral-ligament sprains, signs of effusion are rare.

Signs and Symptoms. Pain is progressively severe and aggravated by the motion of injury, swelling is localized, point tenderness is demonstrable, muscles are spastic, and hemarthrosis may be present. Drawer signs are negative. Postinjury x-ray films may show elongated amorphous shadows near the affected femoral condyle, evidence of hematoma resolution, and possible displacement of the fibula or tibia.

Collateral Ligament Stability Tests. The medial and lateral ligaments provide stability to the knee joint. To examine sideward stability, place the patient supine and flex the knee just enough to free it from extension. To test the integrity of the medial ligament, apply valgus stress to open the knee joint on the medial side. Test the lateral ligament by applying stress to open the knee

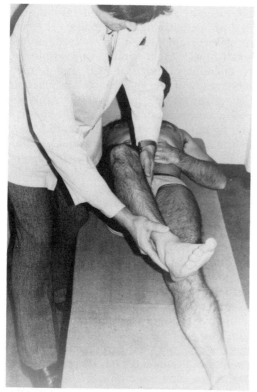

Figure 26.10. Testing lateral collateral ligament by applying varus stress to open the knee joint laterally.

joint on the lateral side. See Figure 26.10. In these maneuvers, secure the ankle with one hand, place the other hand on the opposite side of the knee of the ligaments being tested, and apply pressure towards the ligaments being tested. More knowledge can be gained, however, if the examiner locks the patient's ankle between his arm and chest and uses this hand to palpate the ligaments in question and the underlying joint gap during the test.

Management. The knee should be strapped in complete extension and treated as a severe sprain. Hirata warns that early aspiration or local anesthesia is contraindicated as they both obscure important signs of progress. Straight-leg lifts should be started 36 hours after injury. Effusion arising the first day after injury that subsides 50% or more the second day is an encouraging sign. However, if the swelling reduces and then returns on ambulation, one should suspect related meniscus tear. Early liga-

ment or cartilage tenderness is often obscured by effusion. Once tenderness subsides, graduated resistance exercises may be begun. Once strapping is removed, a brace may be applied which allows flexion but limits lateral motion and full extension. In severe rupture, surgery may be required, but there are no miracles in knee surgery.

The Menisci and Related Ligaments

Almost any sprain that involves rotation will stress the menisci and one or both central cruciate ligaments. However, recent research has shown that the vast majority of knee injuries do not involve severe cartilage damage as once supposed. Several tests help in differentiating true meniscus injury.

Apley's Compression Test. The patient is placed prone with one leg flexed to 90°. The examiner stabilizes the thigh with a knee and grasps the patient's foot. Downward pressure is applied to the foot to compress the medial and lateral menisci between the tibia and femur. The examiner then rotates the tibia internally and externally of the femur, holding downward pressure (Fig. 26.11). Pain during this maneuver indicates probable meniscal damage. Medial knee pain suggests medial meniscus damage; lateral pain, lateral meniscus injury. The incidence of medial cartilage damage is far more common than lateral meniscus injury.

Apley's Distraction Test. Apley designed this test to follow the compression test as an aid in differentiating meniscal from ligamentous knee problems. With the

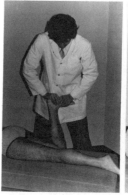 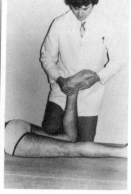

Figure 26.11. *Left*, Apley's compression test for meniscus tear. *Right*, Apley's distraction test.

patient and the examiner in the same position as in the compression test, apply traction (rather than compression) while the leg is rotated internally and externally. This maneuver reduces presssure upon the menisci but stresses the medial and lateral ligaments of the knee.

McMurray's Test. The patient is placed supine with thigh and leg flexed until the heel approaches the buttock. The examiner's one hand is on the knee; his other hand is on the patient's heel. The examiner internally rotates the leg, then slowly extends the leg. Then the examiner externally rotates the leg, then slowly extends the leg. (Fig. 26.12). The test is positive if at some point in the arc a painful click or snap is heared. This sign is significant of menisceal injury. The point in the arc where the snap is heard locates the site of injury of the meniscus; eg, if noted with internal rotation, the lateral meniscus will be involved. The higher the leg is raised when the snap is heard, the more posterior the lesion is in the meniscus. If noted with external rotation, the medial meniscus will be involved. Unfortunately, false-positive and false-negative signs are not uncommon.

Steinmann's Test. In this meniscus sign, tenderness moves posteriorly when the knee is flexed and anteriorly when the knee is extended. This displacement of tenderness does not occur in degenerative osteoarthrosis.

Internal Semilunar Cartilage Injury

Various pathologic factors may produce mechanical derangement within a joint, but trauma is the most common causative agent.

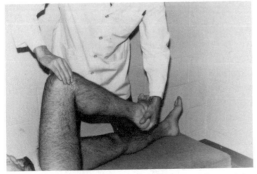

Figure 26.12. Position for McMurray's test for posterior meniscus tear.

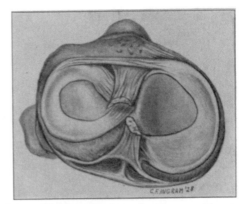

Figure 26.13. Diagram showing superior surface of the tibia, semilunar cartilages, and crucial ligaments.

The anatomic construction of the knee joint predisposes it to attacks of impingement or instability. Injury to either semilunar cartilage may occur at any age, but as trauma received during contact sports is the common cause, men are more frequently affected than women. The injury is most often seen in young adults.

Background. The internal semilunar cartilage is injured 15 times more frequently than the external meniscus. This is because the internal semilunar cartilage is longer than the external, crescentric in shape, and bifurcates at the anterior extremity with the anterior portion of the bifurcation passing across to attach to the external semilunar cartilage. The coronary ligaments that hold the meniscus to the tibia are much shorter than those of its mate and do not permit free play. The external semilunar cartilage ios more circular and thicker than the internal (see Fig. 26.13). It is tied to the tibia by coronary ligaments, as is the internal, but these fibers are much longer and permit more free play than is allowed to the internal cartilage. The external cartilage conforms to the articular surface of the tibia when the bone is extended, but the internal meniscus does not fit snugly in any joint position.

The mechanism of injury which causes internal semilunar stress is also more common—a sudden inward twist of the femur upon the fixed tibia, producing tension and torsion on the anterior border of the meniscus, which may be ruptured or stretched.

Tibial abduction is often associated with torsion and, when present, the mid part of the cartilage may be sucked outward and caught between the femur's inner condyle and tibial tuberosity. Also, abduction widens the medial aspect of the articulation, allowing nipping of the internal meniscus. The posterior border of the internal cartilage may be pinched between the articular surfaces by outward rotation of the femur when the tibia is fixed in extreme flexion (eg, the squatting position). During injury, the meniscus may be contused, subluxated, dislocated, or fractured. Fractures and luxations may be combined during the initial injury or occur after cartilage impingement.

Malpositions. Dislocation of the anterior horn is most common because this part of the meniscus is loosely bound to the internal lateral ligament. After displacement, the anterior border is readily caught between the articulations and may be rolled posteriorly within the joint to cause further displacement or tear. The posterior horn may be loosened and nipped between the back part of the articular surfaces in flexion, preventing full flexion. The central portion may be pulled into the joint when the peripheral attachment is torn. Rarely, the whole cartilage may be detached and avulsed within the joint.

Menisci Fractures. Cartilaginous fractures may be longitudinal, transverse, oblique, or irregular. Bifurcation of the cartilage's anterior border makes this portion particularly easy to split. When the anterior horn is ripped loose and retracted within the joint, the transverse ligament locks the outer edge of the meniscus while traction upon the displaced horn tears the cartilage. The central portion of the meniscus may be jammed between the articulations causing a longitudinal split and displacement of the inner half of the cartilage within the joint (buckethandle type). A similar tear of the posterior horn (posterior tag) may be caused by the same mechanism as dislocation. Transverse fractures are most common where the anterior third of the meniscus joins with the posterior two-thirds. A horizontal "T" or oblique fracture may occur at this point by the cartilage bending without detachment.

Signs and Symptoms. Symptoms reflect the amount of meniscus damage and impingement. The joint may be locked, swollen, and extremely painful. Frequently, there is inability to fully extend the knee, indicating joint locking. The infrapatellar fat pad may be hot and enlarged. Either or both lateral ligaments may be stretched or ruptured. Sometimes swelling does not develop for several hours, upon which tenderness increases over the involved ligament. After recurrent displacement, the picture is not so acute except on rare occasions. A low-grade inflammatory process is related to recurrent displacements associated with proliferative changes in the synovial membrane. Diagnosis is arrived at by the history, along with physical and roentgenographic findings to differentiate arthritis, anomalies, and other causes for the internal derangement and clinical picture

Payr's Sign. The patient is asked to sit flat on the floor with the legs crossed and folded in so that the femurs are internally rotated, the knees are flexed and abducted, and the feet are plantar-flexed. If pain occurs on the medial side of a knee when the examiner applies downward (valgus) pressure on the knee, a lesion at the posterior horn of the medial meniscus is suggested.

Reduction. If the impingement is mild, first flex the knee over counter-leverage pressure with the doctor's fist in the patient's popliteal fossa. Rock the limb gently in this position to loosen the jammed meniscus. The leg is then grasped at the ankle, and the tibia is laterally rocked on the femur to widen the space between the medial condyle of the femur and the tibia's articular surface, thus further freeing the cartilage. The leg is then rotated inward while the patient actively kicks his leg forward and upward. Severe force should never be used. An audible snap is usually heard as the meniscus is repositioned. The test for reduction is the patient's ability to completely extend the knee without assistance. Reduction host be made within 24 hours after injury; if not, effusion causes a loss in meniscus elasticity which prevents it from springing back to its correct position.

Management. After reduction, the injury is treated as a severe sprain. Full weight bearing should be allowed as soon as possible, but motion should be restricted by strapping. The taping procedure is the same as for collateral ligaments. Later, a brace may be applied which allows flexion but restricts rotation. A sole lift is helpful for several months until full strength and stability returns. Competitive activity should never be resumed until all symptoms have subsided and quadriceps strength and tone have returned to normal. Management should also consider strengthening the rotators of the knee.

External Semilunar Cartilage Injury

The mechanism of injury to the external semilunar cartilage is the reverse of that producing internal cartilage damage.

Background. In this type of injury, the foot has usually been fixed upon the ground and the femur rotated outwardly upon the tibia while the knee was simultaneously adducted. The posterior border is ruptured and the cartilage is avulsed within the anterior compartment. The external lateral ligament may also be stretched or torn. The same type of lesions found in internal malpositions are found, but here the whole cartilage is most often displaced because it is thicker and heavier than its mate.

Signs and Symptoms. The symptoms are identical, sometimes milder, to those of medial injury except that they are located at the lateral aspect: locking, local tenderness, and inability to make full extension. Sometimes pain and tenderness are referred medially if the lateral ligament is severely stretched.

Childress' Duck Waddle Test. This is a two phase test: (1) The patient is asked to stand with the feet separated about 12–18 inches apart, assume a "knock-kneed" position by rotating the thighs inward, and then attempt to squat as low as possible. Pain, joint restriction, or a clicking sensation suggest a lesion of the medial meniscus. (2) The test is then conducted, with the patient assuming a "bowed-leg" position, by rotating the thighs outward. Pain, joint restriction, or a clicking sensation when attempting to squat suggests a lesion of the lateral meniscus.

Reduction. The reduction maneuver is the opposite of that used for internal meniscus impingement. The knee is acutely flexed, adducted to open the joint laterally,

and the leg is rotated outwardly while the patient quickly extends the knee. Again, the test for reposition is active full extension of the knee. Management is the same as that for internal meniscus damage.

The Crucial Ligaments

The cruciates may be ruptured by the same mechanisms that produce meniscus displacements.

Background. The anterior cruciate ligament is commonly disrupted when internal rotation of the femur with the knee slightly flexed produces a relaxation of the cruciate ligaments as they untwist. The cruciate ligaments retense with forced external rotation of the femur, and the anterior cruciate gives way because it is weaker than the posterior. Posterior tears are caused by sudden external rotation of the femur with the foot fixed while the knee is forced into abduction, flexion, or by forceful displacement of the tibia backward on the femur with the knee flexed. Another mechanism is a fall onto the knee with the force received on the proximal tibia. Because knee twisting disrupts the meniscus, the coincidence of meniscus and anterior ligament sprain is often seen. Pure A–P shearing stress to the cruciates is rare in sports with the exception of football "clipping" injuries. Crucial sprain is often involved in "the unhappy triad" of (1) medial collateral ligament sprain, (2) medial fibrocartilage sprain, and (3) anterior cruciate sprain.

Signs and Symptoms. If the anterior crucial ligament is torn, the tibia can be glided forward on the femur (drawer sign) and the knee can be hyperextended. However, this sign must be elicited early before reflex hamstring spasm obscures a possibly positive sign. If the posterior crucial ligament is torn, the tibia can be glided posteriorly on the femur. Both the anterior and the posterior crucial ligaments may be torn. Laxity of the anterior cruciate is especially common, but it is unimportant if functional stability is maintained. There will be no lateral instability unless the collateral ligaments are also involved. After rutpure, the subject is quite apprehensive and insecure. The history is one of the knee "giving way" with slight locking, similar to that seen with stretching of a lateral ligament. In full rupture, severe avulsion or fracture of the bony attachment is usually associated. Stress films exhibit excessive joint motion.

Classification. (1) *Mild*: Pain is elicited by passive stress, and point tenderness and local swelling are exhibited. The joint is stable, and there is no locking or effusion. (2) *Moderate*: There is local swelling, some effusion, constant pain aggravated by passive stress, and locking if a meniscus rupture is related. There may be hemarthrosis. (3) *Severe*: Complete tear with or without avulsion. There is severe disability, instability, extensive swelling, agonizing pain, protective spasms, locking if a meniscus is involved, and probable hemarthrosis. Early surgery, within 24 h, should be considered.

Management. In mild cases, treatment is by activity restriction, cold packs, compression, support, and muscle therapy. In moderate to severe cases, the limb should be elevated and cold packs applied for 24–72 hours. When effusion has completely subsided, heat may be applied. The knee should be pressure-dressed and casted in complete extension and treated as a severe sprain until the ruptured ligament is repaired by fibrous adhesions. Weight bearing should be limited and ultimately a program of muscle reeducation initiated. A brace may be applied which allows flexion but inhibits lateral motion. Rehabilitation should emphasize the strengthening of the extensors in the last 10–15°. Management should also consider strengthening the rotators of the knee. In severe rupture, surgery may be required, especially if there is evidence of bone damage.

The Meniscus-Coronary Ligament Relationship

The importance of this relationship was recently emphasized by Dr. John M. Nash.

The menisci of the knee are held firmly at their peripheral boundary to the plateaus of the tibia. This is accomplished by a series of short fibers known as the coronary ligaments. Normally, these fibers perform in such a manner that positional stability is afforded the menisci without interference to the shifting that is mandated by the functional design of the articular surfaces.

Meniscus Shifting

Normal menisci must be able to shift posteriorly during flexion, anteriorly during extension, and concentrically during rotation. During medial rotation of the tibia, the medial meniscus shifts slightly anterior and the lateral meniscus moves posteriorly. Opposite reactions occur during lateral rotation.

This shifting effect is actively performed by the bilateral reflection of the extensor retinaculum (via the meniscopatellar ligament) that attaches to each of the horns of the anterior meniscus. The quadriceps, whose tendon fibers form the extensor retinaculum, performs the extension action at the knee and simultaneously shifts the menisci to ready them for the anterior rolling of the femoral condyles.

In the same manner, the posterior meniscus horns are influenced during the posterior shift that occurs when the knee flexes. The responsible structures are the semimembranosus reflection to the posterior horn of the medial meniscus and the popliteus reflection to the posterior horn of the lateral meniscus. These two knee flexors assist in the posterior directional roll of the femoral condyles during flexion and simultaneously shift the menisci in the proper direction, posteriorly.

If this shifting action should fail to occur, the rolling action of the femoral condyles would traumatize the faulty menisci. Normally, this action just alternately pumps the menisci as an inhibitory influence. This mechanism of shift is therefore responsible for the integrity of the menisci; but in an altered state during activity, it is responsible for demise of the menisci through dessication and traumatic compaction.

The Clinical Picture

The failure of menisci to shift properly is often encountered in patients who will complain of knee pain that has no accompanying swelling and is precipitated by an increase in activity. With knowledge of the shifting mechanisms in mind, the patient must be thoroughly evaluated for any weakness, contracture, coordinative aberration, or nonendurant quality of the dynamics of the knee, leg, ankle, or foot that would discourage normal knee mechanics. The examination will usually demonstrate negative signs during meniscus and ligamentous tests.

An increased activity pattern may be related to either the intensity or duration of effort. It is frequently reported by the novice exerciser who has just started an exercise program or by the trained athlete who has recently accelerated his training. The obvious commonality in each of these cases would be the recent increase in the duration or intensity of activity.

Careful palpation will reveal single or multiple trigger points that are exquisitely tender. Topographically, they are found immediately below the joint line on the tibial plateau. Either the lateral or medial aspects of the knee may be involved, with the medial aspect affected more often than the lateral. The painful sites represent a fibrous scarring reaction in a portion of the delicate coronary ligaments, produced by some minor repetitive biomechanical overstress that appears symptomatically only with the superimposed insult of accelerated activity (duration or intensity).

Management

Treat as any acute sprain during the acute stage. However, to treat the coronary ligaments without regard for the causative entity would merely passify the problem and result in placing the athlete back into competition where he would be vulnerable to identical or possibly greater damage.

Nash describes the treatment of associated trigger points on the coronary ligaments as being deep transverse friction over the painful points for 3–4 minutes, followed by an application of negative high-volt therapy. In the instance of a patient with a low threshold of pain, this treatment should be preceded by 15–20 minutes of ice massage. This regimen will usually accomplish its purpose of re-elasticization and cessation of pain in 1–2 weeks if the therapy is applied three times a week.

Coronary Sprains

Meniscus tear is often confused with an excessively mobile meniscus that results from lax coronary ligaments. The symptoms of coronary sprain mimic mild meniscus sprain with the exceptions that there is no joint locking and point tenderness at the joint line may be more acute. A negative McMurray's sign and Apley's compression sign are found.

Joint Locking

While meniscus tears and lax coronary ligaments may be exhibited in joint locking, there are frequently other causes such as free bodies within the joint which cause a blockage. Transient locking is often the result of recurrent nipping of the alar folds which produces pedunculated tags that are easily caught; hemarthrosis is typically associated.

Because of its anatomic design, the leg cannot be extended without a degree of external tibial rotation on the femur. A maximal rotation of 6° of lateral rotation occurs during the last 10° of extension and the reverse during the first 10° of flexion. This is called the "screw-home" mechanism. The Helfet test determines the integrity of the knee relative to the presence of this normal motion.

Bounce-Home Test. Hoppenfeld refers to an evaluation of full knee extension as the "bounce home" test. the patient is placed supine. The examiner cups one hand under the patient's heel and fully flexes the knee with the other hand. While the patient's heel is grasped, the patient's knee is allowed to passively drop toward the tabletop in full extension, normally with an abrupt stop. If this full extension is not achieved and passive pressure elicits a "rubbery" resistance to extension, a blockage is indicated. This lack of full extension points to a torn meniscus, patellar subluxation, intracapsular swelling, or a loose fragment within the knee joint.

Helfet's Test. This test is designed to detect the presence of a intra-articular "loose body" which disturbs the normal biomechanics of the joint. To test normal knee locking, place a dot with a skin pencil in the center of the patella and another over the tibial tubercle when the knee is flexed. The knee is then passively extended and the motion of the dot relative to the patella is observed. A positive Helfet test occurs when there is lack of full lateral movement of the dot. Palpation of the tibial tubercle during this passive test allows for more subtle determination of disturbed joint mechanics. Aside from intra-articular bodies, both a lack of rotational joint play at the tibiofemoral articulation and imbalance in the tone of the internal and external rotators of the tibia could promote the pathomechanics observed during the test. It should also be noted that all but two of these muscles find their origin in the pelvis.

Osteochondromatosis

Osteochondromatosis is a noninflammatory condition in which pedunculated or loose bodies are formed from the synovial membrane within the joint cavity or in the bursae and tendon sheaths. Traumatic, infectious, and neoplastic etiologies have been put forth. The exact cause is controversial, but the facts tend toward trauma being the primary causative agent.

Pathology. The disorder features villous hypertrophy of the synovial membrane with bony or fibrous bodies forming in the villi. One large cauliflower-like displaced body or several hundred small round or kidney-shaped bodies, closely packed, may be seen free within the joint on x-ray examination. There is some growth after development. Each body contains a cancellous core with fat cells surrounded by a hyaline-like exterior. With time and pressure, large bodies may develop smooth convex facets.

False Locking. While true joint locking can occur from a displaced fragmented cartilage, a false locking may occur where there is stiffening on extension which gives way with persistence. It is more of a painful arc than a true block.

Osteochondritis Dissecans

A bony defect of the articular margin of the femur at the lateral aspect of the medial condyle is referred toas osteochondritis dissecans. This is, however, a misnomer in that it represents a form of compression fracture rather than a dissecting inflammatory lesion. It is frequently related to a history of sports-related trauma.

Incidence. The disorder is essentially an affection of adolescence and young adults (rarely seen in middle age) and almost unknown in later life. It occurs most frequently between the ages of 12 and 25, and males

are more frequently affected than females in a ratio of 15:1. Usually one joint is affected, sometimes bilaterally; and 90% of the time it is the knee. The elbow is next in frequency.

Etiology. Osteochondritis dissecans occurs in the knee (or elbow) at the point of greatest impact; ie, the lateral portion of the surface of the internal condyle adjacent to the intercondylar notch. The cause is unknown, but there are many theories; traumatic, embolic, and constitutional. Most authorities feel that trauma is at least a predisposing agent if not the causative factor. Trauma may act in three ways: (1) by direct force at the point of greatest contact; (2) by direct pull on the anterior attachment of the posterior ligament; and (3) by injury to the arterial supply. Fat embolism or bacterial embolism may also be involved. Aseptic necrosis due to embolism, low-grade bacteria infection, and congenital predisposition of the femoral epiphysis are other typical factors.

Wilson's Sign. The patient is placed supine with the legs in an extended, relaxed position. This is a two-phase test. (1) The knee of the involved side is flexed to a right angle, the leg is firmly rotated internally, and then the knee is slowly extended while maintaining the leg in internal rotation. If osteochondritis of the knee is present, the patient will complain of pain in front of the medial condyle of the distal femur. (2) However, if the leg is then externally rotated, the pain will subside.

Symptoms. The complaint is one of intermittent and mild joint disability. There is usually a low-grade inflammatory process associated with slight effusion, swelling, and joint clicking or locking. Before fragment separation, pain is dull and aching.

Roentgenographic Considerations. Routine A–P and lateral plus a tunnel-view projection are recommended. Whatever the cause, a somewhat crater-like, rarefied, and conical-shaped depression on the border of the condyle involving subchondral bone is characteristic (Fig. 26.14). This may require months or years to develop. Giammarino reports that the most frequent site of the lesion is in the medial femoral condyle near the intercondylar notch. On the surface of the condyle, a punched-out irregular trian-

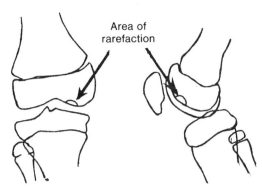

Figure 26.14. X-ray tracing of osteochondritis dissecans.

gular notch of varying size appears. The loose body or sequestra may be seen in the crater or within the joint space. If the body is not completely detached, it may be seen lying in the cavity and separated from the underlying bone by a clear-cut line of demarcation. If detached, it will appear as an oval shadow in the joint. If it is cartilagenous, it may not be visible. As a line of cleavage is formed, the cavity and loose body are covered with fibrocartilage, becoming rough and irregular. It later releases and falls into the joint cavity where it is ground into small fragments by weight pressure, each of which usually continues to increase in size. The fragments may be small or large, round, oval, or irregular.

Management. Mild manipulation, traction, and various forms of physiotherapy will usually ameliorate the symptoms. Mechanical traumatic arthrosis may result if a joint "mouse" repeatedly sets up irritation. As in Legg-Calve-Perthe disease, revascularization of an undisplaced fragment in osteochondrosis dissecans of the knee in children appears to progress with reasonable rapidity in some cases if the joint is protected from bearing weight for about 6 months. If a fragment is caught and unable to be dislodged, or if a loose body is present within the joint, surgery may have to be conducted. In spite of symptom absence, some authorities advise surgery to prevent osteoarthritis. Surgery is normally reserved only for those cases in which clinical and roentgenographic improvement cannot be demonstrated or if displacement occurs repeatedly.

Nerve Injuries

Peroneal Nerve Contusion. The peroneal nerve, a terminal branch of the sciatic nerve, is exposed to injury especially as it winds about the neck of the fibula. In addition to lacerations, it is frequently injured in fracture of the neck of the fibula and occasionally by pressure of poorly-padded supports. A typical "foot drop" results. Treatment is the same as with other nerve injuries, with special attention given to support of the foot in the right-angle position.

Peroneal Nerve Compression. This is a compression syndrome of the common peroneal nerve near the head of the fibula or as the nerve enters the anterior compartment. There is usually a history of recurrent ankle and/or foot injury. The typical complaint is pain on the lateral aspect of the leg and foot, which is initiated or aggravated with pressure over the trunk of the common peroneal nerve. This pressure pain usually radiates into the sensory distribution of the nerve. Neurologic tests indicate motor loss characterized by weak ankle and toe dorsiflexion and weak foot eversion. As in any case of nerve compression, the cause must be determined and corrected. If conservative therapy fails, referral for surgical exploration is indicated.

Lust's Sign. When the external branch of the sciatic nerve, the peroneus communis, is struck with a percussion hammer, the reflex produces dorsal flexion and abduction of the foot. This is best practiced by following the nerve below the bifurcation of the great sciatic nerve, especially an an oblique position outwardly along the outer portion of the popliteal space. This pathologic reflex is indicative of spasmophilia.

Westphal's Sign. This term represents loss of any deep reflex, thus indicative of lower motor neuron involvement. It is especially applied to loss of the patellar quadriceps reflex.

Lasegue's Hysteria Sign. This sign reflects a functional nervous disease, especially hysteria. When hysterical anesthesia of an extremity occurs, the patient will be unable to move the affected part with the eyes closed. With the eyes open, however, volitional movement can be made when attention is directed to the involved extremity, thus simulating a loss of muscle sense. This frequently occurs in hysteria and rarely in other highly emotional states. It is seen more frequently in women.

Subluxations

When a subluxation exists between the distal femur and the proximal tibia, it may be attributed to either bone. We have elected the tibia in the following descriptions, and the reader should realize that this has been an arbitrary decision. Thus, a listing for an externally rotated tibia may be described by another as an internally rotated femur, for example, or a lateral tibia subluxation may be rightfully described as a medial femur subluxation.

Because the articulation between the femur and tibia is so complex, an array of subluxation possibilities exist. The tibia may be translated solely in one direction; eg, medially, laterally, posteriorly, or anteriorly in relation to the femur. In addition, rotatory instability may produce a displacement in the anteromedial, anterolateral, posteromedial, or posterolateral direction. Therefore, astute evaluation of these displacement possibilities and the integrity of the associated soft tissues must be made before a proper adjustment can be made.

Externally Rotated Tibia Subluxation

Associated features are medial capsular pain and tenderness, genu valgum, promi-

nent medial tibial condyle and plateau, tightness of the pes anserine tendons, chondromalacia patellae, and restricted internal tibial rotation.

Adjustment. The patient is placed prone with the involved knee flexed at 70°. Stand at the side of the involved tibia, and place your cephalad knee on the patient's distal femur for stabilization. Grasp the patient's distal tibia and fibula with your fingers interlocking on the anterior aspect. Apply upward traction to the leg, and make a firm but gentle internal rotation manipulation of the leg (Fig. 26.15, *left*). Evaluate the integrity of the semitendinous, semimembraneous, gracilis, sartorius, and popliteus muscles.

First Alternative Adjustment Procedure. The patient is placed supine. Stand on the side of involvement facing the patient. Place your medial foot on the table with your knee against a pad in the patient's popliteal space for countertraction, and place the patient's ankle under your medial axilla. Your lateral hand grasps the anterior surface of the patient's leg just above the ankle, and your medial hand is moved under the patient's leg so that you can grasp your lateral arm. The patient's leg rests within your cubital fossa for support. Apply traction to the leg while simultaneously manipulating the leg with internal rotation (Fig. 26.15, *right*).

Second Alternative Adjustment Proce-

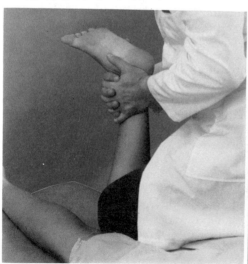 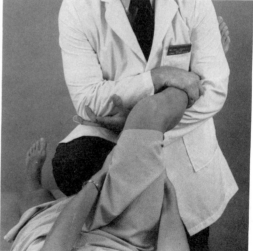

Figure 26.15. *Left,* technique position for adjusting externally rotated tibia. *Right,* first alternative adjustment position.

dure. Stand on the side of involvement of the supine patient. The patient's hip should be flexed about 60° and his knee flexed about 110°. Grasp the patient's lower leg with your medial contact hand, and place your lateral hand on the patient's knee to stabilize the patella (Fig. 26.16). The adjustment is made by flexing and internally rotating the patient's leg.

Internally Rotated Tibia Subluxation

Associated features are lateral capsular pain and tenderness, genu varum, promi-

nent lateral tibial condyle and plateau, tightness of the iliotibial band and lateral hamstring tendons, chondromalacia patellae, and restricted external tibial rotation.

Adjustment. The patient is placed prone with the involved knee flexed about 70°. Stand at the side opposite the involved tibia, and place your cephalad knee on the patient's distal femur of the involved limb for stabilization. Grasp the patient's distal tibia and fibula with your fingers interlocking on the anterior aspect (Fig. 26.17, *left*). Apply upward traction to the leg, and make

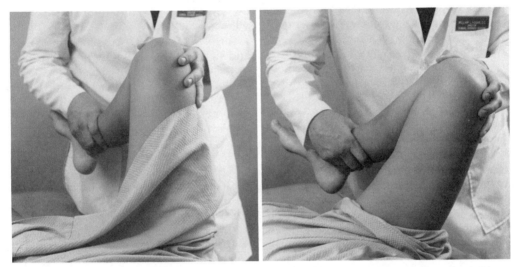

Figure 26.16.   Second alternative adjustment positions for adjusting externally rotated tibia.

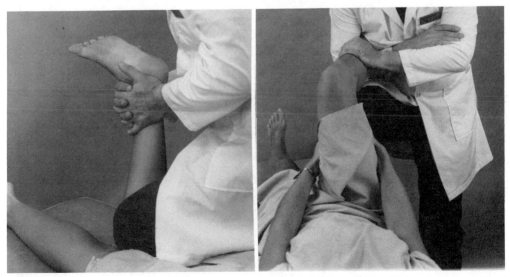

Figure 26.17.   *Left*, technique position for adjusting internally rotated tibia. *Right*, alternative adjustment position.

the adjustment by externally rotating the patient's leg. Evaluate the integrity of the biceps femoris (both heads) and tensor fascia lata.

Alternative Adjustment Procedure. The patient is placed supine. Stand on the side of involvement facing the patient. Place your medial foot on the table with your knee against a pad in the patient's popliteal space for countertraction, and place the patient's ankle in your axilla. Your medial hand should grasp the anterior surface of the patient's leg just above the angle, and your lateral hand is moved under the patient's leg so that you can grasp your medial arm. The patient's leg rests within your cubital fossa for support (Fig. 26.17, *right*). Apply traction to the leg while simultaneously manipulating the leg with external rotation.

Posterior Tibia Subluxation

Associated features include popliteal fossa tenderness, posterior cruciate ligament tenderness, posterior drawer sign, patella tendon hypotonicity and depression, and restricted anterior tibia motion. A history of anterior tibial trauma is usually involved.

Adjustment. Place the patient prone with his knee flexed 70°. Squat at the end of the table, and place the patient's involved leg against your medial shoulder. Interlock

both of your hands on the posterior aspect of the tibial condyles (Fig. 26.18, *left*). Apply traction while simultaneously making a strong adjustment to bring the tibia anterior. Evaluate the integrity of the vastus intermedius, rectur femoris, and hamstrings.

Anterior Tibia Subluxation

Associated features include patellar tendon tenderness, anterior drawer sign, anterior cruciate tenderness, patellar tendon hypertonicity or tendinitis, and restricted posterior tibial motion. The history usually involves a blow to the back of the upper leg (eg, clipping tackle) or a fall backward over a low obstacle.

Adjustment. Place the patient supine, and stand on the side of involvement. Take contact with our cephalad hand against the patient's proximal anterior tibia. Place your caudad hand under the patient's calf to support the weight of the leg and to apply traction during the adjustment (Fig. 26.18, *right*). As traction is made, simultaneously make a short A–P thrust. Evaluate the integrity of the hamstring and quadricep muscle group.

Medial Tibia Subluxation

Subluxation is frequently consequent to medial collateral ligament sprain with re-

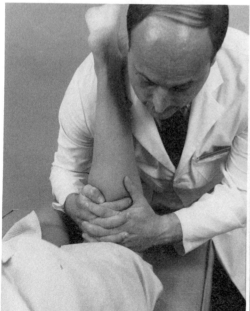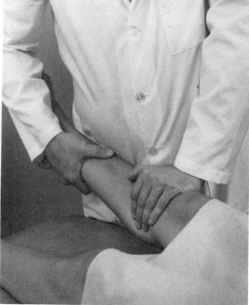

Figure 26.18. *Left*, position for adjusting posterior tibia subluxation. *Right*, anterior tibia.

stricted lateral motion. Trauma to the lateral upper tibia is usually involved.

Adjustment. Place the patient supine with the involved knee extended and the ipsilateral hip flexed about 45°. Stand on the side opposite to involvement, and place your cephalad contact palm against the patient's upper media tibia. A pisiform contact is taken against the medial tibial condyle (Fig. 26.19, *left*). Wrap your caudad hand under the patient's calf so that you can grasp your contact wrist. This will support the weight of the patient's leg. Slightly flex the patient's knee, apply traction to the leg, and simultaneously make a short thrust that is directed from the medial to the lateral. Evaluate the integrity of the tensor fascia lata, hamstrings, gracilis, and sartorius.

Lateral Tibia Subluxation

Subluxation is frequently consequent to lateral collateral ligament sprain with restricted medial motion. Trauma to the medial upper tibia is usually involved.

Adjustment. Place the patient supine with the involved knee extended and the ipsilateral hip flexed about 45°. Stand on the side of involvement, and place your cephalad contact palm against the patient's upper lateral tibia. A pisiform contact is taken against the lateral tibial condyle (Fig. 26.19, *right*). Wrap your caudad hand under the patient's calf so that you can grasp your

contact wrist. This will support the weight of the patient's leg. Slightly flex the patient's knee, apply traction to the leg, and simultaneously make a short thrust that is directed from the lateral to the medial. Evaluate the integrity of the tensor fascia lata, hamstrings, gracilis, and sartorius.

Superior Fibula Subluxation

Subluxation is often consequent to eversion sprain. Features include tenderness about the fibular collateral ligament due to jamming, restricted inferior fibula motion, and a possible slight foot-drop sign.

Adjustment. Place the patient supine with knee extended and hip flexed at about 45°. Stand at the end of the table with the patient's foot placed on your anterior thigh. Grasp the ankle with your lateral hand, and take a web or capitate contact at the proximal aspect of the lateral malleolus. With your medial hand, overlap the contact wrist for stability (Fig. 26.20). Apply traction, and simultaneously make a short inferiorly directed thrust. Evaluate the integrity of the biceps femoris, peroneus group, tibialis anterior and extensor digitorum longus.

Inferior Fibula Subluxation

This subluxation can be the result of inversion sprain and is often associated with tenderness about the collateral ligament of

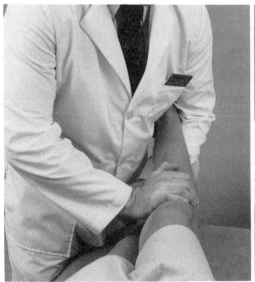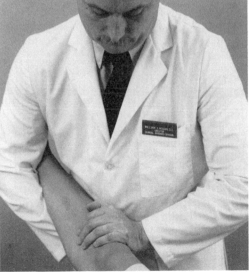

Figure 26.19. *Left*, position for adjusting medial tibia subluxation. *Right*, lateral tibia.

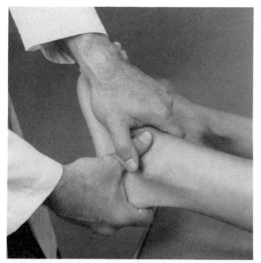

Figure 26.20. Position for adjusting superior fibula.

the fibula and restricted superior fibula motion.

Adjustment. The patient is placed in the lateral recumbent position with the affected side up and the medial aspect of the affected foot resting relaxed on the table. Stand at the foot of the table in line with the longitudinal axis of the patient's affected leg. Take a capitate contact with your medial hand against the inferior aspect of the lateral malleolus, with your lateral hand grasping your contact wrist for stability. Apply pressure, and simultaneously make a short thrust directed superiorly along the vertical axis of the fibula. Evaluate the integrity of the biceps femoris, peroneus group extensor hallucis longus, and extensor digitorum longus.

Posteroinferior Fibula Subluxation

Associated features include pain at the fibular head, lateral collateral ligament pain at the ankle, lateral hamstring complaints, and restricted anterosuperior fibula motion. Subluxation is often the result of inversion ankle sprain.

Adjustment. Place the patient supine with affected knee flexed. Stand lateral to the involved limb with your cephalad hand within the popliteal fossa with thenar-pad contact against the fibular head. For leverage, grasp the anterior aspect of the patient's lower leg with your caudad hand (Fig.

26.21). Apply oblique pressure with your stabilizing hand to flex the knee and push the leg superiorly, while simultaneously sharply lifting the fibular head anteriorly with your contact hand. Evaluate the integrity of the biceps femoris, peroneus group, extensor hallucis longus, and extensor digitorum longus.

Posteromedial Fibula Subluxation

This subluxation is often consequent to inversion sprain, hamstring pull, trauma to the anterolateral knee, and genu valgum. Anterolateral fibula motion is usually associated.

Adjustment. Place the patient prone with leg flexed. Squat at the end of the table, facing the patient, so that the patient's leg rests on your shoulder for stability. Grasp the leg by interlacing fingers around the posterior aspect of the patient's proximal leg (Fig. 26.22, *left*). Make specific pisiform contact with your lateral hand against the medial aspect of the fibular head. Apply traction, and simultaneously rotate the fibula anterolaterally. Evaluate the integrity of the biceps femoris, peroneus group, and extensors hallucis longus and digitorum longus.

Anterolateral Fibula Subluxation

Subluxation is often the result of lateral hamstring strain, eversion sprain, and trauma to the posterolateral aspect of the knee, characterized by lateral hamstring

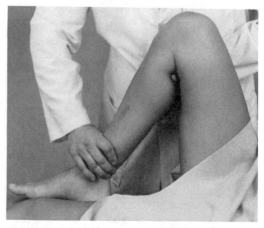

Figure 26.21. Position for adjusting posteroinferior fibula.

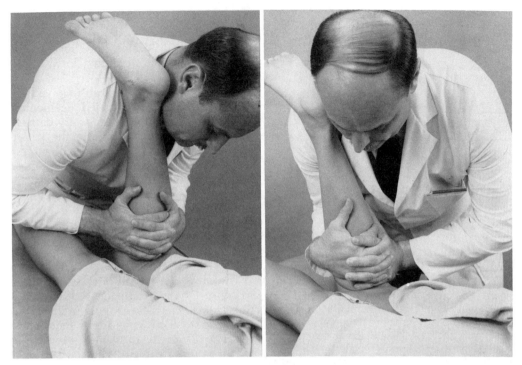

Figure 26.22. *Left*, position for adjusting posteromedial tibia. *Right*, anterolateral fibula.

tendon tenderness, genu varum, excessive pronation, and restricted posteromedial fibula motion.

Adjustment. Place the patient prone with leg flexed. Squat at the end of the table, facing the patient, so that the patient's leg rests on your shoulder for stability. Grasp the leg by interlacing fingers around the posterior aspect of the patient's proximal leg. Make specific pisiform contact with your lateral hand against the anterolateral aspect of the fibular head (Fig. 26.22, *right*). Apply traction, and simultaneously rotate the fibula posteromedially. Evaluate the integrity of the biceps femoris, peroneus group, extensor hallucis longus, and extensor digitorum longus.

Fractures

If fracture is suspected, great care must be made to avoid soft-tissue damage during movement. Supracondylar or intracondylar fractures are rare in the young and during athletics but are quite frequent in the elderly with minimal trauma. The fracture site may be stable, displaced, or comminuted.

The injury mechanism is usually a side-ways blow just above the knee or a direct anterior blow when the knee is fully flexed (eg, hard-surface fall on the knee). Larcher points out that football helmet "spearing" to stop a runner frequently occurs by hitting laterally and anteriorly at the junction of the fibula, tibia, and femur articulations. "This osseous impact is so traumatic that it frequently immobilizes the player to the extent of a fractured extremity, ruptured collateral ligament and meniscus, or severe contusions and hemorrhaging of infra- and supra-patellar synovial sacs and tendinous attachments". Yet, according to statistics, knee fractures are rare in sports.

Distal Femur Fractures. Comminuted lower femoral osteochondral fractures may result from jumping compression forces which may produce bony fragments that are difficult to view on x-ray films. On axial or tangential views, ossicles of the tibial tubercle may project over the femoral margins or patella and be confused with an osteochondral fracture or a loose body of bone. See Figure 26.23.

Proximal Leg Fractures. After a violent twisting of the knee followed by pain local-

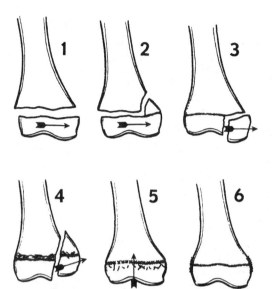

Figure 26.23. Salter-Harris classification of growth-plate fractures: *1*, fracture through the growth plate only; *2*, fracture through part of the metaphysis and growth plate; *2*, fracture through the epiphysis and growth plate; *4*, fracture through the epiphysis, growth plate, and metaphysis; *5*, comminuted fracture of the growth plate; *6*, perichondral fracture. Types *3* and *4* are intra-articular injuries.

ized near the proximal fibula, fracture and upper fibula dislocation should be anticipated. Chronic subluxations or post–traumatic arthritis of the proximal tibiofibular joint are frequent complications. As in the forearm, fractures of the bones in the leg often involve both bones. Sometimes, however, these bones do not fracture at the same level. When an x-ray of the leg does not include the entire length of the bones, there is a possibility that a fracture may be missed. When a fracture is seen in only one of the paired bones at a given level, one must be certain to seek other levels for fracture of the other bone. Tibial fractures are rarely seen; when they are, they are usually the result of one running into an obstacle such as a bench.

Dislocations

Dislocations of the knee are rarely seen except in vehicular accidents or falls from great heights, although a few cases have been reported in football and from slight missteps. The diagnosis is usually obvious

when a dislocation of the knee is encountered. Unfortunately, only in rare cases will a completely dislocated knee regain complete A–P motion, according to Sisto and Warren.

Because of the severe pain involved and the probability of associated ligamentous and capsule tears, popliteal artery damage, and/or peroneal nerve injury, the patient should be referred to an orthopedic surgeon immediately for reduction under anesthesia and continuous evaluation of vascular and nerve status. Vascular repair is often unsuccessful if delayed for more than 8 hours.

Selected Disorders

Osgood-Schlatter Disease

The most likely form of osteochondrosis to be met with in athletics is that of the tibial tubercle. It is seen quite frequently in young football backs and runners of either sex. The disorder is misnamed, however, in that it is not a disease. The exact cause is unknown, but it is thought to be a form of osteochondrosis with intrinsic trauma as the inciting factor; eg, sudden contractions of quadriceps femoris concentrated on a portion of an incompletely developed tibial tubercle resulting in an avulsion fracture. The disorder is not often severely disabling and is milder in young girls than boys. The disorder is often bilateral.

Roentgenographic Considerations. Findings of the A–P view are usually negative. In the lateral view, the epiphysis of the tibia is fragmented and irregular in outline and density during the advanced stage (Fig. 26.24). In the early stage, the patellar liga-

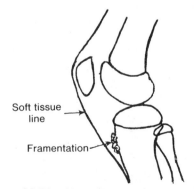

Soft tissue line

Framentation

Figure 26.24. X-ray film tracing of epiphysitis.

ment becomes thickened at its insertion. This is usually evident before osseous changes occur. Williams and Sperryn feel that the anterior tibial tubercle becomes infarcted because of excessive pull from the patella tendon. The primary trauma is followed by numerous lesser injuries which constantly give rise to newer interruption of continuity during the growth period.

Signs and Symptoms. Symptoms depend upon the involvement of the synovial membrane and the mechanical interference of the loose bodies. The complaint is one of pain at the anterior knee, inferior to the patella, especially when the knee is flexed. Repeated attacks of "catching" are common. A hot, red, tender swelling develops over the tibial tubercle when the disorder is active. The patient complains of pain during activity and the inability to kneel. There is also pain on running and climbing stairs. A large tubercle may be palpable. While joint motion may be only slightly affected, crepitation on active and passive motion is typical. Pain is increased by active knee extension against resistance.

Case Management. Immediate rest of the part is indicated. Normalize any existing vertebral motion-unit abnormality if possible, especially those found in the lumbar or sacral area. Normalize muscle tone in the lower back, pelvis, and thigh. A plaster cast, brace, or other means for restricting joint flexion may be necessary to allow the tubercle to fuse: some authorities say always, others say it is never necessary. Ultrasonic therapy helps in increasing vascularization at the appropriate stage. Weight bearing is permitted, but not knee flexion until symptoms subside. Afterwards, weak muscles must be strengthened. Patients responding poorly to conservative measures or who are subject to frequent attacks should be referred for surgical correction. Never overlook a possible aggravating balance defect in the foot or pelvis.

Osteoarthrosis

Osteoarthrosis of the knee is not always a sequel of aging degeneration. It is sometimes seen in the young athlete. Trauma usually initiates symptoms which began, often subclinically, after earlier trauma that was improperly managed (eg, inadequate mobilization and/or muscle reeducation). Heavy weight bearing superimposed on a joint with microcirculation impairment (often of a reflex nature) and congenital defects are two other common predisposing factors.

Surfer's Nodes and Tumors

Surfers frequently present hyperkeratotic skin nodules at the anterior surface over the tibial tubercles and at the bottom of the feet under the metatarsophalangeal joints. These findings are usually associated with a swollen bursa at the proximal aspect of the dorsum of the foot which develops within the synovial sheath of the extensor digitorum longus tendon. These lesions are the result of kneeling on the surfboard during activity. Among surfers, they are more often considered a status symbol than a reason for complaint.

The knee is a common site of occasionally seen giant cell tumors and sarcomata. When discovered, they are usually on a roentgenograph taken to confirm another suspicion.

THE PATELLA

Patellar rupture or tendinitis, quadriceps rupture or tendinitis (jumper's knee), and fatigue fractures of the tibia have a high incidence in basketball. In tendinitis, the pain may be perceived either during and shortly after activity or be chronic. Forceful jumping may result in an avulsive fracture of the patella.

Infrapatellar Fat Pad Hypertrophy

Repeated stress to the knee joint may cause the infrapatellar fat pad or the synovial villi to become hypertrophied. The symptoms are joint weakness or definite locking, joint effusion when acute, pain on the medial aspect of the knee, and tenderness distal and medial to the patella. However, positive diagnosis can only be made upon exploratory surgery. Conservative care is the same as that for severe pain.

Intracapsular Pinches

A sudden joint stress, usually rotational, may cause some soft tissue to be pinched within articular structures during jumping, defensive running, kicking, etc. This is most frequently seen in the knee where the infrapatellar fat pad is nipped, resulting in a degree of effusion and possible hemorrhage. Intracapsular pinches are more common in sports than cartilage injuries.

Signs and Symptoms. Diagnosis is essentially by exclusion. There is no history of external trauma, nor are there signs of joint line tenderness or instability. Discomfort is felt directly behind the patella. A slight effusion may be present and associated with a slight loss in full extension. The sides of the patella and its tendon will feel thick and firm. This mass will be tender, and it will be the *sole* site of tenderness if ligament and fibrocartilage involvement are excluded.

Patella Wobble Sign. A patient in the sitting position is instructed to extend a knee while the examiner cups a palm over the patella. If erratic patellar motion is felt during the last phase of extension, an irregular retropatellar growth or some type of incomplete obstruction is indicated (eg, hypertrophied infrapatellar synovial folds, hardened fat pad).

Management. Management is the same as that for sprain, but active movement is slightly delayed because injured fat is slow to heal. In prognosis, keep in mind that damaged fat is frequently replaced by inelastic fibrous tissue which is readily irritated by stress. Cold packs and compression must be continued as long as there is palpable thickening near the patella and any degree of extension restriction. Despite player objections, no activity should be permitted for 4–7 days.

Surgery may be necessary if the superior portion of the tibia cuts off a large portion of the infrapatellar pad or if the tag later becomes calcified and causes trouble. Surgery is also required in some cases where a pedunculated part may become strangled by adhesions, resulting in torsion gangrene associated with joint locking and hemarthrosis.

Acute Bursitis

"Housemaid's knee" is a bursitis of the prepatellar bursa. Fluctuation, with or without heat and tenderness, that is limited to the prepatellar space is usually diagnostic. Management of an acutely swollen bursa is not difficult if undertaken immediately. Cold packs, rest, and a pressure bandage are usually adequate. On rare occasions, referral for aspiration and steroids may be necessary if swelling does not begin to subside within 24 hours. Graduated activity may begin as soon as the acute phase has resolved.

Knee Effusion Test. If a joint is greatly swollen from a major effusion, place the patient in a relaxed supine position. Relax the limb and slowly extend the knee. Then push the patella into the trochlear groove and release it quickly. This will force fluid under the patella to the sides of the joint and then to return under the patella. This rebound is referred to as a *ballotable patella.* Minimal effusion will not ballot the patella. In cases of minor effusion, it is necessary to "milk" the fluid from the suprapatellar pouch and the lateral side to the medial side of the joint. Once the fluid has been moved medially, tapping over the fluid will return it to the lateral side.

Chronic Effusion

In this state of chronic "water on the knee," the original trauma may not be remembered. It is an inflamed synovial membrane of the knee with escape of fluid into a synovial sac. Causes include trauma, atherosclerosis, flat feet and/or genu valgum, and lymphatic congestion. In some cases, the cause can be traced to psoas dyskinesia from an anterior pelvic tilt and abducted feet producing an increased torque of the knee.

Signs and Symptoms. The picture is one of prepatellar or infrapatellar bursitis with a locally inflamed knee presented (Fig. 26.25). There is little pain except on motion, mild to extensive swelling, and obvious quadriceps atrophy. The knee instability tests may not be strongly positive, yet there may be signs of inhibitions of the neuromuscular mechanisms of the knee and signs of recurrent subluxation of the patella over the lateral condyle.

Management. Chronic strain management and muscle reeducation are usually sufficient; if not, referral for aspiration of fluid, steroids, and possibly antibiotics may be advisable. In competitive sports, there is no absolute cure, and reaggravation can be anticipated. Swimming is beneficial during

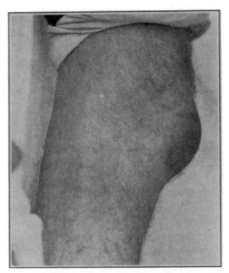

Figure 26.25. Infected prepatellar bursitis. A severe trauma was followed by swelling and eventual suppuration.

recuperation. Protection and compression must be provided during competitive activity until healing is secure in approximately one month. For a hypersensitive knee, standard padding is usually inadequate for football players.

Chondromalacia Patellae

This is a state of rapid erosion and fragmentation of the cartilage of the patella. Incidence is highest in the young (7–25), and genu recurvatum is the typical cause; ie, hyperextension during single-leg stance and the push-off phase of gait.

Background. The cartilage becomes opaque and soft, cracks and fissures appear, and the cartilage becomes thinned. This exposes underlying bone which becomes sclerotic. The exact cause of the syndrome is unknown, although trauma is associated in two-thirds of the cases. In extreme flexion, subpatella pressure may rise to 20 times that of body weight. It may be secondary to recurrent subluxation, quadriceps wasting (especially that of the vastus medialis), pronated or flat feet, Morton's syndrome, postural instability, or a short-leg syndrome.

Signs and Symptoms. Pain arises from the posterior aspect of the patella which is increased by patella compression against the femoral condyles and by strong quadriceps contraction. Tenderness is found at the posteromedial and posterolateral aspects of the patella. Clarke's sign is positive, and a sensation of "giving way," locking, or chronic joint clicking are typical. Stiffness arising after sitting long periods with the knee flexed is relieved by activity. Squatting and the ascending or descending stairs are aggravating. During active knee motion but not passive motion, grating is palpable and usually audible and accentuated with patella compression. Joint effusion and quadriceps atrophy are typical findings. Early x-ray films are negative, but the inner aspect of the patella exhibits sclerosis, roughening, irregularity, a narrowed patellofemoral space, and spurring in late stages.

Clarke's Sign. The supine patient extends the knee and relaxes the quadriceps. The examiner places the web of a hand against the superior aspect of the patella and depresses it distally. The patient then actively contracts the quadriceps as the examiner compresses the patella against the condyles of the distal femur. The sign is positive if the patient cannot maintain contraction without producing sharp pain.

Fouchet's Test. The patient is placed supine with the limbs extended in the relaxed position. If firm pressure on the patella produces pain and focal tenderness at the margin of the patella, chondromalacia of the patella should be suspected.

Perkin's Patella Grinding Test. With the patient supine as in Fouchet's test, the examiner places a firm double hand contact over the anterior knee, leans over the limb, and displaces the patella from side to side while simultaneously applying pressure from the anterior to the posterior. Induced pain or grating (palpable or audible) during this maneuver suggests retropatella arthritis or chondromalacia of the patella.

Management. Treatment is similar to that for chronic sprain. During an acute attack, rest and cryotherapy are advised for at least 48 hours. Adjustments should be given to normalize any associated femoral, tibial, or patellar subluxation/fixations. Check for other sites of related joint restriction (eg, hips, ankles, feet). Therapeutic heat, massage, electrostimulation, and exercise will enhance the healing process if they do not exceed the patient's tolerance.

Strapping is made to restrict excessive motion such as that for sprained collateral ligaments. Most important to healing is restoring of normal vastus medialis function through straight-leg quadriceps reeducation with or without galvanic help. Rehabilitative exercises should include internal and external rotation exercises of the tibia, short-arc quadricep exercises, and static quadricep contractions.

Sinding-Larsen-Johannson Disease

A complaint of knee pain and joint tenderness at the lower pole (rare at the upper pole) of the patella can be attributed to Sinding-Larsen-Johannson disease (*jumper's knee*). Point tenderness is the main feature. Symptoms mimic chondromalacia; eg, pain on kneeling, lower pole thickening and tenderness. It is a self-limited, benign, temporarily disabling, focal tendinitis seen more often in young boys than girls. It is apparently the result of a traction irritation of the tendon at its patella attachment.

Bipartite Patella

A bipartite patella is a congenital deformity characterized by development of the patella as two or more fragments (Fig. 26.26). Two fragments are most frequently seen, usually bilateral. The condition may be discovered incidentally during roentgenography. It is usually asymptomatic unless the components are disrupted. Features usually include a segmented patella with a large crescent-shaped segment located in the superior-lateral quadrant on the A–P view.

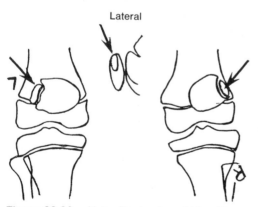

Lateral

Figure 26.26. X-ray film tracing of bipartite patella.

The lateral view may reveal overlapping anomalous segments rather than the normal smooth outline of the patella.

As there may be a history of trauma, distinctive features between such an anomaly and a patella fracture should be recognized. An anomaly usually presents an indefinite history of trauma. A uniform space exists between the surfaces of a fragment throughout its length, and the outline of the fragment is smooth and consists of cortical bone. The defect usually involves the outer-upper qaudrant of the patella. On the other hand, a fracture presents a definite history of trauma accompanied by clinical manifestations of bone injury. It is usually unilateral. There is an absence of uniform space between fragments. The outline of a fragment usually shows serrated edges, and it involves cancellous bone. A fracture less frequently involves the outer-upper quadrant.

Patella Tendon Strain

In sports the patella tendon is subject to partial tears, complete rupture (rare), peritendinitis, and focal degeneration. Chronic strain has a high incidence in high jumpers and runners (eg, basketball, track).

Background.   Partial tears are often misdisagnosed as strain. The picture is one of pain on forced knee extension and during activity, point tenderness, possible extension block and weakness, thickened adjacent tissues, and roentgenographic soft-tissue changes. Differentiation from peritendinitis can only be made during surgery.

Management.   Treat as a severe acute or chronic sprain depending upon the history, with emphasis on rest, heel pads, ultrasound, and deep heat.

Patella Dislocations

In dislocation, a fixed tilt or malposition of the patella or an osteochondral fracture may be noted. Motion will be restricted, and the surrounding tissues will be stressed. Secondary infection may occur.

Roentgenographic Considerations.   Tangential views with the knee flexed about 50° are helpful in showing malposition. The most common patella dislocation is sideward, especially laterally, but proximal shifting may occur. In association with traumatic dislocations, fractures of the medial patellar margin and osteochondrial fracture of the femoral condyles are quite common.

Etiology. The cause may be a congenital or traumatic decrease in the femoral intra-patellar groove, especially at the lateral lip; trauma tearing the ligamentous attachments; inflammation (traumatic or infectious) in the intrapatellar pad which produces an increase in synovial fluid; vastus medialis dystonia; torn collateral or cruciate ligaments; or femoral or tibial dislocation. the patella displaces laterally with vigorous quadriceps contraction. When the person strongly extends the flexed knee with the leg externally rotated, the patella may redislocate.

Signs and Symptoms. The typical acute case preesnts point tenderness, erythema, mild heat, edema, pain aggravated by motion, joint block, patella restriction, and limping. The patella apprehension and bounce-home tests are positive.

Patella Apprehension Test. If a patella is prone to dislocation, any attempt by the examiner to produce such a dislocation will be met with by sharp patient resistance. In testing, the patient is placed in the relaxed neutral supine position, and the examiner applies increasing pressure against the patellar. If a chronic weakness exists, the patients will become increasingly apprehensive as the patella begins to dislocate.

Reduction. The longer reduction is delayed, the more difficult and painful it becomes. Place the patient supine, and provide maximum muscle relaxation by hyperextending the joint (eg, placing the ankle on a pillow). Enhance relaxation of the quadriceps by heat if swelling is not present. Firmly grasp the patella and correct the displacement with steady pressure. Correction will be noted by immediate relief of pain.

Management. If tears are not severe, treatment is by reduction, acute sprain management (eg, cold, compression, felt splints), strapping as for collateral ligament sprain, and quadriceps rehabilitation. Immobilization should be made in 15–20° flexion. X-ray after reduction to determine possible associated bone chips or avulsions, and seek orthopedic consultation. During the early stages, crutches should be used in weight bearing. Recurrence is most common when the patella is small or there is a degree of postural valgus. Each recurrence becomes more difficult to manage even if the dislocation is spontaneously reduced. Preventive strapping during competition is always advisable in such cases. Rehabilitation should emphasize vastus medialis reeducation and active flexion-extension exercises. When tearing is severe, surgery is necessary.

Dreyer's Sign. The patient is placed supine with the legs extended in the relaxed position and asked to raise the involved thigh while keeping the knee extended. If the patient is unable to do this, the examiner grasps the large quadriceps tendon just above the knee to anchor it against the femur, and the patient is asked to try to lift the limb again. If the patient is then able to lift the limb when the quadriceps tendon is stabilized, a fractured patella should be suspected. The reason for this is that the rectus femoris (a primary hip flexor) attaches to the patella by way of the quadriceps tendon.

Popliteal Swelling

There are numerous and variable bursae in the popliteal fossa, and they often fuse to form a large bursa (eg, gastrocnemio-semimembranous bursa). Blits brings out that this is the most common bursa of which the popliteal (Baker's) cyst is a distention. To differentiate this swelling in the popliteal fossa from others, aneurysms, hemangiomas, and neoplasms should be considered. (See Table 26.3.)

Subluxations of the Patella

In athletic knee injuries, the incidence of patella subluxation is secondary only to collateral ligament and meniscus injuries. It should be noted that if the tibia is in a state of fixated external rotation, the patella is especially vulnerable to subluxation or dislocation if the flexed knee is suddenly extended while the leg is rotated externally.

Superior Patella Subluxation

Indications include patellar tendinitis, quadriceps spasm, chondromalacia patellae, and restricted inferior patella motion.

Adjustment. Place the patient supine with the affected knee extended. Stand on

Table 26.3.
Differentiation of Popliteal Swelling

Entity	Primary Characteristics
Aneurysm	Pulsating mass; bruit synchronous with the pulse. Diagnosis is confirmed by arteriography.
Baker's cyst	A soft, nontender collection of synovial fluid that has escaped from the knee joint or a bursa and formed a new synovial-lined sac in the popliteal space (typically the posteromedial or posterolateral aspect). It is often associated with degenerative and other joint diseases.
Hemangioma	Painful, tender, soft swelling. Increased local temperature with superficial vessels dilated. Multipled opacities of calcification confirmed by roentgenography.
Neoplasm	Benign or malignant. Benign tumors are soft, mobile, and well localized. Malignant fibrosarcoma is painful, firm, tender, and fixed to surrounding tissues. The regional lymph nodes may be involved. Diagnosis is confirmed by biopsy.

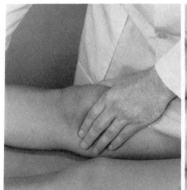 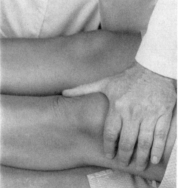 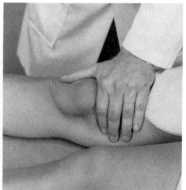

Figure 26.27. *Left,* position for adjusting superior patella. *Middle,* position for adjusting superomedial patella. *Right,* superolateral patella.

the side of involvement. Take a web contact with your cephalad hand against the superior aspect of the patella. Stabilize the patient's leg by your caudad hand grasping the upper shin (Fig. 26.27, *left*). Apply pressure with your contact and make a short thrust directed inferiorly. Evaluate the integrity of the vastus intermedius, rectus femoris, and hamstrings.

Superomedial or Superolateral Patella Subluxations

Associated features include patellar tendinitis, quadriceps spasm, and chondromalacia patellae. Genu varum and restricted inferolateral patella motion are often associated with superomedial subluxations, while genu valgum and restricted inferomedial patella motion are associated with superolateral subluxations.

Adjustment. Place the patient supine with the affected knee extended. Stand on the side of involvement. Take a web contact with your cephalad hand against the involved superomedial or superolateral aspect of the patella. Stabilize the patient's leg by your caudad hand grasping the upper shin. Apply pressure with your contact and make a short thrust directed obliquely to correct the misalignment; ie, inferomedial or inferolateral (Fig. 26.27, *middle* and *right*). Evaluate the integrity of the vastus intermedius and lateralis, rectus femoris, and hamstrings.

Inferior Patella Subluxation

This type of displacement is typically associated with chondromalacia of the patella, blocked superior joint play, suprapatellar tendinitis, and restricted extension of the knee.

Adjustment. The patient is placed supine with the involved knee extended. If full extension cannot be made comfortably, the popliteal space should be supported by one or more rolled towels. Stand on the side of the involvement. Take a web contact with your caudad hand against the inferior aspect of the patella, deep against the patella tendon. Your cephalad hand should grasp the wrist of your contact hand for support and added strength. Apply pressure superiorly so that all joint play is removed, and then make a short thrust to stretch the patella tendon and normalize the position of the patella. Evaluate the integrity of the quadriceps group.

CHAPTER 27

Leg, Ankle, and Foot Injuries

The lower leg, ankle, and foot work as a functional unit. Total body weight above is transmitted to the leg, ankle hinge, and foot in the upright position, and this force is greatly multiplied in locomotion. Thus the ankle and foot are uniquely affected by trauma and static deformities infrequently seen in other areas of the body.

INJURIES OF THE LEG

The most common injuries in this area are bruises, muscle strains, tendon lesions, postural stress, anterior and posterior compression syndromes, and tibia and fibula fractures. Bruises of the lower leg are less frequent than those of the thigh or knee, but the incidence of intrinsic strain, sprain, and stress fractures are much greater.

Various neurologic, orthopedic, and peripheral vascular signs and tests relative to the leg are listed in Table 27.1.

A continual program of running and jogging is typical of most sports. The result is often strengthening of the antigravity muscles at the expense of the gravity muscles—producing a dynamic imbalance unless both gravity and antigravity muscles are developed simultaneously. An anatomic or physiologic short leg as little as an eighth of an inch can affect a stride and produce an overstrain in long-distance track events.

Bruises and Contusions

The most common bruise of the lower extremity is that of the skin, where disability may be great as the poorly protected tibial periosteum is usually involved. Skin splits in this area can be most difficult to heal. Signs of suppuration indicate referral to guard against periostitis and osteomyelitis.

Management. Treat as any skin-bone bruise with cold packs and antibacterial procedures, and shield the area with padding during competitive activity. When long socks are worn, the incidence of shinbone injuries is reduced. An old but effective protective method in professional football

that does not add weight is to place four or five sheets of slick magazine pages around the shin, secured by a cotton sock which is covered by the conventional sock. A blow to the shin is reduced to about a third of its force as the paper slips laterally on impact.

Gastrocnemius Contusion

This is a common and most debilitating injury in contact sports. It is characterized by severe calf tenderness, abnormal muscle firmness of the engorged muscle, and inability to raise the heel during weight bearing.

Management. Treat with cold packs, compression, and elevation for 24 hours. Follow with mild heat and contrast baths. Massage is contraindicated in the early stage as it might disturb muscle repair. The danger of ossification is less in the calf than in the thigh, but management must incorporate precautions against adhesions.

Traumatic Phlebitis

Contusion to the greater saphenous vein may lead to rupture resulting in extensive swelling, ecchymosis, redness, and other signs of local phlebitis. Tenderness will be found along the course of the vascular channel. During treatment, referral should be made upon the first signs of thrombosis.

Management. Management is by rest, cold, compression, and elevation for at least 48 hours. Later, progressive ambulation, mild heat, and contrast baths should be utilized. Progressive exercises may begin in 4–6 days. When competitive activity is resumed, the area should be provided extra protection.

Nerve Contusions

Nerve trauma exhibits palsy, paresthesia, or anesthesia. These signs commonly result from a kick in sports. Trauma behind the knee to the external popliteal nerve features inability to extend the foot. Trauma to the peroneal nerve along the lateral aspect of

Table 27.1.
**Review of Neurologic, Orthopedic, and
Peripheral Vascular Maneuvers, Reflexes,
Signs, or Tests Relative to the Leg**

Buerger's test
Claudication test
Duchenne's sign
Heel walk test
Homan's sign
Hueter's sign
Light touch/pain tests
Lust's sign
Moskowicz's test
Muscle strength grading
Neri's leg sign
Patella reflex
Perthe's test
Pratt's test
Repetitive heel raise test
Strumpell's tibialis sign
Toe walk test
Trendelenburg's vein test

the lower third of the leg may result in a palsy characterized by inability to flex the foot (foot drop). Peroneal symptoms are sometimes associated with asymptomatic loose tibiofibular ligaments. The excessive mobile fibula head, with demonstrated false motion, often "clicks" during gait and tends to irritate the peroneal nerve as it winds around the fibula neck.

Management. Treat as any nerve contusion with emphasis on ice massage or cold packs, followed later by deep massage, contrast baths, and graduated exercises. Heel lifts are helpful in relieving tension on the injured nerve. A loose tibiofibular head can be aided by a sponge pad placed over the area and secured by an elastic bandage. Any case exhibiting a degree of atrophy or sensation loss over a few days deserves neurologic consultation.

Strains

With the increased interest in jogging, musculoskeletal injury is common but usually minor. During middle age, the most common injury is calf-muscle strain, but knee, ankle, and foot sprain, and shin splints do occur frequently. Occasionally, stress fractures will be associated.

A tear of the musculotendinous junction of the medial belly of the gastrocnemius often occurs in tennis, skiing, squash, and track. At the site of tenderness, a palpable gap in the muscle is usually found. It is identified in a radiographic lateral view as an indentation of the soft-tissue margins.

General Management

Heat is helpful to relieve muscle spasm, but cold and vapocoolant sprays have shown to be as effective. Mild passive stretch is an excellent method of reducing spasm in the long muscles. For example, standing on an incline (eg, Flex Wedge) relaxes a spasm through passive stretching. Heavy passive stretch destroys the beneficial reflexes.

Fatigue may increase contractures and produce pain. Spasms are treated by (1) warming the muscle with limbering movements (2) stretching the muscle by resistance to the tightened muscle and its antagonist (3) active stretching in an attempt to fulfull the possible entire range of motion and then by (4) passive stretching to fulfill the possible range of motion. The stretching force must be a careful balance between that of easy performance and that of excessive misuse.

Other methods may prove helpful. Peripheral inhibitory afferent impulses can be generated to partially close the presynaptic gate by acupressure, acupuncture, or transcutaneous nerve stimulation. Isotonic exercises benefit by improving circulation and inducing the stretch reflex when done supine to reduce exteroceptive influences on the central nervous system. An acid-base imbalance from muscle hypoxia or acidosis may be prevented by supplemental alkalinization.

Muscle Rehabilitation

Physiologic elasticity, the ability of a muscle to release tension, is highly important for normal movement. A tired muscle loses some of this ability to relax, thus effecting its elasticity and endurance capacity. A muscle with good endurance readily assumes its maximum length after repeated prolonged contractions, but a tired muscle does not return to its maximum length.

When mechanical elasticity is impaired, muscle tissue does not yield to passive stretch. After injury, this "Contracture Tiegel" is frequently the effect of spasm or prolonged immobilization, or both. For this reason, it is highly necessary in athletics to conduct goniometry in the weight-bearing position. For example, an ankle or knee may record a full range of motion while supine but be severely restricted in the squatting or kneeling position due to residual muscle shortening without actual fibrous contracture.

In most sports, a player should not be allowed to return to competition until the injured muscle becomes as strong as its uninjured contralateral mate. Strength-building exercises should be given just below the fatigue level, keeping in mind that injured muscles fatigue rapidly.

Shin Splints

This syndrome is one of lower leg pain and discomfort after running or walking over-stress that is associated with an aseptic inflammation of the injured muscle-tendon unit. An excessive overstride during running is a typical cause of such irritation. It is a common complaint during early season practice sessions or when the running surface is changed. Keep in mind that the anterior shin muscles warm slowly and cool rapidly because they are squeezed tightly between bone and skin and by fascia. The blood supply of the interosseus membrane is quite limited.

Signs and Symptoms. The term "shin splints" is a catch-all phrase for any discomfort in the anterior leg on exercise. The common cause may be better classified as tibialis anterior or posterior syndrome, tendoperiostosis, or stress fracture. Differentiation is made by mode of onset, site of tenderness, and late roentgenography. A poorly responding case of shin splints with pain even on rest suggests a compartment syndrome. Tenderness is most common over the posterior tibialis muscle, but it is frequently found at the attachment of the anterior tibial muscle to the lateral border of the tibia. The pain is usually throbbing, deep-seated, relieved with rest, but increased at night.

Roentgenographic Considerations. Cortical thickenening of the medical tibia or a minimal periosteal reaction is the roentgenographic counterpart of shin splints, the result of muscle/fascial attachments of the anterior mid or lower leg being torn or stretched. In uncomplicated cases, no evidence may be visible except for slight cortical thickening. The possibility of a stress fracture must always be eliminated.

Management. Once the actual cause has been found, which may be as high as the lower back or as low as the foot, treat as a severe strain with accompanying subluxations. Cryotherapy should be emphasized. After the acute stage, emphasis is on structural alignment, deep heat, analgesic pack, passive massage, heel pad, trigger point therapy, stretching exercises, and good strapping support. The taping or some other type of support should continue for a month after full activity is resumed. Modalities offer unencouraging benefit. An anatomic short leg is often involved that requires a permanent heel lift slightly under actual need.

Some misguided high school coaches recommend that shin splints be "run out." This invariably leads to the development of scar tissue or new bone formation. However, Dayton of Yale feels that most cases will show a history of running "duck footed" with the feet everted and externally rotated, thus stressing the plantar flexors. If this is the case, tenderness and slight swelling will appear at the posteromedial crest where the tibial attachments of the soleus and flexor digitorum longus are located. Dayton feels that strapping the foot in slight inversion and initiating a program of graduated trotting "pigeon toed" is the best regimen to alter the predisposing habit.

Quite frequently, a weak longitudinal arch is involved. A 2 x 2-inch pad of ¼-inch gauze can be secured on the plantar surface of the foot to cover the arch and the anterior third of the heel. Heavy patients may require a double pad. Good support requires taping or bracing high up the lateral and medial leg. Nonyielding tape should never be used. However, the more simple method is to place a 2 x 6-inch piece of ½ inch-thick foam rubber over the shin and secure it with an elastic bandage.

Tibialis Anterior Syndrome

The anterior tibial syndrome is a disabling form of muscle stiffness where intramuscular tension (engorgement) is exaggerated by the unyielding surrounding tissues to a degree that local infarction may occur leading to local massive necrosis or Volkmann's contracture.

Background. Alternately raised muscle fiber tension so alters the muscle's internal frictional resistance that rapid movements are impossible and muscle tearing develops if the whole muscle doesn't go into spasm. The engorged muscle becomes trapped within its fascial compartment and tends to strip from its bony attachments. Circulation of the anterior tibial artery becomes impaired. Most authorities do not attribute any part of the disorder with a local accumulation of lactic acid. On rare occasions, prolonged heavy training or overuse may produce muscle hypertrophy of the lower fibers of the tibialis anterior which causes blocking of the upper extensor retinaculum of the ankle. This "space-occupying" lesion effect produces local symptoms. A blow to the lower leg will have the same result.

Signs and Symptoms. The syndrome features gradually increasing anterolateral leg pain increased on activity, swelling, and restricted motion. Keep in mind, however, that all muscles swell after exercise, and this is particularly true of unconditioned muscles. During the acute stage, and unlike other shin splints, rest offers little relief. Flat feet, tight calves producing plantar flexion, and imbalance between the anterior and posterior muscle groups are commonly associated. That is, the anterior leg muscles are often weaker than the posterior group and this produces a dynamic imbalance which requires special consideration in rehabilitation.

Management. Prevention through properly graduated conditioning and interval training is the best therapy. Of the various possible therapies, ice, massage, elevation, trigger point therapy, stretching exercise, interferential current, and late deep heat are the most effective, but no regimen has proved ideal. If conservative measures are unsuccessful, surgical decompression should be considered.

Posterior Tibial Compartment Syndrome

The cause is similar to that of the anterior tibial compartment syndrome or a crushing injury. Pain, entrapped swelling, and numbness are often severe. The engorged muscle becomes trapped within its fascial compartment and tends to strip from its bony attachments. Signs of tendinitis behind the medial malleolus, deep calf myositis, tenderness in the posteromedial angle of the tibia, pain on use, and foot pronation are commonly associated. A difficult complication is widespread tendoperiostitis which terminates in severe scars and adhesions. Surgical decompression is often required.

Periostitis

Tibial Periostitis. Anterior tibial periostitis is a frequent complication which results from traumatic microelevation of the periosteum by fascial overstress. Severe pain localized at the medial tibial border occurs during activity. A small tender area may be palpable. Conservative measures rarely are helpful other than cold, rest, firm support, and referral for local anesthesia and steroids.

Fibula Periostitis. Fibula periostitis is a frequent complication of blows to the lateral leg, especially at the lower third of the bone. There is persistent soreness aggravated by activity, shaft tenderness, and shaft thickening demonstrated by roentgenography. Crepitus may or not be present. Management should include 1–2 weeks of rest followed by graduated active exercise.

Popliteus Tendon Rupture

A player makes a jump, lands, and feels a "pop" in the calf; a sudden sharp pain develops, and incapacity overtakes the player. This is the typical picture of popliteus tendon rupture which is often confused with meniscal injury, phlebitis, and Achilles rupture or tendinitis. It occurs most often in the middle-aged athlete (eg, basketball, tennis).

Management. Ice, compression, elevation, and rest are the treatment of choice during the early stage, followed by appropriate physiotherapeutic measures. A careful check should be made for associated lower spine, pelvic, hip, or lower extremity subluxations or fixations.

Plantaris Rupture (Tennis Leg)

Although termed "tennis leg" because of its association with overhead forehand over-stress, the disorder is also frequent to football "button-hook" pass receivers and to basketball players during rebound play. It is sometimes confused with soleus or gastrocnemius strain in that its function is to assist these two muscles. In actual plantaris strain, which is rare, there is pain with an explosive onset, tenderness, and an area of indurated tissues located deep at midcalf and lateral to this site when the palm palpates from the popliteal space to the heel. The pain is increased by dorsiflexing the foot against resistance. Bleeding and a deep thrombophlebitis is often associated. Signs of ecchymosis on each side of the Achilles tendon often appear in a few days. Quite frequently, an Achilles sprain and separation of calf fascia are associated.

Management. General strain therapy should include initial cold packs and compression for at least 48 hours. An analgesic pack of menthyl salicylate (buttered and covered under the strapping), deep heat, heel pads, cane support while walking, progressive passive stretching, and whirlpool or shower hydrotherapy at 108°F are helpful. There is always a danger of tendinitis ossificans. Full activity is rarely assumed before 3–4 weeks. When competitive activity is resumed, it should be preceded by deep massage and stretching exercises for 3–5 months after injury. Recurrent symptoms can often be traced to a degree of myositis ossificans.

Gastrocnemius Strain

Strain of the gastrocnemius is the most common strain of the leg in sports and often misdiagnosed as a ruptured plantaris tendon. The onset of symptoms is usually immediate calf cramping, generalized calf spasm, and extreme tenderness at the site of strain. Strain nearer the Achilles tendon is often attributed to running on the balls of the feet. Occasionally, strain occurs at the gastrocnemius heads and is confused with knee injury after a snapping overextension. If this is the case, tenderness will be found deep in the popliteal fossa when the flexed knee is palpated.

Repetitive Heel Raise Test. The standing patient is asked to raise the heels (ie, toe stand) repetitively several times. If this induces ankle pain, instability, a posterior compartment syndrome, or a subluxation complex should be suspected. If this exercise

is unable to be performed because of weakness and ankle pain is absent, a gastrocneiumius weakness or neurologic deficit should be suspected.

Management. Treat as any severe strain, but be forewarned that rehabilitation is difficult. Heat enhances relaxation but increases swelling and pain. Cold reduces swelling but increases cramping. Thus, structural normalization, rest, muscle techniques, electric meridian therapy, and a most gradual program of locomotion are the best therapy.

Soleus Strain

Strain of the soleus independent of the gastrocnemius is rare, but it does occur in sports. It is characterized by a palpably tight and tender soleus but relaxed and nontender gastrocnemius. It is usually a mid-season disability.

Management. As with gastrocnemius strain, management is often frustrating. Rest, structural correction, muscle techniques, acupoint techniques, interferential current, high-volt therapy; and a slowly graduated program of dorsiflexion and stretching exercises are the best aids. It often takes 2 weeks before full competitive strength returns.

Plantar Flexion Restrictions

Limitation of the gastrocnemius or soleus muscle restricting ankle dorsiflexion can be differentiated by the *ankle dorsiflexion* test. Have the patient sit on the examining table with the knees flexed and relaxed. Grasp the foot and flex the knee to slacken the gastrocnemius, then dorsiflex the ankle. If this can be achieved, the gastrocnemius is the cause of the restriction. If the soleus is at fault, it will not be affected by knee flexion; ie, it will be the same in either knee flexion or extension.

Fascial Tears

While fascia tears can occur most anywhere, they are most often seen in the leg following blunt trauma near the tibial crests. Bleeding is more persistent than in typical contusions. After swelling reduces, palpation will reveal the muscle herniating through the fascial defect.

Management. Symptoms are usually

present only during activity where the muscle swells and causes impingement at the hole. This can simply be prevented by an overlaid sponge pad secured by an elastic bandage. While the method may be crude, it is often the choice of the patient over that of surgery which may require a second donor-site incision.

Achilles Tendon Lesions

The tendon of Achilles inserts into the calcaneus and is formed by the common tendon of the gastrocnemius and soleus muscles. It can be readily palpated in the lower third of the calf. Signs of tenderness, swelling, tenosynovitis, or crepitation should be noted. Rupture or tear results in lack of push-off during gait.

Skiers and runners have a high incidence of Achilles tendon injury. In runners, Achilles tendon pain is frequently associated with plantar fascitis, leg or ankle tendinitis, paritendinitis, tendon rupture, or local inflammation. Also frequently associated but overlooked are stress fractures of the

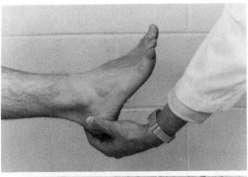

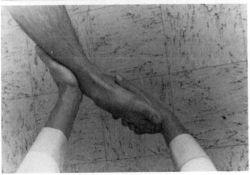

Figure 27.1. *Top*, palpation of Achilles tendon and associated bursae. *Bottom*, position for testing the strength of the tibialis anterior muscle against resistance.

2nd metatarsal and fibula. Other sites of related fatigue fractures include the calcaneus, tarsal navicular, tibia, and femur.

Ruptures

Due to the great tensile strength of the normal Achilles tendon, femoral or calcaneus fractures invariably occur before the tendon ruptures. However, this may not be true when excessive force is applied to a previously injured or diseased tendon. The cause is usually traced to overuse, direct violence during stretch, or a poorly placed injection.

Incidence. The incidence of intrinsic stress injuries is high in middle- and long-distance runners. Complete rupture is exceedingly rare in players under the age of 40 years. Both complete and partial ruptures are most often seen in middle-aged athletes.

Signs and Symptoms. Rupture may be present even if the player can extend the foot against resistance. A gap or area of extreme tenderness in the Achilles is greater evidence. The site of tear is unvariably about 2 inches above its attachment at the heel. Care must be taken to differentiate rupture from partial tear: (1) Rupture is characterized by sharp pain, often accompanied by perception of an abrupt "thud" at the site. The sharp pain soon subsides, but ankle weakness produces a flat-footed gait. Plantar flexion is usually but not always impossible, and passive dorsiflexion is restricted. The onset is always sudden, a tendon deficit is usually palpable, and Thompson's test is positive. The calf muscles retract to a higher position than normal. (2) Partial tear, less common than rupture, is characterized by acute pain during activity which persists until stress can be avoided. When activity is resumed, severe pain returns. A tender swelling is inevitably noted when the site is palpated. The onset of symptoms is usually sudden. The soleus and gastrocnemius test weak during weight bearing. Thompson's test weak during weight bearing. Thompson's test may be positive or negative. Tenderness if often more severe than that in complete rupture.

Roentgenographic Considerations. The lateral x-ray view of the normal ankle shows a lucent triangle of fatty tissue bounded below by the calcaneus, posteriorly by the smooth margins of the Achilles and anteriorly by the posterior tibial muscles. Upon tendon rupture, the smooth margin of the tendon becomes altered at the site of rupture as edema and hemorrhage occur within the tendon and the fatty triangle. Signs of fluid filling the triangle appear.

Thompson's Test. To detect a rupture of the Achilles tendon, place the patient in the prone position or have him kneel on a chair with his feet extended over the ede. Squeeze the middle third of the calf. If the Achilles tendon is ruptured, especially the soleus portion, the squeeze will not cause the normal plantar flexion response.

Simmond's Test. With the patient prone, the knee is flexed to a 90° angle and the foot is plantar flexed and then relaxed. The examiner grasps the upper calf strongly and squeezes the muscles against the tibia and fibula. A slight loss in plantar flexion is seen when the Achilles tendon is ruptured.

Achilles Tap Test. With the patient prone, flex the knee to a right angle and tap with a reflex hammer the Achilles tendon about 1 inch above its insertion into the calcaneus. If pain is induced or the normal plantar flexion reflex of the foot is absent, a rupture of the Achilles tendon should be suspected.

Management. Surgery presents the risk of complications but usually leads to a quicker return to activity (within 3–4 months) than conservative measures. An extensive postoperative rehabilitation program is necessary after casting. Also, tendinitis with healing and repair might precede an episode of complete rupture requiring prolonged casting or surgical repair. In cases of only a few torn fibers, complete immobilization is contra-indicated.

Ossification

In partial tendon tears, ossification may be found in the patellar tendon during roentgenography following hemorrhage. If joint dislocation has occurred, signs of ossification may be found in the soft tissues. After blunt trauma, the soft tissues may show evidence of heterotopic bone formation. Such ossification involves not only the muscle tissue but also occurs within the fascial planes. The typical picture is one of trauma, muscle pain and soreness, and hemorrhage into the soft tissues, with poorly defined ossification developing in 2–5 weeks.

Focal Stess Degeneration

A common site of central-tendon degeneration is at the midpoint between the musculotendinous junction and insertion of the Achilles tendon: the site of poorest blood supply in the tendon. Ischemia appears to be the triggering mechanism. Low-heeled shoes, heel-strike running events, training on hard surfaces, and severe training schedules are causative factors.

Signs and Symptoms. During the early stages, pain is only felt during early warmup and disappears with activity. Later, pain becomes persistent and increases in severity. The onset is gradual. Swelling is characteristic, and tenderness is severe. Somewhere in the range of motion, a painful point in the arc is manifested. Thompson's test is negative.

Management. Of the conservative measures, rest, ultrasound, interferential current, hydrotherapy, and heel padding offer temporary relief, but activity causes relapse. Injections are dangerous. Surgical procedures appear to be the best alternative, and most players are able to return to competitive activity in several weeks.

Tendinitis

Achilles tendinitis is a frequent finding in basketball. The onset of Achillodynia in tendinitis is insidious, and there is severe swelling, tenderness, crepitus, and disability. Thompson's test is negative. The cause can sometimes be traced to tape applied too tightly over the tendon.

Management. Conservative management is extremely long and frequently disappointing; thus surgical decompression is considered the treatment of choice if relief does not occur within 7–10 days. Some relief is obtained by rest, physiotherapy, and heel lifts. Postoperative disability rarely exceeds 6 weeks.

Peritendinitis

In acute peritendinitis, the onset is rapid, there is swelling and a little tenderness, crepitus may or may not be present, and Thompson's test is negative. Chronic peritendinitis presents a gradual onset, swelling may or may not be present, a thickened nontender paratendon is palpable, and Thompson's test is negative.

Management. Conservative management is usually successful unless there are associated fibrosis and strictures of the paratendon. Postoperative disability is about a month.

Tenosynovitis

Tenosynovitis of the Achilles' tendon often produces pain in the tendon area which is increased by use and sometimes associated with palpable crepitus. Other symptoms include pain on motion, tenderness, and a distinct limp. Treat as any inflammatory tendon reaction with emphasis on hydrotherapy and interferential current.

Dry Sheath

This disorder of unknown cause is the result of diminished lubricating fluid within the sheath of the Achilles tendon. Adhesions form binding the tendon to its sheath. Symptoms include a burning pain during and after strenuous activity, inability to raise the heel from the ground during weight bearing, tenderness, mild swelling, and restricted ankle motion. Crepitus is often present.

Management. During the acute stage, immobilization may be necessary. Contrast or whirlpool baths (108–110°F) at least twice daily, analgesic packs, strapping, and vitamin-mineral supplementation are helpful. Bilateral heel pads should be provided to reduce the strain on the tendons. Rehabilitation to full activity usually requires about 2 weeks.

Fractures and Dislocations

Displacement of lower tibia or fibula fracture is usually posteromedial due to the strong action of the gastrocnemius and soleus. Care must be taken not to mistake an incomplete fracture of the distal-medial tibia (Pott's fracture) for a severely inversion-sprained ankle. See Figure 27.2.

Hueter's Fracture Sign. Being relatively dense, bone readily transmits sound waves. Thus, if a fracture of a long bone is suspected (eg, the tibia), the examiner can use a stethoscope to auscultate 2–3 inches prox-

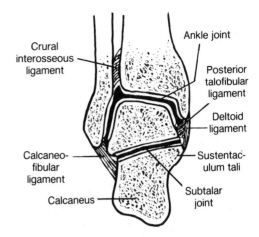

Figure 27.2. Coronal section through the ankle joint.

imal to the suspected site while the skin over the bone is tapped with a percussion hammer or a supported index finger 2–3 inches distal to the suspected site. If the percussion sounds are not transmitted in the involved bone, but are in the contralateral limb, a fracture line inhibiting the flow of the vibration is indicated. A variant of this test is to use a 512-c tuning fork rather than percussion. In addition, either procedure can be used effectively to judge the state of healing of a fractured long bone when roentgenography is either not available or ill-advised.

Lower Tibia Fractures

Inasmuch as the tibial epiphysis does not ossify until the early twenties, epiphyseal fractures are not uncommon in adolescent contact sports. Fatigue stress fractures are characterized by a dull gnawing pain following a run which increases in severity with time and weight bearing.

Lower Fibula Fractures

Most fibula injuries occur at its distal portion. Minor fractures are often missed as the symptomatic picture often resembles a bruise or mild sprain. As the fibula does not carry direct body weight, a player may continue activity long after fracture has occurred and complicate the original injury. Uncomplicated fractures rarely require more than support followed by progressive exercise unless the medial ligaments of the ankle or tibiofibular supports are ruptured.

Fatigue Fractures

With repeated, forceful contractions of leg muscles, lower leg stress fractures are sometimes seen as the result of tibia or fibula "wobble." These are commonly related to track and field injuries and can occur whenever a force exceeds the bone's structural strength. Humans are not the only ones affected by this disorder; greyhounds and racing horses also show frequent stress fractures within the limbs.

Signs and Symptoms. Progressive pain during physical activity is the typical symptom. An early sign is that of a linear periosteal reaction which rarely exceeds 1 cm and may present a local bony tenderness. However, bony tenderness is not common. In time, resorption of the fracture margin produces a lucent linear defect on roentgenography. Soft-tissue views and bone scanning are frequently necessary to determine a stress fracture.

Note: The clinical term stress fracture is a misnomer that is common in use. The term *fatigue* fracture is more accurate biomechanically as all fractures are the result of overstress.

Fatigue fractures of the legs are most always horizontal but occasionally are seen as longitudinal. The first roentgenographic signs are (1) a minute radiolucent tunneling of the cortex as a result of osteoclastic resorption, followed by cortical resorption in a fracture line of one cortex, and (2) a localized haze on the bone surface representing callus or periosteal new bone development. Within the endosteal bony surface, a line of condensation may be seen. Later, an abundant callus may be confused with a neoplasm.

Management. Most stress fractures do not require splinting or casting unless extensive or if the patient is unreliable in providing the necessary rest of the part.

Circulatory Disturbances

Intermittent Claudication

Intermittent claudication and cramps from insufficient circulation through the arteries of the legs may give rise to a sudden "giving way" of one or both legs during running or walking. Power returns after a short rest. In patients at rest, the frequent recurrence of painful cramps may be the only manifestation of the disorder. In other cases, there are various forms of paresthesia such as numbness, prickling, and "hot feet" at night. True claudication, however, is rare in sports. Obliteration of the dorsalis pedis (or larger arteries) by arteriosclerosis is sometimes found in the older patient, but there is reason to believe that local anemia due to vasomotor disturbance or other causes may produce similar cramps such as those seen in athletes after a hard run and in pregnancy. Rarely is Buerger's or Raynauld's syndrome found.

Varicose Veins

Varicose veins, with their eczema and ulcers, are the most common lesions of the lower leg. The soft, twisted, purplish eminences are easily recognized. Hardness in such a vein usually means thrombosis. Chronic ulcers of the lower leg, especially those in front, are usually due to varicose veins and the resulting malnutrition of the tissues. They leave a brown scar after healing.

Saphenous Tests. Palpate the greater saphenous vein close to the groin where it joins the femoral vein. Have the patient cough. A transmitted pulse will be felt if the major valve at this junction is incompetent. Then place your fingers over the largest mass of varicosities on the leg and tap the upper greater saphenous with the fingers or the other hand. Incompetent valves will be indicated if again an impulse is transmitted downward.

Edema

Lymphatic obstruction, venous disease, or acute arterial occlusion may result in ankle edema. Venous disease is the most common cause of pitting on pressure. Trauma or local disease is the usual cause for unilateral swelling. Unilateral edema may be due to thrombosis of a vein, pressure of tumors in the pelvis, or to inflammation. Bilateral edema of the legs is most often due to uncompensated heart lesions (primary or secondary from lung disease), lymphatic disorders, nephritis, cirrhotic liver, anemia, neuritis, varicose veins, obesity, flatfoot, and other causes of deficient local circulation. In some cases, no cause can be found (angioneurotic, essential, hereditary types).

Diagnosis depends on the history and the examination of the rest of the body. Edema is usually greatest in the front of the leg and in the back of the thigh. Tenderness in the lower legs frequently accompanies edema from any cause. It may also be due to neuritis, trichiniasis, or any local inflammation.

Circulatory Tests

Low back pain is one of the most common complaints to be heard in a chiropractic office. Because of this, Whiele points out the importance of recognizing associated problems of neurovascular stenosis in the large arteries of the leg due to L4–L5 irritation and differentiating them from other factors that can produce circulatory insufficiency. For example, thrombosis of the femoral artery can produce the same symptomatic picture as sciatic neuritis. Thus, diagnostic procedures might include, when indicated, plethysmography, unilateral/vertical and bilateral/horizontal blood pressure comparisons, Doppler ultrasound readings, and reactive hyperemia tests in addition to the clinical tests described below.

Homan's Sign. The patient is placed supine with the knees extended in a relaxed position. The examiner, facing the patient from the involved side, raises the involved leg, sharply dorsiflexes the ankle with one hand and firmly squeezes the calf with the other hand. If this induces a deep-seated pain in the calf, a strong indication of thrombophlebitis is present.

Buerger's Test. The patient is placed supine with the knees extended in a relaxed position, and the examiner lifts a leg with the knee extended so that the lower limb is flexed on the hip to about a 45° angle. The patient is then instructed to move the ankle up and down (dorsiflex and plantar flex the foot) for a minimum of 2 minutes. The limb is then lowered, the patient is asked to sit up, the legs are allowed to hang down loosely over the edge of the table, and the color of the exercised foot is noted. Positive signs of arterial insufficiency are found if (1) the skin of the foot blanches and the superficial veins collapse when the leg is in the raised position and/or (2) it takes more than 1 minute for the veins of the foot to fill and for the foot to turn a red-dish cyanotic color when the limb is lowered.

Claudication Test. If claudication is suspected, the patient is instructed to walk on a treadmill at a rate of 120 steps/minutes. If cramping, and sometimes a skin color change, occurs, the approximate level of the local lesion can be identified. The time span between the beginning of the test and the occurrence of symptoms is used to record the "claudication time," which is usually recorded in seconds.

Perthe's Tourniquet Test. This is an excellent test to use in differentiating the extent of superficial and deep lower limb varicosities. An elastic bandage is applied to the upper thigh of a standing patient sufficient to compress the long saphenous vein, and the patient is instructed to walk briskly around the room for approximately 2 minutes. The varicosities are then examined. This exercise with the thigh under pressure should cause the blood in the superficial (long saphenous) system to empty into the deep system via the communicating veins. Thus:

1. If the varicosities increase in their distention (become more prominent) and possibly become painful, it is an indication that the deep veins are obstructed and the valves of the communicating veins are incompetent.

2. If the superficial varicosities remain unchanged, the valves of both the long saphenous and communicating veins are incompetent.

3. If the superficial varicosities disappear, the valves of the long saphenous and the communicating veins are normal.

Pratt's Tourniquet Test. This variation of Perthe's test is used to evaluate the integrity of specific communicating veins. The patient is placed in the supine position with the knees extended position. The limb is raised to about 45° to empty the veins, and an elastic bandage is applied to the upper thigh sufficient to compress the long saphenous vein. A second elastic bandage is wrapped about the limb from the foot to the tourniquet on the thigh. The patient is then instructed to stand, and the examiner carefully observes the varicosities of the leg as the lower bandage is slowly unwrapped from above downward. The tourniquet on the thigh is left in place. As the lower bandage is untwined, the site of an incompetent communicating vein will be indicated by the appearance of a prominently bulging varicosity (blowout). When the first blowout is found, the spot is marked, and the upper bandage is extended to that point. Another bandage is then applied from that site downward, and the test is repeated again and again until all blowouts have been marked. Caution should be taken in this test because severe pain and swelling may arise in the calf if the deep veins are obstructed.

Moskowicz's Tourniquet Test. The patient is placed supine with the knees extended in a relaxed position. The straight limb is then elevated by the examiner to about 45°, an elastic bandage is wrapped around the limb in an overlapping fashion from the ankle to the midthigh, and the elevated limb is supported in this position for 5 minutes. At the end of this time, the examiner quickly untwirls the bandage from above downward and notes how rapidly the skin blushes when the obstruction to the collateral circulation has been removed. If the normal blush is absent or lags far behind the unbandaged area, something interfering with the collateral circulation is indicated (eg, an arteriovenous fistula).

Miscellaneous Pathologic Signs and Reflexes

Strumpell's Tibialis Sign. This test is often used to confirm a pathologic reflex suggesting spastic paralysis in the lower extremity. The patient is placed supine with the knees extended in a relaxed position. The examiner, standing to face the involved limb, lifts the patient's leg, flexes the knee, places his caudad hand against the distal posterior thigh, and grasps the patient's shin with his cephalad hand. The thigh is then flexed on the hip while simultaneously flexing the leg against the examiner's hand held near the popliteal space. If the foot briskly dorsiflexes (and sometimes adducts) on this maneuver, it is a positive sign of an upper motor neuron lesion.

Piotrowski's Sign. Percussion of the tibialis anticus muscle produces sharp dorsiflexion and supination of the foot. When this reflex is excessive, it signifies organic CNS disease.

Oppenheim's Spastic Sign. This reflex is met with in spastic conditions of the legs. With the patient prone, the sign is elicited by striking or goading the midline surface of the leg posteriorly from the upper posterior portion of the tibia downward, which causes contraction of the tibialis anticus, extensor hallucis longus, extensor digitorum communis, and, in some instances, also the peroneal muscle. It has Babinski implications.

Neri's Leg Sign. In organic hemiplegia, while the patient is in the supine position and the affected straight leg is lifted, the sign consists of spontaneous flexion of the knee.

INJURIES OF THE ANKLE

Except for a few sports such as rowing, kite flying, and auto racing, the base of an athlete's activity is provided by the soft tissues and osseous complex of the ankle and foot. Ankle injuries in sports are close in incidence to that of knee injuries. One study has shown that 50% of ankle injuries during all athletics at one college occurred in basketball. Soccer also presents a high incidence.

Various neurologic and orthopedic signs and tests relative to the ankle are listed in Table 27.2.

Table 27.2.
Review of Neurologic, Orthopedic, and Peripheral Vascular Maneuvers, Reflexes, Signs, or Tests Relative to the Ankle

Abadie's sign
Achilles reflex
Achilles tap test
Ankle tourniquet test
Chaddock's ankle reflex
Draw sign
Hoffa's sign
Lateral (eversion) stability test
Light touch/pain tests
Medial (inversion) stability test
Muscle strength grading
Range of motion tests
Repetitive heel raise test
Simmond's test
Talar slide test
Thompson's test
Tinel's foot sign

Bruises

Ankle bruises are usually bone bruises which readily respond to cold, elevation, a dressing, and an elastic ankle bandage or strap for 2–4 days. Resumed activity should be safeguarded with a protective pad for 2–3 weeks. The incidence of ankle contusions without sprain is highest in hockey from stick and puck blows.

Effects of Chronic Pronation

In-roll of the talocalcaneal articulation is not an uncommon condition, and it can show its effects high in the spine. A shin-splint syndrome often arises in the flexor group and often is isolated to the posterior tibial muscle. Many patients suffer from the effects of a unilateral or bilateral foot pronation problem, especially if they spend the greater part of the day on their feet. The most common cause of excessive pronation is foot-muscle fatigue. A weak foot is hypermobile.

Biomechanics

Abnormal pronation is characterized by the superior aspect of the calcaneus tilting and rolling toward the midline carrying the talus with it. This releases the navicular from its arthrodial articulation with the talus permitting it to roll toward the midline. As the navicular is the keystone of the medial longitudinal arch, its downward subluxation results in collapse of the arch and the beginning of a progressive distortion that may extend onto the occiput. When viewed from the rear, observation of the exposed Achilles tendon shows deviation with the inward tilting of the calcaneus. An associated tendon inflammation may be associated with abduction strain, characterized by motion restriction, pain, tenderness behind the medial malleolus, and crepitus on rare occasions.

As the inward tilting of the foot includes the talus which supports the tibia, unusual and downward tilting of the articulating surface of the talus causes an inward rotation of the tibia which extends onto the femur. This brings the greater trochanter forward and outward, stretching the piriformis muscle. The piriformis muscle inserts into the apex of the trochanter and is placed on a windlass-type stretch. The origin of the piriformis is at the anterolateral aspect of the S2–S4 segments. Thus, the sacrum may be pulled into a subluxated anterior and inferior position. In compensation to this, the gluteus maximus muscle contracts to resist the downward and forward pelvic tilt. Because this muscle finds its origin on the outer lip of the posterior third of the iliac crest, the innominate at its iliac portion is rotated posteriorly and thus produces a typical pelvic distortion. With the sacrum thus drawn into an anteroinferior position, the L5 vertebral body gravitates and rotates toward the low side according to Lovett's law and establishes the beginning of a structural scoliosis. Thus, the effects of pronation can be witnessed as high as the occiput.

Signs and Symptoms

The problem expresses fundamentally as an inward roll of one foot or both, with a resultant lengthening of the foot with an automatic stretching of the plantar muscles. This in itself produces many reflex patterns that evidence themselves as sciatic pain, numbness, tingling and various other paresthesias, all of reflex origin. But as the foot pronates and rolls inward, it also produces an inward roll of the talus, and this inward roll continues to have an inward torque on the tibia. Ordinarily, the fibula follows suit with the torque continuing through the knee joint, producing a sustained torque to the femur which then allows the lesser trochanter to move in a rotary fashion backwards and laterally, possibly causing a microavulsion of the trochanteric attachment of the iliopsoas muscle. Thus, if the psoas tests weak, a foot pronation problem is usually associated. The thigh abductors and neck flexors will usually test weak on the side of a weak iliopsoas, and a lower inner longitudinal arch will usually be found on the side of the weak iliopsoas. When the arch rolls inward (pronates), the tibia twists, the knee strains, the femur rotates, the pelvis tilts forward, and the curves of the spine are affected.

Associated foot and ankle signs include lateroinferior cuboid, medioinferior navicular, posterocalcaneal torque, internally rotated tibia, inferior tarsals, inferior 2nd–4th metatarsals, superior 1st and 5th metatarsals, lateral deviation of the Achilles tendon during weight bearing, and flattening of the longitudinal arch. A corn at the 2nd metatarsal head, a tailor's bunion on the lateral 5th metatarsal head, Haglund's deformity, and bunion are typical findings.

Insert an index finger under the inner longitudinal arch to a point midway under the foot and palpate the plantar fascia for tension. Rotate the foot to its outer border and the knee laterally, then repeat plantar palpation. Tenderness on pressure and "fiddle string" fascia that disappears when the foot is rotated to its outer border indicate pronation in an apparently normal foot.

Drop a plumbline from the center of each patella. Normally, the bob will be in the approximate midline of the ankle. In pronation, the bob will be near the medial malleolus. Remove the patient's shoes and inspect A-P and P-A foot posture and the degree of inward pronation or outward suppination.

To record the effects of foot pronation, measure the amount of knee rotation. Place a mark with a skin pencil in the middle of each patella and measure the distance between marks. Then roll feet to outer borders and measure the distance between patella

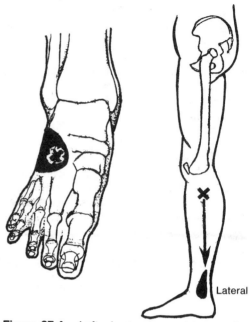

Figure 27.4. *Left*, short extensor trigger point; *X*, common site. *Blackened areas* indicate typical sites on referred pain. *Right*, peroneus longus trigger point.

marks: pronation causes inward rotation of the knees.

Strains

Most ankle strains will involve the peroneus or posterior tibial muscle units. Symptoms often arise a day or two after injury. Strains must be differentiated from sprain, referred trigger point pain (Fig. 27.4) and fatigue fractures.

Peronei Strain and Inflammation

The peronei tendons pass behind the lateral malleolus. They are best palpated during active eversion and plantar flexion. The peronei are the primary foot everters and help in plantar flexion. An aseptic tendon inflammation is often involved. If stenosis of the tunnel in which the tendons run occurs, the peroneal tubercle will feel tender and thick. Tenderness here also suggests bursitis or fracture of the styloid process in severe sprain.

When an associated peroneal tenosynovitis or tendovaginitis is associated with strain it is characterized by acute tenderness, pain, motion restriction, swelling of the sheath, a

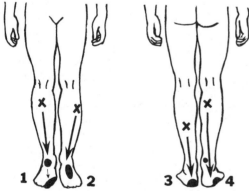

Figure 27.3. *1*, Tibialis anticus trigger point; *X*, common site. *Blackened areas* indicate typical sites of referred pain. This point refers pain chiefly to the front ankle and great toe. *2*, Extensor digitorum longus trigger point. This point refers pain more laterally in the ankle and to the dorsum of the foot in the area of the 4th metatarsal. Points *1* and *2* are common trigger areas in ankle pain. *3*, Soleus trigger point. *4*, Gastrocnemius trigger point.

probable squeaking crepitus or joint movement, and possible ecchymosis.

Management. Treatment is similar to that for an acute strain, with cold packs, rest, strapping or aircasting for 8–12 days, and graduated active exercises. Tendovaginitis is stubborn to manage and often requires referral for tendovaginotomy.

Peroneoextensor Spasm

Peroneoextensor spasm produces a spastic flat foot characterized by pain at the lower lateral leg and ankle, especially after cross-country runs. There is little or no area tenderness, but dorsiflexion and inversion are restricted. Spasm in eversion may become quite marked and may indicate an eversion subluxation.

Management. Management consists of muscle techniques, passive peroneal stretching, interferential current, high-volt therapy, and progressive mobilization.

Posterior Tibial Tendon Strain

While tendons of the peronei run behind the lateral malleolus, the tendon of the posterior tibial muscle passes behind the medial malleolus. The clinical picture is similar to that of peronei strain and inflammation—tenderness, sheath swelling, crepitus, possible ecchymosis.

Trigger Point Ankle Pain

Pain referred chiefly to the front of the ankle and big toe is frequently caused by a trigger point located in the upper anterolateral aspect of the leg in the tibialis anticus muscle. Firm sustained pressure at this trigger point sets off an aggravating ache. At other times, a trigger area just lateral to this located in the extensor digitorum longus muscle will refer pain more laterally in the ankle and to the dorsum of the foot in the area of the 4th metatarsal bone.

Management. If the area of pain is sprayed with a vapocoolant, the pain will be relieved only momentarily, but spraying over the trigger area may abolish the pain, the restricted motion, and deep tenderness in the reference zone for many hours, if not permanently.

Ankle Instability

Ankle instability results when inversion or eversion sprains stretch or rupture supporting ligaments. Always test and compare bilaterally. Screen tests for active range of motion can be made by toe walking to test plantar flexion and toe motion, heel walking to test dorsiflexion, lateral-sole walking to test inversion, and walking on the medial borders of the feet to test eversion. In testing passive subtalar inversion and eversion, stabilize the distal end of the tibia with one hand and firmly grip the heel with the active hand. Alternately invert and evert the heel. Pain during this maneuver suggests subtalar arthritis that is possibly from an old fracture.

Draw Sign

Tenderness along the course of the anterior talofibular ligament points to sprain damage. Tears in this ligament allow the talus to slide forward (subluxate) on the tibia. To test for instability and subluxation of the tibia and talus, place one hand on the anterior aspect of the sitting patient's lower tibia and grip the heel within your other palm (Fig. 27.5). When the calcaneus and talus are pulled anteriorly and the tibia is simultaneously pushed posteriorly, the anterior talofibular ligament should allow no forward movement of the talus on the tibia. The test is positive if the talus slides anteriorly from under cover of the ankle mortise. Sometimes the abnormal bone movement can be heard as well as felt during the maneuver.

Lateral or Medial Instability Tests

Gross lateral instability results when both the anterior talofibular and calcaneofibular ligaments are torn. To test lateral instability, stabilize the patient's leg and invert the heel back and forth, noting if the talus rocks loosely in the ankle mortise. Medial insta-

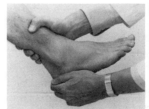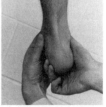

Figure 27.5. *Left*, position to elicit the anterior draw sign to evaluate the integrity of the anterior talofibular ligament. *Right*, position for testing passive foot eversion and inversion.

bility results from a tear or stretch of the deltoid ligament. To test medial instability, stabilize the patient's leg and evert the heel back and forth, noting any gapping at the ankle mortise.

Talar Slide Test

This test evaluates ankle joint play (translation) in the horizontal plane. With the patient in either the prone or supine position, the doctor stands to the side and faces the ankle to be tested. The examiner's cephalad hand grasps the patient's lower leg just above the malleoli and the caudad hand grasps the heel just below the malleoli. A pull is made with the upper hand on the lower leg while the lower hand pushes the heel horizontally. Then a push is made with the upper hand while the lower hand pushes the heel. Excessive lateral or medial motion with pain indicates ligamentous instability.

Sprains

As with knee sprain, ankle sprain produces a wide variety of damage depending upon which ligaments are stretched and the degree of tear. Isolated tears are rare, and many severe ruptures are associated with lower leg fracture.

The most common form of tarsotibial sprain is created by twisting the leg in varus; ie, inversion and internal rotation, especially when the foot is plantar flexed with the heel off the ground. This injures the talofibular bundle of the lateral ligament. Tears are usually at attachments, with or without avulsion, rather than at the middle of the ligament. Isolated tenderness is usually most acute over the anterior talofibular ligament or less often over the calcaneofibular ligament if stress occurs when the ankle is at a right angle. During inversion stress, we see a class-one lever amplifying the external force (five or six times) far above the resistance limit supplied by the bones and ligaments. See Figure 27.6.

Lateral sprain often produces an indirect lesser tenderness in the deltoid ligament area from impaction. After eversion sprain, this area will exhibit primary tenderness with secondary tenderness from impaction on the lateral aspect. Hyperextension sprain exhibits lateral, medial, and sometimes posterior tenderness and swelling.

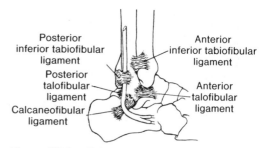

Figure 27.6. Schematic of major anterior and posterior ankle ligaments.

Incidence. According to several studies, capsular ankle sprain appears the most common injury within sports—especially basketball, occurring under the backboard while attempting to recover a rebounding ball. As the result of consistent quick stops and turns, tears of the capsule and the ligaments covering the back of the talonavicular joint are invariably involved. Nearly all participants in hang-gliding and parachuting present some degree of ankle injury as the result of poor landings. With the exception of contusions, ankle sprains and muscle tears near the ankle and knee are the most common injuries in lacrosse. Overlong shoe spikes and studs in football and other field sports render the ankle unstable and contribute to ankle sprain.

Signs and Symptoms of Inversion Sprain. The symptoms and local manifestations are mild to severe pain and swelling beneath the affected tendons and ligaments, tenderness, possible ecchymosis, hypermobile inversion, and spastic functional impairment. The lateral malleolus, talus, and cuboid will palpate as prominent. The talus is usually subluxated from the ankle mortise. In mild cases, only the lateral sulcus is filled with effusion. To support your diagnosis, check for draw sign, judge lateral and medial instability, and use Thompson's test. Acute traumatic arthritis of the ankle following severe sprain is produced by rupture or stretching of the ligaments of the joint by direct or indirect violence.

Signs and Symptoms of Eversion Sprain. Low fibula bone damage is more the rule than are isolated medial ligament tears because of the strength of the deltoid. If the inferior tibiofibular ligament tears, the fibula and tibia will separate at the ankle mortise. This widening produces instability leading to degenerative changes. Local manifestations include pain, tenderness, swelling, possible ecchymosis, eversion hypermobility, and inversion motion restrictions. See Figure 27.7.

Management. Poorly treated initial injuries invariably lead to chronic states. Good management requires time and patience. Structural alignment, cold water immersion, elevation, and pressure strapping should be applied as soon as possible after injury to prevent swelling. Strapping or aircasting should be made with slight eversion in lateral sprain or inversion in medial strain. After strapping over a protective underwrap, walking is encouraged, as functional use facilitates recovery. Keep in mind that the greater the support, the greater the atrophy. Pain relief is enhanced by placing a 2 × 2-inch gauze pad that is about ¼-inch thick within the longitudinal arch prior to taping. Double pads are necessary for heavy patients. During the acute hyperemic stage, positive galvanism, interferential current, high-volt therapy, mild ultrasound, rest, and possibly elevation are also indicated. An application of hyaluronidase is helpful to reduce tissue swelling and edema if used with iontophoresis. Swelling should subside in 36 hours.

After 72 hours, passive congestion may be managed by contrast baths, light massage, gentle passive manipulation, sinusoidal stimulation, heel lifts, and ultrasound. During the stage of consolidation, local moderate heat, moderate active exercise, bracing, moderate range of motion manipulation, and ultrasound are beneficial. In the stage of fibroblastic activity, deep heat, deep massage, vigorous active exercise, toe walking, inversion and eversion walking, negative galvanism, ultrasound, and active joint manipulation speed recovery and inhibit postinjury effects. Active rehabilitative exercises should not begin until walking gait is normal and painless. In preventive strapping, the anterior talofibular ligament which runs from the distal fibula to the talus is the most important ligament to protect for lateral stability, especially protecting the anterior limb of the deltoid after medial sprain. During rehabilitation, a lateral heel wedge is helpful in lateral instability; medial heel wedge, in medial instability. Vitamin C and manganese are helpful during care.

Vapocoolant Technique in Grade I Ankle Sprains. Place the patient supine with pillows under the knee and ankle. Spray the painful ankle area, and gently assist and resist the patient in ankle flexion-extension. As the pain shifts position, spray the affected area. Once relief has been obtained in flexion-extension, add inversion, eversion, and toe flexion-extension, spraying painful sites as necessary between movements. Have the patient attempt to walk, and spray the painful area if necessary. If possible, have the patient stand on his toes and bend forward with his heels on the floor. Once relief is obtained, correct any subluxations isolated, strap the ankle, and instruct the patient in home exercises, 1–2 minutes each half hour during the waking hours. Begin resistance, stretching, and weight-bearing exercises as soon as logical. These should include toe standing, soleus muscle stretching, and eversion standing.

The Gibney Taping Method. This is one of the more time-consuming but stable methods. It also allows for swelling without constriction. The foot and leg are shaved and the foot is held at a right angle to the leg while the dressing is being applied. A

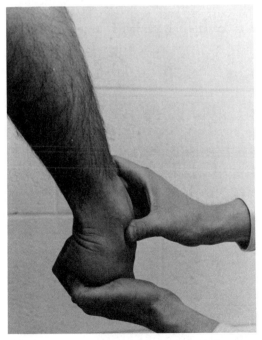

Figure 27.7. Palpating the deltoid ligament area.

strip of 1½- or 2-inch-wide adhesive plaster is placed against the outer aspect of the leg, passed downward over the outer malleolus, under the heel, making firm upward pressure against the arch by traction as the remainder of the strip is applied to the inner aspect of the leg. A second strip is placed at a right angle to the first, beginning on the outer aspect of the foot over the cuboid bone, passing on the medial side of the foot over the internal cuneiform bone. Successive strips are placed alternately about the leg and foot until the ankle is encased. Semicircular strips of tape are used about the anterior foot and leg to retain the dressing.

Subluxations

Lateral Talus Subluxation

Characterisitics associated with this subluxation are inversion ankle sprain, excessive pronation, pain anterior to lateral malleolus, and anterior talofibular ligament tenderness.

Adjustment. The patient is placed supine. Sit at the foot of the table, facing the patient. Place the third finger of your medial contact hand over the anterolateral margin of the talus with your thumb on the plantar surface. Your lateral stabilizing hand supports the heel. Apply traction with your stabilizing hand to separate the calcaneus from the talus while simultaneously making a lateral to medial torque adjustment towards yourself. Follow correction by evaluating the integrity of the muscles involved in excessive pronation: tibialis posterior and anterior, peroneus longus, flexors digitorum longus and hallucis longus, abductor hallucis, soleus, gastrocnemius, and intrinsic foot muscles.

Alternative Adjustment Procedure. The doctor-patient position is the same as above. Internally rotate the patient's leg, and make a double-thumb contact on the lateroanterior aspect of the talus. Your lateral hand grips the calcaneus, while your medial hand grasps the anterior surface of the tarsals. Apply pressure with your double-thumb contact, slightly invert the foot, apply traction, and simultaneously make a short, sharp pull towards yourself.

Medial-Inferior Talus Subluxation

This subluxation is often found in association with eversion ankle sprain exhibiting tenderness at the deltoid ligament.

Adjustment. This is essentially the opposite of the adjustment for a lateral talus. The patient is placed supine. Sit at the foot of the table, facing the patient. Place the third finger of your lateral contact hand over the anteromedial aspect of the talus with your thumb on the plantar surface. Your stabilizing hand supports the heel (Fig. 27.8). Apply traction with your stabilizing hand to separate the calcaneus from the talus while simultaneously making a medial-to-lateral torque adjustment towards yourself. Follow correction by evaluating the integrity of the tibialis anterior and posterior.

Anterior Talus Subluxation

Indications include pain and tenderness at the anterior aspect of the ankle, inversion sprain that occurs with plantar flexion, exostosis of the dorsal talonavicular articulation, and excessive pronation.

Adjustment. The patient is placed supine. Sit at the foot of the table, and face the patient. Interlock fingers across the anterior ankle with thumbs placed on the plantar surface and your elbows moderately flexed. The third fingers should make spe-

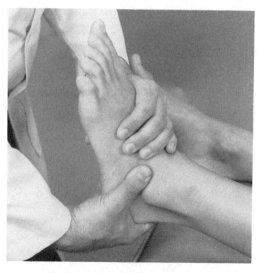

Figure 27.8.   Position for adjusting medial-inferior talus.

cific contact over the anterior aspect of the talus. Apply traction to separate the calcaneus and talus while simultaneously snapping your wrists and elbows inferiorly in a scooping fashion to move the talus from the anterior to the posterior. Evaluate the integrity of the tibialis anterior and extensor digitorum longus.

Fractures and Dislocations

The patterns of ankle injuries can be classified according to direction of primary and secondary forces such as external rotation, abduction, adduction, and vertical compression.

External Rotation Injuries

The most common mechanism involved in ankle injury is that of external rotation plus abduction. The classic fracture of this type is an oblique fibular line directed from the anterior-inferior to the posterior-superior aspect which is frequently comminuted along the posterior cortex. Foot pronation is the usual mechanism, associated with a deltoid tear. The interosseous ligaments are usually spared if the foot is in supination rather than pronation. An oblique transverse fracture of the medial malleous at or beneath the tibial articular surface may occur, with fragments displaced inferiorly by the pull of the deltoid ligament and tearing of the anterior tibiofibular ligament. A small posterior malleolar fracture may result from the rotating fibula.

Abduction and Adduction Injuries

An abduction fibula fracture is typically oblique, short, often with comminution of the lateral cortex. As external rotation injuries, abduction injuries produce transverse malleolar fractures or deltoid tears. This fibula fracture usually occurs below or within the syndesmosis. It may occur above the syndesmosis if it ruptures. When external rotation is a secondary force added to abduction, the fracture is usually higher on the fibula and/or more oblique. In abduction injuries, the lateral fibular cortex may be comminuted, small dorsal tibial and fibular avulsions may be noted, and diastasis is more common because the syndesmosis is ruptured. A horizontal fracture of the medial malleolus or torn deltoid, a high fibula fracture, and a complete rupture of the syndesmosis (called a Dupruytren fracture-dislocation) is an unstable injury resulting from abduction and lateral rotation.

Adduction ankle injuries frequently result in distal fibular horizontal fractures at or below the articular surface. Frequently associated is a vertical fracture of the medial malleolus projecting above the articular surface that is often related with a fracture of the lateral aspect of the talar dome. Diastasis is not associated with adduction injuries, but post–traumatic arthritis may result from comminution of the articular surface. Fractures to the posterior margin are not common.

Vertical Compression Injuries

Vertical compression injuries are subdivided by Dalinka into posterior marginal fractures, anterior marginal fractures, and supramalleolar fractures.

Posterior Marginal Fractures. These types of fractures may occur (1) with significant vertical compression of the articular margin or (2) without vertical compression. External rotation injuries, with or without an abduction factor, may produce small posterior marginal fractures. Vertical compression with external rotation force is more likely to produce large fragments. When the posterior articular fragment is large, the incidence of posttraumatic arthritis and chronic instability is high. Posterior marginal fractures seldom occur as isolated injuries, thus the proximal fibula must also receive careful evaluation. Rips of the anterior tibiofibular ligament are frequently associated.

Anterior Marginal Fractures. This type of fracture, frequently isolated, may be comminuted. It usually occurs in the dorsiflexed foot.

Supramalleolar Fractures. This fracture, invariably associated with fracture of the fibula, is of the distal 4 cm of the tibia above the ankle (Malgaine fracture). It is typically open, severely comminuted, and related to high-impact forces in the direction of axial compression.

Roentgenologic Considerations

Lateral, A-P, and oblique x-ray views are standard for evaluation of a possible ankle fracture, and sometimes tomography or stress views during inversion and eversion are required.

Severe Ankle Injuries in Children

The area of greatest weakness in children during ankle trauma is at the growth plate. Epiphyseal separations are more common than fractures, as the ligaments attach to the epiphysis. The Salter and Harris classification is widely applied to ankle injuries in childhood.

Type I. Fractures occurs through the zone of provisional calcification where the entire epiphysis may be separated or the growth plate widened. Although views may appear normal, the periosteum may be either intact or torn on one surface. Swelling and tenderness are frequent. The mechanism is usually one of inversion or abduction force. This type of injury is uncommon to the tibia, but common to the fibula. Because the germinal layer is intact, prognosis is excellent. Diagnosis is confirmed in 2 weeks after injury by noting periosteal new bone formation.

Type II. Epiphyseal separation plus a small metaphyseal fragment (Thurston-Holland sign) is seen. Plantar flexion and eversion result in fracture produced by lateral displacement. The periosteum is intact on the side of the metaphyseal fragment, and ischemia of the foot may be noted if the fracture is severely displaced. With this tibial injury, a green-stick fibula fracture is frequently associated. Prognosis is excellent as the germinal layer remains with the epiphysis and the separation is through the zone of provisional calcification.

Type III. An intra-articular epiphyseal fracture is seen at the lateral aspect of the tibial epiphysis. The mechanism is one of lateral rotation or shearing injury (Tillaux fracture). The lateral part of the tibial epiphysis is attached to the fibular metaphysis by the anterior tibiofibular ligament, and it is the pull of this ligament which avulses the lateral or anterolateral part of the tibial epiphysis. The medial part of the tibial epiphysis fuses at 13–14 years. There is usually little or no displacement. In spite of damage to the growth plate, prognosis is good if growth has ceased.

Type IV. This is a rare fracture across the epiphysis and the growth plate with a small metaphyseal fragment. Premature growth cessation in the fracture area may result.

Type V. This is a rare compression injury of the growth plate, usually medially, that does not exhibit abnormality in the ossified epiphysis. Premature growth cessation in the fracture area results.

Severe Ankle Injuries in Adults

Ankle fractures are frequently associated with severe ligament injury. One report states that rupture of one or more syndesmotic ligaments occurs in more than 90% of malleolar fractures. Ligamentous injury is always indicated in displaced malleolar fractures. One of the more common fracture sites occurs when the talus is displaced in the ankle mortise, shifting the talus and fibula laterally. When this happens, a slight widening of the distal interosseous space between the tibia and fibula (indicating interosseous membrane rupture) will be noted.

Fractures of the calcaneus are the most frequent. They usually result from falls where the victim leads stiff legged on his heels. Fracture of the calcaneus may be obvious with a widely separated fracture line and grossly disturbed positioning of fragments or it may be quite discrete with little obvious change visible. Frequently, normal structure is disturbed consequent to crushing of the spongy bone and deformity of outline. The survey should include the posterior halves of both heels. In later views, the fracture line is seldom seen. These injuries are frequently accompanied by compression fractures in the lumbar or lower thoracic regions from force traveling up the legs to the spine. Thus, it is always a good rule to x-ray the thoracolumbar region when crushing fractures of the heel are found.

For the purpose of accurate diagnosis, the utilization of *Boehler's angle* is recommended (Fig. 27.9).

Fracture of the talus and cuboid are next in frequency to those of the calcaneus. Bilateral films are helpful to rule out a tri-

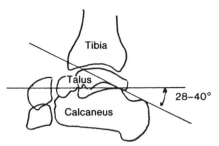

Figure 27.9. Boehler's angle. For the normal calcaneus, a line drawn from the posterosuperior margin of the talocalcaneal joint through the posterosuperior margin of the calcaneous makes an angle of about 35–40° with a second line drawn from the posterosuperior margin of the talocalcaneal joint to the superior articular margin of the calcaneocuboid joint. Boehler's angle of less than 28° is definitely abnormal and indicates poor position from a functional standpoint.

gonum, the posterior extension of the talus occasionally occurring as a separate bone. Another anatomic variation which sometimes leads to interpretative error is the presence of a separate ossification center at the base of the fifth metatarsal which is usually bilateral.

Fractures also commonly occur in the posterior or midportion of the talus. This area may be the site of avascular necrosis, viewed as a lucent crescent under the articular margin of the talus. In advanced cases, the superior portion of the talus may show collapse of its articular margins. This is best observed on the A-P view as the overlapping malleoli cloud the picture in the lateral position. Care must be taken to not confuse a sharp or rough-edged fracture fragment at the posterior talus with a rounded-edged accessory ossicle (os trigonum). Fractures secondary to impact of the talus are oblique and frequently comminuted, while those secondary to ligamentous avulsion are horizontal. The obliquity of the fracture line is determined by the direction of force. It should be kept in mind that as little as 1 mm of lateral displacement reduces the area of tibial-talar contact by 42%.

Gait Clues

During the stance phase, note heel strike, foot flat, midstance, and toe push-off of each extremity. When the foot slaps down sharply after heel strike, weak dorsiflexors

should be suspect. On the other hand, the fused ankles will prevent a midstance flat foot. Failure to hyperextend the foot during push-off is a sign of arthrosis. A flat-footed calcaneal gait during push-off is symptomatic of weak gastrocnemius, soleus, and flexor hallucis longis muscles.

During the swing phase, note acceleration, midswing, and deceleration of each extremity. If the hip is flexed excessively to bend the knee and thus prevent the toe from scrapping the floor as in a steppage gait, weak ankle dorsiflexors are the usual cause. The foot will have trouble clearing the floor if the ankle dorsiflexors are weak or the knee is unable to flex properly.

Selected Disorders of the Ankle

The pulse of the posterior tibial artery is often difficult to locate, even when the ankle is relaxed. This artery lies between the tendons of the flexor digitorum longus and the flexor hallucis longus muscles. If the pulse is noted, it should be compared bilaterally. The tibial nerve follows the course of the posterior tibial artery and is located just behind and lateral to the artery. A ligament binds the neurovascular bundle to the tibia creating the tarsal tunnel which has the same implications as the carpal tunnel in the wrist.

Tarsal Tunnel Syndrome

This is a nerve compression syndrome of the neurovascular bundle under the medial malleolus. The disorder is characterized by burning sensations of the toes and plantar surface. Pain is often referred along the posterior tibial nerve as high as the buttocks. Deep palpation posterior to the medial malleolus initiates or aggravates pain in the sensory distribution of the nerve. When the neurovascular bundle is percussed, a positive Tinnel's sign is elicited with radiating pain. In the chronic stage, claw toes develop which restrict extension.

Tinel's Foot Sign. With the patient prone, flex the knee to a right angle and tap, with a reflex hammer, the tibial nerve as it passes just behind the medial malleolus. If paresthesiae arise that radiate to the foot, a tarsal tunnel syndrome is suggested.

Ankle Tourniquet Test. The patient is placed supine in a relaxed position, a sphygmomanometer cuff is wrapped around the ankle of the affected side, and the cuff is inflated to just above the systolic level and maintained for 90 seconds. An exacerbation of pain in the ankle or foot is indicative of tarsal tunnel syndrome.

Management. The cause of the compression must be found. This may be traced to the effects of chronic subluxation, scar and adhesion formation, tenosynovitis, venous engorgement, valgus deformity of the foot, etc. Recurrent trauma is usually involved. If symptoms fail to respond to conservative care, referral to exploratory surgery is indicated.

Spurs

Two common posttraumatic abnormalities are talonavicular spurs and narrowing of the subtalar joint. These are most common from chronic stress to the talonavicular ligament in sports requiring constant speed, jumping, and rapid changes in direction such as seen in basketball, tennis, soccer, and field hockey.

Bowler's Spurs. Degenerative changes or fracture may result in spur formation of the posterior talus that may irritate the posterior margin of the tibia's inferior articular surface. Once formed, the spur becomes constantly irritated by forced ankle flexion. Conservative care is often frustrating when activity is continued. Deep heat, interferential current, ultrasound, and graduated exercises bring the best results, but referral for surgery to remove spurs or loose bodies may be required. Progression into osteoarthrosis is a common complication.

Football Ankle. This disorder consists of a traumatic osteitis that is sometimes confused with chronic sprain. There is general ankle pain, minimal swelling, and soreness which is aggravated by kicking the ball. Roentgenography shows new bone formation on the margins of the inferior articular surface of the tibia, but the joint surfaces are not involved as in osteoarthrosis. Conservative care incorporating rest, physiotherapy, and graduated active exercises will usually suffice. If not, the spurs must be removed surgically.

INJURIES OF THE FOOT

The foot is caught between forces from both above and below. Even minor traumatic disturbances can greatly inhibit optimal athletic performance. In addition, one study has shown that while 99% of all feet are normal at birth, 8% develop troubles by the first year of age, 41% at age 5, and 80% by age 20.

During running on a level surface, the force on the support foot is about three times body weight. This increases to four times body weight during downhill runs. Added to this stress is the effect of unyielding surfaces.

The patellar tendon reflex tests the integrity of the femoral nerve and the L2–L4 segments, while the Achilles tendon reflex reflects the function of the tibial nerve and the L4–S1 pathways. Various neurologic and orthopedic signs and tests relative to the foot are listed in Table 27.3.

Table 27.3.
Review of Neurologic, Orthopedic, and Peripheral Vascular Maneuvers, Reflexes, Signs, or Tests Relative to the Foot

Achilles reflex
Abadie's sign
Ankle tourniquet test
Babinski's plantar sign
Chaddocks's ankle sign
Crossed extension sign
Drawer sign
Duchenne's test
Gonda's sign
Gordon's toe sign
Heel walk test
Hirschberg's sign
Hoffa's sign
Light touch/pain tests
Mendel-Bechterew's sign
Morton's test
Muscle strength grading
Neuroma squeeze test
Oppenheim's spastic sign
Oppenheim's hemiplegic sign
Patellar reflex
Piotrowski's reflex
Plantar tension test
Range of motion tests
Rossolimo's sign
Schaeffer's sign
Strunsky's test
Thompson's test
Tinel's foot sign
Toe walk test

Postural Foot Alterations

The foot does not necessarily have to be painful to be the cause of postural imbalance and the resulting nerve and muscular tensions in other parts of the body. It is also well to keep in mind that a painful foot results in a protective posture and gait that has gross biomechanical implications.

Frequently, a progressive distortion begins in the foot and moves upward or is reflected into the foot from above. Weight-bearing distortions in time may produce such symptoms as generalized fatigue, dull leg and knee aches, and back pain at any vertebral level. To show the relationship between foot and pelvic mechanics, palpate the greater trochanters while rolling the feet medially and laterally. Femur rotation can be felt with minimal foot rotation.

Postural foot alterations produce and maintain far-reaching effects both in spinal and pelvic distortions as well as distant somatic or visceral disturbances. When these changes are overlooked, symptoms referred to other parts of the body continue because their cause, being in the feet, has failed to be properly diagnosed and removed.

Flat Arch

Often the feet of the same patient may vary to an amazing degree. One foot may have a good arch and be in a straight-line position while the other foot is flat and toed-out. Many times the patient with an apparent short leg has a greater pronation or inward roll on that leg, and the arch may be lessened.

"Flatfoot" is a breaking down or weakening of the normal arch of the foot. The cause may be congenital, atrophic, traumatic, or from obesity or ill-fitting shoes. There may or may not be changes in the sole-print. There may be pain and tenderness near the attachment of the ligaments and often higher up on the leg, but many cases appear symptomless. Some track stars present completely flat arches without any discomfort.

Signs and Symptoms. A convex medial border of the foot is a sign of an extremely flat arch. Check for foot pronation which may be associated with a fallen arch but is a separate deviation. Note the existence of hammer toes or marked deviation of the large toe toward the midline of the foot (hallux valgus). In a flat foot, the head of the talus drops down and medially from under the navicular and stretches the tibialis posterior and spring ligament which obliterates the longitudinal arch and causes a callous to form under the talar head. There is usually a pronated gait, joint stiffness, loss of spring in the step, disability during gait, excessive eversion during weight-bearing, and peroneal muscle spasm. The pain may be local in the arch or extend to the medial malleolus, knee, hip, or lumbar area.

Supports. A longitudinal arch that is absent in both the standing and nonweight-bearing position is rigid and may be aggravated by an arch support. A longitudinal arch that is absent in the weight-bearing position but present in the nonweight-bearing position may be aided by longitudinal arch supports. The human foot can be held up in an arched position only by the power of the muscles acting coordinately the instant weight is borne. This is anticipating that there is nothing to hinder the component bones from taking their normal position and that the Achilles tendon is not short.

Toe-in

Excessive toeing-in, especially in children, may be the result of excessive internal rotation of the tibia caused by a fixed point at either end of the tibia. Common points of fixation are at the malleoli in the ankle or the tibial tubercle below the knee. The ankle mortise normally faces 15° externally; but in internal tibial torsion, the ankle mortise faces anteriorly or internally.

Bruises and Wounds

Contusions and Abrasions. Most foot contusions can be traced to cleat wounds or bone bruises. A blow to the lateral ankle occasionally dislocates the peronei tendons anteriorly from their normal position behind the malleolus.

Bone Bruises. A bone bruise affecting the 2nd or 3rd metatarsal head, and sometimes the transverse arch, is referred to as a "stone bruise." It is most common in track and the result of running fullweight onto some small, hard object without adequate shoe support.

Puncture Wounds. A puncture wound

of the sole of the foot presents a special problem. In spite of proper care, some may develop cellulitis, osteomyelitis or arthritis of the foot. Upon the first signs, surgical referral should be made for debridement and antibiotics.

The Heel

Palpate the dome of the calcaneus from above plantarward. Examine the area of the medial tubercle lying on the medial plantar surface of the calcaneus and check for spurs in adults or signs of epiphysitis in children.

Hoffa's Sign. The patient is placed prone with the relaxed feet and ankles hanging over the edge of the table. A positive sign of an avulsion fracture of the calcaneus is found if the examiner by deep palpation finds that (1) the Achilles tendon is lax, (2) relaxed dorsiflexion is greater, and, possibly, (3) a bone fragment is felt behind either malleolus on the involved side.

Bruises

Heel bruises are seen affecting the plantar surface of the os calcis. This is often seen in track where the shoes are often heelless, flexible, and ultrathin (eg, long-distance runners, jumpers, hurdlers). Prolonged stress from heavy heel landings displaces the fat pad and causes rupture of the fibrous septa under the calcaneus. The area will be tender and often feel thick and boggy.

Management. Initial treatment must be quick to minimize bleeding and swelling through cold, compression, elevation, and rest. Padding, often specially designed, should be worn as long as tenderness persists. During recovery, mobilization, local heat, ultrasound, and massage may be applied to relieve related soreness. Heel cups are helpful in prevention and during healing. Chronic cases, often leading to spurs, usually require surgical excision of new bone, necrotic fibers, and granulations.

Bursitis

Palpate the area of the retrocalcaneal bursa located between the anterior surface of the Achilles tendon and the top of the heel. Lift the skin away from the tendon with one hand while you palpate anterior to the tendon. Then check the calcaneal bursa situated between the insertion of

Achilles tendon and the skin. Both of these bursae are subject to inflammation from pressure or friction from poorly fitting shoes, especially football shoes with their heavy counters. Care must be taken not to confuse heel bursitis with avulsion of the Achilles insertion.

Management. Treat as any bursitis, with initial emphasis on cryotherapy. During nonactivity, heelless sandals or slippers are recommended. During activity, low-cut shoes and heel padding throughout the counter area are recommended to avoid recurrent swelling.

Spurs

Soccer players especially present chronic ankle complaints, spurs, and degenerative changes as a result of kicking the ball with the dorsum of the foot. The activity of fast running with sudden stops, quick changes of position, and jumping account for chronic ankle and foot stress. About a third of the time in professional basketball players, roentgenography shows bony spurs of the anterior or dorsal talus. Trauma is but one of the causes; focal infections, metabolic disturbances, and contracted plantar fascia may be involved.

A heel spur usually forms at the inferomedial aspect of the calcaneus from chronic traction of the plantar fascia upon calcaneal periosteum (Fig. 27.10). The symptomatic picture presents a distinct limp, constant pain only during weight bearing, tenderness increased in dorsiflexion, and mild swelling along the medial aspect of the os calcis or plantar fascia attachments at the calcaneal tuberosity.

Management. Minor conditions can be aided by heel pads any taping or orthotic procedure that supports the arches of the foot.

Plantar Strain and Fascitis

In palpating the plantar surface of the foot, the plantar aponeurosis should feel smooth, without areas of tenderness. These strong bands of fascia have the origin at the medial tubercle of the calcaneus, fan across the sole, and insert near the metatarsal heads. See Figure 27.11. True plantar fascitis is rare in sports, but when it occurs, it is often confused with sprain of the spring

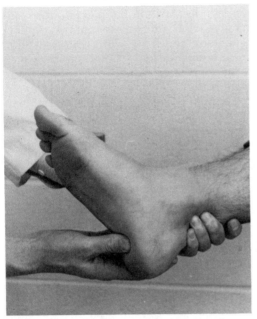

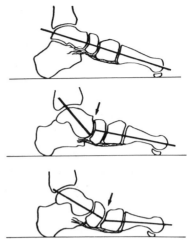

Figure 27.12. *Top diagram*, the normal longitudinal arch. *Middle diagram*, flattened arch due to talonavicular subluxation. *Bottom diagram*, flattened arch due to naviculocuneiform subluxation.

Figure 27.10. Seeking signs of a heel spur that may affect the heel-strike phase of gait.

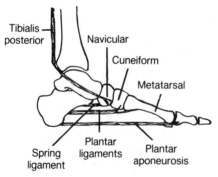

Figure 27.11. Schematic showing the major structures responsible for maintaining the longitudinal arch of the foot.

ligaments in the arch. See Figure 27.12. It is usually the result of chronic pronation or fascial tears from dorsiflexion overstress or it may be associated with calcaneal stress fractures. The cause can usually be attributed to chronic pronation, landing hard on the ball of the foot, or injury during quick running starts or stops.

Signs and Symptoms. There is pain upon running due to plantarfascial stretch with tenderness found just distal to the calcaneal tubercles. Palpable stiff cords or nodules within the fascia suggest plantar fascia spasm or Duputyren's contactures tender under deep pressure or plantar warts

tender to pinching. A slight degree of swelling may be palpable. Tight plantarfascia raises the longitudinal arch. Callosites, like contractures, are tender to pressure but not to pinching. In acute cases, a slight degree of ecchymosis and severe tenderness may be exhibited at attachments, especially at the heel. Early roentgenograms are negative, but calcification may appear on later films.

Plantar Tension Test. The patient is placed supine and the involved foot and toes are dorsiflexed so that the plantar fascia is tensed. If pain occurs or if bead-like swellings and irregularities are found as the examiner deeply runs his thumb vertically along the plantar surface, plantar fasciitis is suggested.

Management. Check carefully for possible cuboid or navicular subluxation. Adjunctive care consists of cold packs, deep massage, trigger point therapy, and ultrasonics. A temporary longitudinal arch support (or taping) and crutches are helpful during initial healing. Chronic low arches do not appear to be a precipitating factor.

Anterior Compartment Syndrome

Tissues of the anterior compartment should normally feel soft and yielding; tautness suggests pathology (eg, anterior compartment syndrome). The sinus tarsi area is often involved in ankle sprains wherein its normal concavity is swollen and tender (see Fig. 27.13). Deep tenderness suggests arthritis, myositis, fracture, or spastic-foot syndrome.

The pulse of the dorsal pedal artery can be felt between the extensor hallucis longus and extensor digitorum longus tendons of the dorsum of the foot. Being surrounded by bone, tendons, and fascia, it has difficulty in expanding and often leads to swelling within the anterior compartment that progresses to necrosis of vessels, muscles, and nerves creating foot-drop or an anterior compartment syndrome.

Sprains

Rearfoot Sprains. These are usually chronic in nature and characterized by progressive pain and minimal swelling in the rear half of the foot during activity. Talar subluxations and restrictions are often associated. In some cases, the cause will be traced to a low-grade tarsal synovitis from poor foot support on hard ground during strenuous activity.

Calcaneocuboid Sprain. This is usually the result of forceful internal rotation of the foot on the talonavicular joint when the foot is inverted. There is immediate severe pain, swelling over the calcaneocuboid area, and great disability.

Spring Ligament Sprain. Overstress of the plantar calcaneonavicular ligament is often associated with navicular subluxation. Symptoms of medial aching pain and tenderness deep within the plantar arch commonly arise after cross-country running when soft shoes are worn. Differentiation must be made from plantar fasciitis, which is more posterior and usually of a more acute nature.

Forefoot Sprains. Distal ache with tenderness under the 2nd and 3rd metatarsal heads is often the result of postural stress (see Fig. 27.14). As a consequence of severe eversion or inversion strain, avulsion of the insertion of the tibialis posterior may feature acute styloid tenderness.

Management. Correct any subluxations isolated and apply general sprain management with emphasis on rest, contrast baths, and ultrasound. During rehabilitation, arch strapping, passive mobilization of the entire foot, intrinsic exercises, sole padding, and improved foot support are helpful.

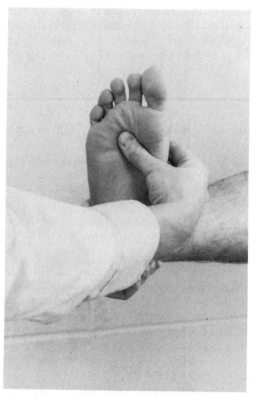

Figure 27.14. Palpation of the metarsal heads with the thumb on the plantar surface and the forefinger on the dorsal surface of the foot. Each joint is palpated individually. Morton's neuroma is occasionally located, especially between the 3rd and 4th metatarsal heads.

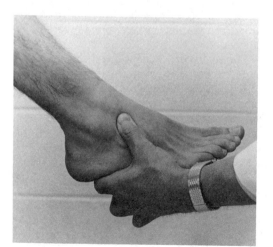

Figure 27.13. Palpation of the sinus tarsi.

Metatarsalgia

Morton's syndrome (metatarsalgia) exhibits pain at a small spot near the proximal end of one of the three outer toes. It is especially debilitating in track and almost always associated with compression of the foot by tight shoes resulting in pinching of the external plantar nerves between the metatarsal bones. The syndrome triad consists of (1) a 1st metatarsal bone that is shorter than the 2nd, (2) hypermobility at the naviculocuneiform and medial- and inter-cuneiform articulations, and (3) posteriorly displaced sesamoids. Differentiation must be made from postural strains, neuroma, march fractures, subluxations, exostoses, and tendon avulsions. See Figure 27.15.

Signs and Symptoms. There are toe pains, foot fatigue, and pronation complaints that are often associated with plantar callous patterns, bunion, corns, and inter-metatarsal neuroma. The sesamoids are displaced posteriorly, there is hypertrophy of the 2nd metatarsal joint, the foot is pronated and the arch flattened, and there is abnormal weight balance and distribution.

Strunsky's Test. This test is designed essentially for the recognition of lesions of the metatarsal arch. Under normal conditions when the toes are grasped and quickly flexed, the procedure is painless. Pain results if there is any inflammatory lesion of the metatarsal arch.

Morton's Test. In metatarsalgia, transverse pressure across the heads of the metatarsals causes a sharp pain, especially between the 2nd and 3rd metatarsal.

Management. Adjunctive care includes joint mobilization, ultrasound, padding beneath the tongue of the shoe, and transverse arch support. A metatarsal crescent can be applied to the sole of the shoe or a felt pad placed just behind the plantar metatarsal heads involved. In either case, the object is to slightly lift the stress joints during weight bearing. The player should be advised to lace the foreshoe loosely. Graduated tiptoe walking and walking on the lateral edge of the foot are most helpful during rehabilitation. Poorly responding cases may require referral for cortisone and anesthetic injections.

Plantar Neuroma. A rare cause of met-

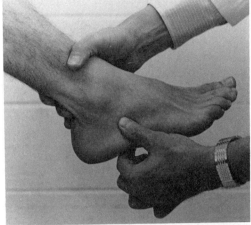

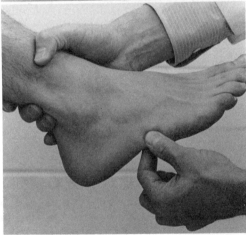

Figure 27.15. *Top*, palpation of the peroneus longus and brevis muscle tendons as they cross the peroneal tubercle. *Bottom*, palpation of the styloid process of the 5th metatarsal.

atarsalgia is Morton's neuroma—painful round "beads" found between the heads of the 1st through 4th metatarsals, especially between the 3rd and 4th. They are thought to be the effect of excessive foot rolling where the plantar nerve is chronically impinged on taut fascia or bone and hypertrophy of the nerve sheath develops. There is an accompanying digital artery disorder. The shooting distal pain and sometimes numbness are severe but quickly relieved when the shoeless foot is rested. Roentgenographs are negative. The disorder is rare in athletics but must be differentiated from postural strains and tendon avulsions that produce forefoot pain and plantar tenderness (see Fig. 27.14).

Neuroma Squeeze Test. If needle-like shooting pains occur when the forefoot is slowly squeezed, the probability of neuroma should be considered.

Exostoses. Bony overgrowth rarely forms at the head of a metatarsal, especially the 1st metatarsal. Treatment is usually by exostectomy. However, what may appear to be an overgrowth during palpation (a knuckle-like prominence) is actually a metatarso-cuneiform subluxation when demonstrated by roentgenography.

Subluxations

Subluxations of the cuboid are one of the most frequent subluxations found and frequently involved in a wide variety of reflex manifestations. William Locke, MD, of Ontario, Canada built a world-wide reputation in the 1930s adjusting this articulation especially.

Lateral Cuboid Subluxation

This subluxation is usually associated with inversion sprain, lateral longitudinal arch pain and tenderness, and excessive pronation.

Adjustment. Place the patient supine, stand at the foot of the table centered to the involved limb, and face the patient. Grasp the anterior ankle with your medial hand so that the thumb is on the lateral aspect of the cuboid. Your stabilizing hand is placed palm up against the lateral ankle so the thumb of the contact hand is between the thenar and hypothenar pads of the stabiliz-

ing hand. While maintaining this contact, stand closer to the patient so that the foot is between your thighs, and assume a crouching position. Apply traction by thigh pressure, and simultaneously make a thrust directed medially with the stabilizing palm against the contact thumb. Follow correction by evaluating the integrity of the peronei and the muscles involved in excessive pronation.

Alternative Adjustment Procedure. The doctor-patient position is the same as above. Contact is made with the web of the lateral hand, with the fingers on the anterior ankle surface and the thumb on the plantar surface (see Fig. 27.17). The medial hand stabilizes the metatarso-cuneiform region by grasping the medial forefoot with the thumb on top and the fingers wrapped around the distal arch. Apply traction, and simultaneously make a scissors-type adjustment by thrusting medially with your lateral contact hand and laterally with your stabilizing hand.

Inferior Cuboid Subluxation

Associated features of inferior cuboid subluxation are lateral longitudinal arch pains and excessive pronation or supination.

Adjustment. Place the patient prone, and stand at the foot of the table latero-oblique to the involved limb. Locate the

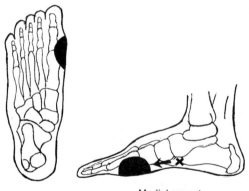

Plantar aspect   Medial aspect

Figure 27.16. Abductor hallucis trigger point; *X*, common site. *Blackened areas* indicate typical sites of referred pain.

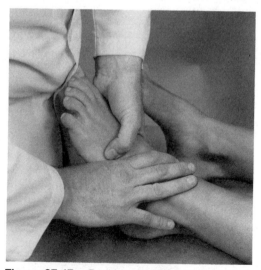

Figure 27.17. Position for the alternative adjustment procedure for a laterally subluxated cuboid bone.

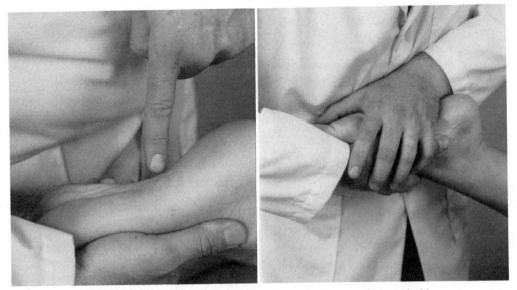

Figure 27.18. Technique positions for adjusting an inferior cuboid.

plantar aspect of the cuboid. A contact is made with the pisiform of your cephalad hand with the fingers wrapping around the lateral aspect of the foot (see Fig. 27.18). The patient's anterior foot rests in the palm of your caudad stabilizing hand. Apply traction to the forefoot with your stabilizing hand with emphasis upon the 5th metatarsal, and simultaneously make a short, sharp thrust toward the floor. Follow correction by evaluating the integrity of the peronei and the muscles involved in excessive pronation.

Alternative Adjustment Procedure. Place the patient prone, and stand at the foot of the table latero-oblique to the involved limb. Locate the plantar aspect of the cuboid. A contact is made with the thumb of your caudad hand with the fingers wrapping around the anterior aspect of the foot for support. Make pisiform pressure over your contact thumb with your cephalad hand. Apply traction, and simultaneously make a thrust towards the floor with a drooping motion aided by bending your knees.

Posterior Calcaneus Subluxation

This subluxation is usually associated with tarsal tunnel syndrome, excessive pronation, and pain sited inferior and slightly posterior to the medial malleolus.

Adjustment. Place the patient prone, and stand at the foot of the table facing the involved limb. With your medial hand, grasp the patient's anterior ankle with your fingers and place the thumb firmly against the distal plantar calcaneus. With your lateral hand, cup the heel with firm pressure against the posterior aspect of the calcaneus. The adjustment is made with a snapping force by the thumb of the contact hand superiorly while the stabilizing hand rotates the calcaneus towards your body (Fig. 27.19). Both hands must work in unison. Evaluate the peroneus longus, tibialis posterior, and flexor digitorum brevis.

Anterior Calcaneus Subluxation

Associated features for an anterior calcaneus subluxation include excessive supination and pes cavus.

Adjustment. Place the patient prone with involved knee flexed. Stand on the side of involvement. Your caudad hand contacts the anterior plantar aspect of the calcaneus with a web contact, while your cephalad hand stabilizes the talus, tibia, and fibula by grasping the posterior ankle with a web contact. Apply pressure with your contact hand against the calcaneus, and simultaneously make a short, sharp thrust that is directed from the anterior to the posterior (Fig. 27.20). Evaluate the peronei

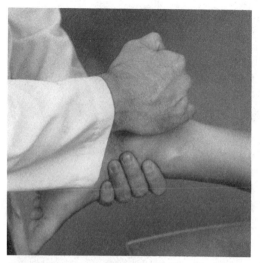

Figure 27.19. The adjustment procedure for adjusting a posterior calcaneus.

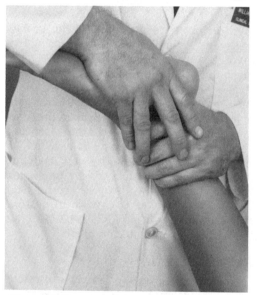

Figure 27.20. Position for adjusting an anterior calcaneus subluxation.

and muscles involved in excessive supination.

Inferior-medial Navicular Subluxation

This subluxation is associated with medial longitudinal arch pain, excessive pronation, and inversion or eversion ankle sprain.

Adjustment. Place the patient prone with the involved knee slightly flexed. Stand at the foot of the table on the side of involvement. Grasp the anterior surface of the patient's foot with your caudad hand so that your 2nd and 3rd fingers are hooked over the inferomedial aspect of the navicular. With your cephalad hand, take a pisiform contact over your contact fingers. Apply traction, and simultaneously thrust obliquely lateral towards the floor. Evaluate the tibialis anterior and posterior, peroneus longus, abductor hallucis, and flexors hallucis longus and digitorum longus.

Inferior Metatarsal or Tarsal Subluxation

These subluxations are associated with arch pain, ankle sprain, and excessive pronation or supination.

Adjustment. Place the patient prone with the knee slightly flexed. Stand at the foot of the table facing the patient and centered at the involved side. Take a double-thumb contact on the involved inferior tarsal or metatarsal bone with your fingers extending around to support the anterior aspect of the foot (Fig. 27.21). Apply steady plantar flexion to the foot, and simultaneously make a snapping thrust with your contact thumbs directed towards the floor. Evaluate the muscles involved in excessive pronation.

Alternative Adjustment Procedure. Place the patient supine with the foot at a right angle to the leg. Stand at the foot of the table facing the patient and centered at the involved side. Take a double-thumb contact on the involved inferior tarsal or metatarsal bone with your fingers extending around to stabilize the anterior aspect of the

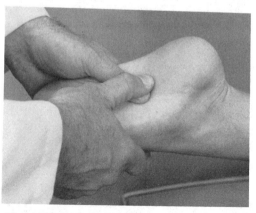

Figure 27.21. Position for adjusting an inferior metatarsal or tarsal subluxation.

foot. Apply steady plantar flexion of the forefoot by finger pressure towards your body, and simultaneously make a short, quick adjustment by thrusting your thumb contacts cephalad by snapping your elbows foreward. Your fingers, thumbs, wrists, and elbows must work in unison.

Superior Proximal Metatarsal or Tarsal Subluxation

Associated features for these types of subluxations are pain on the dorsum of the foot, inversion sprain resulting in a 1st metatarsal displaced superiorly, pronation syndrome with superior 1st and 5th metatarsals, and excessive supination.

Adjustment. Place the patient supine. Sit at the foot of the table facing the patient. Grasp the patient's lateral foot with your lateral hand so that the superiorly subluxated bone is under the proximal or medial phalanx of your third finger and the thumb stabilizes against the plantar surface. Your medial hand is interlaced over the contact hand so that the third finger is on top of the contact hand's finger and the thumb stabilizes against the plantar surface. See Figure 27.22, *left*. Remove any foot inversion or eversion present. Apply traction with firm contact pressure, and simultaneously make a sharp pull towards yourself to move the subluxated bone caudally. Evaluate the integrity of the muscles involved in excessive pronation or inversion sprain.

Inferior Distal Metatarsal Subluxation

This type of subluxation is commonly associated with excessive callus formation across the metatarsal heads, plantar forefoot pain, and excessive pronation.

Adjustment. Place the patient supine. Sit at the foot of the table facing the patient. Grasp the patient's lateral foot with your lateral hand so that the inferiorly subluxated bone is under your thumb and your fingers extend around the medial aspect and rest upon the anterior surface of the foot. With the thumb of your medial hand, contact the phalanges of the involved metatarsal. Remove any foot inversion or eversion present. Apply traction to the phalanges, and simultaneously make a short thumb thrust cephalad to move the subluxated bone superior. See Figure 27.22, *right*. Evaluate the integrity of the transverse head of the abductor hallucis and muscles involved in excessive pronation.

Orthotics

Foot orthotics—the field of knowledge relating to protecting, restoring, aligning, or improving function of the foot and ankle—has made great technologic strides in recent years. A proper appliance has shown to be a distinct advantage in the treatment, rehabilitation, and prevention of many vertebral and lower extremity disorders.

One company has recently developed stabilizers that greatly reduce bone shock at

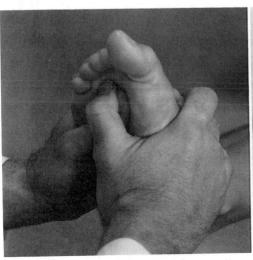
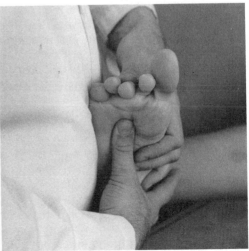

Figure 27.22.　*Left*, position for adjusting a superior proximal metatarsal or tarsal subluxation. *Right*, inferior distal metatarsal.

heel strike—a factor vitally important to the treatment of many athletic injuries of the lumbar spine, pelvis, and lower extremities. This is possible by constructing the stabilizers with Sorbothan II, a viscoelastic polymer that has the ability to accept pressure, shear, and torque forces synchronously without parmanent distortion. For further information, write Foot Levelers, Inc, 1901 Rockdale Road, P.O. Box 272, Dubuque, Iowa 52004-9998.

Fatigue Fractures and Cysts of the Foot

March fractures are characterized by point tenderness and sometimes a palpable callus. The onset of symptoms may be rapid or gradual. Diagnosis is made early by exclusion and late by roentgenographic findings. Management is similar to that for metatarsalgia: rest and support. This rare condition is not common to athletes but is occasionally found in unconditioned joggers who run on hard surfaces. The second metatarsal is the site of the most common fatigue fractures seen in the foot. Various congenital or acquired factors such as Morton's toe, warts, and bunion may be the underlying factor in symptomatic runners.

Bowerman points out that chronic stress of the talus may produce marginal degenerative cysts similar to those seen in other weight-bearing joints (eg, knee, hip). Usually, but not always, the joint space near the cyst will be narrowed.

Circulatory Disturbances

Skin color normally darkens in the weight-bearing position. An elevated pink foot that markedly deepens in color in the standing position suggests arterial insufficiency or vascular disease. Note the venous filling time on the dorsum of the foot at the same time. The collapsed veins should fill within 12 seconds upon standing. If pulses are absent in a limb, check the most distal palpable pulse and auscultate for an audible bruit suggesting the site of obstruction. Apply finger pressure to the medial dorsal area of the foot and note time for the white spot to disappear; then rotate weight to outer border and repeat test. Blanching time is delayed in cases of pronation and arch weakness due to circulatory interference.

Erythromelalgia (red neuritis of the extremities) is most common in the feet. The toes (or fingers) are red, hot, tender, and painful. In Raynaud's disease, the digits are cold and painless or anesthetic. The attacks are aggravated by heat and not, like those of Raynaud's disease, by cold. Such attacks are probably akin to the condition of "hot feet" often seen in the arteriosclerosis of elderly people. The patient kicks off the bed clothes from his feet at night on account of the burning sensations. Other evidences of insufficient arterial blood supply (eg, clubbing, intermittent claudication, cramps, gangrene) may coexist.

Buerger's disease (thromboangitis obliterans) exhibits inflammatory changes in the small and medium-sized arterioles and veins that manifests as a nonsuppurative panarteritis and/or panphlebitis, typically in a segmental pattern. Early associated features include cold feet, pallor on elevation, intermittent claudication, paresthesiae, Raynaud's phenomenon, and impaired or absent pedal artery pulsations. Local ischemia develops from arterial occlusion disease, which may be accentuated by degrees of arteriospasm and minor venous thrombosis, and leads to trophic changes and latter to gangrenous ulcers. This disorder of unknown etiology is predominantly seen in males, aged 20–40, who are heavy smokers.

Miscellaneous Pathologic Signs and Reflexes

Duchenne's Test. The patient is placed supine with the lower limbs extended in a relaxed position. The examiner's thumb is placed on the plantar aspect of the head of the 1st metatarsal on the involved side, and the patient is instructed to plantar flex the foot. If during this action the head of the 1st metatarsal offers little or no pressure against the examiner's thumb, the medial border of the foot dorsiflexes while the lateral border plantar flexes, and the arch disappears, the test is positive for peroneus longus paralysis (L4–S1).

Abadie's Sign. This manifests as a loss of deep pain during strong pinching of the Achilles tendon. It is an early sign of tabes dorsalis.

Babinski's Plantar Sign. Stroking the sole of the foot with a moderately sharp instrument, from the outer side of the heel toward the small toe for about 2 inches, will usually result in rapid plantar flexion of all toes. When the small toes fan into the plantar flexion slowly and the great toe strongly dorsiflexes, a positive sign occurs that indicates pyramidal tract disease. A Babinski response is the most constant of all pathologic reflexes.

Rossolimo's Sign. This late inconsistent pathologic plantar reflex, a Babinski variant, occurs when the great toe of the paralyzed side is lightly percussed or stroked upon its plantar surface and extension or abduction of the toe results.

Hirschberg's Sign. This pathologic sign is exhibited by internal rotation and adduction of the foot when friction is applied to the lateral aspect of the plantar surface.

Oppenheim's Hemiplegic Sign. The examiner grasps the anterior-external aspect of the tibia, making firm pressure with the thumb and fingers from above downward, causing the great toe to plantar flex in cases of organic hemiplegia.

Chaddock's Ankle Sign. Stroking the lateral-distal leg just behind and under the external malleolus with the handle of a reflex hammer will elicit a Babinski-like sign.

Schaeffer's Sign. This reflex occurs in organic hemiplegia. When the middle portion of the Achilles tendon is firmly pinched, plantar flexion of the foot and dorsiflexion of the toes, especially the great toe, results in a Babinski-like fashion.

Gordon's Toe Sign. A Babinski-like dorsiflexion of the great toe, and possibly others, occurs when sudden kneading pressure is made upon the deep flexor muscles of the calf when the pyramidal tracts are involved.

Gonda's Sign. This Babinski-like reflex response is elicited by pressing downward on the third toe and suddenly releasing it with a snap, causing an upward movement of the great toe.

Mendel-Bechterew's Sign. In organic hemiplegia or cerebellar tract disease, plantar flexion of the lateral toes results from percussing the dorsum of the foot in the area of the cuboid. Under normal conditions, dorsiflexion of the lateral four toes occurs. In pathologic states, plantar flexion is produced.

Crossed Extension Sign. The patient is placed supine with both knees slightly flexed. Stimulation of the plantar surface of one foot produces extension of the contralateral knee.

INJURIES OF THE TOES

Contagious and traumatic-related skin diseases of the foot and toes have been discussed previously. Here we shall consider the deeper musculoskeletal and related disorders.

Gait Clues

Pain in a foot during midstance may be caused by corns, calluses from a fallen transverse arch, rigid pes planus, or subtalar arthritis. Pushing off with the lateral side of the front of the foot is usually seen in disorders involving the great toe. Sharp pain in push-off is often caused by corns between the toes or metatarsal callosities. Inability of a foot to heel strike is an indication of a heel spur and associated bursitis.

Restrictions

In testing flexion and extension toe motion, first test the great toe. To test motion of the 1st metatarsophalangeal joint, stabilize the foot with one hand while the active hand flexes and extends the joint. Restricted movement in this joint frequently produces a protective gait restricting push-off. Flexion is the only motion of the great toe's proximal interphalangeal joint. In the lesser toes, flexion and extension occur at the proximal and distal interphalangeal joints and the metatarsophalangeal joint. Restricted extension of the proximal and distal interphalangeal joints and restricted flexion of the metatarsophalangeal joints are a feature of claw toes. Restricted flexion of the distal interphalangeal joint and metatarsophalangeal joint with restricted extension of the proximal interphalangeal joint are features of a hammer toe.

Claw Toes

Claw toes, usually associated with pes cavus, feature flexed proximal and distal interphalangeal joints and hyperextended metatarsophalangeal joints. An early sign is the formation of callosities over the dorsal surface of the toes, on the tips of the toes, and on the plantar surface under the metatarsal heads.

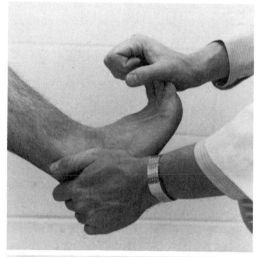

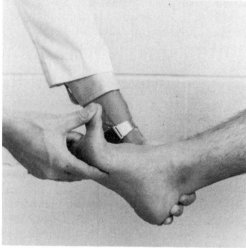

Figure 27.23. *Top*, position for testing the strength of the digitorum longus muscle. *Bottom*, testing the flexion strength of the great toe against resistance.

Hammer Toe and Mallet Toe

A hammer toe presents flexion of the proximal interphalangeal joint and hyperextension of the metatarsophalangeal and distal interphalangeal joints. It is usually singular and associated with a callosity on top of the proximal interphalangeal joint. Predisposing factors include forceful plantarflexion of the metatarsal, pes cavus, short metatarsal, forefoot valgus, trauma, or pronation imbalance.

A mallet toe is a distal interphalangeal joint flexion contracture which usually occurs in the smaller toes. It is less common than a hammer toe.

Hallus Rigidus

This disorder is characterized by pain, tenderness, stiffness, and limited motion of the 1st metatarsophalangeal joint. Incidence is higher in females during youth but higher in males during adulthood. Contrast baths, a rigid insole, and passive foot mobilization are helpful. Stubborn cases require phalangeal osteotomy.

Hallux Valgus and Bunion

This is a state of lateral deviation of the great toe, usually found in conjunction with a hypermobile pronated foot and the wearing of pointed-toed shoes producing abuse to the medial aspect of the front toe. The 1st metatarsal becomes fixed in abduction and the hallux subluxates laterally. In time, the abductor hallucis becomes fixated in lateral displacement beneath the metatarsal head. The muscle becomes ineffective in maintaining abduction.

Adjustment. Place the patient supine. Stand at the foot of the table facing the patient and centered to the involved limb. With our medial contact hand, grasp the great toe with your third and fourth fingers extended along the plantar and medial aspect of the foot and the thumb placed against the anterior aspect of the involved joint (Fig. 27.24). Your lateral stabilizing hand grasps the wrist of the contact hand

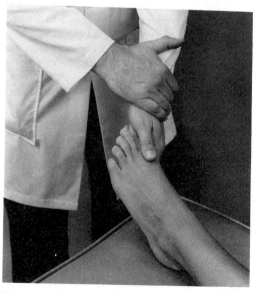

Figure 27.24. Position for adjusting a hallux abducto valgus subluxation.

for support. Apply traction, remove the valgus deviation, and make a short pull towards your body. Evaluate the integrity of the abductor hallucis and the muscles involved in excessive pronation.

Bunion. A bunion is an effect of prolonged hallux valgus where the great toe displaces laterally with rotation about the long axis so that the nail faces medially. The sesamoid enlarges, and the soft tissues on the lateral aspect of the great toe enlarge. An adventitious bursa forms which often becomes tender and inflamed (Figs. 27.25 and 27.26).

Toe Sprains

The most common sprain of this area is that of the great toe, especially at the metatarsophalangeal joint as the result of forced plantar flexion or dorsiflexion. Sideward sprains are rarely witnessed. Swelling may be severe, but bony tenderness or crepitus is absent. Disability is severe because weight bearing is predominantly on the hallus. Sprains of the toes are managed similar to finger sprains.

Selected Disorders

Circulatory Disturbances

To evaluate the capillary filling time of the toes, compress a selected toe until it

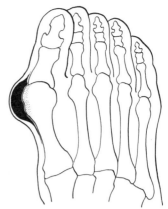

Figure 27.26. Hallux valgus with inflamed bursa on the medial side of the 1st metatarsophalangeal joint.

blanches white, then release pressure quickly. Normal color should return within 6–10 seconds. Tenderness along the transverse arch is common in aseptic necrosis from a circulatory disturbance.

Black Heel

Pigmented areas on the posterior aspect of the heel secondary to petechial hemorrhage are sometimes seen in athletes. Heel pain following activity is the common complaint, but it is frequently asymptomatic. The disorder is most often associated with tennis, badminton, basketball, and soccer.

Tennis Toe

A chronic complaint of pain in one or more of the longer toes is frequently associated with hemorrhage, usually horizontal, under the toenails (tennis toe). The cause, seen in several sports, is felt to be from sudden stops, quick changes of direction, and the severe forward motion of the body which propels the long toes against the front of the inside shoe. If the hemorrhage is longitudinal, the disorder is easily confused with the splinter hemorrhages associated with subacute bacterial endocarditis after a recent illness.

Ungual Injuries

As with finger nailbed injuries, toe nailbed injuries are common in sports where shoes require little or no toe protection. The degree of injury may vary from slight nail

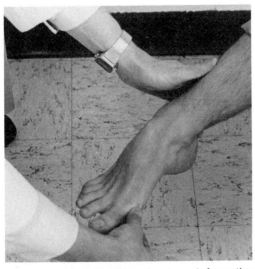

Figure 27.25. Checking for bursal formation over the head of the 1st metatarsal and the metatarsophalangeal joint.

splits to painful complete nail avulsion to the base with tears in the nailbed. As the nailbed is contiguous with the periosteum of the underlying bone, bleeding may be associated with phalanx fracture or a crush injury. Crushing injuries, however, are much more common than nailbed avulsions.

Management. In uncomplicated avulsions apply cold to reduce bleeding and swelling. An avulsed nail should be repositioned and a light pressure bandage applied to keep it from snagging socks or other objects until it painlessly separates by itself. Care must be taken not to bandage the distal end so tightly as to restrict drainage. A longer shoe may be temporarily necessary to allow for protection without increasing pressure. If a painful subungeal hematoma develops from lack of drainage, referral is necessary for relief.

Sesamoiditis

Deep palpation within the flexor hallucis brevis tendon may locate the two sesamoids where signs of sesamoiditis exist. Sesamoid necrosis under the head of the 1st metatarsal within the flexor hallucis longus tendon may show roentgenographic signs.

Management. Strapping, rest, physiotherapy, sole padding, and improved footwear are beneficial. Progressive exercises may be started immediately afer the acute stage has subsided.

Closing Remarks

Nash points out that the physician who deals with athletes must be skilled in the general examination procedure in preparation for the special examination that is unique to each individual sporting event. This special procedure will encompass evaluative measures that are unique to the sport and more specifically to the position for which the athlete will train. Each position will have special demands and skill drills necessary for developing reactively precise performance. These demands, while resulting in better performance, often produce injuries when applied to a susceptible individual under certain circumstances.

It is the duty of the valuable physician involved in treating athletes to discover those factors that constitute susceptibility—frequently an intuition resulting from an understanding of the athlete, equipment, apparatus, courts and fields. Prevention, which results from this understanding, is the greatest challenge given the doctor dealing in sports, and it should be the most satisfying reward of his contribution. In essence, he must have full knowledge of the anatomy and biomechanics involved in the specific athlete and athletic event.

Suggested Readings: Part 4

CHAPTERS 19-27

Aarons, MW et al: *Applied Kinesiology, Pressure Point, and Pain Control Technics*, Lombard, IL, National-Lincoln School of Postgraduate Chiropractic Education, 1974.

Albright, JA and Brand, RA: *The Scientific Basis of Orthopaedics*, New York, Appleton-Century-Crofts, 1979.

Albright, JP et al: Head and Neck Injuries in Sports. In Scott, WN, et al (eds): *Principles of Sports Medicine*, Baltimore, Williams & Wilkins, 1984, pp 40-85.

Anderson, LD and D'Alonzo, RT: Fractures of the Odontoid Process of the Axis, *Journal of Bone and Joint Surgery*, 56A:1663, 1924.

Andreoli, G: Neurological Implications of Sports Injuries, *New England Journal of Chiropractic*, Winter 1979.

Andriacchi, T et al: A Model for Studies of Mechanical Interactions Between the Human Spine and Rib Cage, *Journal of Biomechanics*, Vol 7, 1974, pp 497-507.

Appley, AG: The Diagnosis of Meniscal Injuries, *Journal of Bone and Joint Surgery*, 29:78-84, 1946.

Arthur, PB: General Management of On-Field Injuries, *ACA Journal of Chiropractic*, August 1979.

Aston, JN: *Textbook of Orthopaedics and Traumatology*, ed 2, Toronto, Canada, Hodder and Stoughton, 1976.

Bailey, HW: Theoretical Significance of Postural Imbalance, Especially the 'Short Leg', *American Osteopathic Association Journal*, Vol 7, February 1978.

Barnvinchack, E: An Evaluation of an Acute Closed Head Trauma, *ACA Journal of Chiropractic*, January 1982.

Basmajian, JV (ed): *Therapeutic Exercise*, ed 3, Baltimore, Williams and Wilkins Co., 1978.

Bennett, TJ: *A New Clinical Basis for the Correction of Abnormal Physiology*, Burlingame, CA, published by author, 1960.

Berkman, EH: The Troublesome T.M.J., *ACA Journal of Chiropractic*, June 1971.

Berkow, R (ed): *The Merck Manual*, 13th edition, Rahway, NJ, Merck, Sharp & Dohme Research Laboratories, 1977.

Betge, G: *Physical Therapy in Chiropractic Practice*, Via Tesserete 51, Switzerland, published by author, 1975.

Blits, J: Ortho-Differential Diagnosis of Popliteal Swelling, *Ortho-Briefs*, 5(1):5, April 1983.

Bolton, PS: Torticollis: A Review of Etiology, Pathology, Diagnosis and Treatment, *Journal of Manipulative and Physiological Therapeutics*, 8:29-31, March 1985.

Bormann, WR: Applied Kinesiology of the Hamstring Muscles and Related Factors, *Wisconsin Chiropractic Association Journal*, 28:15, April 1975.

Bowerman, JW: *Radiology and Injury in Sport*, New York, Appleton-Century-Crofts, 1977.

Brewer, BJ: Aging and the Rotator Cuff, *American Journal of Sports Medicine*, 7:102-110, 1979.

Brunarski, DJ: Chiropractic Clinical Decision Making and Low Back Pain, *ACA Journal of Chiropractic*, July 1983.

Brunarski, DJ: Functional Considerations of Spinal Manipulative Therapy, *ACA Journal of Chiropractic*, May 1980.

Bryan, EC: The Traumatic Cervical Root Syndrome, *ACA Journal of Chiropractic* April 1967.

Cailliet, R: *Soft Tissue Pain and Disability*, Philadelphia, F.A. Davis Company, 1977.

Carpenter, SA et al: An Investigation into the Effect of Organ Irritation on Muscle Strength and Spinal Mobility, *Bulletin of the European Chiropractors Union*, 25:2, 1977.

Carrick, FR: Cervical Radiculopathy: The Diagnosis and Treatment of Pathomechanics in the Cervical Spine, *Journal of Manipulative and Physiological Therapeutics*, 6(3):129-136, September 1983.

Cichoke, AJ: Athletic Injuries, Inflammation, and Proteolytic Enzyme Therapy, *Journal of the ACA Council on Sports Injuries*, 1(2):15-16, April 1982.

Cipriano, JJ: *Photographic Manual of Regional Orthopedic Tests*, Baltimore, Williams & Wilkins, 1985.

Claypool, DS: Cervical Rib, *Roentgenological Briefs*, Des Moines, IA, Council on Roentgenology of the American Chiropractic Association, date unknown.

Cooper, VH: Analytical, Manipulative and Supportive Procedures Affecting the Knee, *ACA Journal of Chiropractic*, April 1981.

Copass, MK and Eisenberg, MS: *The Paramedic Manual*, Philadelphia, W.B. Saunders Company, 1980, chapter 2.

Cowen, AR: Emergency Care of Spinal Injuries: A Field Approach for Chiropractic Physicians, *ACA Journal of Chiropractic*, June 1979.

Cox, JM: Mechanism, Diagnosis, and Treatment of Lumbar Disc Protrusion and Prolapse: A Statistical Evaluation, *ACA Journal of Chiropractic*, Part I, September 1976; Part II, October 1976.

Craig, TT (ed): *Comments in Sports Medicine*, Chicago, American Medical Association, 1973, pp 18-20.

Crawford, JP et al: Vascular Ischemia of the Cervical Spine: A Review of Relationship to Therapeutic Manipulation, *Journal of Manipulative and Physiological Therapeutics*, 7(3):149-154, September 1984.

Cyriax, J and Russell, G: *Textbook of Orthopaedic Medicine*, Vol II, Baltimore, Williams & Wilkins, 1977.

Dalinka, MK: Ankle Fractures and Fractures and Dislocation about the Shoulder, in Feldman, F (ed): *Radiology, Pathology, and Immunology of Bones and Joints*, New York, Appleton-Century-Crofts, 1978.

Daniels, L and Worthingham, C: *Therapeutic Exercise*, ed 2, Philadelphia, W.B. Saunders Company, 1977.

Daube, JR and Sandok, BA: *Medical Neurosciences*, Boston, Little, Brown, and Company, 1978.

Davis, BM: Spondylolisthesis and Spondylolysis, *Roentgenological Briefs*, Des Moines, IA, Council on Roentgenology of the American Chiropractic Association, date unknown.

DeBoer, KF et al: Reliability Study of Detection of

Somatic Dysfunction in the Cervical Spine, *Journal of Manipulative and Physiological Therapeutics*, 8(1):9–15, March 1985.

Dolan, JP and Holladay, LJ: *First-Aid Management: Athletics, Physical Education, Recreation,* ed 4, Danville, IL, Interstate Printers & Publishers, Inc, 1974, chapter 7, 11.

Drum, DC: The Nature of the Problem: A Functional Concept of Vertebral Subluxations, *The Kentucky Chirogram,* 36:78.

Eriksson, E: Sports Injuries of the Knee Ligaments: Their Diagnosis, Treatment, Rehabilitation, and Prevention, *Medical Science and Sports,* 8:133–144, 1976.

Feldman, F (ed): *Radiology, Pathology, and Immunology of Bones and Joints: A Review of Current Concepts,* New York, Appleton-Century-Crofts, 1978.

Fox, TF: A Review of Cervical Spine Reference Lines, *Orthopedic Brief,* ACA Council on Chiropractic Orthopedics.

Fromelt, KA et al: Activities Causing Injury to the Lumbar Spine: A Computer Study, *ACA Journal of Chiropractic,* March 1983.

Galway, R et al: Pivot Shift: A Clinical Sign of Symptomatic Anterior Cruciate Insufficiency, *Journal of Bone and Joint Surgery,* 54B:763–764, 1974.

Gatterman, MI: Indication for Spinal Manipulation in the Treatment of Back Pain, *ACA Journal of Chiropractic,* October 1982.

Gertler, L: *Illustrated Manual of Extravertebral Technic,* ed 2, Bayside, NY, published by author, 1978.

Giammarino, MA: The Adolescent Knee, *Roentgenological Briefs,* Des Moines, IA, Council on Roentgenology of the American Chiropractic Association, data unknown.

Gillet, H: Feet, Hands, Cranium, etc, *Bulletin of the European Chiropractors Union,* date unknown.

Gillet, H: Movement Palpation—Measurements, *Bulletin of the European Chiropractors Union,* 23:2, 1974.

Goodheart, GJ: *Collected Published Articles and Reprints,* Montpelier, OH, Williams County Publishing Co., 1969.

Goodheart, GJ: Reactive Muscle Patterns in Athletes, *ACA Journal of Chiropractic,* April 1982.

Goodrich, TM: Analysis and Treatment of Common Lesions of the Knee, *ACA Journal of Chiropractic,* January 1963.

Goodwin, PN et al: *Physical Foundations of Radiology,* ed 4, New York, Harper & Row Publishers, 1970.

Gorman, BD: Ophthalmology and Sports Medicine. In Scott, WN, et al (eds): *Principles of Sports Medicine,* Baltimore, Williams & Wilkins, 1984, pp 87–96.

Grant, JM: Carpal Tunnel Syndrome: A New Concept in Conservative Chiropractic Management, *ACA Journal of Chiropractic,* February 1979.

Grant, WF and Cinotti, AA: Eye Problems, in Haycock, CE (ed): *Sports Medicine for the Athletic Female,* Oradell, NJ, Medical Economics Company, 1980.

Green, L: The Adjustment in Acute Lumbosacral Disc Lesions, *ACA Journal of Chiropractic* May 1967.

Greenawalt, MH: Feet and the Dynamic Science of Chiropractic, *ACA Journal of Chiropractic,* May 1983.

Greenawalt, MH: *Spinal Pelvic Stabilization,* ed 2, Dubuque, IA, Foot Levelers, Inc, 1978.

Grossman, RB and Nicholas, JA: Common Disorders of the Knee, *Orthopaedic Clinics of North America,* 8:619–640, 1977.

Grove, AB: *Chiropractic Technique: A Procedure of Adjusting,* Madison, WI, Straus Printing & Publishing Co, Inc, 1979.

Gunn, CC and Milbrandt, WE: Early and Subtle Signs in Low-Back Sprain, *Spine,* September 1978.

Hains, G: *Post-traumatic Neuritis,* Trois-Rivieres, Quebec, Canada, published by author, 1978.

Hariman, DG: Lumbosacral Instability, *Roentgenological Briefs,* Des Moines, IA, Council on Roentgenology of the American Chiropractic Association, date unknown.

Hasemeir, RR: The Elbow, Part II, *Roentgenological Briefs,* Des Moines, IA, Council on Roentgenology of the American Chiropractic Association, date unknown.

Hass, RG: Cervical Strain, *Ortho-Briefs,* ACA Council on Orthopedics, Winter 1982, pp 8–10.

Hasselberger, FX: *Uses of Enzymes and Immobilized Enzymes,* Chicago, Nelson-Hall, 1978.

Hazel, RH: Iliotibial Band Syndrome, *The Journal of the Council on Sports Injuries (ACA),* 1(4):12–14, September 1983.

Heilman, KM et al: *Handbook for Differential Diagnosis of Neurologic Signs and Symptoms,* New York, Appleton-Century-Crofts, 1977.

Helfet, AJ: *Disorders of the Knee,* 2nd edition, Philadelphia, J.B. Lippincott, 1982.

Helfet, AJ and Gruebel Lee, DM: *Disorders of the Lumbar Spine,* Philadelphia, J.B. Lippincott Company, 1978.

Hibbard, D: Effects of manipulation on gait muscle activity, *ACA Journal of Chiropractic,* October 1983.

Hirata, I, Jr: *The Doctor and the Athlete,* ed 2, Philadelphia, J.B. Lippincott Company, 1974, chapters 8–9, 11–13.

Homewood, AE: Innervation of the Shoulder Joint, *The Chirogram,* April 1974.

Hoppenfeld, S: *The Physical Examination of the Spine and Extremities,* New York, Appleton-Century-Crofts, 1976, p 194.

Howe, JW: Determination of Lumbo-sacral Facet Subluxations, *Roentgenological Briefs,* Des Moines, IA, Council on Roentgenology of the American Chiropractic Association, date unknown.

Howe, JW: Frequently Missed Fractures, *Roentgenological Briefs,* Des Moines, IA, American Council on Roentgenology of the American Chiropractic Association, date unknown.

Illi, FW: *The Vertebral Column: Life-Line of the Body,* Lombard, IL, National College on Chiropractic, 1951.

Insall, JN: Patellar Pain, *Journal of Bone and Joint Surgery,* 64A:147–152, 1982.

Iversen, LD and Clawson, DK: *Manual of Acute Orthopaedic Therapeutics,* Boston, Little, Brown, and Company, 1977.

Jackson, RB: The Neurovascular Compression Syndromes, *ACA Journal of Chiropractic,* March-May 1963.

Jacobs, MD: Preventive Spinal Hygiene and the Human Machine, *ACA Journal of Chiropractic,* August 1980.

Jacobus, AW: Lumbar Spondylosis and Its Treatment, *ACA Journal of Chiropractic,* September and October 1966.

Janse, J et al: *Chiropractic Principles and Technic,* Chicago, National College of Chiropractic, 1947.

Janse, J et al: *Principles and Practice of Chiropractic,* Lombard, IL, National College of Chiropractic, 1976.

Jaskoviak, PA: A Look at the Sprained Ankle, *Journal*

of Clinical Chiropractic, Special Edition: Athletic Injuries, 1:6, 1974.

Jaskoviack, PA and Schafer, RC: *Applied Physiotherapy*, prepublication manuscript, Arlington, VA, American Chiropractic Association, scheduled to be released in 1986.

Jeffreys, E: *Disorders of the Cervical Spine*, Boston, Butterworths, 1980.

Jessen, AR: Chiropractic Is the Treatment of Choice of Bursitis, *ACA Journal of Chiropractic*, May 1967.

Jessen, AR: The Sacroiliac Subluxation, *ACA Journal of Chiropractic*, September 1973.

Johnson, AC: *Chiropractic Physiological Therapeutics*, Palm Springs, CA, published by author, 1977.

Kaplan, HA: Head Injuries, in Haycock, CE (ed): *Sports Medicine for the Athletic Female*, Oradell, NJ, Medical Economics Company, 1980.

Kendall, HO et al: *Muscles Testing and Function*, ed 2, Baltimore, Williams & Wilkins 1971.

Kennedy, JC and Fowler, P: Medial and Anterior Instability of the Knee, *Journal of Bone and Joint Surgery*, 53A:1257–1270, 1971.

Kettelkamp, DB: Management of Patellar Malalignment, *Journal of Bone and Joint Surgery*, 63A:1344–1347, 1981.

Kimmel, EH: Barre-Lieou Syndrome, *Ortho-Briefs*, ACA Council on Orthopedics, Winter 1982, p 11.

Kirby, JD: *Essentials of Physical Diagnosis*, North Hollywood, CA, Chiropractic Business Services, 1978.

Klyop, GW et al: Iliotibial Band Syndrome, *The Physician and Sports Medicine*, 9(10):13, December 1981.

Larcher, AC: Football Helmet Injuries, *Journal of Clinical Chiropractic*, Special Edition: Athletic Injuries, 1:6, 1974.

Logan, AL: *Clinical Application of Chiropractic Low Back and Pelvis*, Westminster, CA, West-Print, 1977.

MacIntosch, DL: The Pivot Shift and the Anterior Cruciate. Paper presented at the New York State Orthopaedic Society Meeting, New York, 1979.

Macnab, I: *Backache*, Baltimore, Williams & Wilkins, 1977.

Malik, DD et al: Effectiveness of Chiropractic Adjustment and Physical Therapy to Treat Spinal Subluxation, *ACA Journal of Chiropractic*, June 1983.

Markovich, SE: Painful Neuro-Muscular Dysfunction Syndromes in the Head: A Neurologist's View, American Academy of Cranio-Mandibular Orthopedics Meeting, New Orleans, September 1976.

Marshall, J and Rubin, R: Knee Ligament Injuries, *Orthopaedic Clinics of North America*, 8:651–665, 1977.

Marshall, J et al: The Anterior Drawer Sign: What Is It?, *American Journal of Sports Medicine*, 3:152–158, 1975.

Maurer, EL: Osteochondritis Dissecans, *Success Express*, 9(4):41–45, published by Goals Unlimited International, Dubuque, IA.

Maurer, EL: The Thoraco-Costal Facet Syndrome with Introduction of the Marginal Line and the Rib Sign, *ACA Journal of Chiropractic*, December 1976.

Mayes, GT: Forget-Me-Nots, *Parade*, August 25, 1985, p 24.

McAndrews, JF: Spinal Motion Examination, *ACA Journal of Chiropractic*, May 1969.

Mennell, JMcM: *Joint Pain*, Boston, Little, Brown and Company, 1964.

Michelle, AA and Eisenberg, J: Scapulocostal syndrome, *Archives of Physical Medicine and Rehabilitation*, 49:383–387, 1968.

Miller, DR: The Shoulder Joint, *ACA Journal of Chiropractic*, February 1976.

Mouk, SL: Sacro-Occipital Technique, *The Texas Chiropractor*, April 1978.

Nash, JM: personal correspondence, Pasadena, TX, 1985.

Ng, SY: Sacroiliac Lumbar Mechanism, *ACA Journal of Chiropractic*, April 1983.

Ng, SY: The Significance of Psoas Myospasm in the Lordotic Compared to the Kyphotic Sacrolumbar Spine, *ACA Journal of Chiropractic*, October 1978.

Ng, SY: Skeletal Muscle Spasm: Various Methods to Relieve It, *ACA Journal of Chiropractic*, February 1980.

Nisonson B et al: The knee. In Scott, WN, et al (eds): *Principles of Sports Medicine*, Baltimore, Williams & Wilkins, 1984, pp 270–337.

Nobel, CA: Iliotibial Band Friction Syndrome in Runners, *American Journal of Sports Medicine*, 8:232–234, August 1980.

O'Donoghue, DH: *Treatment of Injuries to Athletes*, 3rd edition, Philadelphia, W.B. Saunders, 1976.

Ogden, JA: Subluxation and dislocation of the proximal tibiofibular joint, *Journal of Bone and Joint Surgery*, 56A:145, 1974.

Olsen, RE: Acute Lumbosacral Angle, *Roentgenological Briefs*, Des Moines, IA, Council on Roentgenology of the American Chiropractic Association, date unknown.

Olsen, RE: The Traumatized Shoulder, *ACA Journal of Chiropractic*, April 1965.

Orringer, MB: Chest Injuries in the Athlete. In Schneider, RC, et al (eds): *Sports Injuries: Mechanisms, Prevention, and Treatment*, Baltimore, Williams & Wilkins, 1985, pp 826–827.

Owen, JD: Lower Extremity Problems Relating to Back Problems, *ACA Journal of Chiropractic*, February 1971.

Pamer, T: The Frozen Shoulder Syndrome, *ACA Journal of Chiropractic*, July 1975.

Parkes, JC: Common Injuries About the Elbow in Sports. In Scott, WN, et al (eds): *Principles of Sports Medicine*, Baltimore, Williams & Wilkins, 1984, pp 140–154.

Pashby, TJ and Pashby, RC: Treatment of Sports Eye Injuries. In Schneider, RC, et al (eds): *Sports Injuries: Mechanisms, Prevention, and Treatment*, Baltimore, Williams & Wilkins, 1985, pp 572–591.

Paul, L and Johl, JH: *Essentials of Roentgen Interpretation*, New York, Harper and Row, 1965.

Pecoraro, A, Jr: What to Look for When Examining a Wrestler, *ACA Journal of Chiropractic*, January 1982.

Phillips, RB: The Irritable Reflex Mechanism, *ACA Journal of Chiropractic*, January 1974.

Phillips, RB: Upper Cervical Biomechanics, *ACA Journal of Chiropractic*, October 1976.

Pinkenburg, CA: A Study of the Sacroiliac Articulations, *ACA Journal of Chiropractic*, November 1978.

Radin, EL et al: *Practical Biomechanics for the Orthopaedic Surgeon*, New York, John Wiley & Sons, 1969.

Reed, RC: On Field Management of Athletic Injuries, *ACA Journal of Chiropractic*, July 1981.

Rehberger, LP: Reversal of Normal Cervical Curve, *Roentgenological Briefs*, Des Moines, IA, Council on Roentgenology fo the American Chiropractic Association, date unknown.

Rehberger, LP: Spondylolisthesis, *Roentgenological Briefs*, Des Moines, IA, Council on Roentgenology of the American Chiropractic Association, date unknown.

Roaf, R: Rotation Movements of the Spine with Special Reference to Scoliosis, *Journal of Bone and Joint Surgery*, 40B:312–332, 1958.

Roaf, R: Study of the Mechanics of Spinal Injuries, *Journal of Bone and Joint Surgery*, 42B:810–823, 1960.

Rothman, RH and Simeone, FA: *The Spine*, Vols I and II, Philadelphia, W.B. Saunders Company, 1975.

Salter, RB: Injuries of the Ankle in Children, *North American Clinical Orthopaedics*, 5:147, 1974.

Sante, LR: *Principles of Roentgenological Interpretation*, Ann Arbor, MI, Edwards Brothers, Inc, 1961.

Schafer, RC: *Clinical Biomechanics: Musculoskeletal Actions and Reactions*, Baltimore, Williams and Wilkins, 1983.

Schafer, RC: *Symptomatology and Differential Diagnosis*, prepublication manuscript, Arlington, VA, American Chiropractic Association, scheduled to be released in 1986.

Schafer, RC (ed): *Basic Chiropractic Procedural Manual*, ed 4, Arlington, VA, American Chiropractic Association, 1984.

Schafer, RC: *Chiropractic Physical and Spinal Diagnosis*, Oklahoma City, OK, American Chiropractic Academic Press, 1980.

Schneider, RC: *Head and Neck Injuries in Football*, Baltimore, Williams & Wilkins, 1973.

Schneider, RC et al (eds): *Sports Injuries: Mechanisms, Prevention, and Treatment*, Baltimore, Williams & Wilkins, 1985.

Schoenholtz, F: Conservative Management of Costovertebral Subluxation, *ACA Journal of Chiropractic*, July 1980.

Schoenholtz, F: Conservative Management of Selected Shoulder Problems, *ACA Journal of Chiropractic*, October 1979.

Schultz, AL: *The Shoulder, Arm, and Hand Syndrome*, Stickney, SD, Argus Printers, 1969.

Scott, WN et al (eds): *Principles of Sports Medicine*, Baltimore, Williams & Wilkins, 1984.

Shanks, SC and Kerley, P: *A Textbook of X-ray Diagnosis*, Philadelphia, W.B. Saunders Company, 1959.

Shephard, WD: Subluxation Compensation or Strain? *The Texas Chiropractor*, June 1975.

Sisto J, and Warren R: Complete Knee Dislocation. Paper presented at the American Orthopaedic Society for Sports Medicine, Anaheim, CA, March 1983.

Slocum, D et al: Clinical Test for Anterolateral Rotatory Instability of the Knee, *Clinical Orthopaedics*, 118:63–69, 1976.

Smillie, IS: *Injuries of the Knee Joint*, 5th edition, New York, Churchill Livingstone, 1978.

Smith, DM: Vertebral Artery, *Roentgenological Briefs*, Des Moines, IA, Council of Roentgenology of the American Chiropractic Association, date unknown.

Solheim, RN: Cerebral Contusion Syndrome with Post-Traumatic Headaches, *ACA Journal of Chiropractic*, November 1965.

States, AZ and Hildebrandt, RW: *The Science and Art of Specific Spinal Manipulation*, Lombard, IL, National-Lincoln School of Postgraduate Education, 1974.

Steindler, A: *Kinesiology of the Human Body Under Normal and Pathological Conditions*, Springfield, IL, Charles C Thomas, 1955.

Steingisser, AR: "Chiropractic Orthopedics in General Practice", *New England Journal of Chiropractic*, Winter 1979.

Stonebrink, RD: Palpation for Vertebral Motorcity, *ACA Journal of Chiropractic*, February 1969.

Stonebrink, RD: Thoraco-Costal Adjustments and Related Supine Techniques, *ACA Journal of Chiropractic*, May 1975.

Straus, H: *Sports Medicine and Physiology*, Philadelphia, W.B. Saunders, 1979.

Swiss Chiropractors' Association, *Annals*, Vol VI, Geneve, Switzerland, 1976.

Synder, D: Chiropractic on the Field, *Journal of Clinical Chiropractic*, Special Edition: Athletic Injuries, 1:6, 1974.

Torg, J et al: Clinical Diagnosis of Anterior Cruciate Ligament Instability in the Athlete, *American Journal of Sports Medicine*, 4:84–92, 1976.

Triano, J: Significant Lumbar Dyskinesia, *ACA Journal of Chiropractic*, February 1980.

Tullos, HS and Bennett, JB: The Shoulder in Sports. In Scott, WN, et al (eds): *Principles of Sports Medicine*, Baltimore, Williams & Wilkins, 1984, pp 110–138.

Tullos, HS and King, JW. Throwing Mechanism in Sports, *Orthopedic Clinics of North America*, 4:709–720, 1973.

Turek, SL: *Orthopaedics. Principles and Their Application*, ed 3, Philadelphia, J.B. Lippincott Company, 1977.

Turner, EA: Spondylosis—Spondylitis—Spondylolysis, *Roentgenological Briefs*, Des Moines, IA, Council Roentgenology of the American Chiropractic Association, date unknown.

Wax, M: Procedures in Elimination of Trigger Points in Myofascial Pain Syndromes, *ACA Journal of Chiropractic*, October 1962.

Weed, ND: When Shoulder Pain Isn't Bursitis, *Postgraduate Medicine*, 73(3):97–104, September 1983.

West, HG: Vertebral Artery Considerations in Cervical Trauma, *ACA Journal of Chiropractic*, December 1968.

White AA, III and Panjabi, MM: *Clinical Biomechanics of the Spine*, Philadelphia, J.B. Lippincott Company, 1978.

Whiting, RJ: Cervical Spondylosis, *Roentgenological Briefs*, Des Moines, IA, Council on Roentgenology of the American Chiropractic Association, date unknown.

Wiehe, RJ: The Importance of Peripheral Vascular Diagnosis, *The Chiropractic Family Physician*, 2(4):12–15, May 1980.

Williams, JGP and Sperryn, PN (eds): *Sports Medicine*, ed 2, Baltimore, Williams & Wilkins 1976.

Wilson, FC: Fractures and Dislocations of the Ankle, in Rockwood CA Jr and Green DP (eds): *Fractures Philadelphia*, Lippincott, 1975, p. 1361.

Wolf, M and Ransberger, R: *Enzyme Therapy*, New York, Vantage Press, 1972.

Yashon, D: *Spinal Injury*, New York, Appleton-Century-Crofts, 1978.

Zange, LL: Sesamoiditis: A Sesamometatarsal Lesion, *ACA Journal of Chiropractic*, February 1982.

Zatzkinn, HR: *The Roentgen Diagnosis of Trauma*, Chicago, Year Book, 1965.

Zuidema, GD et al: *The Management of Trauma*, ed 3, Philadelphia, W.B. Saunders Company, 1979.

INDEX